During the 1940s and 1950s, tens of thousands of Americans underwent some form of psychosurgery; that is, their brains were operated upon for the putative purpose of treating mental illness. From today's perspective, such medical practices appear foolhardy at best, perhaps even barbaric; most commentators thus have seen in the story of lobotomy an important warning about the kinds of hazards that society will face whenever incompetent or malicious physicians are allowed to overstep the boundaries of valid medical science. *Last Resort* challenges the previously accepted psychosurgery story and raises new questions about what we should consider to be its important lessons.

Through an extensive study of patient records, professional correspondence, and the day's medical literature, Jack D. Pressman establishes that lobotomy occurred, not at the periphery of medical practice, but at its center – a finding that engenders a different set of historical problems. To account for why so many reasonable and trusted physicians might have supported psychosurgery's validity, the book reconstructs the particular challenges facing the psychiatrists of the time and the kinds of disciplinary tools that were available to them. The new lesson that emerges from the psychosurgery story, then, is that our usual models of understanding how medicine progresses are deeply flawed. The success of a research venture in medicine is never a safe bet, and the evaluation of therapeutic success is not an absolute measure, being relative to time and place. The standard of what constitutes valid medical science is itself never fixed, but evolving.

T0268992

# Last Resort

# Cambridge History of Medicine

Edited by

CHARLES ROSENBERG, Professor of History and Sociology of
Science, University of Pennsylvania

COLIN JONES, University of Warwick

## Other Titles in the Series:

*Continued on page following the index*

# Last Resort
## Psychosurgery and the Limits of Medicine

JACK D. PRESSMAN
UNIVERSITY OF CALIFORNIA, SAN FRANCISCO

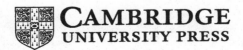

PUBLISHED BY THE PRESS SYNDICATE OF THE UNIVERSITY OF CAMBRIDGE
The Pitt Building, Trumpington Street, Cambridge, United Kingdom

CAMBRIDGE UNIVERSITY PRESS
The Edinburgh Building, Cambridge CB2 2RU, UK
40 West 20th Street, New York NY 10011–4211, USA
477 Williamstown Road, Port Melbourne, VIC 3207, Australia
Ruiz de Alarcón 13, 28014 Madrid, Spain
Dock House, The Waterfront, Cape Town 8001, South Africa

http://www.cambridge.org

© Jack D. Pressman 1998

First published 1998
First paperback edition 2002

*Typeface* Sabon.

*A catalogue record for this book is available from the British Library*

*Library of Congress Cataloguing in Publication data*
Pressman, Jack David.
Last resort: psychosurgery and the limits of medicine
/ Jack D. Pressman.
p.      cm. – (Cambridge history of medicine)
ISBN 0 521 35371 8 (hardback)
1. Psychosurgery – United States – History.   I. Title.   II. Series.
[DNLM: 1. Psychosurgery – history – United States. WL 11 AA1 P935S
1998]
RD594.P655   1998
616.89′1–dc21
DNLM/DLC
for Library of Congress
97-14074   CIP

ISBN 0 521 35371 8  hardback
ISBN 0 521 52459 8  paperback

Gentle, clever your surgeon's hands
God marks for you many golden bands
They cut so sure they serve so well
They save our souls from Eternal Hell
An artist's hands, a musician's too
Give us beauty of color and tune so true
But yours are far the most beautiful to me
They saved my mind and set my spirit free.

– Written by Lobotomy Patient #68,
ca. 1942 (from the archives of
James W. Watts III, M.D.)

# Contents

# Figures and Tables

## Figures

## Tables

# Acknowledgments

This project began a long time ago. In the time that has passed since its earlier incarnation as a doctoral dissertation, I have had the good fortune to continue to draw upon the wise counsel and support of my former teachers Henrika Kuklick, Charles Rosenberg, and Rosemary Stevens, and to have cultivated new mentors as supremely helpful as Gerald Grob. I want to express my special thanks to John Burnham and Don Herzog, who closely read the entire manuscript and made excellent suggestions in both form and content; a similar debt is also owed to Henrika Kuklick, David Barnes, Elizabeth Haiken, and Caroline Acker, who provided comments on individual chapters.

During my time as a postdoctoral student at the Rutgers Institute for Health, Health Care Policy, and Aging Research, I was also fortunate to have been surrounded by an engaged group of social scientists who prodded me into systematic analysis of patient records. I thank them for their camaraderie as well as for their advice. I also want to thank the National Institute of Mental Health, whose support during this traineeship allowed me to pursue in-depth this avenue of research.

Since arriving in the Bay Area, I have entered a rich community of intellectual and professional resources. A special note of thanks is reserved for my department chair and colleague, Guenter Risse, who invested a considerable amount of his own time and scholarly resources in the nurturance of a fledgling scholar. A number of able individuals have at some point assisted in the research and preparation of this manuscript, including Rebecca Ratcliffe, Andrea Richardson, Patricia Zimmermann, Deirdre O'Reilly, and Halle Lewis in our own office; Jeff Mifflin at McLean Hospital; and our graduate students Mita Giacomini, Caroline Acker, and Colin Talley. I also want to thank our truly dedicated departmental staff, Elizabeth Murray and JoAnne Lopez.

Any historical endeavor that is based upon extensive use of archival records, such as this one, depends upon the dedication of the archivists who make it possible to find the necessary materials. I thus want to express my deep appreciation of the efforts made on my behalf by the staff

at the Yale University Library, Yale Medical School Library, Rockefeller
Foundation, American Psychiatric Association, College of Physicians of
Philadelphia, Gertrude Himmelfarb Library of the George Washington
University Medical School, Institute of Pennsylvania Hospital, Massa-
chussetts Mental Health Center, Menninger Foundation, Archives of Psy-
chiatry, Columbia University Manuscripts, Library of Congress, National
Archives, National Academy of Sciences, Illinois State Archives, Ohio
State Historical Library, and Countway Library at Harvard Medical
School. I want to single out here Terry Bragg, Archivist at McLean Hospital, whose efforts toward preserving psychiatric records and making them
accessible to historians are unparalleled; if it were not for Terry, a significant portion of this project would not have been possible. I want also to
thank Walter J. Freeman III, who made available to me a copy of his
father's unpublished autobiography.

My most heartfelt thanks of all, of course, go to my family, Wendy, Abe,
and Zoe, who put up with a heck of a lot.

This journey really began even longer ago, when as an undergraduate
major in biology I was unable to reconcile my unhappiness with the
privations of laboratory work with my growing fondness for dusty books.
A single course with Will Provine – whose infectious enthusiasm for the
scholarly life and commitment to teaching are legendary – pointed the way
to an alternative career: through the study of history, a fondness for both
science and culture could be connected. It is thus to Will Provine that I
dedicate this work.

San Francisco, May 1997

# Jack D. Pressman

## An Appreciation

### Gerald N. Grob

The publication of a first book – particularly one that makes a major contribution – is generally an occasion marked by joy and satisfaction. The years of preparation are more than compensated by the appearance of a book incorporating arduous labor and sustained thought.

In this case, however, the author did not live to see his creation. A few days after sending the copyedited manuscript to Cambridge University Press, Jack Pressman died suddenly on the morning of June 23, 1997. For the world of scholarship the loss was self-evident. For his wife and two young children, his parents and sister, the event was a personal tragedy for which words are inadequate to describe.

I first became acquainted with Jack more than a decade ago. He had just completed his dissertation on the origins of psychosurgery under Professor Charles E. Rosenberg at the University of Pennsylvania, and had accepted a National Institute of Mental Health postdoctoral fellowship at the Institute for Health at Rutgers University, with which I am affiliated. When I read his dissertation, I was astonished at its originality and penetrating insights into the origins and deployment of a therapy long since consigned to the dustbin of medicine.

Shortly after his arrival at Rutgers our relationship underwent a sharp metamorphosis. We went beyond the role of mentor and student, and quickly developed a close and trusting friendship marked by collegiality and mutual respect. He was one of those rare persons who combined scholarly originality with a warm and engaging personality and a subtle yet delightful sense of humor. I can recall our many conversations that, no matter how time-consuming, ended all too quickly. Although I had been working on the history of American psychiatry for more than twenty-five years, I found myself learning from my younger friend who had taken a familiar subject and analyzed it in an entirely novel and persuasive way.

After a year and a half at Rutgers, Jack accepted a position in the history of medicine at the University of California in San Francisco, one of the nation's premier medical institutions. Separated by distance, we nevertheless remained close. I urged Jack to revise his dissertation and submit it for publication; I did not see the necessity for major changes. Wisely, Jack pursued his own strategy: He did a great deal of additional research and eventually produced a book that bore only a schematic resemblance to what had been an outstanding dissertation. In retrospect his decision to defer rapid publication was correct. Historians of medicine and psychiatry are the beneficiaries of his determination not to be caught up in the race to publish prematurely.

When Jack first began his research, psychosurgery for severe mental disorders had achieved an odious reputation as a cruel and barbaric intervention. Yet if such was the case, why had it achieved some measure of approval and accolades in the 1940s? Were those who had been recruited into psychiatry and neurology uncaring and ignorant persons who thoughtlessly adopted a radical invasive procedure and remained oblivious to its consequences? Indeed, the criticisms of psychosurgery that became so pervasive during and after the 1960s often hinted that those who sanctioned and performed various types of lobotomies actually were either evil or ignorant individuals masquerading as physicians. The characters so graphically portrayed in Ken Kesey's *One Flew Over the Cuckoo's Nest* are perhaps symbolic of the simplistic perception of psychosurgery that has prevailed in the popular mind.

To Jack's everlasting credit, he did not follow the prevailing conventional wisdom that was so contemptuous and dismissive of psychosurgery. Instead of writing a jeremiad, he began with several deceptively simple questions that in truth required complex and sophisticated responses. What were the medical and scientific origins of psychosurgery? Why did key individuals in neurology and psychiatry become involved with this therapy? What standards were employed to measure therapeutic efficacy? How could individuals with a psychodynamic perspective endorse an extreme somatic therapy? In brief, he addressed questions that had implications not merely for psychiatry and neurology, but for virtually all of medicine.

Too often the history of medical therapies has been written in terms of progress. Scholars and physicians alike have been prone to overlook the obvious fact that the overwhelming majority of medical therapeutics (even in the recent past) have proven less than efficacious. What makes *Last Resort: Psychosurgery and the Limits of Medicine* such an important and enlightening work is its author's refusal to portray the history of psychiatry and medicine in stark terms that pits good against evil, enlightenment against ignorance, and science against charlatanism. Medical science, however impressive its achievements, exists within a larger social system and is thus susceptible to the same contingencies that shape all human activities. In this respect *Last Resort,* in illuminating the rise and fall of psychosurgery, offers a sobering lesson to those who herald every new therapy as a fundamental breakthrough; it renders firm moral judgments about the history of therapeutics more problematic. Above all, *Last Resort* should be an antidote to the perennial human tendency to view medicine in purely technical terms or to fall into the Faustian fallacy of defining its goal as the final conquest of disease.

I cannot close before expressing my own sadness at Jack's untimely passing. I think of the books that he might have written, of the students he might have taught, and of the contributions that he might have made to the wider world of scholarship. Recalling how Jack's eyes would light up when recounting to me the latest news of his family, I think of the loss that his wife, Wendy, and his young children, Abe and Zoe, have sustained. Yet I hope that those who were closest to him can find meaning and a measure of consolation in a life that was all too brief, but one that left a rich personal and scholarly legacy.

# Introduction
## A Stab in the Dark

Error which is not pleasant is surely the worst form of wrong.
> T. H. Huxley (1888)

"The knife passed as usual. . . . On the whole, I think this case should be a satisfactory section."[1] With these casual words, dictated in 1947, a surgeon described an afternoon's handiwork in which he performed a major brain operation upon a thirty-three-year-old woman. First, the patient's head was partially shaved and then immobilized against a modified dental chair. After a local anesthetic was given, a burr hole was drilled into each of her temples and the buttons of bone removed so that the surgeon could observe the exposed brain. (The patient was conscious during the operation and could answer questions.) Into one of these holes he slowly inserted a blunt-edged scalpel and then swept it back and forth, severing the connections between the front portion of the brain and its deeper centers. The procedure was then repeated on the other side. Satisfied that no major blood vessels were inadvertently cut, he finished the operation by meticulously sewing up the surface layers of the brain. Lastly, he replaced the pieces of bone removed earlier.

What makes this particular story different from the usual dramas of heroic medicine was the unlikely reason why this young woman had become a candidate for brain surgery. The surgeon was not, as might be expected, removing a life-threatening tumor or cleaning out an abscess caused by a runaway infection. In fact, the best medical instruments of the time would have indicated that the patient's cerebral tissues were perfectly normal. The brain looked healthy enough – at least prior to surgery.

The reason this young woman was in the surgical chair that day had little to do with the known condition of her brain. More to the point was her social status. A proven failure in life, the young woman had become a permanent resident on a mental hospital ward. A bitter divorce was evidence of her incapacity to fulfill the traditional role of a housewife; and with no occupation or career in sight, the patient was unable to live independently. Throughout her life, the patient had seemed unable to establish the "right" kinds of social bonds (in this regard, her sexual liaisons with other women did not help her case). The patient herself had little hope that she might ever become a fully functioning citizen, and bouts of depression, hallucinations, and other grave mental afflictions eventually led to a string of suicide attempts. Her relatives saw no choice other than to commit her.

The patient's fate thus fell into the hands of a series of psychiatrists who saw only further problems ahead. To them, the patient's life history and clinical signs were all too evocative of a kind of severe mental deterioration they had seen many times before. When the usual modes of treatment and counseling had failed to change her situation, these physicians had come to their own wits' end. Convinced of the need for more direct intervention, they recommended that a lobotomy – a new kind of brain operation – be tried in the hope of turning her life around. In a calculation that seems rather startling to us today, these doctors believed that by destroying a portion of this patient's brain they might make life for her more bearable as well as transform her into a better person. Desperate circumstances, they told themselves, justified drastic acts. If pressed, the patient's doctors would have had to admit that they had little idea of the exact neurophysiological mechanism by which the operation worked. For example, even one of its supporters went so far as to depict the use of lobotomy as being little more than "a stab in the dark" – literally, as well as figuratively.[2] Psychosurgery had become their treatment of last resort.

This patient's story was not unique. Although these psychiatrists were unsure about the procedure's physiological action, they were certain that it would have a dramatic effect on the course of their patients' lives. And so it happened that the drama above was played out in America time and time again. Between the procedure's initial introduction in 1936 and its decline in the mid-1950s, at least twenty thousand such operations were performed in the United States.[3] Lobotomy had become the latest technological solution for a range of problems that as yet had no good answers.

This book is about hope and despair, about our faith in the powers of science to deliver us from the reality of human tragedy. Its central concern is with the story of medical progress, the process by which advances in scientific knowledge presumably leave us individually and collectively better off. In particular, it is about those fateful moments of convergence when a discovery concerning the inner workings of the body is perceived as having a profound significance for human welfare.

Customarily, the saga of medical science has been told through detailed expositions of medicine's most visible successes – the kinds of innovations that placed their creators in the pantheon of Nobel prize winners. Such case studies suggest themselves as the likeliest place in which to examine the development of modern medicine. In this manner, my own historical strategy in this book is to explore the life course of a particular therapeutic innovation as it made its way from early experimental trials to full-fledged dissemination as a valued therapy. However, the specific subject that I have selected for such a case study – that of psychosurgery in America – does not present itself as an obvious choice.

At first glance, the idea of analyzing the trajectory of medical progress by studying the fate of lobotomy seems a peculiarly wrongheaded, if not perverse, place to begin. If anything, psychosurgery now connotes an image exactly *opposite* to that of mainstream medicine, its reputation firmly established as something that occurred on the far periphery of accepted practice. An argument could even be made that it has become our most visible icon for everything that is dangerous and bad about uncontrolled medical science, about the havoc that can ensue when evil (or perhaps simply misguided) individuals masquerade as competent scientists or doctors. A steady production of popular books, movies, and plays – *One Flew Over the Cuckoo's Nest, Planet of the Apes,* and *Frances,* to name a few – have forcefully explored this point. As a result of these gripping and often lurid portrayals, we have become morbidly fascinated by lobotomy's potential to transform its victims into robots or "vegetables," individuals no longer able to disturb the powers that be and, in so doing, to destroy that which is most sacredly human within us.

During the heated political debates of the 1970s, in which various aspects of medicine were criticized as forms of social control cloaked in the ideology of science, lobotomy was denounced by the laity and professionals alike as an indefensible form of domination. Bioethicists, for example, found in psychosurgery an almost ideal subject with which to prompt debates on where to draw the line between individual and societal interests in medicine, a balance continually upset by emerging technologies. Neurophysiologists and other researchers joined in such attacks, happy to point out the superior status of their own scientific methods as compared to the barbarism of the receding past. And as a result of the popular outcry, an unusual federal commission was created to construct guidelines for its regulation.[4]

Over time, the meaning of *psychosurgery* has thus become restricted to that of a "cautionary tale" of science gone awry, a "morality play" to instruct eternal vigilance. We tell ourselves that this was by no means the first time that a therapeutic fad was driven forward by a cadre of physicians who overstepped the boundaries of good medicine; and that, should we drop our guard, it will certainly not be the last. What could this ugly story possibly have in common with those that recount *true* medical triumphs?

While the mad-doctor characterizations make for great polemics and for spine-tingling science fiction, as history they are often just plain wrong. In the best account to date of lobotomy's rise, Elliot Valenstein recently noted that psychosurgery was "not an aberrant event but very much in the mainstream of psychiatry."[5] Indeed, even a cursory examination of the day's medical reports will show that the psychiatrists who recommended the procedure, the neurosurgeons who performed the operations, and the scientists who justified it, all came from the highest ranks. To be sure, most lobotomies were performed on patients in the back wards of the remote state hospitals, a fact consistent with the most negative scenarios. This statistic only reflects, however, the reality that the majority of the nation's mentally ill happened to reside within the state hospital system. Lobotomies were also performed in most of the elite research institutes, in the (then) well-equipped and staffed veterans' hospitals, and even in the richly endowed private asylums.

The simple truth was that one could grow up in a socially powerful family, consult the most respected physicians in the nation, and enter the finest mental institutions money could buy – and still end up with a lobotomy. Such was the case of the young woman described at the beginning of this introduction, who received her brain operation in a private mental hospital that was ranked as one of the best. Her surgeon was Dr. W. Jason Mixter, at the time one of the most prominent neurosurgeons in the world. There is also the unexpected news that Egas Moniz, the Portuguese neurologist who invented lobotomy, was awarded the Nobel Prize in 1949. Psychosurgery *was* in the pantheon, after all.

Ironically, a reappraisal of psychosurgery that faithfully depicts its former centrality within mainstream psychiatry raises more problems than it dispels. As in the case of other popular treatments whose initial therapeutic esteem eventually soured, psychosurgery's about-face in clinical fortune poses a troubling enigma: why would reasonable, well-meaning physicians and scientists at first value a procedure so highly, only to abandon it later as obviously meritless and inhumane? As Roger Cooter has argued in discussing the nineteenth-century faith in phrenology, it is insufficient to state that proponents simply acted unthinkingly until that inevitable time when they "came to their senses." This kind of response does not confront the question but merely redescribes it.[6] We are left with two variant story lines, equally disturbing: (1) that something so dubious as lobotomy was on a pedestal alongside the likes of anesthesia and x-rays, if only for a limited time, or (2) that membership in science's supposedly eternal hall of fame is revocable.

The transitory nature of medical convictions also bedeviled contemporaries. The confidence of these practitioners was sorely tested by the realization that, one day, the shifting sands of scientific knowledge would bare the foundations of their own therapeutics. None of them were immune from future ridicule. In 1941, the colorful psychiatric statesman C. C. Burlingame expressed this quandary in an intimate after-dinner speech irreverently entitled "Quacks But No Ducks." "What then," he asked his brethren, "of our vitamin capsules, our electric therapies, our ultra violet lamps, our short wave treatments and our shock therapies . . . ?" He continued:

> Do we use these as empirically as our predecessors did their leeches and their bleedings? . . . Are we, in the light of others who come after us, going to be accused of being users of stupid, bizarre or crude methods? Will they think us no better than quacks? . . . Will they read our shock therapy methods with horror and say, "Why, they should have used baseball bats – it would have been just as productive of results"?[7]

As it so happens, within a few years of this speech the biggest such bat in Burlingame's own medical repertoire was in fact psychosurgery. How are we to resolve this tension between past and present to reach a perspective from which to understand – and perhaps judge – our medical heroes, fallen or otherwise?

At issue is our understanding of how medical science evolves. Typically, the explanation of how a new treatment achieved widespread acceptance by the medical profession reduces to this: it was effective, spectacularly and undeniably so. Diphtheria antitoxin saved a young girl's life on Christmas Eve, 1895; penicillin prevented countless thousands of gangrene-related amputations during the Second World War; and so on. The usual parade of such examples reinforces belief in the supposition that the life course of a medical innovation is determined mostly by that treatment's inherent soundness. Procedures that work, fly and are assured their place in the medical record; those that do not, crash and appropriately find only oblivion. The true value of any particular therapy is thus assumed to be a quality that is both immediate and yet transcendent, equally visible across the decades.

It is precisely this assumed timelessness of medical potency that has distorted our historical vision. Charles Rosenberg observed not too long ago that historians of medicine have been accustomed to considering the subject of therapeutics "an awkward piece of business" and have generally "responded by ignoring it," especially in regard to medicine as it was practiced before the advent of the laboratory. In his diagnosis, the problem lies in our preoccupation with applying the standards of modern medicine to the methods of yesteryear's physicians. When examining a particular mode of therapy, the first question has always been "Did it work?" – a criterion, Rosenberg notes, more physiological than historical. Within such a framework, the sensibilities of the physician and the historian have converged: as there were indeed few treatments of any scientifically proven merit until the late nineteenth century (other than, say, digitalis, quinine, or vaccination), it is no wonder there has been a dearth of interest in telling the story of apparently worthless medicine. Curiously, historical accounts of the postscientific era of medicine have likewise been hobbled within this framework.[8] As the matter of what are the great medical triumphs is already known, the essential narrative of the story is virtually prefabricated. All that remains for the historian to do is interview the extant researchers as to what, in their recollection, led to the fateful discoveries.

The model of medical science that is generated by all this attention paid to the stories of laboratory success is also directly responsible for our tortured historical paradoxes. Medical innovation is at root a risky, perilous venture, a drama that has been obscured by the focus on only those instances where everything went right. To assume that when physicians consider a new treatment they somehow are guided by a special insight into its true clinical value – a value not yet determined – is to impose an unwarranted, although heartening, teleology.

Similarly, our understanding of what determines the trajectory of a medical innovation after the first experimental reports have been published has also been distorted by exclusive attention devoted to the best-case exemplars of medical science. In such stories, the consideration of a treatment or diagnostic device's efficacy happens only once: in the initial stage of discovery. The technology itself is tracked as a kind of black box, the inner aspects of which are divorced from further analysis; its path into widespread clinical practice is reduced to a matter of political economy – another instance of "technological momentum" in play. A generation of political scientists, economists, and sociologists have thus plotted the diffusion of EEG machines, intensive-care units, CAT scanners, and the like in the United States, with the rate of adoption being determined by such indices as the number of hospitals and the mode of funding.[9] In this manner, medical technologies are reified into discrete, stable entities that are somehow insulated from the overall historical process; lost along the way is any consideration that the functions of a given treatment or instrument may be multiple, not single, and in a process of continual flux.[10]

New approaches to the issue and a way out of the resulting paradoxes can be found, however, by deliberately examining the story of therapies that have *not* stood the test of time.[11] For Rosenberg, the lesson that traditional therapeutics (i.e., the prescientific practices of the nineteenth century and before) offers historians of medicine is their invitation to a more anthropological reading of how medicine functions: things work not just within a human body but within a prevailing culture. Traditional therapeutics were judged successful by lay and professional groups, Rosenberg argued, because these interventions were consistent with a conceptual system that linked the two communities.[12] In the prelaboratory era, the classic treatments didn't fail because they were revealed to be inadequate. Rather, the world itself had changed in the interim, altering the inner cultures upon which the previous system of therapeutics had ultimately depended. Cast in this manner, the history of medicine was thus reintegrated into broader historical currents. To explain why physicians reached consensus that a particular treatment appeared worthwhile, the historian now looked to the sensibilities of the time, not just to the laboratory results; moreover, the history of medicine itself was promoted into an unusually valuable resource for reconstructing past cultures.

Rosenberg's article heralded a wave of similar investigations into the social meaning and structure of earlier periods of medical practice.[13] Even so, historians of medicine have generally shied away from applying such lessons to therapies in the scientific era. As Rosenberg himself pointed out, the modern period is characterized by a cleavage between scientific and lay cultures. Moreover, it is one thing to argue that the evaluation of a traditional therapy was dependent upon cultural factors at a time when *none* of the participants could scientifically ascertain its actual clinical value. It is quite a different challenge to make such a claim stick in modern times, when the true efficacy of a treatment is presumably knowable to those on the scene.

For the scientific era, it is in the stories of failed medical technologies that new avenues into the problem can be found. Their baroque charms notwithstanding, such episodes are valuable in that, as case studies running counter to expected form, they test comfortable assumptions concerning the introduction, evaluation, and diffusion of therapeutic innovation. (One might say that they are historical "control" samples.) As evidence mounts that supporters of many ill-fated treatments were not acting outside of accepted medical practices, the claim is weakened that their more fortunate counterparts succeeded because of a careful adherence to the standards of good scientific medicine. Any connections made between what a treatment *really* does and its subsequent life course must be proven, not assumed. In short, medical treatments do *not* possess an inherent clinical attractiveness in the way that physical objects possess mass. Rather, clinical assessment is a contingent historical product. The foundation of medical belief thus becomes, in its own right, an important subject for historical explanation.[14]

In the story before us, how was the connection made that operating on the brain was a likely route to improved mental health? What conditions existed at the time that made such a drastic response appear necessary for so many? Why were the changes exhibited by patients after lobotomy interpreted as bona fide clinical gains? Why did psychosurgery work – then?

Answering these questions for the case of lobotomy will illustrate the kinds of social and professional factors that shape the evaluation of medical therapies – factors that are rooted in specific moments and hence are vulnerable to change.

To chronicle the rise of psychosurgery is to follow two narrative lines. On one hand, it is a case study of the origin, adoption, and diffusion of a particular medical technology, a story that was played out over two decades and that moved between elite research laboratories and numerous clinical sites scattered around the nation. At the same time, it is an account of what happened within the medical specialty of psychiatry in a period roughly bounded by World War I and the Korean War. My goal here is to demonstrate the importance of weaving both kinds of narratives into a single story, and for this purpose, the topic of lobotomy provides an excellent opportunity for analyzing how the power of medical knowledge becomes directed toward particular areas of concern.

Although the first lobotomies occurred in America in 1936, the proper place to begin the story of its acceptance is at the turn of the century when Adolf Meyer outlined a new vision of psychiatry, one that might join the separate fields of the asylum physician, the elite neurologist, and the general practitioner into a single medical specialty. Within Meyer's monistic philosophy of psychobiology, all distinctions were to be collapsed among the various approaches toward understanding mind and body; and by replacing the reigning concept of insanity with that of maladjustment, the reach of the modern psychiatrist was to extend into the concerns of everyday life. Chapter 1 describes how, as a result of the stimulus of World War I and the calculated patronage of the Rockefeller Foundation, Meyer's framework was established as the primary platform for remaking the domain of mental health in America. Within the new framework, it was hoped, psychiatry might emerge as the one field that might link all the disparate studies of humankind, from neurophysiology to urban sociology. For the moment, a special premium was placed on any investigation that promised to link the world of the laboratory with grave problems of human living.

Left unsettled, however, was where the new gains would first emerge. Would the remote state hospitals become centers of scientific advance, or would elite academic medical centers find a way to bring the study of mental disorders within their doors? As the constituencies within each domain held to widely differing conceptions of what was valid therapeutic practice or research, the future shape of psychiatry itself was considered to be at stake in the issue. Such tensions were muted in the 1930s, however, when an expansive model of medicine prevailed, allowing all of the fractious elements of the new psychiatry to coexist – for a time. With insanity redefined as a problem of mental disorder and maladjustment, it was even left an open possibility that the latest advance in psychiatry would come not from psychiatrists but from elsewhere.

By all accounts, the specific link between neurosurgery and mental disorders was forged at the Second International Neurological Congress held in London in 1935. Egas Moniz, a Portuguese neurologist, happened to be in the audience when John F. Fulton, a distinguished Yale neurophysiologist, described the interesting results of his brain experiments on chimpanzees; Moniz returned home from the meeting convinced about the possibility of psychosurgery. Chapter 2 explores how the standard account of the origin of psychosurgery – a familiar story of serendipity in science – is both less and more true than at first reading. On the one hand, that the chimpanzee experiments would be interpreted within a psychiatric framework at Yale was not a product of mere happenstance, for they occurred within a program that was one of the showpieces of the new psychobiology. On the other hand, the direct role of Fulton's research as an intellectual stimulus to Moniz has been overstated at the same time that his indirect role as its most significant patron, in convincing others to invest in the procedure's future, has remained hidden.

The subsequent change in lobotomy's status from that of an experimental technique of uncertain merit, to a perception that it was of widespread utility and certain benefit, is the subject of Chapter 3. Moniz's technique was targeted at first mostly on patients with agitated depressions. The immediate cessation of the patient's misery deeply impressed the first psychosurgeons; such visible results convinced other medical observers to follow suit. H. D. Banta has observed that the uses of a medical technology often change once the technique moves away from its initial trials into larger field studies, where new possibilities arise.[15] So too with psychosurgery. When the lobotomy studies shifted from the office-based practices to mental hospitals, the operations were found to have a positive effect on a different group of patients, the chronic schizophrenics. Although the gains in such cases were not considered as impressive as those achieved with the original class of depressives, this discovery had a profound impact on lobotomy's later course. This latter class of patients constituted the most pressing problem for the mental hospitals, in that no adequate treatments were yet available for their condition. Psychosurgery was thus introduced into a realm of almost limitless horizons, having no real competitors.

In the years immediately following World War II, the use of psychosurgery reached its heyday, peaking at over five thousand such operations performed in 1949 alone. A large number of psychiatrists had found in lobotomy a tool that altered human character to an extent unmatched by any other resource in their armamentarium. For them, psychosurgery clearly worked. The next three chapters explore the reasons why the procedure was viewed so positively: lobotomy worked on several levels simultaneously. Chapter 4 documents the acute crisis facing the nation's vast system of overburdened state mental hospitals. Professional leaders desperately sought means of motivating the public to reinvest in the mental health infrastructure, as well as of shoring up the profession against further demoralization. They settled upon a strategy of selling a vision of what psychiatry might accomplish if it were sufficiently medicalized, equal in stature and resources to the best of the other specialties. Lobotomy, the most visibly medical intervention of the day, was seized upon as exactly the kind of "active treatment" that might bring results to the profession of psychiatry as well as to the individual patient.

Lobotomy did not cure any patients of a specific disease. More accurately, it transformed them into persons whose characteristics, physiological as well as psychological, were quite different than they had been before the operation. The challenge is to explain why such effects were interpreted as a true medical benefit, and why such a drastic procedure was considered necessary in the first place – and even humane. Even its most vocal advocates advised that lobotomy was to be used only as a treatment of last resort, and that recipients "paid a price" in unfortunate side effects. Psychosurgery was a form of human salvage, not rescue.

The reason lobotomy programs rose to such prominence, Chapter 5 argues, lies in the special circumstances of the day that had placed so many patients within this category of last resort, and that had framed the matter of mental health in such a manner that the operation's benefits were amplified and its drawbacks minimized. It is hard, decades later, to appreciate the enormity of the clinical challenge facing psychiatrists in the 1940s. When physicians figured the therapeutic calculus according to the time's harsh realities, even the marginal gain that resulted from the operation in the average patient was interpreted as sufficient justification to proceed. Moreover, beginning in the late 1930s, institutional psychiatrists invested their hopes in a series of somatically based therapies. Thus began a new era of "heroic" therapy in psychiatry, as the use of insulin coma, metrazol convulsion, and electroshock stormed onto the hospital wards. Even as hopes were raised by psychiatry's newfound potency, however, the problem of what to do with those patients who resisted cure was increasingly problematic. Psychosurgery, which offered the promise that now no mental patient might slip outside the reach of medical intervention, thus became the capstone to the modern psychiatric system.

The question of lobotomy's perceived efficacy leads to another historical dilemma. Psychosurgery often was considered necessary not just from the perspective of the patient's welfare but from that of the harried institutions. Lobotomy was also an administrative cure. Some patients, it is clear, received a lobotomy primarily because their obnoxious behaviors made life difficult for everybody else around them. How is it possible that the lobotomists saw no contradiction between their responsibilities as healers and the need to maintain order on the wards? Indeed, recent critics of psychiatry have characterized this latter role as proof that psychiatrists were more concerned with their mission as enforcers of social control than with the guidelines of valid medical practice.

Chapter 5 also explores how such easy distinctions are anachronistic. Thanks to the long legacy of psychiatry's institutional locus, and to the interjection of Meyer's more recent model of maladjustment, lobotomy's ability to render the unmanageable more manageable was interpreted as a direct clinical gain and not just hospital expediency. In the 1940s, a patient's restoration to citizenship was in fact the highest criterion of mental health. Moreover, the dual responsibility of preserving the public as well as individual health was exactly the combined service role Meyer had carved out for the modern psychiatrist.

How the *individual* patient came to be selected for the procedure is the focus of Chapter 6. By re-creating in some detail the population of an entire mental hospital for a selected year, it is possible to reconstruct the kinds of considerations that targeted particular persons for the procedure. The winnowing process was neither random nor fixed, but specified in the interaction of local circumstances and generalized knowledge; the challenge of clinical decision making also involved an array of considerations not usually associated with narrowly defined images of medicine. The story of psychosurgery thus becomes an occasion to reexamine the human boundaries and limitations of the art of medicine. Taken together, these three chapters reconstruct why lobotomy made sense to psychiatrists – around 1949.

Even as the use of lobotomy accelerated, establishing it as a significant feature of psychiatric practice, the unease generated by such a drastic intervention was growing in proportion, not dissipating. Although the odds of an individual being reduced to a "zombie" were low, it did happen frequently enough to prevent complacency. Fears were also spreading that perhaps the lobotomy enterprise, which now offered as many different kinds of procedures as there were neurosurgeons, had somehow grown beyond the limits of neurophysiological knowledge. Chapter 7 recounts the heated battles that ensued in the search for a better lobotomy, one that was physiologically justified and that might yield the best results without any of the frequent ill-effects.

Chapter 8 reveals that even at the height of its acceptance the technique of psychosurgery became embroiled in the contradictions that were enveloping all of psychiatry. As lobotomies were considered the first treatment in psychiatry that might result in irreversible harm, critics as well as proponents of the procedure were eager to assess just what it was that the operations did. In such attempts, psychiatrists discovered that the tools available for determining lobotomy's precise clinical value were thoroughly inadequate. Even worse, they learned, the same could be said of *any* psychiatric therapy then in use. The experience of submitting psychosurgery to a high level of scrutiny taught American psychiatrists that their entire system of therapeutics was equally vulnerable to criticism. Freudian analysts and advocates of shock therapy were all in the same leaky boat together.

Much to their chagrin, psychiatric leaders thus found that the issue of scientific validation of psychiatric therapy no longer could be avoided. Until this moment, the matter of therapeutic assessment had been left up to the judgment of the individual clinician. In general medicine, however, a new trend was under way that subordinated an individual practitioner's opinion concerning a particular drug or procedure to the findings of controlled experiments, and psychiatry's laissez-faire arrangement was threatened by obsolescence. In addition, the rapid growth and success of psychiatry as a medical specialty meant that the rest of medicine looked to it to act accordingly; only recently had its professional organization become responsible for policing the borders of accepted psychiatric practice. Moreover, in the wake of the wartime experience, a fundamental shift had occurred in the role that the federal government played in the support of academic science in America. Indeed, with the creation of the National Institute of Mental Health in 1946, psychiatric leaders for the first time were asked to rank the research requests of their diverse membership in ways that were justified by some defensible scientific standard. Unlike the previous era when private philanthropy reigned, such decisions were no longer in the hands of only an aristocratic few and were becoming part of an increasingly public process.

Postwar developments intensified other internal crises. Meyer's expansive vision of a single medical specialty that might range from psychoanalysis to neurophysiology, and from the state mental hospitals to elite office practices, was severely strained by the unfolding history of the profession's shift away from the institution as the core of its disciplinary identity. Fault lines appeared as somaticists fought psychotherapists and hospital psychiatrists battled urban analysts. The specific events of World War II further fractured the overall political structure of the profession. In a replay of what followed World War I, a motivated and seasoned vanguard emerged from the military psychiatry program intent upon remaking the profession in civilian life. At war's end, psychiatry's professional organizations thus became the new battleground. In sum, as psychosurgery represented the gravest therapeutic decision facing contemporary psychiatrists, it occasioned the first significant attempts toward upgrading the scientific methodology of the profession. And as the technique was the most controversial treatment of the day, discussions about its suitability were politicized into forums in which the warring factions jockeyed for the future of the profession. In the subject of psychosurgery, issues of scientific control and professional control merged.

If the story of psychosurgery appears so opaque to us today, it is not because the participants involved were somehow lesser mortals than we. The source of our puzzlement lies not in any widespread defect of their character or intellect that sets them apart but in the manner in which we construct our stories of how medical practices evolve.

From today's perspective, there was nothing in Moniz's initial report that need have compelled other medical investigators to follow his brazen lead. If anything, it seems, they should have known better and let his example pass them by. Medical innovators, however, have no special faculty that allows them to anticipate with any certainty which new research opportunity will succeed and which will fail. Instead, they consult with their peers and mentors to see if a particular venture fits within the overall trend of research. In the 1930s, several disciplines were in fact converging upon the exact research terrain demarcated by the brain operations. In the brave new world of the science of mental disorder, lobotomy appeared as good a bet as any for extending the power of the laboratory into the domain of psychological well-being. Moreover, a retelling of the tale of Moniz and Fulton's chimps reveals that the classic accounts of scientific discovery are often wrong – and not by accident. Constructed around a central narrative of intellectual cause-and-effect, these fables misdirect our attention away from looking too closely at the actual social process by which medical scientists reach consensus that a new research opportunity is worth the gamble. Such decisions are a lot messier than they are usually portrayed, framed as much in contemporary social and professional concerns as in the timeless logic of science.[16]

The particular pattern of psychosurgery's diffusion, in which the primary diagnostic category of patients selected for the procedure quickly crossed over from what were considered the best candidates, such as the agitated depressives, to mediocre ones, such as the chronic schizophrenics, makes little sense when judged according to any rational hierarchy of clinical appropriateness. Rather, the extent to which a treatment flourishes is directly dependent upon the specific features of the day's clinical landscape. In the long haul, viability is a matter of ecology, not virtue.[17]

When psychosurgery reached its heyday and the psychiatric profession had extensive opportunity to witness the mounting number of operative failures, why did some medical investigators choose to redouble their efforts to develop new forms of lobotomy rather than use this as an occasion to mount a strategic retreat? To have abandoned the enterprise at this stage, however, would have been for them an abdication of their responsibilities as medical scientists. Indeed, it is precisely those treatments that yield satisfying results only some of the time which afford the best opportunities for further research; this is what science often does best – improve upon its mistakes. An examination of this second wave of psychosurgery also attracts attention to the normally unseen tensions that exist between physicians on the front lines of clinical work and their counterparts in the academic laboratories when the need arises to improve an existing therapy. Although such tensions can erupt into overt hostility (as when Walter Freeman trumpeted his infamous "ice-pick" method of mass lobotomy to scientist John Fulton), the two domains are in fact more interdependent than members of either would care to admit.

Moreover, one might also have expected that the growing doubts associated with the lobotomy programs should have prodded the relevant psychiatric authorities into actively curtailing them. Yet this kind of professional enforcement apparatus simply did not exist at the time. And even if it had, it is unlikely that psychosurgery would have triggered any such action. For there did not yet exist any methodological techniques that might separate out the worthless psychiatric therapies from the bona fide – at least in a way that meets today's standards of scientific clarity. Indeed, friends as well as foes of the procedure were frustrated by the inability of existing scientific tools to resolve the conflict between them.

Most puzzling of all is the dramatic reversal in the verdict concerning the procedure's clinical effectiveness. From the perspective of medical science, observers past and present cannot both be right: either the procedure worked or it did not. What constitutes the medical ideal should not be confused with everyday reality, however. Rather, as I suggest in this book, the more we adhere to a narrow laboratory-science image of medicine as the defining basis of the profession, the less will be known about what it actually means to be a physician in the modern world.

The efficacy of a medical treatment is often explained in terms of a "lock and key" analogy: the right drug or tool will unlock the specific physiological mechanism that is wreaking so much bodily havoc. Medicine is never confined to the world beneath the skin, however. The conception of every disease entity, to be sure, has a biological dimension that refers to a constellation of physiological signs and symptoms. Yet, inasmuch as any illness affects a person's social relations, its meaning also reflects a particular pattern of social considerations – a dimension that is no less real. Something is always at stake, for the individual and for society, whenever a diagnosis is made. A given disease, Rosenberg notes, "necessarily reflects and lays bare every aspect of the culture in which it occurs." Doctors do not just fix up this or that broken organ, the way an auto mechanic patches up a faulty carburetor. Rather, they are asked to solve *problems* – problems that are generally ascribed to bodily defect, and that erupt in the home, community, or workplace.[18]

A physician's success is therefore not wholly dependent upon the actual physiological status of the ailment under treatment but is linked to the perception that the problem has been resolved: thus medicine itself is embedded within the larger social system. As the life of a modern citizen is comprised of a series of overlapping social roles, identities, and environments, each with its own set of responsibilities and expectations, so the introduction of a treatment cuts across each of these settings and is judged simultaneously from the perspective of the institutions in which it is given, the medical professional who administers it, the research discipline that investigates it, the patient who receives it, the family that pays for it, the employer to whom the patient returns, and other segments of society that observe and comment upon it. Sometimes, a particular medical innovation is perceived within each of these domains in a positive light, appearing as a solution to a series of pressing problems or tensions that may or may not even be related. When this kind of concordance occurs, a treatment becomes imbued with a reputation as an important social asset and thereafter flourishes.

Indeed, at every turn, physicians confront the changing social boundaries of their tasks. The perception that a medical crisis is present and requires intervention, the evaluation that a given therapeutic goal is worth its risks, the judgment that a cure has been effected – these important elements of medical practice are all rooted in the specific needs and values of the day. And as such factors are themselves direct products of historical circumstance, the employment of a particular therapy is intelligible only in a given context. When times change, as they must, the factors that once were all neatly lined up in support of a treatment realign and the issue of a treatment's efficacy becomes open for reassessment. In short, the fact that psychosurgeons seem so bizarre to us today is an indication that even in the recent past the world itself has changed substantially. The multiple "locks" that psychosurgery once were meant to open have already faded away and the particular frames with which the participants viewed the procedure's results have since been discarded.[19]

The conventional accounts of lobotomy in America assume that the historical significance of the procedure lies in its standing as an exemplar of the outside limits of bad medicine. The core narrative of such stories is based upon the putative deviation of the psychosurgeons *away* from the standards of good medical practice. Their hope is that a proper examination of the tale of psychosurgery – an unparalleled occasion in which a handful of overambitious physicians, left unregulated and unsupervised, were able to instigate a broad catastrophe – will lead to more effective checks and balances within the medical system, and thus ward off future such disasters. This is the common wisdom.

A more instructive approach, however, comes from the recognition that the psychosurgeons (for the most part) differed from their colleagues, not because of any professional behavior that marked them as unique, but because a particular change in historical circumstances has since made the normally hidden aspects of their medical practice uniquely exposed. Indeed, it is precisely the direct parallels that can be drawn to the *rest* of medicine, as practiced everyday and everywhere, that make the case of psychosurgery such a valuable historical subject.

If there is a single set of lessons to be learned from the story of psychosurgery, it is that the success of a research venture in medicine is never a safe bet; the evaluation of therapeutic success is not an absolute measure, but is relative to time and place; and the standard of what constitutes valid medical science is itself never fixed, but evolving. The discovery of human nature, it appears, is ineluctably embedded within the human nature of discovery. Consequently, the route to progress in medical science and practice is no less problematic than it is in any other endeavor in which people are involved.

And if there is a warning to be derived from medicine's cautionary tales, it is to beware of relying upon simplistic morals. In the case of those physicians of the past who stand before us today in shame and disgrace, it is all too easy to explain away their actions as the consequence of reckless judgment – no doubt something that right-minded persons (like us) can recognize and avoid when facing similar challenges, now and in the future. It would be ironic indeed should it turn out that we have cultivated our own hubris in identifying theirs.

# 1

## Psychiatry's Renaissance
### The Problem of Mental Disorder, 1921–1935

The eminent psychiatrist Adolf Meyer announced in 1921, "Today we feel that modern psychiatry has found itself." To his colleagues as well, it was clear that something dramatic had indeed happened to the field of mental medicine, which the public until then had associated with the isolated, stigmatized world of the asylum. The nation, it seemed, had become fascinated with madness. The following year Albert Barrett stated, in his presidential address to the American Psychiatric Association: "There was never a time in the world's history when there was such a widespread interest in the mind and its disorders in their relation to human life." For evidence, he declared, one only had to look as far as the latest cultural innovation, the "psychological novel and the psychological play," or to the daily papers' infatuation with all forms of mental strangeness. The avant-garde's flirtation with the recent import of psychoanalysis provided an additional cachet. Likewise, the profession as a whole was engaged in an energetic revival. The psychiatric literature was replete with optimistically titled articles such as "The Broadening Field of Mental Medicine" and "The Newer Psychiatry."[1]

Located at the nexus of converging historical currents within medicine, science, politics, and society, by the end of the 1930s the field of psychiatry was riding a wave of popular and professional interest. Psychiatry had not only found itself, it had been discovered and nurtured by a widening coalition of physicians, researchers, academicians, social reformers, philanthropists, and government leaders. As one participant proudly noted, a "psychiatric renaissance" was under way in America.[2]

### The American School of Psychiatry

Adolf Meyer (1866–1950) himself had played a pivotal role in this transformation.[3] The profession of psychiatry as we know it is a relatively recent construction. As late as World War I, the province of mental health belonged to no single group of physicians in the way diseased eyes be-

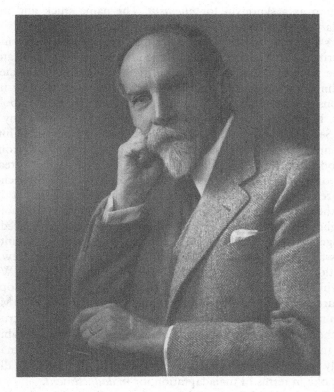

Figure 1.1. Adolf Meyer, 1910. (Source: Archives of the American Psychiatric Association)

longed to ophthalmologists, sick babies to pediatricians, and parasitic infections to tropical disease experts. What we recognize today as the domain of psychiatry was, at that time, scattered among asylum-based physicians (known then as *alienists*), private-practice neurologists, and general practitioners. These three groups of medical workers were deeply divided by differences in the location of their worksites and by who their patients were (and what were their complaints), as well as by fundamental disparities in training, career paths, and medical orientation. Although Meyer began his career as a narrowly focused neuropathologist within the state hospital system, his great accomplishment was to articulate a vision of a single profession united in theory, education, and practice that might hold its own as a respectable medical specialty. Meyer sold this framework under the name *psychiatry*, a European term that in America had come into fashion as a synonym for *alienism*. The name stuck and in time became largely synonymous with Meyer's vision.[4]

Meyer's blueprint consisted of a series of sweeping, linked reforms. His first priority was to reestablish the study and treatment of the insane as a bona fide medical enterprise by importing up-to-date clinical methods into asylum practice and by arguing for the full integration of mental institutions into the emerging systems of university medical schools and hospitals. Psychiatrists were to act, think, and be trained like any other doctors. Second, Meyer sought to redress the sins of dualism, an intellectual principle that had separated the scientific study of the mind from that of the body, and thus psychology from biology. He offered instead the doctrine of *psychobiology*, a monistic philosophy in which psyche and soma were considered not as antithetical entities but as different dimensions of the same thing. In Meyer's school of thought, psychopathologists thus might study mental illnesses from either viewpoint, as needs and knowledge arose. An individual's personality, not his or her faculties or organs, was to be the primary object of study. Third, Meyer drew upon the functionalist teachings of John Dewey, Albion Small, and William James, which were transforming education, sociology, and philosophy, to reconfigure the medical and social meaning of mental disease.[5] In Meyer's system, a mental disturbance was no longer considered to be a structural defect either of mind or of body, but a lowering of an individual's ability to function in the struggle for existence – a struggle that for modern man was intimately bound up with his success in social relations. Instead of disease, Meyer spoke in terms of maladaptation, or *maladjustment*.

The new conceptual framework provided intellectual legitimation for the fourth plank of Meyer's platform: the construction of an altogether different professional and social role. In reorienting the field from its basis in mental disease to that of mental disorder, Meyer provided the means for overriding the conceptual barriers that had stood in the way of a merger among the various medical factions concerned with mental health. In his maladjustment model, differences between normality and abnormality, between severe psychoses and the minor neuroses, were not qualitative but a matter of shades of gray. In principle, then, the same physician might care for the withdrawn catatonic, the troubled neurotic, and the worried well; the doctors who treated mental disorders in the state hospital, the clinic, or the office were envisioned as all being members of the same medical specialty.

At the same time that the maladjustment model called for a redesign of medicine's internal professional structure, it also invited a reconfiguration of the physician's external relations to both patient and society. The Chicago school of sociology, which heavily influenced Meyer, had promoted the idea of society as a complex organism constructed out of an interlocking web of differentiated social roles and institutions; our collective health depended upon the ability and willingness of each citizen to fulfill these necessary functions. As a derivative of this philosophy, Meyer's maladjustment concept thus construed mental disorder directly in terms of the individual's social failure: the status of a person's mental well-being commingled with his or her standing as a good citizen. By combining the troublesome as well as the troubled into a single medical framework, Meyer's vision created a powerful justification for extending the reach of the physician into such nontraditional contexts as the home, the workplace, the school, and the legislative floor. Henceforth, physicians in the Meyerian world would bear a dual responsibility: to maintain societal as well as personal fitness. In sum, Meyer's genius was seeing in the form of a combined neurologist, alienist, and general practitioner – one who adhered to the guidelines of psychobiology and the maladjustment paradigm – the possibilities for a new kind of medical worker who might inhabit the social space generated in the intersection of private and public health. Such a physician became known as the psychiatrist.

Invited to write a chapter on the subject of insanity for the *Encyclopaedia Britannica* in 1926, Meyer was so confident as to pen instead an obituary for the concept, as well as for the entire system of mental medicine it had legitimated. Instead of being limited to the world of the remote asylum, "The wider field of psychiatry now includes mental and behavior problems outside as well as inside hospital walls." In place of the outdated notions of lunacy, Meyer explained, "we speak today of mental *disorders,* of psychoses and psychoneuroses, viewed as problems of adaptation of the individual to his environment."[6] Indeed, Meyer's conception of maladjustment would become the master paradigm that formed the "American School" of psychiatry in the 1930s.

## The Problem of Civilization Itself

To some extent, the various groups concerned with mental health had already been converging as each had been beset by inner tensions that challenged the status quo. Alienists, looking outward from their besieged institutions, found themselves imprisoned professionally as well as intellectually. Derided as the most backward of specialists, they desperately sought means of reintegration within the field of medicine. The alienists' more successful cousins, the neurologists, had unexpectedly stumbled upon a truth that undermined their own enterprise. Nervous conditions, they learned through humbling experience, were attributable not just to nerves but to problems within the mind. Internists, for their part, were riding a wave of success that radiated outward from the laboratory and the public health clinic. Here too, however, dramatic attainments had yielded unanticipated problems. Paradoxically, the public expected ever higher levels of cure and mastery, presumptions that were always one step beyond what regular medicine could deliver.

At the same time, the advance of laboratory analysis allowed physicians to see, in startling focus, the real limits of their own curative powers. Thus, the problem of what to do with the patient who stubbornly resisted cure (even after repeated consultations with wave after wave of expert specialists) was further compounded by the obverse need to account for those mortifying instances when individuals were ostensibly cured by healing cults and folk medicaments, even though medical science had certified such methods as worthless. Thus prodded into action, reformist members within each camp looked to new models of body and mind, of health and disease, and of treatment and healing, to reconstitute their own medical authority. They found common ground in an emerging psycho-pathology movement that extended categories of mental disease to include problems outside of the institution, that postulated a direct interaction between mental and physical events, and that also rediscovered the physician's power to heal simply through suggestion and his own commanding presence.

Meyer found strong support for his professional reforms within this band of fellow travelers as well as from the broader Progressive Era movements that had identified psychiatric services as a valued part of modern society. Through his personal influence on a vanguard of professionals he either taught or supervised, on the National Committee for Mental Hygiene (NCMH, founded in 1912), and on reform-minded state legislatures, important parts of Meyer's campaign were in fact put into place, if partially.[7] Such innovations included individualized case files, staff conferences, psychopathic institutes, and psychiatric social services. Lasting change, however, would require nothing less than a transformation of the public's understanding of insanity, as well as a total reworking of the professional realities that maintained a wide breach between private-practice neurologists and hospital alienists. Such deeply entrenched social forms, however, are notoriously difficult to alter.

## Over There

The missing catalyst was provided by the Great War, when an acute social need and a distinct medical challenge merged. With the nation's attention riveted on the triumphs and tragedies of this awesome conflict, the realm of nervous and mental disorders escalated into a matter of national concern as reports of "shell-shocked" soldiers mounted in frightening numbers. The appointment of Thomas Salmon (1876–1927), the chief medical officer of the NCMH, as director of the army's program in mental medicine brought Meyer's blueprint for professional reform to a crucial test. Salmon saw in the war effort a unique opportunity to prove the modern psychiatrist's worth to his skeptical medical colleagues overseas, as well as to an engaged public at home.

When Salmon arrived, he found the neurologists and the alienists divided into two distinct camps, each with its own separate responsibilities and independent chains of command. Neurologists were assigned as consultants to the hospital wards that dealt with the organic wounds, while psychiatrists were assigned more exclusively to traditional insanity cases and to the frontline situations. Thanks to the special circumstances of war, however, Salmon had been given the mandate to preside over *all* of the army's nervous and mental cases, and was thus able to achieve by military order what was politically impossible back home. Within the newly formed "Department of Neuropsychiatry," the neurologists and psychiatrists were integrated into a joint service. The seven-week-long boot camps became an occasion to indoctrinate hundreds of young alienists and neurologists alike into the Meyerian brand of interpretive psychobiology. This intensive training was followed up at the front lines, where both kinds of physicians were forced to serve side-by-side, treating head wounds one day and war neurotics the next. "These men," the officers boasted, "were indeed neuropsychiatrists."[8] Ironically, the first prototype of a modern American psychiatrist thus appeared, not in some urban U.S. setting, but in the foreign environment of the Argonne forest and the base hospital.

The putative success of the war neurosis model and of Salmon's cadre of neuropsychiatrists signaled a new era in the lay and professional community's understanding of insanity and the social role of psychiatry. In particular, it forcefully demonstrated that mental diseases could be provoked by situational stresses, not by biology alone, and suggested that something positive could be done through prompt and expert medical psychotherapy. Sanity was revealed as a fragile state that might come undone in anyone – at any time and anywhere – whenever the burdens of life proved overwhelming. After the war, the model was transferred to civilian experience when practitioners made direct analogies between the stresses of the battlefield and those of modern society: the same psychical processes were said to be at work, only in a different scale of time or intensity. Moreover, through the massive screening program that Salmon had put into place, the troops and the general public were educated for the first time about the reality of the "psychoneuroses" that had gone undiagnosed in civilian life. As a consequence of the intense publicity generated by the war effort, the public was ready to welcome the neuropsychiatrist as a new kind of medical worker, whose services were of great value to each citizen's personal pursuit of "health, happiness, and efficiency."[9]

A second lesson of the war, however, was the utility of the neuropsychiatrist as an adjunct to military administration – someone available for consultation whenever a behavioral problem cropped up in the platoon that proved recalcitrant to the usual methods of persuasion and coercion. Henceforth, neuropsychiatrists were looked to explicitly for their expertise in managing the unmanageables, a service role that legitimated a greatly expanded presence in postwar America. If industrial unrest, juvenile delinquency, and social strife were all traceable to mental disorders, then an immense opportunity lay ahead in the peacetime economy for Salmon's band of war-trained physicians, who would bring solutions to the factory floor, the courts, and the schools. Psychiatry answered to a public mission as well.

Perhaps the most important result of the wartime experience derived from the effect of having both functions performed by a single set of medical professionals. Indeed, the most radical aspect of Meyer's vision was the reshaped professional role of the physician, in which the doctor was to serve simultaneously the interests of the individual client and those of society. Production of such an entity was possible only if the existing roles of the neurologist and the alienist, with their separate roots in private practice and government control, could somehow be united – a daunting prospect at the time. A major effect of the war, however, was precisely the conjoining of the domains of private and public health, a state of affairs that proved advantageous for the realization of Meyer's vision of professional transformation.

Salmon's neuropsychiatrists solved the difficult political problem posed by those who could or would not fulfill their social obligations. As confidants and trusted physicians, these doctors might guide each broken or confused soldier through the strains and pitfalls of his passage to citizenship; as deputized representatives of the military machine, they would at the same time ensure that the necessary social functions were being fulfilled. (One might say that the trained instincts of the reassuring neurologist and of the officious asylum administrator thus met in happy union.) The astonishing aspect of the war was its poignant demonstration of how the root of all this disturbing nervous pathology was traceable precisely to these individuals' failures to make peace with their social role. The issues of physical disorder and citizenship, of private and public health, thus all converged in a single heated moment. Meyer's dual-role physician was launched.

## Over Here

If Meyer was the architect of the new psychiatry, Salmon was its project engineer.[10] Significantly, it had taken a physician with no formal psychiatric training or responsibilities to bring Meyer's vision into being. With a background neither in neurology nor in alienism, Salmon was perceived as a neutral by both sides. A bacteriologist by training, who had risen from the ranks of the United States Public Health Service, Salmon was untainted by direct association with the treatment of the insane and thus was able to speak about mental disease in the language of medicine that the rest of the general medical community might find palatable. And through his experiences and high profile as a government health officer, Salmon was able to guide the development of psychiatry forward as a subset of public health in concert with Meyer's expansive conception. By war's end, Salmon had acquired the organizational savvy, public visibility, and professional contacts within government, medical, and philanthropic circles to bring to fruition what Meyer himself could not.

The corps of neuropsychiatrists who emerged from the war were well poised to remake the mental health care professions from within and to exploit opportunities for an expansion directly into social affairs.[11] Overnight, what had been Meyer's agenda for slow professional reform became the basis of a comprehensive overhaul of the medical specialty. The most conspicuous example of how the professional world of mental health was altered came in 1921 when the American Medico-Psychological Association was rechartered as the American Psychiatric Association (APA), its current designation. For the first time, an organization that had been the exclusive province of the asylum-bound alienists now admitted members from the ranks of private-practice physicians (most notably neurologists) and from other nonasylum locations as well. Salmon's own election to the presidency of the APA two years later testified to the depth of this reconfiguration: he was the first member so honored who had never held a post inside a mental institution.[12]

To Salmon, the war had provided a rare opportunity for psychiatry to prove its true medical value in a context that was relatively untainted by harsh prejudices. In allowing neuropsychiatrists to work alongside regular physicians, Salmon noted, the war experiences "went far toward breaking down the isolation of mental medicine." Or, as another firsthand observer noted, "through the exigencies of war" neuropsychiatry had taken its "proper place in the domain of medicine." After the war, one of Salmon's primary objectives was to build upon the newfound respect for psychiatry, extending its reach throughout the medical infrastructure. His immediate task was to address the needs of the repatriated wounded, of which approximately 20 percent or more were considered mental casualties. Salmon strove to create a large national system of veterans' facilities and hospital wards to care for the projected tens of thousands of serviceman; he re-created within this system the neuropsychiatric structures of the war. Next, Salmon turned his attention to the inadequacies of professional training, a painful lesson uncovered by the army campaign. Salmon recognized only one hundred and fifty "true" neuropsychiatrists in all of the United States, and he began to lobby powerful philanthropists to underwrite the costs of upgrading the teaching of psychiatry in the nation's university medical schools. Not only would this path be necessary for the training of the modern psychiatric specialist, he hoped it would also enable every medical student of whatever orientation to gain a credible working knowledge of modern psychiatric principles and practice. In this manner, psychiatry's future as a regular partner of modern medicine might be assured.[13]

As for his own career, Salmon accepted a faculty position at Columbia University's medical school in New York City, where he pioneered in bringing the teaching of psychiatry into the second year of medical school (a topic as a rule relegated to later years). He was also instrumental in bringing the New York State Psychiatric Institute onto the Columbia campus, where it was integrated into the rest of the medical school's programs of therapy, research, training, and social service. When it opened in 1929, it was cited as the most impressive professional moment in the current history of American psychiatry. At its dedication, officials unveiled a tablet bearing the promise that the new facility would typify "the integration of psychiatry with general medicine."[14]

At the same time the war experience provided an opportunity to change the inner culture of medicine, it provided a fulcrum from which to budge society's conception of mental illness. The highly publicized and extensive war efforts achieved a degree of public education that public health exhibits and pamphlets alone could not. Among the messages successfully delivered were the ones that mental health was an issue of vital importance to the nation's continued well-being; that this field referred to far more than the hopeless insanities befalling an unfortunate few, as it also included the resolvable problems of living that might afflict anyone; and that the psychiatrist who treated these problems was in fact a new kind of expert whose knowledge was applicable to a broad range of social ills. In proving themselves as guides for those citizen-soldiers who had lost their way on the battlefield, the neuropsychiatrists were assuming responsibility for a similar role at home, to heal the breaches in the social contract wherever they appeared. In the words of Stewart Paton, the war had been an "opportune moment for democracy to demonstrate that successful control of human energies can be entrusted only to those who understand the mechanism by which life is adjusted." Discussions of maladjustment also became a proxy for debates that touched upon an individual's obligations in a free society. "The nihilist anarchist, the parlor Bolshevik, the cubist, and the free love doctrinaire," Austin Riggs explained, "are examples of essentially maladjusted and discontented people."[15] Civilization needed to be defended from its discontents, and the discontents from themselves. The modern psychiatrist would do both.

The profession's expansion was tied directly to this broader definition of psychiatry. The reorganization of the APA, for example, which opened up the profession to nontraditional career paths, was portrayed in precisely these terms. The first leader of the new association, Albert Barrett, justified these changes in his 1922 presidential address. Psychiatric problems, Barrett declared, no longer were limited to the conditions that formerly concerned the psychiatrist "*either in institutional work or in private practice.*" Rather, psychiatrists now dealt with all the factors that disturbed the path of social progress. A new epoch had begun, he declared, in which psychiatry would extend its interests to include "all that concerns mental disorders in their widest relationships." In Barrett's words, the new mission of psychiatry was to intervene whenever such malcontents were "disturbing the smooth course of social progress."[16] In the merging of the interests between self and society, modern psychiatry had discovered its mission.

In a 1926 article entitled "The Newer Psychiatry. Its Field – Training for It," William Healy announced that the domain of psychiatry "has extended beyond all anticipations of a generation ago." "A vast new world," he added, "has been opened to the psychiatrist and indeed, very largely by him." As chair of an APA panel that had been created to address the question of whether psychiatry should commit itself to so broad a service role, Healy announced that "it seemed to be the unanimous opinion that psychiatry is not an art or a science confined to the study and treatment of mental disease, whether it be psychosis, psychopathy, psycho-neurosis or defect." "It was very strongly expressed," he continued, "that it is exactly the psychiatrist's proper business to take over the problems of mental adjustments that are so immediately and overwhelmingly involved in the problems of personality, of family and other social maladjustments, of misconduct, of vocational dissatisfactions, of educational misfittings in primary or secondary school or college." These kinds of problems surfaced in divorces, guidance centers, juvenile halls, industry, courts, social agencies – the list was endless.[17]

In short, Meyer's original plan to interject the psychiatrist into all areas of social life had been galvanized by Salmon's wartime demonstration of the role of neuropsychiatry and of the potential of the maladaptive model of mental disorders. The "failures in human adaptation" that had appeared so conspicuously on the front lines were indeed striking examples – so the argument went – but no more prevalent or ultimately significant than those that appeared in every facet of civilian life. After the war, it was common for psychiatrists to describe how psychiatric work results in "the location of a patient in his proper place in society." "Society, or the State," explained S. I. Franz, "strives through education to fit individuals into the niches which they may best occupy, but at present this is poorly accomplished." Such failures must be "reconstructed" so that they become "capable of behaving like the normal people in [their] environment." Indeed, "the end of the re-education of the psychotic is to return him to his family and to the community as a working member." Within this new framework, patients thus were not cured of a particular disease so much as they were *restored* as functioning citizens. "It would be best if the patient could be called something other than 'patient,'" Franz boldly argued, "something which would always convey to him, to his family, and to his friends, the fact that he is being fitted to take up his life work again."[18]

Although a stroke in 1927 cut short Salmon's life, he had had sufficient time to oversee psychiatry's expansion into a multitude of niches. Even before the war, he had been influential in arranging for the appointment of what were the first psychiatrists employed in private industry and inside the prison system. Capitalizing upon his postwar status as a psychiatric statesman, Salmon had been able to convert the Meyerian blueprint into tangible reality. Salmon was eulogized in the *New York Times* as the "foremost exponent of the new school" of thought regarding mental disorders, one who "lifted psychiatry out of its state institutional setting and made it a living, dynamic thing of service to normal and abnormal alike." Moreover, the rapid development of psychiatric clinics in general hospitals, courts, prisons, "industrial establishments and social agencies," as well as "the origin and development of child guidance work throughout the country during the last ten years," were all directly attributed to Salmon's leadership.[19]

## Good Citizens

In adopting Meyer's new standard, psychiatrists had found a confident voice with which to counsel citizens on right living and to advise policymakers and agencies on how to make their citizens live right. Moreover, thanks to the framework's equation of mental health with good citizenship, the psychiatrist who emerged in the postwar decades was uniquely situated to take advantage of a nation searching for new models of social cohesion and for useful forms of expert intervention. As Elmer Southard put it, the psychiatrist had become nothing less than "the modern specialist in Unrest."[20] Political frameworks that might reach past the polar choices of laissez-faire individualism and of statist autocracies – reviled by many as dogmas of the past – drew special attention. Meyer's maladjustment model, with its balanced choreography of individual and social obligations, thus fit the bill in its presentation of how an enlightened society, full of free-acting but imperfect citizens, might overcome errors of biology and culture to forge a united nation. Indeed, in the 1920s and 1930s, a third political model entered the scene, that of technocracy, which claimed to navigate between individualism and collectivism. In this worldview, human society was perhaps like an organism, but it was in part an artificially designed one, open to continual tinkering and improvement through scientific expertise.

The new heroes were the engineer and the manager, the academician and the enlightened policymaker. But respect for the power of rational control was bounded by a newfound appreciation of the depths of human irrationality. It appeared that man was more than a machine after all. The human element in industrial production, in all forms of social intercourse, and even within the profession of medicine itself was now rendered problematic, in need of an altogether different kind of expert assessment and control.[21] Indeed, if sociology was becoming medicalized, medicine itself was becoming sociologized – concern being centered on the connections between disease and social status, on the relations between physicians and their patients in the age of specialization, and on the proper training of the medical student in so human an enterprise. "If medicine is a science," Henry Sigerist declared to George Sarton in a famous rebuttal, "then it is a social science." His argument rested upon the true social function of medicine, which he defined in precisely Meyerian terms: the physician's goal, he noted, was "to keep his fellowmen socially adjusted or to readjust them if necessary."[22]

Meyer's vision of the modern psychiatrist was thus geared to meet the needs of a growing cadre of reformers, policymakers, and professional leaders. In Barrett's words, psychiatry had entered a new epoch when it positioned itself as the "liaison science between medicine and social problems." Or, as W. A. White (Meyer's heir apparent as the scholarly leader of American psychopathology) stated in 1933: "One must realize that the field of psychiatry . . . is no less than the problem of civilization itself."[23]

## New Foundations

Any lasting change in the mental health care infrastructure would, of course, require large investments of capital. The sad irony of the wartime success, for Salmon and his band of neuropsychiatrists, was the fact that their overseas triumph was dependent upon a set of circumstances very different from those at home. Returning stateside, these physicians found the asylums just as impoverished and isolated as when they had left, and the medical schools just as apathetic. Indeed, the broad gap between what modern psychiatry might accomplish under ideal circumstances and its grim reality as the poorest specialty in medicine soon drew the attention of influential philanthropies. In the period between the two world wars, organizations such as the Carnegie Foundation, the Rockefeller Foundation, and the Commonwealth Fund were shouldering the responsibility for financing the buildup of science and scientific medicine in the United States, if not the world. The latter two were no strangers to the field of mental health in general, nor to Thomas Salmon in particular. In the years during which Salmon was an executive officer of the NCMH, the Rockefeller Foundation paid his salary; it also financed his initial overseas tour of the shell-shocked Allied soldiers. The Commonwealth Fund, at Salmon's request, had underwritten the expenses of the child guidance movement.[24]

Following its reorganization in 1929, the Rockefeller Foundation (the single largest private philanthropy of the day) made the deliberate decision to replace its policy of "scientific" charity with a direct investment in science itself. In accordance with its prime directive – "to promote the well-being of mankind" – medical science was given the highest priority; and within medicine, the field of psychiatry was chosen as the primary target. In explaining their strategy, the trustees noted that psychiatry was "the most backward, the most needed, and the most probably fruitful field in medicine."[25] Lasting roughly twenty years, the campaign in psychiatry and the human sciences consumed approximately sixteen million dollars, a vast sum at the time. Due to the foundation's policy of investing in human potential, the largest share went into the creation of entire departments of psychiatry and new research institutes, with the goal of training the next generation of leaders in psychiatry and psychiatric-related research. The rest of the money was spent on small grants-in-aid spread over such topics as epilepsy, delinquency, conditioned reflexes, constitutional medicine, neurosurgery, industrial psychology, schizophrenia, genetics, neurophysiology, and sex.[26]

The campaign had multiple goals. First, the overarching purpose of the foundation's funding efforts was "the advance of knowledge, with research as the chief tool." A foundation officer's fondest hope was to approve funding for a researcher or project that might result one day in a miracle cure. One had only to look at the nation's overflowing state hospital system to know that in the case of psychiatry the potential for such rewards was enormous. Psychiatry's peculiar position as the liaison science between society and medical science, however, made it attractive to the foundation for additional reasons. In the opinion of some foundation officials, a crisis had arisen within the field of medicine itself. Since 1880, they explained, thanks to cellular pathology and bacteriology, medical progress had progressed dramatically, but at the cost of "something approaching neglect of the patient as a person." President Raymond Fosdick himself declared that, in spite of medicine's newfound scientific image, the physician's office remained "a confessional of spiritual as well as physical disability." "Mankind's eternal cry is for release," he continued, "and the physician must answer it with something more than a test tube." The new psychiatry, it was hoped, would reconstruct the importance of the patient–physician relationship; to bring psychiatry back into the medical fold was to shore up medicine itself.[27]

Another of the Rockefeller Foundation's closely held motivations was not just to cure the physical ills of mankind but also to advance social stability. Even in the prewar period, the threat of continuing labor strife (which resulted in such disasters as the 1913 Ludlow massacre) had prompted the Rockefellers to support the search for more effective means of social understanding, which someday might obviate the need for such direct confrontations between workers and managers.[28] When the foundation subsequently reorganized, its explicit mission was to "rationalize human behavior," with the aim of "control through understanding." Alan Gregg, the charismatic director of the foundation's medical sciences program, explained that physicians increasingly "are being looked to for knowledge that will help in interpreting as well as in guiding the behavior of man." Because "medicine lacks sufficient basic data in these fields to meet such a demand," he continued, what was needed was the knowledge of the "ideal psychiatrist" that might speak to these kinds of "economic, moral, social, and spiritual losses."[29] Such concerns stayed true to the Baptist values that influenced the foundation officials, especially when they agonized over the potential threat posed to the social order by the very sciences they funded. (Even in these preatomic years, the new dawn of science raised the spectre of another, even more dangerous, Fall.) Psychiatry stepped forward as the last hope modern man had to ensure that the awesome power of the laboratory might remain yoked to human need, that the tools of our potential self-destruction would not be deployed before mankind was sufficiently mature. What was necessary, they thought, was to discover some means of uniting the world within with the world without, of connecting the human drive for knowledge with a new search for knowledge about humans.

Gregg found in Meyer's paradigm of maladjustment a psychiatry that might simultaneously alleviate human suffering, patch up a medical establishment sapped by the unanticipated consequences of its own success, and even provide a vantage point from which to guide human affairs under the cover of medical authority. His own model psychiatrist derived directly from the philosophy of psychobiology, with its presumed unity of mind and body and its doctrine that psychopathology consisted of a single spectrum that extended between the "uncontrollable manias of the madhouse" and the "trivial fears and . . . petty foibles of everyday life." Gregg also could argue that this brand of psychiatry would in fact encompass all of the foundation's ambitious and diverse programs. Inasmuch as the domain of mental disturbances corresponded to the problem of social maladjustment, the new science of man, Gregg maintained, was necessarily interdisciplinary, ranging from anatomy to psychology and anthropology.[30] Meyer's expansive vision of the psychiatrist as the lone medical specialist who stood in the overlap between individual and public health – and who might make use of *any* scientific discipline – was tailormade for the foundation's need to articulate a coherent but broad programmatic vision.

### Psychosomatic Medicine

The success of the psychobiology campaign was by no means assured, even given the Rockefellers' vast resources. In the final analysis, psychiatry's fate ultimately depended upon its standing as a bona fide medical science. Unfortunately for Gregg, the standards of what constituted valid medical knowledge had shifted significantly since Meyer's (and even Salmon's) heyday. When Meyer began his mental health care reforms at the turn of the century, the laboratory appeared to him as part of the problem, not the solution. In his judgment, the relentless search for this or that brain lesion or blood assay only drew attention away from where the real difficulty lay – the patient's inability to get on in life. Instead, he emphasized the importance of studies that were performed at the bedside and in the field.

By the 1930s, however, a stance that had originally been welcomed as a fresh vision in psychiatry appeared to be hopelessly shortsighted. A whole spectrum of medical activities, ranging from diagnostics to pharmacology, and from surgery to disease control, were viewed by the educated public and professionals as being dependent upon the insights of laboratory-based investigations. A series of celebrated achievements provided compelling evidence of what the future would bring once medicine was grounded in a scientific understanding of the body. These included the introduction of Salvarsan for the treatment of syphilis (1910), insulin for diabetes (1922), and liver extract for pernicious anemia (1926). A steady barrage of newspaper and magazine stories on research into such matters as genetics, hormones, vitamins, nerve impulses, or metabolism whetted the public's expectation that the secrets of the human body were at last being unlocked. Indeed, it seemed only a matter of time before the medical scientist, lionized in such popular works as Sinclair Lewis's *Arrowsmith* (1925) and Paul de Kruif's *Microbe Hunters* (1926), would usher in an era of unprecedented medical advances.

In developing a treatment for general paresis (the final stage of syphilis), experimental medicine had already produced a striking example of what could be accomplished in psychiatry. Known colloquially as "softening of the brain," in which patients invariably developed ever more severe neurological and psychiatric disorders, this dread disease accounted for as much as 20 percent of the mental hospital population. In 1917, an Austrian doctor suggested that paretic patients be inoculated with malaria in the hope that the ensuing high fever might weaken the microorganism that caused syphilis. Malaria therapy was found to be successful in arresting the further progress of the disease, and its inventor received the 1927 Nobel Prize in Medicine – the first ever awarded for the treatment of a disease with psychiatric complications. Here was proof that psychiatric conditions, too, might benefit from scientific investigation.[31]

The plain reality was that, for any medical specialty to be considered scientific, some form of visible anchor to the laboratory domain now had to be demonstrated. Alan Gregg's plan to remake psychiatry through a commitment to a program of psychobiology was thus in jeopardy even before it began. In 1930, the dean of Harvard Medical School, David Edsall, was invited by the Rockefeller trustees to comment upon its proposed initiative in the medical sciences. Edsall delivered a harsh judgment. After outlining the substantial changes that general medicine had undergone in the previous thirty years or so, he declared that "no such change has come" about in psychiatry, as it was largely dominated by "the speculative, the imaginative, the descriptive." There was a critical need, he continued, to "displace the present point of view in psychiatry," replacing it with "such a change as has been made in medicine itself." Edsall concluded that progress would not ensue until such time as "forcible laboratories" were built, and the experimental method was absorbed in its entirety.[32]

Gregg found the crisis in psychiatric authority to be indeed vexing. From his perspective, although social experts offered important insights into human society, they lacked the requisite scientific methodology to make a lasting impact. Bench investigators, in contrast, held the full imprimatur of science but were inherently myopic when examining human beings in vivo. This problem of psychiatric authority was further compounded by the case of the psychoanalysts, who in spite of their meagre laboratory credentials assumed a disproportionately high ranking at the top of the professional hierarchy, thanks to their learned European backgrounds and to their storied successes in treating some types of intractable neuroses. The problem was not just a matter of finding the right personnel, it was one of location as well. Institutional psychiatry in America had developed in the state hospitals; almost as a rule these were located in rural areas far removed from university medical centers. In consequence, there had been few opportunities to develop within them any kind of experimental tradition. University medical centers and hospitals, for their part, had little or no interest in treating or studying insane patients. At the first sign of a mental disturbance, a patient would be shipped off to what was considered a more appropriate facility. The culture of medicine, Gregg realized, had to be changed from within if a scientific psychiatry were to emerge that might respond to the kinds of criticism Edsall raised.

Gregg's creative response was to refabricate Meyer's doctrine of psychobiology in such a way that the laboratory was given center stage, resulting in a new framework that he made famous in America as *psychosomatic* medicine. His goal was to break down, through the largesse at his command, the institutional, professional, and conceptual barriers that so far had hampered the scientific investigation of mental disturbances. The future of the field, in his opinion, depended on initiatives that might bring the experimental study of mental disorders into the university hospitals and research institutes, where a broad range of patients, exhibiting symptoms from minor to severe, might be studied from an equally diverse mix of perspectives ranging from psychoanalysis to endocrinology. Gregg successfully sold his psychosomatic doctrine to the Rockefeller Foundation trustees, the psychiatrists at the vanguard of professional change, and eventually the rest of general medicine. Thanks to Gregg's heavy-handed but astute leverage, the neuropsychiatrist of Meyer and Salmon – updated to include an emphasis on laboratory research – appeared prominently at the forefront of the profession in such programs as Harvard's Massachusetts General, the Institute of Pennsylvania Hospital, the Chicago Institute of Psychoanalysis, Yale University's Institute of Human Relations, Washington University in Saint Louis, and the Montreal Neurological Institute.

Each of the major research sites Gregg funded had at its core a commitment to the collapse of disciplinary borders and a faith in psychobiological unity. At the Montreal Neurological Institute, Gregg's first major initiative, psychiatric progress was linked to the union of neurology, neurophysiology, and rare state-of-the-art neurosurgical facilities. Gregg supported a large grant to the psychiatry department at Yale because of its unique location within the Institute of Human Relations, an interdisciplinary complex of medical, social, and behavioral science facilities that incorporated everything from psychoanalysis to primate neurophysiology. In Chicago, Gregg underwrote the cost of one of the first psychoanalytic training institutes in America precisely because its director aggressively promoted a distinct psychosomatic orientation. Perhaps no better illustration of the Rockefeller orientation can be found than in the example provided by the researchers at the Chicago Institute of Psychoanalysis who made electroencephalographic recordings of their patients before and after analytic sessions.[33]

Gregg also labored to construct a department of psychiatry that would be located in a general hospital and under the supervision of a major university medical school – that is, a flagship facility that might be of sufficient national and international prominence to influence a generation of practitioners in their attitudes toward the medical relevance of psychiatry. As few medical centers boasted the requisite professional leverage, Gregg's choice was an easy one. It was made even easier by the availability of Harvard's Stanley Cobb as its director, a man whom Gregg characterized as possessing "unusually excellent leadership." Cobb, a prominent professor of neuropathology and neurology in the prime of his career, had expressed an interest in expanding his work at Massachusetts General to include psychosomatic disorders of adolescents and psychiatry in general. Beginning in 1933, the Rockefeller Foundation assumed the costs of maintaining Cobb and his group, support that would last more than fifteen years – easily Gregg's longest continually funded project. The special mission of the Harvard program was to "link psychiatry to the rest of medicine" by demonstrating that a teaching and research unit in psychiatry was an essential part of a general hospital. Gregg could not have found a stronger proponent for his psychobiological program. Within Cobb's service one would find a mixture of state-of-the-art laboratory facilities, clinicians trained by the finest internists, and residents exposed to psychoanalytic methods. No one approach dominated; all were integrated. Neuroses, for example, were analyzed in terms of the autonomic nervous system as well as social maladjustment. Years later, Gregg was able to claim that the Harvard model was indeed being emulated across the country, with many directorships filled by Cobb's former students.[34]

Meyer's framework of maladjustment had depended upon a prevailing theory of *habits* to connect cerebral function with educability and social performance. At the turn of the century, habits were posited as the meeting place of nervous physiology, the subconscious, socialization, and individual willpower. "Habit," wrote Edward Taylor in 1898, "constitutes the very essence of a well-organized and effectual life." As we age, we become "more and more subservient to the power of continually repeated acts, until finally we become, in great measure, automatic." Adult man, in fact, is little more than "bundles of habit." In a famous analogy, William James likened the nervous system to a field in which well-worn paths are eventually cut by daily walks; what is "plastic" at an early age is not so easy to change at a later date. The emphasis on habits coincided with a shift to brainwork as the most important aspect of human evolution. "We need poets and scientific investigators and artists, rich in imagination, even more than soldiers and backwoodsmen, strong of limb," declared psychopathologist J. J. Putnam in 1909. And if an individual's capacity to adapt to the environment is the key to evolutionary success, it is the brain itself that provides this facility; as Llewellys Barker declared in 1908, the brain *is* "the great organ of adaptation." When it came time to identify the exact mechanism by which the theory of maladjustment operated, the Meyerians simply appropriated the habit model. Habits, redefined thusly as "a new form of adjustment acquired during the lifetime of an individual," became the foremost preoccupation of the modern psychiatrist. Whereas few people were blatantly insane or mentally ill, nearly everyone could stand to have his or her repertoire of daily habits fine-tuned.[35]

By the time Gregg came forward to survey the mental health scene, the faithful habit model had been superseded by recent developments in neurophysiology that had begun to fill in the picture of what the prior model was content to leave unspecified. A new generation of investigators, such as John F. Fulton at Yale and Stanley Cobb at Harvard (who were inspired by the British scientist Sir Charles Sherrington), were in fact building a model of cerebral function that integrated behavior, sensation, and emotion into a single dynamic system of hierarchically ordered neural networks. The connection between the nervous system and socialization was no longer assumed, but had to be established anew. Habits were not enough. Instead, the psychosomaticists seized upon the recent conceptual breakthrough of the Russian physiologist Ivan Pavlov. The great promise of Pavlov's model of conditioned reflex was that of establishing experimental physiology as the master discipline for the study of the human organism. In the early 1930s, Pavlov himself suggested a direct application of his model to the domain of psychopathology, coining the term *experimental neurosis.* The matter of abnormal human behavior, it seemed, was now open to laboratory investigation and control. Instead of resituating laboratory scientists within the remote world of the asylum or troubled home, Pavlov had provided a means of bringing the psychiatric domain itself into the laboratory.[36]

Gregg at once saw the Pavlovian model's importance for the effort to place the study of mental disturbances on a defensible scientific footing. At Cornell, for example, Gregg funded Liddell's research on conditioned reflex in pigs, arguing for its potential to illuminate "some of the fundamental biological processes in human maladjustment, through studies of animals whose lives are carefully controlled and conditioned." There, he explained, Liddell "substitutes non-social laboratory conditions for the social factors with which the physician is compelled to deal." Another grantee of special importance was Robert Yerkes and his group at the Yale Laboratory of Comparative Psychobiology, who pioneered in the experimental analysis of primate behavior and placed special emphasis on those projects with direct relevance to human psychopathology. Indeed, it was not long before one of the Rockefeller grants led to a report by Carlyle Jacobsen, one of Yerkes's staff of experimental psychologists, delivered before the New York Academy of Science's Section on Neurology and Psychiatry – in 1935, an almost unprecedented disciplinary crossover. Jacobsen was lauded by the physicians present for having established, with concrete experimental evidence, that the frontal lobes were that part of the primate brain responsible for "the ultimate adjustment of the individual organism to the environment."[37] In the new theories of brain and behavior, Meyer's maladjustment model had found a second life.

## The American School of Psychiatry

Psychiatry's further progress was now placed in the hands of those programs that crossed over from brain to behavior, from laboratory to society, and from animal to man. In Gregg's view, two opposing lines of inquiry had found a point of intersection. From one perspective, the 1920s and 1930s were a period when sociology rose to prominence within academic and policy circles; the nation's future seemed bound up with what might be learned when sociologists made survey expeditions to the gambling dens, church groups, gang centers, and stock exchanges. From another perspective, though, the power of science lay instead in its *inward* excursions into the glands, the cells, and especially the brain. Gregg's hope was that by updating the maladjustment model into an experimentally based framework, psychiatry would step forward as that medical specialty best able to close the breach that had arisen between the internal and external investigations of man.

The "American School of Psychiatry" that came to dominate the field in the 1930s – represented by the likes of William A. White, Edward Strecker, Earl Bond, the Menningers, and Nolan D. C. Lewis – drew renewed strength from the interdisciplinary framework of Meyer's psychobiology as updated by Gregg's vision of psychosomatic medicine. Putatively brought within a single profession were the erudition of the psychoanalyst, the clinical experience of the ward physician, the social utility of the urban consultant, and the solid rigor of the laboratory investigator. In substituting the new experimental models of human behavior for Meyer's reliance on habits, Gregg reinvigorated the framework of maladjustment as a means of holding together this diverse range of perspectives and methods.

Knowledge of humankind's internal aspects, whether of mind or body, all seamlessly interconnected with the growing literature on its external features. In this manner, the study of psychoanalysis, which in the viewpoint of many contemporary physicians looked distinctively nonmedical, was not so much repudiated as it was assimilated and kept in reserve as a useful resource for explaining the causative processes that resulted in mental disturbances. The modern psychiatrist might consider himself "psychodynamic" in orientation, but this stance did not imply that his practice was based on dream interpretation or transference.[38] At the same time, this group of medical professionals was just as happy to resort to neuroendocrine models to justify the use of the latest glandular extract, or to sociological mappings that linked increased psychosis to urban decay. The catchwords were *pragmatism* and *eclecticism:* whatever worked was fine. Thus, it was entirely consistent that the same university course might teach the principles of neurophysiology and of unconscious ideation, or that workers at the prestigious government hospital for the insane at St. Elizabeth's (Washington, D.C.) might pioneer both fever therapy and psychoanalysis.

Emboldened by the Rockefeller Foundation's entrance and by Gregg's personal commitment to Meyer's and Salmon's expansive vision of modern psychiatry, a growing vanguard of psychiatric reformers and leaders took up the challenge to remake the profession. Confidently setting up programs of neuropsychiatry at such prestigious locations as the Institute of the Pennsylvania Hospital, Harvard, McLean Hospital, and the Hartford Retreat, a new generation of psychiatrists took upon themselves the task of building a medical specialty that broke through all the traditional barriers that still divided the mental health field. With some excitement, for example, Edward Strecker at the Institute in Pennsylvania set about putting in place a single program that linked laboratory studies and clinical experience, the study of minor neuroses and severe psychoses, Freudian perspectives and somatic treatments – all within an urban facility that served both the institutionalized mentally ill and normal schoolchildren. Working within the maladjustment model that provided a scientific justification for everything from endocrine studies to vocational guidance, Strecker was so bold as to open a private consulting room in a downtown office building, thus earning credit for becoming the first psychiatrist in a wholly nonmedical setting.[39] The future seemed unbounded.

## The Problem of Mental Disorder

In the two decades that followed the rechartering of the American Psychiatric Association in 1921, the various components of Meyer's vision came together. The doctors who staffed the state hospitals, the private-practice offices, the clinics, and the social service agencies might all legitimately claim to be members of a single profession: psychiatry. The new psychiatry gained a foothold in the medical school curricula and the wards of the university hospitals, thanks to the influence of the Rockefeller Foundation's calculated philanthropy. In these progressive sites, students of all specialties were taught a passably unified system of psychiatric diagnostics, nosology, and etiology. And with the introduction of Bleuler's conception of schizophrenia, which drew from both Freudian and Kraepelinian frameworks, psychoses and neuroses were at last joined into a single system of classification and mental dynamics.[40] The new "dynamic psychiatry," as it was popularized, embraced a disparate array of therapeutic interventions that ranged from psychotherapy and occupational instruction to glandular treatments and colon surgery. The conceptual justification for this unabashed eclecticism was found in Meyer's philosophy of psychobiology, which wove organs, consciousness, and social actions into a seamless web.

In 1934, representatives from the American Medical Association, the American Neurological Association, and the APA hammered out an agreement to form the American Board of Psychiatry and Neurology, thus formally signifying the formation of an independent, bona fide medical specialty. In a startling reversal of roles, the senior and previously more powerful field of neurology now played second fiddle to its upstart cousin – its name trailed not by accident. As one observer noted in 1943, although 48 percent of diplomates received certification only in psychiatry, and another 47 percent in both specialties, only 5 percent were so brave (or foolhardy) as to try to base a career on neurology alone. The woeful state of neurology consumed the interest of the profession's leaders.[41] (One publicly lamented that for a neurologist to make a go of it, he would have either to moonlight as a violinist or take up psychotherapy.) As to the fate of the term *neuropsychiatry*, once the reconfiguration of psychiatry was in fact complete, when its rootedness in alienism was displaced by the new definition, the prefix *neuro-* was quietly abandoned.

By the middle of the 1930s, the field seemed poised for tremendous expansion, drawing strength from each of its diverse roots. With its massive base in the asylums, psychiatry was in control of an enormous service role that was only growing larger every day. The lines of financial support, however meagre, were guaranteed for the foreseeable future. From the neurological tradition, the new psychiatry gained a license to traffic in the lucrative business of the urban dweller, whose minor depressions and neuroses provided an inexhaustible reservoir of clinical income. And the extension into the clinics, agencies, guidance centers, and other nontraditional locations of medical authority gained for psychiatry a voice in personal and social affairs, large and small, that was complemented by a growing presence in magazines, newspapers, and advice books that fed the obsessions of a public hungry for personal guidance.[42] Lastly, its rehabilitated status as a legitimate branch of medicine cloaked the field of psychiatry in the aura of scientific progress, thus promising ever more fantastic accomplishments.

Flushed with a renewed sense of professional success and social prestige, psychiatrists sought their fortunes in all directions. Indeed, the Rockefeller program in psychosomatic medicine proved remarkably successful in establishing the subject of mental disturbances as a field ripe for experimental investigation; in the 1930s, research into psychiatric problems blossomed across a wide variety of subfields, including genetics, constitutional medicine, intelligence tests, blood sugar and metabolism studies, pathology, endocrinology, urinalysis, pharmacology, epidemiology, nutrition, and neurophysiology – not to mention the wide variety of competing psychologies. So conspicuous was the upswing in such investigations that reports in the psychiatric literature for the first time began to chronicle this trend as an important subject in itself.[43] Moreover, the multiplicity of methods and approaches broached by modern psychiatry was rivaled only by its diversity of social roles, which included those of researcher, clinician, guidance counselor, hospital administrator, social theorist, and a proxy for the legal system. It was all psychiatry.

## Psychiatry's Future

Although all of these groups identified themselves as parts of the same profession, this facade does not imply that the field was harmonious or devoid of internal strife. To the contrary, even with all of its professional gains, psychiatry remained a fractious and heterogeneous medical specialty. Somaticists still battled psychologists, hospital psychiatrists tussled with their private-practice counterparts, laboratory-based researchers retained their smug condescension, and everybody had a bone to pick with the Freudians. The crucial point, however, was that now there existed a framework in which all of these factions might link their futures in a common enterprise, providing a front that, if not completely united, hung together well enough for public display. Psychiatry, it might be more accurately stated, was a *confederation* of disparate subgroups that – for the time being, at least – saw more opportunity in collective than in individual efforts.

Perhaps Meyer's most fateful move was his strategy of reconfiguring psychiatry as the medical specialty that dealt, not with insanity, but with mental disorder. In the prior framework, the physician had been restricted in subject matter to events that transpired mostly within the confines of the body, and in professional reach by an unfortunate historical legacy that kept him tethered to the asylum. In the new system, however, the physician's concern shifted from curing disease to solving problems, broadly construed, thus opening up a range of clinical and research opportunities that stretched to an almost infinite horizon. So defined, the need for the psychiatrist's expert intervention was apparent wherever a person's emotional structure or personality might affect his or her performance – namely, everywhere. And in the context of post–World War I America, the matter of social functioning was promoted to center stage. Mental health was discovered to be an issue of vital importance to the individual, to society, and to managers at every level in between. The payoff of any future advance in psychiatric knowledge thus seemed immense. The vast social burden presented by the severely disturbed in the state hospitals was still in need of a solution; and now added to this were the manifold problems that appeared in the urban consulting rooms, general hospital wards, guidance centers, social welfare bureaus, prisons, the workplace, and the home.

The wide response provoked by Meyer's and Gregg's invitation to explore the domain of mental disorders stemmed not just from the size of the potential rewards but from the special way in which psychiatry was mapped by them. In effect, the pair had redrawn the world of mental health as a dimensionless space in which all preexisting boundaries among disciplines were erased, and in which an investigator pursuing one type of research might meet up with a colleague of a very different stripe. A researcher who was examining the function of the inner brain of a primate thus might cross paths with a doctor writing up a case history of a paranoid on the wards, or even with a sociologist at work on a participant observation of a Chicago slum – within this framework, it was all essentially the same enterprise. Indeed, the dissolving of boundaries between self and society, between the internal environment and the external, led to a slew of bold medical formulations. In the psychobiological world, refitting an individual to society was to be achieved not only by sociological means. Indeed, the rise of plastic surgery in the 1930s is but one example of how physicians seized hold of the new opportunities by using the maladjustment model to reconceptualize their work. Before, these medical specialists were limited to restoring to natural shape tissue that had suffered gross pathological destruction by disease or accident. Now, however, a large but otherwise "healthy" nose was pathologized as a focal point of an individual's inferiority complex, a source of maladjustment that was surgically remediable.[44] In sum, it was all terra incognita once again, ripe for prospecting by adventurers and workers in a dizzyingly diverse range of locations.

A truly open frontier, the psychobiological world thus allowed for a broad range of disciplines to coexist. Those already located within one of the subgroups of mental health care were encouraged to redouble their efforts at clinical or bench research, and were at the same time willing to grant prospecting rights to the other clans, so long as their own were respected and unfettered. A different tactic was followed by those who put their faith directly in the psychobiological program, believing that multidisciplinary research alone would find the answer. These were the band of elite neuropsychiatrists who, equipped and funded by the deep pockets of the Rockefeller Foundation, staked out their claims in the psychiatric "borderlands."[45] In this context, the otherwise constant drumbeat of internal strife within the various psychiatric subfields was muted or ignored in the rush to claim the nearest rewards. Clan hatreds could wait.

As exciting as were the opportunities afforded by the new psychiatry, Meyer's vision at all times remained vulnerable to an array of grave challenges. To begin with, Meyer himself realized that much had been achieved on the basis of a promise that was as yet unfulfilled. If perceptions shifted to the conclusion that psychiatry had been oversold, the backlash would doom any further progress.[46] Second, the successful remedicalization of the field drew attention from powerful scientific quarters that until this time had safely ignored it. In building bridges to the rest of medical science, psychiatrists in effect had opened up their field to poachers from the outside. Mapped by Meyer as a borderless domain, the subject area had become unpatrollable. Ironically, psychiatrists thus might have become scientific only to lose control of their field to established scientists. Lastly, the confederation of disciplines and subfields would hold together only as long as two conditions pertained. On the one hand, there had to exist a shared scientific language and framework that might translate between all of their sundry interests and claims. Meyer's maladjustment model, as reinvigorated by Gregg, played this vital role; how long it would pass muster was unknown. On the other hand, the overall conception of what constituted valid scientific or medical knowledge had to remain sufficiently expansive to allow all of the diverse parties – whether informed by neurophysiology, psychoanalysis, or sociology – to continue to march together under the same banner of modern medical science.

Such was the state of affairs facing the entire medical and psychiatric community in the 1930s when the National Research Council, with the aid of the Carnegie Foundation, commissioned a high-profile meeting with delegates from all of the relevant fields. According to its organizers, the purpose of this conference on "The Problem of Mental Disorder" was to ascertain the status of psychiatry as a scientific pursuit. Noting the existence of multiple forms of mental medicine, the roster of speakers was deliberately pluralistic in scope, including Adolf Meyer on psychobiology, Lawrence Kubie on psychoanalysis, and Abraham Myerson on physiological psychiatry. Other invitees included H. S. Jennings on genetics, Joseph Jastrow on clinical psychology, A. L. Kroeber on anthropology, C. V. Cowdry on neurocytology, and Leta Hollingworth on education, to name a few.[47]

As diverse as were the individual approaches, a common thread was found in the participants' unfaltering focus on man's "maladjustive disorders." All were convinced of the immense potential of the field, which included the "stupendous problem of caring for hundreds of thousands of hospitalized patients and for more hundreds of thousands of unhospitalized persons unfit for making their way and their living in the community." "A vast host of the restrained psychotic and of the unrestrained neurotic," wrote the organizers, "afflict themselves, distress their families, trouble the local community, disturb business and profession, and create an enormous economic loss." In addition, there was the matter of "the queer, the vagrant, the flighty, the incorrigible, the suspicious, the irascible, the unstable, and the reclusive." "All these," it was noted, "are social hazards . . . incapacitated for effective living and for that measure of contribution to society which its members are called upon to make in the well-ordered state or community."[48]

For psychiatric leaders such as Adolf Meyer, the conference was a bittersweet affair. To be sure, the close attention paid by the rest of the biological and human sciences to the domain of psychiatry was proof positive of the gains that had been made since the start of his reform campaign. In designating the new psychiatrist as the medical expert who was responsible for the realm of mental disorder, Meyer had billeted his foot soldiers precisely at the vortex of converging social, scientific, and political currents. Experimentalists were looking outward from their laboratories, hoping to connect their petri plates and microscope slides to the larger social issues of the day; a number of social scientists met this gaze from the other direction, seeking to anchor their own global models in hard biological truths; and in the middle were the physicians, trying to straddle both knowledge domains in a quest for more social authority and a wider service role. Meyer's vision of mental disorders was precisely the realm in which all of these interests collided. The arrival of the large philanthropies and the heightened interest of the public provided an additional groundswell of support that carried forward psychiatry's momentum.

The same forces that hastened the growth of the profession, however, threatened to consume it at any time. It was difficult enough to construct a professional and disciplinary identity which might be shared by all of the various combative factions that comprised psychiatry. Any one of these subgroups might just emerge powerful enough to cannibalize the rest from within. At the conference, for example, Lawrence Kubie expounded upon the breadth and depth of the Freudian revolution that was overturning every discipline's conception of human nature; at the same time, neuropathologist Walter Freeman declared his faith that only chemical research would at last "dissolve the mists that surround the one irresistible conclusion that faulty cortical function is synonymous with psychosis."[49] Moreover, the new attention paid to mental disorders by the rest of the scientific establishment posed its own dangers from without. The fact that neither of the organizers of the conference had been psychiatrically trained or employed – one being a psychologist, and the other a cytologist – was in itself a source of great consternation to Meyer. His fears were hardly assuaged when the pair, in summarizing the conference, declared that it was high time for psychiatrists to bring their unsolved problems to the endocrinologist, the biochemist, the psychologist, and the physiologist.[50]

The entrance of the psychologists into the mental health care field was especially worrisome for psychiatric leaders. The redefinition of insanity as maladjustment had unintentionally opened the way for nonmedically trained professionals to claim expertise as restorers of mental health. At the time of the conference, the threat posed by the psychologists who had "invaded the clinical field" was already serious enough to warrant strongly worded attacks by APA presidents.[51]

Would psychiatry succeed? The campaign by Meyer, Salmon, and then Gregg was, in effect, a promise that the center could hold, that the many perspectives on the human organism and its social affairs were commensurable, and that one medical specialty might combine the social functions of healer, educator, manager, and producer of knowledge. The doctrine of psychobiology and the model of maladjustment were indeed powerful conceptual structures by which to integrate all of these varied information systems and social roles. Scientists, physicians, social reformers, and the public all looked to the problem of mental disorder as a domain of vast importance. Within this domain, such disparate groups had identified a common target at which they might aim in unison; at the same time, they espoused a unified purpose, that of restoring unproductive and suffering individuals to society as fully functioning citizens.

The success of the new psychiatry, however, ultimately depended upon the actual integration of what had been the separate worlds of the asylum, the urban agency or clinic, and the university laboratory. To some extent, each of these perspectives had been merged within the overall conception of psychiatry, advanced by Meyer the hospital clinician, Salmon the public health administrator, and Gregg the entrepreneur of experimentalism. And thanks to the selective seeding of the Rockefeller Foundation, highly visible demonstration projects sprung up around the nation where the psychobiological program was put into motion, collapsing disciplinary boundaries.

Nonetheless, the crucial issue of what was to be the next location of psychiatric advance, or what might be the future shape of the profession, remained unknown. It was not at all clear, for example, which would prove easier: to bring the problem of mental disorder into the controllable confines of the elite laboratory or to relocate the scientist within the remote world of the asylum. Each domain had its own distinct culture, perspective, priorities, and work practices, a disparity that militated against the unification of disciplines, regardless of how they might be brought together conceptually or organizationally. Moreover, whether or not the diverse kinds of problems that existed in the field really were fundamentally connected remained an open question: the chronic schizophrenic on the back wards of the mental hospital might prove *not* to have that much in common with the psychoneurotic in an urban clinic or the juvenile delinquent in a truant hall.

The organizers of the Conference on the Problem of Mental Disorder were acutely aware of these dilemmas. Their doubts centered specifically on the continuing rift that existed between the world of the clinic and that of the laboratory, one that the new psychiatry had perhaps simply papered over. For example, Madison Bentley (one of the conference organizers) called attention to the simple truth that workers in the physical, biological, and even psychological fields had limited contact with psychiatric patients, and that psychiatrists, for their part, were only crudely aware of what is involved in good science. One should therefore not expect too much of psychiatry's recent attempt, Bentley cautioned, to link "fundamental knowledge" with "the field of curative art."[52]

This stipulated, it was also clear that the momentum was to push ahead regardless of such doubts. In the face of the dire consequences posed by the existence of mental disorders, something had to be done soon. "It is necessary to face the problem in hand," Bentley concluded, "to invent solutions, and to provide adequate knowledge and means of relief." This was not something that might be left fallow until better circumstances arrived, for "the family, the neighborhood, and the state are all desperate."[53]

To the psychiatrists on the sidelines, the future was equally uncertain and yet in need of resolution. While the avant-garde within the profession celebrated their success in remaking psychiatry's self-identity, the everyday problems of what it meant to be a working professional were only worsening. The widening gap between reality and ideal hastened the drive for new kinds of solutions that might finally liberate the profession from its unfortunate past.

# 2

## Sufficient Promise
### John F. Fulton and the Origins of Lobotomy

> In science, just as in art and in life, only that which is true to culture is
> true to nature.
>
> Ludwik Fleck (1935)

One would be hard-pressed to locate a more nurturing environment for
the "new science of man" than Yale University in the 1930s, when –
courtesy of the Rockefeller philanthropies – many millions of dollars were
flowing in for the endowment and operation of the Institute of Human
Relations (IHR), an ambitious "experiment in total science." The time
had arrived for all of the human sciences, then scattered about the academic landscape, to be integrated into a single organizational structure. A
revolutionary transformation of knowledge would surely follow – or so
was the common belief among university reformers. Even the institute's
architectural design and building site, a series of interconnected facilities
situated at the heart of a medical school campus, spoke eloquently of the
need to overcome traditional disciplinary boundaries and barriers. Studies
on religion, law, industrial relations, sociology, economics, anthropology,
and psychology were envisioned as melding with ongoing medical ventures such as bacteriology, neuroanatomy, obstetrics, and child psychiatry. The resulting complex was named the "Human Welfare Group."[1]

The placement of the institute within the Sterling Hall of Medicine was
an important complement to Dean Milton Winternitz's efforts to reform
the Yale Medical School, a project also funded by foundation monies. As
he believed that "physical well-being is no less dependent upon psychic
and social than upon physical factors," Winternitz's strategy was to promote interdisciplinary research, for "there are no boundary lines to demar-
cate exactly the interests of biologists, psychologists, and sociologists."[2]
The fields of neurophysiology, neuroanatomy, and neuropathology were
given by him special emphasis, as scientific breakthroughs within them
might lead to a dramatic reconfiguration between the laboratory and
society. Throughout the entire complex the goal was the study and modi-

47

fication of human behavior, the method was research and the training of
new investigators, and the theme was cooperation among disciplines.[3]

Students of the behavioral sciences will easily recognize the names of
many of the prominent investigators whose work flourished at the institute. The long list includes Malinowski, Hull, Hilgard, Child, Dollard,
Sears, Sapir, Thomas, and Erikson; their output was to influence a generation of research on the subjects of motivation, aggression, socialization,
learning, culture, and personality.[4] One interdisciplinary study in particular, however, a project that merged neurophysiology, psychology, and
comparative biology, would profoundly affect American psychiatry.

### "The Face That Lopped Ten Thousand Lobes"

To contemporary observers, the intellectual origin of psychosurgery was
never much in doubt. By all accounts – then or now – Portuguese neurologist Egas Moniz was prompted to perform the first such operation by a
research paper that emerged from the internationally renowned laboratory of Yale physiologist John F. Fulton, whose facilities were a centerpiece of the Sterling Hall of Medicine. When Egas Moniz was awarded the
1949 Nobel Prize in medicine and physiology, less controversy was engendered by the prize committee's choice of scientific advance than by its
selection of whom to honor. Several observers held that Fulton was the
true "father" of psychosurgery and should have shared the prize.[5] These
sentiments were based on a well-known story which intimates that
Moniz's specific inspiration to perform such an operation stemmed from
his attendance at the Second International Neurological Congress, held in
London in August 1935, where he listened to a paper jointly delivered by
Fulton and a junior research associate, Carlyle Jacobsen.[6] In Fulton's own
encapsulated version of the events, Moniz had heard a description of how
brain operations altered the intellect and behavior of two chimpanzees,
Becky and Lucy. In particular, Becky had been a highly emotional animal
with a low tolerance for frustration. Failure in an experimental task triggered a tantrum in which Becky rolled on the floor, defecated, or flew into
a rage. After neurosurgery, however, Becky was keenly different, no longer
prone to such behavioral disturbances. In Jacobsen's words, it was as if the
animal had joined a "happiness cult" or had "placed its burdens on the
Lord!" According to the usual story, Moniz, in the public discussion
period, startled Fulton by asking whether these experimental findings in
chimpanzees might be applicable to the treatment of depressed human
patients. Fulton replied that there was a theoretical basis but as yet the
operation probably was "too formidable" to justify its use.[7]

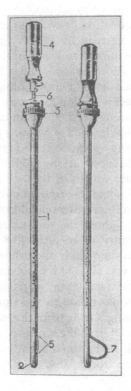

Figure 2.1. The Moniz leucotome. (Source: Walter Freeman and James Watts, *Psychosurgery,* 2d ed., 1950. Courtesy of Charles C. Thomas, Publisher, Springfield, Illinois.)

Moniz was referring, however, to the possibility of a much less extensive operation. Instead of completely severing the frontal lobes, as in Becky's and Lucy's *lobectomy,* Moniz was contemplating the destruction of small areas of this region, or *leucotomy.* Upon his return to Lisbon, he at once pressed forward, persuading psychiatrists at the government mental hospital to provide suitable candidates and a young but distinguished neurosurgeon, Almeida Lima, to undertake the operation. A series of twenty operations was commenced on 12 November 1935. At first, the patients had their brain tissue destroyed through the injection of absolute alcohol; in the remaining patients, Moniz switched to the use of a plunger-activated corer (see Figure 2.1). The best results were obtained in cases of agitated depression and involutional melancholia, of whom the majority were "greatly improved"; of seven schizophrenics, only two improved. Moniz soon named his innovation "psychosurgery."[8]

Moniz's initial report was read by Walter Freeman, an enterprising American neurologist, who immediately set out to repeat the experiment, assisted by his colleague, neurosurgeon James Watts. The pair in turn kindled interest in the United States. Due to failing health and a weakened political base, Moniz himself was soon forced to abandon such work and was content to let the Washington, D.C. team carry the day. Within six months of when they had first learned of Moniz's procedure, Freeman and Watts had performed as many operations as had their Portuguese counterparts; several years later their operations would total in the thousands.[9]

Later, when the procedure was in its heyday, Fulton proudly noted in his diary that "the operation had its origin in our lab." Harvard neurologist Stanley Cobb, in his 1949 presidential address to the American Neurological Association, highlighted the procedure's remarkable development. "Seldom in the history of medicine," Cobb remarked, "has a laboratory observation been so quickly and dramatically translated into a therapeutic procedure." It was clear to those in attendance whose laboratory deserved credit for the instigation of psychosurgery. At the same meeting, Cobb paid facetious tribute to the significance of Fulton and Jacobsen's work by projecting a slide of Becky, captioned "The face that lopped ten thousand lobes." Or, in the words of another observer, it was evident that "the shot fired" by Fulton into the frontal lobes of Becky was ultimately "heard round the world."[10]

## A Question of Paternity

There are serious flaws in the contention that John F. Fulton was somehow the father of psychosurgery. To begin with, it is highly doubtful that the dramatic public exchange between Moniz and Fulton ever occurred. Every account of this alleged meeting invariably refers back to the description penned by Fulton a full decade after the original event. No independent verification or memory of this event exists. Furthermore, this reconstruction differs from an earlier, unpublished account of his, in which Fulton refers to some passing comments made in a brief private encounter between the two. In either actuality, the notion that Fulton and Jacobsen's findings were the deciding factor for Moniz is farfetched. To begin with, Moniz's own testimony downplayed the significance of the animal experiments in his fateful decision. Even should one suspect Moniz's powers of recollection or veridicality, however, the historical record undermines Fulton's version of events. From a reconstruction of the clinical and research context of the time, it will become evident that Fulton's findings were certainly not necessary for Moniz to reach his fateful decision; and furthermore, whatever psychiatric significance Fulton saw in the chimpanzee findings was thoroughly lost on Moniz.[11]

In the mid-1930s, a broad array of investigators reaching across many medical and scientific disciplines were in hot pursuit of the mystery of frontal lobe function, lured by a conspicuous experimental challenge. The dominant scientific model of neurophysiology held that within the nervous system a component's function was dependent upon its date of evolutionary appearance. Newer parts, such as those appearing in mammalian as opposed to reptilian brains, were more complex in function and higher up in control than lower, earlier systems. The most recently evolved part of the nervous system – and thus by inference the most dominant control center in the cerebral hierarchy – were the frontal lobes of the human brain. What is evident in theory, however, is not always easily demonstrated in the lab.

Modern neurophysiology was born in the late nineteenth century when researchers, guided by the model of hierarchical dominance, feverishly began to map out the nervous system through a combination of advances in anatomical staining, direct electrical stimulation of brain tissue, and neurosurgical attack in man as well as animal. Yet even as the explorations penetrated ever deeper into the brain's "dark" structures, researchers were unexpectedly confounded by their inability to determine, experimentally, just what the frontal lobes did. Investigators could stimulate it electrically, or remove large sections of it, without any visible change in an animal's behavior. As a result, this portion of the unmapped brain became known sardonically as "the silent lobe."[12]

The first substantive reports emerged in the decade or so following World War I when the battlefield carnage produced numerous head injuries, many of which resulted in interesting neurological complications. In addition, neurosurgical technique had advanced to the degree that bolder operations were attempted for the removal of tumors or focal epilepsies in man and for localization studies in experimental animals.[13] The assorted clinical reports of frontal lobe damage slowly condensed into a behavioral syndrome known as "Witzelsucht" in which the victims were characterized by hilarity, euphoria, and childishness. The special elusivity of frontal lobe function became clearer when it was realized that injury to one frontal lobe (unilateral deficit) might be compensated for if the frontal lobe on the opposite side of the brain remained healthy.

The modern understanding of the frontal lobes is usually traced to the work of Italian neurologist Leonardo Bianchi and his publication in 1922 of a lengthy monograph on the subject. His research, which was based on frontal lobectomies in dogs, foxes, and monkeys that were *bilateral* (on both sides), strongly suggested that the intellectual basis of civilization was in fact localizable to the frontal lobes. Bianchi's findings were not considered to be without fault, however. They conspicuously lacked scientific rigor, were based more upon picturesque case histories of the injured animals rather than upon experimental protocols, and were mired in the kinds of rhetorical excesses that were endemic to the Italian academy.[14]

The pace of frontal-lobe research rapidly picked up after the first bilateral frontal lobectomies in man, which were performed for the removal of a rare kind of brain tumor. Walter Dandy performed the first such operation at Johns Hopkins in 1930, which was reported by neurologist Richard Brickner at the 1932 meeting of the Association for Research in Nervous and Mental Disease. The most astonishing aspect of "Patient A" was his apparent normality upon casual inspection. Brickner illustrated this point by describing how A accompanied two unsuspecting neurologists on an hour-long tour of the facilities at the New York Neurological Institute. Neither physician detected anything unusual about their tour companion, and Brickner was forced to conclude that the "frontal lobes are not 'centers' for the intellect" in any obvious sense. John Fulton, in the audience, commented upon some striking similarities between Patient A and a few experimental animals of his. Brickner's report was soon followed by a similar one, in which neuropsychiatrist Spafford Ackerly described the effects of an analogous operation performed in 1934 on a patient of neurosurgeon R. G. Spurling.[15]

Scientific and medical interest reached a new peak at the Second International Neurological Congress in London when a long session, presided over by the distinguished French neurologist Henri Claude, was devoted to the frontal lobes. Claude opened the session with a comprehensive overview of current knowledge, an account that drew upon a wide spectrum of clinical and experimental research from several countries (including the work of Fulton and his colleagues James Watts, Margaret Kennard, and Henry Viets). The literature suggested, Claude noted, that "altering the frontal lobes profoundly modifies the personality of subjects." In the session that followed, stimulating reports were filed by neurosurgeons, neuroanatomists, psychologists, and neurologists, including Richard Brickner's latest update on Patient A. Fulton and Jacobsen's paper was delivered in a separate session devoted to papers on physiology; here, too, four papers were devoted to issues of the frontal lobe. What distinguished the Yale report, "The Functions of the Frontal Lobes: A Comparative Study in Monkeys, Chimpanzees and Man," was its direct linkage of animal with human reports.[16] In sum, by the time of his trip to

London, Moniz had available to him a rich and interconnected body of research on the significance of the frontal lobes.

Moniz seems an unlikely innovator. He came to medicine late in life, having first pursued a colorful career in national politics, including a stint as Portugal's foreign minister (he had signed the Treaty of Versailles on behalf of his country). Although based in Lisbon, Moniz was by no means isolated from the world medical community, and he rapidly acquired an international reputation in neurology. His renown was due chiefly to his contributions to cerebral angiography, a method of rendering arterial circulation of the brain visible through x-ray opaque dyes. Assuming the mantle of Portugal's only statesman of science, Moniz maintained high visibility through an active membership in the French Academy of Medicine and through an international correspondence that included neurophysiologist John Fulton and neurologist Walter Freeman.[17]

To Moniz, the idea of using brain surgery to treat the mentally ill, although novel and controversial, was not unprecedented. In his preliminary communication on leucotomy, he did expect that some physicians would deride his "audacity" and condemn the treatment as "excessively daring." But such potential criticism left Moniz undaunted. The positive results, he argued unapologetically, were sufficient vindication. Just as important, however, were the theoretical justifications. "We did not perform surgical interventions in the mentally ill at random," he declared. First was the matter of clinical orientation. Apparently, when Moniz attended the London congress he was already mulling over the possibilities of brain operations. History, Moniz wrote, argued for the organicist's direct approach to insanity. One by one, the functional or psychological diseases would fall by the wayside as their true physiological nature was understood. Next was the matter of choosing a potent means of attack. Moniz had been impressed by the clinical reports that had described profound personality changes following damage to the frontal lobes. When these reports were combined with existing neurophysiological information, it was clear that the frontal lobes figured in the very highest centers of brain function. This was not to say that such higher functions were specifically localizable, for "it is not conceivable that we can discover a center of intelligence, of memory, of personality, of conscience, and of will."[18] Mental pathology could not be surgically removed with the ease and certainty with which neurosurgeons excised cancerous tissue. Medicine was not helpless, however. Moniz's proposal was to follow through on the logical implications of traditional neurological doctrine, which held that personal habits of behavior and mind, if constantly repeated, somehow become neurologically "fixed." Was it not possible, Moniz argued, that much of mental pathology was due to instances where such brain wiring had become excessively rigid? If so, might not surgical intervention somehow free a patient's brain from enslavement to those circuits that dominated consciousness with their interminable, pointless reverberations?

Moniz's initial plan of attack, then, was to sacrifice a portion of the bundles of long fibers that connected the cells of the frontal lobes with other brain centers, thus sparing the gray cell bodies on the surface. Patients thought to be most appropriate for such an operation were those who suffered from a fixed idea, intractable emotion, or persistent delusion. Moniz was aware that a surgical attack on the frontal lobes would yield adverse side effects, including the possibility of "puerility, change of character, loss of social and moral sense, instability, etc." Nevertheless, Brickner's and others' case studies demonstrated, Moniz argued, that "all these disorders are not total. . . . The patient can still understand simple elements of intellectual material." "In other words," he continued, "even after the *extirpation* [destruction] of the two frontal lobes, there remains a psychic life which, although deficient, is nevertheless appreciably better than that of the majority of the insane."[19] And as his operation left untouched the majority of the frontal lobes, Moniz felt considerably assured in the reasonableness of his operation.

It is clear that clinical reports were the crucial factor in Moniz's decision to venture forth on the new treatment in psychiatry. Moniz, it is true, did make considerable reference to the animal studies under way. Indeed, in his landmark monograph *Tentatives Opératoires dans le Traitement de Certaines Psychoses* (1935), Moniz declared in the introduction that animal experimentation was the necessary first phase in the acquisition of new therapeutic knowledge. And in the body of the text, he quotes at length from Henri Claude's synopsis of animal studies on the frontal lobes that gave particular emphasis to the work of Fulton and his colleagues who established, among other things, the existence of connections between the frontal centers and the diencephalic (lower) centers.[20] The animal studies were especially important for proving the necessity of bilateral surgery, Moniz also noted. Later in his monograph, he singled out Fulton and Jacobsen's work for establishing that the capacity for recent memory and reeducation had been altered (though not eliminated) in surgery on the frontal lobes alone.

To Moniz, though, the animal studies were of only limited relevance in the study of psychiatric maladies, as "it is not possible to obtain experimental subjects among animals." There simply existed too "great a difference between the psychic life of man and that of animals, even among those most elevated in the zoological scale."[21] The story of Becky had been helpful to Moniz, but only to a point. The Yale primate studies were for him more a source of confirmation than of inspiration; to a large extent, he missed the point of what the chimpanzee experiments were about. Whereas Moniz was searching for a neural basis of emotions with a model based largely on the nineteenth-century framework of habits, Fulton and the Yale group focused on cognitive or neurological performance, employing a more recent model of dynamic neurophysiology. Fulton's claim to a direct paternal role in the origins of lobotomy thus seems stretched, at best. It is quite likely that, even without Fulton's contribution at the Second International Neurological Congress, Moniz – and then Freeman – would have proceeded as they did.

## Science Fictions

Now that the classic account of Moniz's discovery appears doubtful – the intellectual origins of leucotomy are not so easily attached to the primate laboratory at Yale – what are the consequences of this knowledge for the overall story of psychosurgery? And, in light of the fact that Fulton and Moniz have nonetheless been so effectively yoked together over the decades, what additional doubts are raised about our *other* such narratives of scientific discovery?

Ironically, the parable of Becky and the frontal lobes should not be fully repudiated, for there is a hidden truth lurking somewhere within it. It is the contention here that although Fulton's direct contribution to psychosurgery was less than what is implied in the standard narration, his indirect contribution was far greater. Fulton's true role in furthering the development of the procedure in fact has been overlooked, an omission that itself derives from a flawed conception of how science normally progresses. The historical puzzle presented by the story of psychosurgery thus invites a reassessment of our usual habits of storytelling in science.

In the first place, the question of whether Fulton and Jacobsen's paper really was or was not the factor that precipitated Moniz's fateful decision is a red herring, as is any attempt to pin the development of psychosurgery on a single research contribution. Traditional history of science has trained us to focus on the issue of who was the "father" of a particular technical innovation, school of thought, or mode of practice. Such an approach is appealing for its romanticization of the scientific process but lacks something in academic rigor, for the task of establishing the true genealogy of any scientific idea is more chaotic than we have been led to believe. Mental products are infinitely plastic things. With a little creative effort, one can make a case all too plausibly that any set of ideas A, B, C, and so on, did or did not influence idea Y.

The problem lies with the assumption that typically there exists a single "Eureka!" moment when a discovery bursts fully formed into a researcher's consciousness. More often, a researcher (or perhaps a scattered group of investigators) becomes intrigued by an interesting set of experimental phenomena and begins to reshape available theories and definitions to fit the unexpected results. The process is a continuing one, with new conceptions being shuffled and reshuffled among old ones until all the clunkers are discarded and a stable new framework survives. When a scientific community reaches consensus that a discovery has indeed occurred, after an interval of often considerable duration, its first action is to certify which experiments or ideas were the crucial stepping-stones that led to the current triumph.[22] The lone surviving framework thus becomes a template with which to reorganize the prior scientific record into a coherent, rational tale of progress, a means of identifying which researchers managed to get a piece of the puzzle "right."

Such narratives of discovery, although edifying and ennobling, are an invitation to bad history. Rarely do the certifiers encounter only a single possible pathway to resurrect. Just as troubling, the very notion of discrete steps to discovery is itself misleading. Ideas do not necessarily occur in distinct quantum leaps. Rather, they slowly evolve, containing some parts old and some parts new. Thus any attempt to date, say, the scientific discovery of oxygen or the medical innovation of penicillin to a single experiment is as wrongheaded as the quest to pin down the exact moment on the evolutionary continuum when "man" first appeared.[23] This kind of bad history is not without purpose or effect, however, as will become evident below.

The conventional search for a "father" of this or that medical innovation is misleading in other important ways. The dissemination of a new procedure, no matter how serendipitous its origins or favorable its outcomes, occurs within a particular medical community at a specific historical moment. If a medical innovation is to be considered plausibly useful and of scientific merit, there must exist a shared conceptual framework and a technical language that can encompass and explain its clinical effects, integrating them into the accepted scientific record. Moreover, medical communities have a definite social structure as well. If a new procedure is to gain attention, the findings of early experiments or clinical trials must be published in important journals, presented before prestigious societies, and demonstrated to potential practitioners; such activities require the support of influential figures within the professional

hierarchy. Success at all levels – intellectual, disciplinary, and professional – is necessary for a medical innovation to invite significant experimental trials.

Indeed, other physicians, in emulating Moniz, did not necessarily follow his particular theories or convictions. Although Moniz was quick to
publish enthusiastic accounts of the brain surgery in several languages,
setting off a flurry of clinical trials worldwide, the procedure's eventual
acceptance as a standard psychiatric therapy was largely due to the
dogged efforts of the American team of neurologist Walter Freeman and
neurosurgeon James Winston Watts.[24] In short, undue attention devoted
to the matter of who fathered the original idea of psychosurgery has
obscured the more salient issue of why the astonishing claims of Moniz (as
modified by Freeman and Watts) were adopted by so many in the wider
medical community. Pyschosurgery did not germinate in a historical
vacuum.

That Moniz and Freeman were successful in enlisting others to their
cause is not proof of a mass delusion among researchers but an occasion
to analyze the normal process by which investigators reach consensus that
an opportune moment has arrived. In particular, Fulton may not have
been psychosurgery's father, but he played a more important role as its
most significant *patron* in providing the scientific justification as well as
the professional support that guided the new procedure through its tentative first few years. The challenge, then, is to reconstruct why in the 1930s
it looked like a reasonable bet to pursue a psychiatric cure through neurosurgical means, and why so many leading physicians and scientists gave
credence to Fulton's opinion.

Indeed, it was no accident that the experiments used to justify psychosurgery originated in Yale's Human Welfare Group. The reason that Freeman's and Moniz's proposal was positively viewed by the broader community of scientists and physicians lies embedded within the prior history
of Fulton and his laboratory; the fate of psychosurgery in its early years
became wrapped up in the excitement surrounding a new science of man
that had coalesced at Yale. From the perspective of this band of investigators, what the new procedure might accomplish extended far beyond its
effects on a handful of the mentally ill. It also represented the unlimited
potential of an innovative kind of scientific research, one that promised a
new alignment between the laboratory and the clinical world.

In following this historical strategy, a better understanding will be
gained as to why – in its initial experimental phase, anyway – the brain
operations of Moniz and Freeman were judged as having "sufficient
promise," representing a venture worth the investment of research efforts

and their attendant risks. In so doing, an opportunity will appear to reassess the general manner in which laboratory knowledge and clinical utility come to be joined – for successes as well as failures.

The key to the puzzle of psychosurgery's early years thus lies nestled within the deeper meaning of Becky's tale. Although one can discount Fulton's own interpretation of what were the direct consequences of his research on Moniz's actions, the reasons behind Fulton's later fabrication are not to be dismissed so lightly. Novels and other fictions often reveal a deeper truth than objective, journalistic accounts. Sometimes this adage also pertains to the stories of science.

### John F. Fulton

There was something about John Fulton that destined him for a life of professional success and gracious living. Born into a midwestern doctor's family of modest means, Fulton graduated from high school at age sixteen. Following army service in World War I, he entered Harvard University where he showed early promise as a scientist (he had published six papers by 1921, the year of his graduation). Awarded a Rhodes Scholarship to Oxford, Fulton spent the next few years in the laboratory of Sir Charles Sherrington, then the world's leading neurophysiologist; in 1923, Fulton was promoted to University Demonstrator in Physiology. After two more years (with his publication count already pushing thirty), he returned to enter Harvard Medical School. At Harvard, Fulton came under the wing of Harvey Cushing, the patrician surgeon who was pioneering the new field of neurosurgery (known then as neurological surgery), and in the year after his graduation in 1927, Fulton was granted a post as Associate in Neurological Surgery at Peter Bent Brigham Hospital. As the protégé of both Harvey Cushing and Sir Charles Sherrington, Fulton had been groomed to become an international figure in medicine as well as in science.

With his marriage to the wealthy Lucia Wheatland in 1923, Fulton was assured a life of comfort and privilege that most scientists in America could only dream about. A true bon vivant – lover of gourmet food, expensive wines (1848 Madeira was his favorite such indulgence), tasteful clothes, and all of the finer things that money could buy – Fulton made the most of his good fortune. A scientist's lot is often not a happy one, but Fulton found a genteel way to temper the demands on his time and energies. Visits to international congresses every year, for example, were made that much more bearable by traveling first class on the *Queen Mary* (Fulton and Lucia sat at the captain's table, hobnobbing with movie stars).

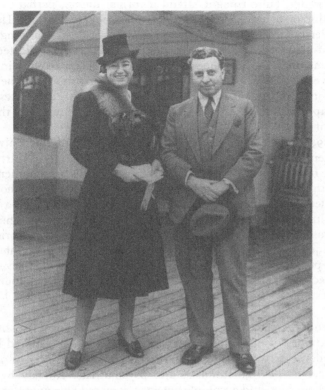

Figure 2.2. John Fulton and Lucia Wheatland Fulton on holiday, 1939. (Source: John Farquhar Fulton Papers, Yale University, Harvey Cushing/John Hay Whitney Medical Library)

Most fortunate of all, Lucia's wealth allowed him to satisfy his passion for book collecting: his collection would eventually become the centerpiece of one of the world's great libraries in the history of science and medicine.

Somehow, his indefatigable energies and interests all blended together. A day might start with Fulton tending to his herculean correspondence, a task that utilized one of the first dictating machines and the services of five secretaries. In the late morning, he might operate upon one or two chimpanzees and then preside over a graduate student's thesis defense, or hold a seminar on physiology for medical students. After a lunch date with some medical school bigwigs, there was perhaps a historical lecture on seventeenth-century science to deliver, a chapter to write for a medical textbook, or a few hours on the phone wrangling with a book dealer. And in the evening, Fulton might attend a formal dinner, perhaps with an ambassador or a luminary such as his neighbor, playwright Thornton Wilder. Personally, Fulton was always the perfect host, charming, attentive, good-humored, and loyal to a fault. He and his wife dedicated themselves to making a second home for those who had come to work in or visit New Haven. Those who knew him felt that he had "touched" their lives. Whether it was a student at the outset of a career or an elder statesman of science approaching retirement, all trusted their futures to the wise counsel of Fulton.[25]

In 1929, John F. Fulton assumed the chairmanship of Yale University's Department of Physiology at the remarkably young age of thirty – the youngest full professor in the university. As Fulton's appointment coincided with the physical reconstruction of the Yale Medical School, this young scientist had the good fortune of launching a career with a laboratory outfitted to his exact specifications. Visitors universally commented, Fulton was able to boast in 1933, that Yale's physiology laboratories were the best equipped in the country.[26] From its inception, Fulton's laboratory drew top postdoctoral students and researchers from around the world. In its first decade, the laboratory hosted sixty-two investigators, fourteen of them prestigious Rockefeller fellows, and published several hundred papers.

This is not the place to do justice to Fulton's professional rise. Involved in the activities of numerous professional societies, he centered himself within a dense network of research-oriented physiologists, neurologists, neurosurgeons, neuroanatomists, and psychiatrists. Already by 1935, Fulton's reputation and accomplishments prompted Sherrington to name him as his successor at Oxford and convinced Alan Gregg, director of the Division of Medical Sciences of the Rockefeller Foundation, to consider him as head of the Rockefeller Institute of Medical Research, America's leading center of scientific medicine. Fulton declined both offers (much to the relief of the Yale trustees), believing that his post at Yale provided a better vantage from which to transform neurophysiology. In 1938 Fulton published *The Physiology of the Nervous System,* a text that was eventually translated into six languages and established him as perhaps his generation's leading authority on neurophysiology. In 1946, he took over as editor of the fifteenth edition of *Howell's Textbook of Physiology,* extending his authority into general medicine as well (within two editions it was renamed *Fulton's Textbook*). A close observer later described Fulton as one who truly represented "global medicine" in vision and stature. Others identified him as the American scientist who should be credited most for revitalizing interest in neurophysiology.[27]

Fulton's scientific lifework was the construction of a coherent model of

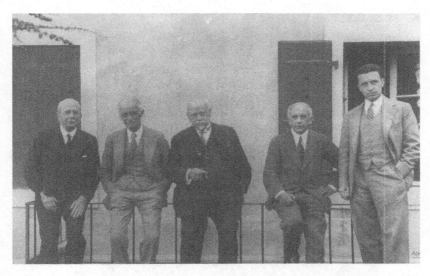

Figure 2.3. John Fulton and patrons, 1931. *Left to right,* Sir Charles Sherrington, Harvey Cushing, William Welch, Graham Brown, and John Fulton. (Source: John Farquhar Fulton Papers, Manuscripts and Archives, Yale University Library)

the nervous system. His specific research interest concerned the "encephalization" of the mammalian central nervous system, the evolutionary process by which the control of various intellectual, sensory, and autonomic functions shifted from "lower" brain systems to newer, "higher" systems. Fulton was deliberately extending to the entire central nervous system Sherrington's depiction of the hierarchical, integrated systems found in spinal cord reflexes. Experimental strategy remained the same. To reveal the dynamic relations among neural systems, the investigator would sever the connecting pathways in progressively higher neuroanatomical levels of the system. When a lower level is thus deprived of the communication from a higher system, it becomes "disinhibited," and will reveal itself through an unusual neurological sign or change in reflexes. To discern the function of a specific brain region, the area in question was removed and the animal was studied to see what faculty was lost or which new physiological conditions were imposed. This research strategy required proficiency in both neurosurgery and experimental physiology, an unusual combination of skills and knowledge that Fulton had obtained through his hybrid training. An immediate implication of this model was the need to experiment on animals more advanced on the evolutionary scale than

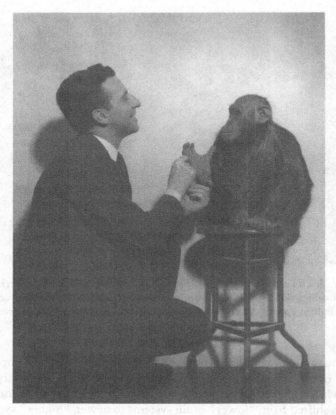

Figure 2.4. John Fulton and chimpanzee. (Source: John Farquhar Fulton Papers, Yale University, Harvey Cushing/John Hay Whitney Medical Library)

the cat or dog, the staple research subjects of most physiology laboratories. For this reason, Fulton insisted upon the construction of animal facilities that might support a wide range of primate research and set out to organize the first laboratory of primate physiology in the United States.[28]

Initially, the research plan worked well in the mapping of various motor, sensory, and autonomic systems. Advances in neurosurgical technique, such as Fulton's introduction of barbiturate anesthetic for operations on animals, encouraged researchers to study evolutionarily higher animals and the more complex brain regions such as the frontal lobes.[29]

When Fulton targeted the problem of frontal-lobe function as his laboratory's primary focus, however, unexpected hurdles arose. Destruction of
higher cerebral tissue yielded effects far more difficult to analyze than
those seen when studying the lower centers, which produced only simple
reflexes or neurological deficits. "Turning to questions involving perception, learning, memory and other higher intellectual faculties," Fulton
wrote in 1933, "objective data are far more difficult to obtain." Study of
neurophysiological function, it appeared, was inevitably merging with the
study of behavior. Fulton looked to Pavlovian conditioning experiments,
which were based on objective, quantifiable methodology, to complete the
analysis of cerebral function. Fulton pointed out how Sherrington had
foreseen, as early as 1906, that neurophysiologists of the future would
have to combine methods of experimental physiology with those of comparative psychology, when they would study the effect of cerebral lesions
on animals that had been trained to perform specific tasks.[30]

Resourcefully, Fulton developed close ties to Robert Yerkes's Laboratory of Comparative Psychobiology at Yale, where psychologists were
advancing precisely the kinds of animal studies recommended by Sherrington. In 1931, Fulton discovered that a recently hired psychologist,
Carlyle Jacobsen, was performing behavioral analyses of frontal lobe
function, and he "jumped" at the opportunity for collaboration. By 1935,
Fulton's frontal-lobe project was well under way. By the time of the London meeting, the work at the Yale laboratory on the subject was recommended to Claude as the very best in the world.[31]

### Jacobsen and the Psychopathology of Animal Life

Carlyle Jacobsen designed the experiments for which Fulton performed
operations on Becky and Lucy. Jacobsen's investigations were the direct
culmination of a well-planned program of research that explored the
problem of functional localization in the mammalian brain, a line of
inquiry that grew out of his work as a graduate student in psychology
under Karl Lashley. In Jacobsen's opinion, methodological flaws had
tainted earlier investigations. For example, he characterized the body of
research instigated by Leonardo Bianchi as haphazard and subjective, for
it relied upon such intangible criteria as the investigators' impressions of
the animals' "sense of shame." Others, such as S. I. Franz, he felt, had
pointed the way to a truer, more objective analysis by constructing "problem boxes" that tested the learning skills of cats and monkeys before and
after removal of selected brain tissue. Here, too, work was confused, as

poor surgical technique had resulted in lesions of uncertain extent and location. "The history of the problem," Jacobsen wrote, "is full of contradictory results, futile speculations, denials and counter-denials."[32]

Yale's unique combination of resources enabled Jacobsen to overcome these limitations. Supervised by Robert Yerkes, Jacobsen developed problem boxes of greater sophistication. At the same time, he had the full run of Fulton's Laboratory of Primate Physiology, where he acquired invaluable neurosurgical and neurophysiological expertise. Jacobsen soon produced a series of landmark papers that delineated subtle differences in intellectual and motor performances, functions related to specific cerebral areas across several primate forms. The most significant results came from his "delayed response test" (see Figure 2.5). In this test a monkey watched as the experimenter placed bait under one of two cups. An opaque screen was then lowered, blocking the animal's view. After an interval of varied length, the screen was raised, allowing the subject to choose a cup. Unlike the situation in earlier problem boxes, animals had to solve such experimental challenges by relying upon short-term memory rather than immediate sensory cues alone. When portions of their frontal lobes were removed bilaterally – and only bilaterally – animals failed the new test even with delays of only a few seconds. Yet the removal of analogous amounts of tissue in other areas of the brain produced no such effect. Jacobsen had established, in defensibly quantifiable and objective terms, that neuroanatomically precise removals of frontal-lobe tissue would indeed result in the loss of a specific faculty. He concluded from his elegant series of experiments that the frontal lobes, though not the fabled "organ of intelligence," provided an ability to integrate the experience of the recent past into current actions. Fulton wrote in his diary that Jacobsen's work represented "a brilliant deduction from experimental studies."[33]

Although Jacobsen's primary goal was the mapping of particular intellectual functions to discrete cortical sites, on occasion he did pay attention to changes in the animals' emotional behavior following the brain operations. Even before the reports on the chimpanzee Becky, for example, he noted that several postoperative monkeys no longer appeared to "worry" over mistakes and seemed impervious to frustration.[34] Such observations were useful for legitimating the expensive primate research programs; because direct clinical analogies could be drawn between neurological syndromes in man and those in animals, such investigations were likely to shed light on future issues of human neurophysiology. For example, Jacobsen compared Becky's and Lucy's conditions as exactly analogous to the few well-studied clinical cases of human frontal-lobe damage, especially to the patient described by Richard Brickner.[35] When he first reported upon the effects of frontal lobectomies in chimpanzees, at a meeting of the

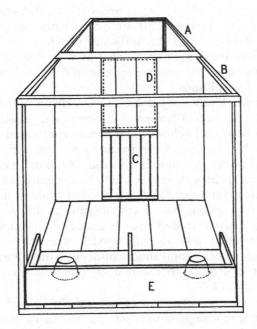

Figure 2.5. Diagram of apparatus used in delayed-response test. (Source: *Comparative Psychology Monographs*, 1936. Courtesy of The Johns Hopkins University Press.)

New York Neurological Society in January 1935, Jacobsen declared that the resulting behavioral disturbances were "strikingly similar to those described in man." Frederick Tilney, a prominent neurologist, saw in Jacobsen's presentation a "great deal of significance for clinical interpretation." Other than forming a few scattered impressions, however, Jacobsen did not explore the matter further. He remained leery of scientific investigations into personality or temperament, as such enterprises in his opinion were invariably undermined by their subjective components. Jacobsen clearly stated at the outset of his research that attempts to localize emotional functions must wait until a suitably "objective criterion" could be devised.[36]

It comes as a surprise, then, to discover that Jacobsen's findings were in fact interpreted as having broad *psychiatric* significance, and might serve as a neurophysiological rationale for lobotomy. How was it possible that his objective, scrupulously scientific approach to the study of animal behavior could refer to the richly subjective world of human mental disorders? An illustration of this difficulty was Jacobsen's recourse in likening postoperative Becky to a member of a "happiness cult," an uncharacteristically subjective analogy for one so dedicated to assailing the sins of anthropomorphism.

The psychiatric relevance of Jacobsen's work stemmed from a scientific model then in vogue, that of "experimental neurosis," which promised to unite the study of animal behavior and human psychopathology. Pavlov had fashioned this concept in the 1920s to account for occasional instances when laboratory animals suffered apparent "nervous breakdowns." Behavioral abnormalities in animals, he discovered, might result from a traumatic natural event such as a flood or from artificially induced stress such as that arising from a conditioning experiment in which a laboratory subject was forced to attempt sensory discriminations beyond its faculties. In either instance, the model of experimental neurosis brought the study of behavioral abnormalities into the laboratory context as reproducible occurrences that were open to modification, experiment, and ultimately control.[37]

During the 1930s, a movement to expand the role of experimental investigation in American psychiatry popularized the Pavlovian model. In 1937 the NRC's Inter-Divisional Committee on Borderland Problems of the Life Sciences met to ascertain what efforts should be made to advance "the scientific study of behavior problems." Psychiatry's dependency on mere clinical investigation, committee members agreed, had placed limits on its scientific productivity. A special committee was created, the Committee on Problems of Neurotic Behavior, to sound out the feasibility of attacking behavioral disorders through a coordinated program of multidisciplinary experiments. Experimental neurosis provided the committee with a unifying theme, and a Conference on Experimental Neuroses and Allied Problems was organized. A far-reaching intellectual synthesis, the model provoked much intellectual excitement as a new foundation for studying human behavior. Experimental neurosis, defined by the conference participants not as a disease entity but as a method of producing pathological mental states, was held to encompass the entire psychiatric domain, psychoses included. The model also symbolized a particular vision of the relations between laboratory science and clinical medicine, in which psychiatry would become objective not by bringing the experimenters into the world of the asylums but by redefining the laboratory as an environment in which psychiatric problems would become visible. Jacobsen himself participated in this conference and contributed to its report.[38]

Experimental neurosis was analyzed in the rat, cat, dog, goat, and sheep; Jacobsen's observations on primates extended this growing literature several steps closer to man. At first glance, his colorful remarks about Becky's behavior simply painted a vivid picture of the animal's unexpected behavioral transformations. But placed within the framework of the Pavlovian model, such comments were suffused with a deeper significance. Jacobsen reported that Becky's violent preoperative behavior, when elicited by the delayed reaction test, was "as complete an 'experimental' neurosis as those obtained by Pavlov's conditioned reflex procedures." Excision of Becky's frontal lobes had produced a startling effect: even though she now made far more mistakes, extensive testing with difficult problems did not evoke even a hint of experimental neurosis.[39] Within this intellectual context, Jacobsen's experimental findings inadvertently joined neurosurgery, neurophysiology, psychology, and psychiatry into a compelling combination ready for direct application to the problem of human mental illness.

Jacobsen's interdisciplinary investigations fulfilled the precise mission of the university's unique Human Welfare Group and its primate research program. The primate lab resulted from the combined interests of Robert Yerkes, who had been responsible for the presence of temporary animal quarters at Yale since 1925 and who was devoted to establishing a vigorous program of primate psychobiology; Fulton, whose desire to study the evolution of cortical dominance in the higher primates led him to designate such facilities as a non-negotiable item in his contract; and Dean Milton Winternitz, who was eager to prod the Yale Medical School into intensive research efforts on the central nervous system and its relation to human behavior. In 1931, Yerkes and Fulton exchanged memos concerning Jacobsen's studies; psychological equipment would be obtained from Yerkes's laboratory and surgical facilities would be provided by Fulton. Both Yerkes and Fulton viewed these experiments as a concrete symbol of the intimate connection between their two laboratories and of the interrelation of their fields. Within the decade, Fulton's program grew in stature to become America's most prominent location for investigations into the functions of the brain, drawing an unusual mix of young, talented researchers working at the boundaries of neurosurgery, neurophysiology, neurology, and behavioral science. Such a rich program, Fulton observed in 1933, was made possible by Yale's "peculiar combination of facilities and interests." By 1935 he was able to boast that more papers on primate brain function had been produced by the Yale laboratory than by any other medical school.[40]

The distinct institutional mission that made Jacobsen's studies possible also reflected an environment in which the potential psychiatric implications of his work would receive maximum consideration.[41] The Yale complex was one of the major beneficiaries of the calculated patronage of the Rockefeller Foundation, which as mentioned previously was redirecting the attention of medical researchers to psychiatric issues. In addition to its conspicuous funding of the IHR, the foundation endowed the Yale Medical School's "fluid research fund," the account from which Fulton maintained his expensive primate facilities. When his laboratory faced grave financial difficulties because of growing requests for research fellowships, Fulton approached the foundation for supplemental aid. Between January 1934 and June 1938, the foundation allocated approximately $25,000 to Fulton, which amounted to more than half of his total budget for the acquisition and care of primates. His laboratory was viewed by the foundation as a training center for young researchers who some day might revolutionize psychiatry and clinical neurology. Fulton's program fitted well with the Rockefeller Foundation's overall strategy of rebuilding American psychiatry; Jacobsen's research was a natural extension of Fulton's program. As early as 1933, Fulton was extolling the possible impact of Jacobsen's work on psychiatry.[42]

Psychiatry at the IHR Human Welfare Group had a special meaning, one that had little reference to traditional mental hospital practice, the mainstay of the psychiatric profession in America. Here, the study of mental disease was overshadowed by an orientation toward the problem of mental *disorder,* the approach of the mental health reformers outlined earlier. It was not expected that the next breakthroughs in psychopathology would necessarily be achieved by psychiatric researchers. The group looked instead to any of a number of scientific disciplines, ranging from neuroanatomy to sociology, that were investigating new models for understanding the psychobiological functioning of the organism in society: Newton's *Principia* was considered as fundamental a text as was Freud's *Interpretation of Dreams.* Pavlov's model of experimental neurosis perfectly exemplified this orientation. (Not insignificantly, the 1938 NRC committee on experimental neurosis would convene at the IHR.)

In short, the core mission of the IHR was to investigate the "failures of man to make satisfactory adjustments to his environment." Dean Winternitz focused the research efforts of the medical school on a similar goal. It is within this particular context that Jacobsen's contributions, framed within the Pavlovian model of mental disorder, would acquire a meaning especially relevant to psychiatry. In January 1935, when Jacobsen first reported his findings on the behavioral changes of chimpanzees to the New York neurologists and psychiatrists, he was congratulated for demonstrating that the frontal lobes could no longer be regarded as silent. In the audience's view, Jacobsen had discovered the region of the brain directly responsible for adjusting the organism to the environment. Becky's "maladjustment," they perceived, had been alleviated through experimentally verifiable methods. Whereas Yale had demonstrated an innovational institutional arrangement for extending laboratory studies into the social realm, Jacobsen's paper had provided an intellectual means for bridging the gap in practice.[43]

### Fulton's Radiations

Fulton and his laboratory at Yale had other important direct ties to the origins of psychosurgery in America. In a letter to Gregg, Fulton confided that he thought his most lasting contribution to science and medicine would stem from his role as a teacher, not from any personal scientific discovery. Emulating the great physiologists Carl Ludwig and Sir Michael Foster, Fulton sought to "pick the right men," those who "through force of character and originality [would] make their mark and come ultimately to occupy influential positions in the field."[44] Fulton nurtured with special care the career of James Watts, a young neurosurgeon who spent 1932-3 as an Honorary Research Fellow in the Yale laboratory.

Watts brought to Yale an impressive list of credentials, having trained under Percival Bailey at the University of Chicago, William J. Mixter and Henry R. Viets at Massachusetts General Hospital in Boston, and Ottfried Foerster in Breslau, all the while publishing a substantial number of research articles.[45] Although Watts's southern drawl, lethargic manner, and seriousness at first delayed his acceptance into the Fulton team, his neurosurgical skill and scientific style eventually won him general admiration. In Watts's most notable paper produced at Yale, he demonstrated a then unknown connection between the hypothalamus and gastric function. At the conclusion of Watts's fellowship, Fulton enthusiastically supported his application for a prestigious neurosurgical post at the University of Pennsylvania School of Medicine under Francis Grant and Charles Frazier. Fulton wrote to Grant:

> I have watched him closely this year and I have come to the conclusion that he has one of the most beautiful pairs of hands that I have ever seen work at an operating table. It is really quite extraordinary. He goes slowly, handles tissue with a Halstedian touch. . . . Scientifically he is independent, careful, slow to reach conclusions, and I think in consequence that he would never go halfcocked in any form of work.[46]

After Watts left for Philadelphia, Fulton closely monitored his career. For example, he orchestrated Watts's appearance before leading scientific

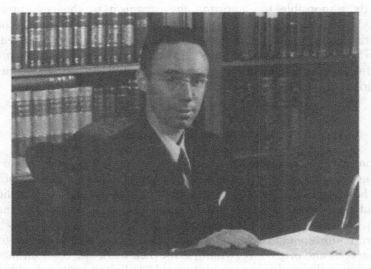

Figure 2.6. James W. Watts at Yale, 1933. (Source: John Farquhar Fulton Papers, Manuscripts and Archives, Yale University Library)

societies such as the 1934 meeting of the American Medical Association in Cleveland. Watts made good use of Fulton's aid. In Cleveland, he buttonholed the neurologist Walter Freeman about the climate for a neurosurgical career in Washington, D.C. This query soon led to Watts's directing his own neurosurgical service at the George Washington University Medical School in conjunction with Freeman's Department of Neurology. Watts wrote gratefully to Fulton that, although the starting salary was low and it would take several years to build up a profitable practice, "I know one thing, I am going to have the finest service in the country somewhere sometime."[47] Fulton felt personal as well as professional pride in Watts's continuing success.

Watts's career is but one example of how Fulton, by launching young investigators on fruitful research projects and then using his professional standing to advance their careers, was extending his influence through a new generation of rising neurosurgeons, neurophysiologists, and neurologists. Walter Freeman saw in Watts's appointment the growing significance of Fulton's role. "One might speak of a rather large grain of radioactivity," he wrote to Fulton, "centering in yourself in New Haven with secondary radiations emanating from those whom you have activated."[48] Only a short time later Freeman himself would be drawn directly into discussions with Fulton when beginning trials of a bold new therapy.

## Walter Jackson Freeman

At the time of Watts's recruitment, Walter Freeman was just entering the peak phase of a career in neurology and neuropathology that combined the many responsibilities of educator, researcher, clinician, and administrator. Appointed professor of neurology at George Washington University (GWU) in 1927, Freeman was given free rein to build up a clinical service, educational program, and laboratory facility. GWU had been under academic probation to upgrade its medical school, and thus Freeman was encouraged by the dean to develop the department as he saw fit. The District of Columbia itself, Freeman recalled, was a "neurologic vacuum" and open to innovation.

Freeman's clinical duties included making rounds at a number of local hospitals. In addition to teaching at GWU, he also lectured at Walter Reed and Georgetown, becoming known for his captivating pedagogical style, which included such flourishes as drawing anatomical sketches on the board with two hands simultaneously. A born showman, Freeman awed audiences with an uncanny ability to adopt the exact mannerisms of a patient with any kind of neuropsychiatric syndrome. The addition of Watts enabled Freeman to introduce a joint neurological/neurosurgery service and to start up a laboratory effort at GWU. A tireless investigator, Freeman maintained a steady stream of research reports, soon winning a university prize for a paper on multiple sclerosis. His 1933 monograph, *Neuropathology: The Autonomic Foundation of Nervous Diseases*, one of the first on the subject in the English language, was instantly regarded as a medical classic. Always up on the latest technical advances, Freeman credited himself as the first in the D.C. area to introduce into clinical practice carotid arteriograms, cistern puncture, thorotrast meningograms, and malaria therapy for general paresis.[49]

Freeman also moved in local and national professional medical circles, holding prominent appointments. His most visible role, however, was that of founding secretary of the influential American Board of Psychiatry and Neurology, which was established as the sole certifying body of the specialty's elite corps. Between 1934 and 1945, Freeman personally supervised the rigorous examinations of a generation of applicants, earning himself the sobriquet "the son of a bitch" of American psychiatry and neurology. In reward for his efforts, he was named president of the board in 1946. A pragmatic activist who loved a good fight, Freeman wanted to get things done, whether in the laboratory, clinic, or professional organization.[50]

Success came hard to Walter Jackson Freeman even though, in his own words, he was born with "the proverbial [silver] spoon in my mouth."

The eldest son of a respected Philadelphia family, he was given every social advantage. Childhood revolved around riding lessons, dance classes, and good boarding schools, as his mother prepared all seven of her children for the travails of high-society life. His classical education followed him through life, a knowledge of Greek coming in handy in his later professional training; his autobiography is also sprinkled with references ranging from Kipling to Rabbi Ben Ezra. The family's fortune and social standing rested upon the distinguished career of his maternal grandfather, William Williams Keen (1837–1932), widely regarded as one of the nation's foremost surgeons – and perhaps the first ever successfully to remove a brain tumor. His father, a well-liked otolaryngologist, apparently was more adept at medicine than he was at managing the family finances. During the Depression, both patriarchs passed away, shattering the family's comfortable existence. There was no longer any suggestion of joining high society. As for all the childhood preparation, Freeman soberly reflected, "such efforts were wasted." In personality, Freeman described himself as "never easygoing" and a loner; or, in Kipling's phrase, "the cat who walks by himself."[51]

Freeman entered college at Yale in 1912 with little ambition or direction. Much to his family's relief, he eventually decided upon a career in medicine. Indeed, at the Medical School of the University of Pennsylvania, Freeman finally found his calling. When World War I interrupted his studies, he landed a position as a medical intern at Camp Dix through the intervention of his grandfather. Although Freeman never saw warfare, the deadly flu epidemic of 1918 baptized him into medicine's grimmer aspects. Ministering to the nighttime needs of sixty young soldiers in a tent, Freeman watched as death would empty half of the cots by morning. Masks afforded little protection, as the physicians personally had to pipette blood samples by mouth. Daytime duties involved autopsying the same soldiers, a grisly, repetitive business of weighing lung after lung frothy with blood and other fluids. Upon his return to school, Freeman shifted his studies in the direction of neurology and research, mentored by William Spiller. Freeman's romance with medicine thus took root in the autopsy and pathology rooms, where he worked long hours in an attempt to improve upon some histological stain or neuropathological diagnosis.[52] The work was laborious, exactingly disciplined – and to him exciting. Freeman had found a lifelong outlet for his restless energy, where his love of tinkering might find full expression. In his senior year, he won the prize for best undergraduate research and had a paper published in the *Archives of Neurology and Psychiatry*. He graduated in 1920, second in his class.

Postgraduate training cemented Freeman's career choice of neuropathology. After working under N. W. Winkelman in Philadelphia, he set out for a European tour with letters of introduction from Keen that opened the doors of the best laboratories. His stops included the workshop of Pierre Marie in France, Giovanni Mingazzini in Rome, and Otto Marburg in Vienna. Acquiring along the way a working knowledge of French, Italian, and German, Freeman opportunistically bounced from project to project, examining brain tissues in everything from human fetuses to zoo elephants. Whereas others sent home pictures and travelogues, Freeman was just as likely to publish a paper on some new staining technique or histological observation as a souvenir of his time abroad.

The tour was cut short in 1924 when Freeman received a cable informing him that he had been selected as the new director of the Research Laboratories of the Government Hospital for the Insane in Washington, D.C. (informally known as St. Elizabeth's), a coveted post that had been arranged through yet another benevolent act by Keen. Returning home, Freeman quickly plunged into the work, found a bride, and fathered four children within forty months.[53] In 1931, Freeman believed that he had arrived professionally. As chairman of the AMA Section on Nervous and Mental Disease, he happily presided over its session at the association's annual convention, which just happened to meet that year in his hometown of Philadelphia. Adding to this, his scientific exhibit was awarded the bronze medal. Freeman proudly stood next to his grandfather, age ninety-four, when Keen received an ovation at his last public appearance. Following the meeting, Freeman was invited to join an executive committee of the AMA, a post that directly involved him in the creation of the American Board of Psychiatry and Neurology, and which established him as a national figure in American neuropsychiatry.

## The Riddle of Psychiatry

Freeman's entry into psychiatry was pure happenstance. The duties at St. Elizabeth's were akin to what one might expect in a busy pathology department at a very large general hospital. In his first few years, Freeman explored standard neuropathological matters, publishing articles on Parkinson's disease, brain tumors, encephalitis, and neuroanatomy. As mental institutions were filled with inmates who were in exceptionally poor health, and who also were routinely abandoned by their families, they provided a rich source of clinical cases that might be followed up at autopsy. Freeman mined this material for his monograph on neuropathology.[54]

Characteristic of his tendency to exploit whatever research opportunity

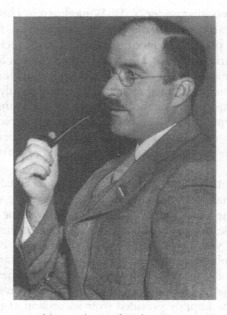

Figure 2.7. Newspaper publicity photo of Walter Freeman, 1935. Caption states, "Knows His Endocrines – Dr. Walter Freeman, of Washington, grandson of Philadelphia's late great Dr. W. W. Keen, upset some of the theories of endocrine gland control in human beings." (Source: *The Evening Bulletin* [Philadelphia], 30 April 1935. Courtesy of Urban Archives, Temple University, Philadelphia.)

happened to appear nearby, Freeman inevitably was drawn to a new frontier in the problem of mental disorders. Quite naturally, his initial research strategy was to apply familiar neuropathological and histological techniques in a search for definite physical signs that might identify insanity. In spite of arduous labors, including the analysis of 1,400 autopsies, Freeman confronted a string of negative results. He sardonically remarked that, when performing autopsies at St. Elizabeth's, if he encountered an especially "normal" brain, he was inclined to make the diagnosis of psychosis. Freeman later recognized that during this period his regard for the inmates had been limited to their value as a source of material for laboratory analysis, and consequently he had paid little attention to their suffering. An insane asylum was not where he had expected his career to begin. He explained, "On first visiting a mental hospital I had about the same reaction, I think, as most; a rather weird mixture of fear, disgust and shame." Yet, slowly transformed by daily contact with psychiatric patients, Freeman eventually became interested in their plight.[55]

With his sympathy thus engaged, Freeman set out to discover practical means of treatment. A true organicist, Freeman had little patience for psychotherapy, a treatment that was enjoying great popularity at the time. In his opinion, it was not idle chatter that was needed but a clear, understandable medical procedure that might get patients out of the hospital and back into society. He was chagrined to discover, however, that the popular organic models of psychiatry were just as impotent. As a spin-off of his massive pathological study of insane patients, Freeman tested the accuracy of Nolan D. C. Lewis's claim that schizophrenic hearts were smaller than normal hearts; they were not. Similarly, Freeman investigated whether variance in the endocrine glands might account for the distribution of mental diseases, a theory then dominating psychiatric research. Here too the conclusion was disheartening. One by one the current theories and practices were disposed of, and he abandoned the quest, mildly disgusted.[56]

Freeman was thus realistic about the possibilities of new psychiatric therapies, as when he delivered a 1935 paper titled "The Mind and the Body." "Changing the Constitution of the United States is child's play," he bemoaned, "in comparison with changing the constitution of man." In the same address, in a more philosophical tone, Freeman noted that:

> It does seem a pity that a patient who has been an inmate of the institution since you and I were born should come to necropsy and reveal what appears to be a perfectly normal brain in a reasonably healthy body. There is a riddle somewhere, and neither psychology nor psychiatry nor psychoanalysis, on the one hand, nor morphology nor pathology nor bacteriology, on the other hand, has gone any distance at all in its solution.

Frustrated, Freeman was looking to new vistas. "Perhaps the new field of electrophysiology, of cerebral action currents, so promising in the realm of epilepsy, will open vistas of cerebral activity that at present are closed to us," he wrote. "Even more promising," he stated, "is the exploration of the central vegetative [evolutionarily primitive] centers in the interbrain. . . . The behavior disturbances following relatively localized disease of this region as in encephalitis and syphilis give hope that *we may be able to influence behavior in a significant manner by destroying certain localized portions.*" The potential of brain surgery thus was clearly something Freeman had already pondered.[57]

In any event, for Walter Freeman neuropathology had run its course professionally as well as intellectually. He left St. Elizabeth's in 1933 to devote his full energies to a career at George Washington University and to cultivate his private neuropsychiatric practice. His continued interest in the treatment of mental illness was also a matter of economics, the need to support his growing family. Neurology as a lucrative specialty was in decline by the 1930s, and like so many others in his position, Freeman discovered in psychiatry a vast clientele. In 1936, he was forty-one years old, an ambitious and proud researcher who was determined to forge a medically productive if not profitable career. In the young neurosurgeon Watts, Freeman had found an ideal colleague to share new adventures, one who was also trained in research and even more concerned about the need to develop a clinical practice. The 1930s were a period in which it still took "courage" for a young surgeon to limit his practice to neurosurgical cases.[58]

When abstracting papers for a review of neurology in the spring of 1936, Walter Freeman happened upon Egas Moniz's preliminary communication in the relatively obscure journal *Lisboa Medicina*. Freeman had already been well acquainted with Moniz and his work. For some time, he had been experimenting with Moniz's technique of cerebral angiography. Indeed, at the Second International Congress the summer before, Freeman mounted a poster exhibit based on angiography only to discover, to his delight, that Moniz himself was stationed in an adjacent booth. Freeman came away from the encounter awestruck by what he described as the "sheer genius" of the Portuguese statesman-scientist. Had it not been for this chance meeting, he later commented, it is unlikely that he would have given Moniz's latest work serious consideration.[59]

Freeman wrote to Moniz, at the end of May 1936, that for some time past he had been contemplating such a brain operation, but now, "having your authority I expect to go ahead." Moniz, in reply, promised to send his more detailed monograph as soon as it was published and suggested that in the meantime Freeman should order a leucotome (the device designed by Moniz to cut brain tissue) from his French instrument makers. In August, upon return to Washington from a cross-country camping vacation, Freeman picked up the correspondence. He breathlessly wrote to Moniz that he had risen at five in the morning to finish reading the monograph, which he had received in his absence, and to fire off a positive review of it for the *Archives of Neurology and Psychiatry*. Freeman was certain that it would "prove epoch making in the scientific approach to mental disorders."

In the unsigned review, Freeman stated that "its importance can scarcely be overestimated." He boiled down Moniz's theory to the following argument. Although in the brains of the mentally ill "the cell bodies may remain normal," and "their processes [connecting trunks] show no anatomic alterations," the areas of multiple connections may contain "fixation of certain patterns of relationship among various groups of cells." This accounted for the "persistent ideas and delusions characteristic of certain morbid psychic states." To Freeman, Moniz's conjectures were a tour de force, representing the first viable solution to the vexing riddle of why persons with obviously deranged nervous systems nevertheless have normal-looking brains. The decades-old approach of attempting to localize the pathological brain "lesion" or cellular abnormality was fundamentally in error. The brain tissue itself was healthy – it was the functional wiring that was at fault. The problem was finally diagnosed and a workable solution presented. Freeman himself recognized that, when pressed on details, Moniz's theory was "naive." Nevertheless, here was "something tangible, something that an organicist like myself could understand and appreciate."[60] What was left to work out was simply a matter of optimizing the procedure by determining which were the best circuits to cut and which kinds of mental disturbances were most relieved by doing so. This was exactly the kind of straightforward challenge upon which Freeman thrived.

### The First Few Cases

By the beginning of September 1936, Freeman had both convinced Watts to join him in a trial of the Moniz technique and obtained the first surgical prospect, patient "A.H." A middle-aged woman with severe agitated depression, A.H. had complained of nervousness, insomnia, depression, and a constant feeling of insecurity and anxiety. As a girl, she had been a "nervous child." In the last ten years, she stated, she had not had a decent night's sleep. Over last few months, however, she had been increasingly despondent and apprehensive, worrying over trifles, "turning things over and over in her mind until she felt as though she would 'go crazy.'" She had always been rather vain about her looks and was depressed about effects of growing old; during the observation period at the hospital, she would pose nude before a mirror and make faces at it. Shortly before admission, "she exposed herself before the window, and urinated upon the floor." The patient reported that she had entertained thoughts of suicide but had lacked sufficient courage to go through with it. The family was convinced that permanent institutionalization lay just ahead.

The idea of trying the operation was discussed with both patient and husband, and consent obtained. (The patient agreed only after receiving

assurance, false, that her hair would not be shorn during the operation.)
Apparently, the family did not approve the operation without first seeking
additional information about the Washington team. The patient's son-in-
law was a midwestern physician who sought counsel from Karl Menninger, head of the famous Menninger Clinic (soon to become America's
most illustrious psychiatrist). In particular, the son-in-law asked for a
judgment concerning Freeman's care. Shortly thereafter, Menninger related the incident to Freeman: "He [A.H.'s son-in-law] said that you
contemplated an interesting brain operation for the relief of what I took to
be an agitated depression." Menninger was happy to inform Freeman that
"Of course, I was glad to tell him how well we knew you and how highly
we regarded you."[61] The green light had been given, and by an impressive
independent voice.

The operation was performed on 14 September 1936, with a leucotome
that Freeman had ordered earlier from Paris. As Freeman narrated the
events: "Four hours later, as the anesthetic was wearing off, she was not
the least bit excited and declared that she felt 'much better.' . . . The
following day the patient was propped up in bed, put out her hand and
greeted her physician alertly but unconcernedly."

Freeman: Are you content to stay here?

Patient: Yes.

Freeman: Do you have any of your old fears?

Patient: No.

Freeman: What were you afraid of?

Patient: I don't know; I seem to forget.

Freeman: Are you sad?

Patient: No.

Freeman: Are you happy?

Patient: Yes.

Freeman found it significant that she allowed her husband to leave the
room, remaining perfectly composed, whereas previously his exit would
have incited an outburst of anxiety. The results were dramatically visible
to Freeman and Watts, leaving an intense memory. "I knew from the
first," the former would later write, "that here was a stroke at the fundamental aspect of the personality, that part that was responsible for much
of the misery that afflicts man. . . . "[62]

One week after the operation, Menninger wrote to Freeman that the
son-in-law had called and informed him that the patient was much improved immediately following the operation. Menninger added, "Natu-

rally, I am extremely interested in this and would appreciate it very much if you would have time to write me a little more in detail about the theory and practice of this new treatment." In closing the letter, he stated that he, as well as his brother Will (also a leading psychiatrist), sent their "best regards and congratulations on the success of this interesting work."[63]

Freeman and Watts rushed to present their case before the local medical society and immediately published the results. They wrote:

> A month after operation, the patient asserted that she was no longer inclined to worry, that she could follow out a trend of thought without distraction, that she could enjoy the company of a very energetic friend whose company formerly she could scarcely endure without exhaustion, and that she was content to grow old gracefully. She was well dressed, talked in a low natural tone, volunteered relatively little, but upon questioning showed excellent appreciation of her changed condition. Her husband asserts that she is more normal than she has ever been.

Freeman, on a cautionary note, concluded that it was unknown what would be the "permanent residuals of frontal lobe deficit." Nevertheless, "the agitation and depression that the patient evinced previous to her operation are relieved." Emboldened by the positive results, Freeman and Watts proceeded to do another five surgeries in quick succession. After the third such operation, on 20 October, Freeman happily described to Moniz more good results, though he noted that during the last operation the leucotome broke. He again congratulated Moniz for "having driven an entering wedge into successful treatment of certain of the psychoses."[64]

The first real professional hurdle came at the November meeting of the Southern Medical Society in Baltimore, when results of their first six cases were presented to prominent representatives of the neuropsychiatric community. Struggling to put into words precisely what the operation accomplished, they stated that it was "as if the 'sting' of the psychoses had been drawn." On the other hand, "We do not wish even to mention the word cure." "In all of our patients there was a substratum, a common denominator of worry, apprehension, anxiety, insomnia and nervous tension, and in all of them these particular symptoms have been relieved to a greater or lesser extent." They concluded:

> we wish again to define our position in regard to the operation. We have undertaken it as a measure of relief from symptoms that were causing great distress to the patients and to their families. . . . These symptoms have tended to subside following operation, and the patients have become more placid, more content, and more easily cared for by their relatives. The symptomatic relief has been almost immediate, and has persisted to the present time.[65]

Freeman and Watts were not so bold as to proclaim that the procedure should be used wantonly. "We wish to emphasize also that indiscriminate use of the procedure could result in vast harm," they declared, and added that they were extremely doubtful whether chronic, deteriorated patients would benefit from it. "Moreover," they warned, "every patient probably loses something by this operation, some spontaneity, some sparkle, some flavor of the personality, if it may be so described."

In Freeman's recollection, this meeting held special significance for the further development of the operation, as Adolf Meyer himself, the dean of American psychiatry, rose from the floor to declare, "I am not antagonistic to this work, but find it very interesting." Caution must be preserved, Meyer went on to note, and no promises should be made to relieve common distraction and worries by surgery, lest the presenters inflame "an epidemic of hasty human experimentation." It was essential that the public "should not be drawn into any unwarranted expectations." This said, "the available facts are sufficient to justify the procedure in the hands of responsible persons." As the procedure was in the care of Freeman and Watts, he declared, "I know these conditions will be lived up to."[66] Freeman later stated that Meyer's positive evaluation had a tremendous effect on his willingness to persevere.

Not all comments were as favorable. Dexter Bullard, director of the psychoanalytically oriented Chestnut Lodge in Maryland, where Freeman had acted as a consulting neurologist, was so infuriated by the idea of using brain surgery on mental patients that he tried to shout down Freeman and Watts. Balancing Bullard's attack – which was not published in the proceedings – were the comments of a physician from New Orleans who congratulated the pair on their attempt "to give comfort, courage and hope to patients suffering as these were."[67]

Freeman wrote at length to Moniz, heartened by this positive turn of events. He mentioned Meyer's support and then added that Ackerly at the meeting related how his own patient, who had had a large portion of his frontal lobes removed bilaterally to fight a tumor, was nonetheless able to survive well in society. Brickner was unable to attend the meeting, Freeman continued, but visited the next day to inspect personally four of their patients. Brickner left impressed and had started to make his own plans to operate. Several months later, Ackerly, too, would personally inspect several of their patients and leave with an idea to begin similar work.[68]

In the course of the following year, Freeman and Watts presented their findings to professional societies across America from New York to Los Angeles. It was not just the psychoanalysts, they discovered, who expressed grave doubts about the medical validity of operations on patients whose brain tissues demonstrated no visible abnormalities. Against criticism that was often heated, and occasionally vicious, the two held their ground. At the same time, they were developing a core of supporters and advancing both the theory and the technique of the operation.[69]

In February of 1937, Freeman traveled to Chicago, where he described their results in a series of twenty patients of varying diagnostic categories. Similar to Moniz's findings, he reported that the agitated depressives fared the best, whereas five out of six schizophrenics were unimproved. Psychological considerations were explored in greater depth than in their earlier communications. Apparently, constructive imagination and synthetic ability were impaired to a greater degree than more "fundamental" thought processes. "Patients can name colors rapidly, add columns of figures correctly, remember recent and remote events exceptionally well and concentrate on tasks with less effort than before," he reported. Moreover, "agitation is reduced in all cases." "The outstanding result," he concluded, "is reduction in the obsessive nature of the painful ideas." It was clear that "signs of intellectual deficit are not pronounced and do not handicap the patient for ordinary occupations of routine nature."[70]

Freeman knew that the paper was hastily pieced together and informally delivered, yet the harshness of the response still surprised him. The first comments were targeted at the issue of whether these positive results could be attributed to the operation's psychological as opposed to its physiological effects; perhaps the drama of a brain operation itself influenced these patients, acting as a not-so-benign form of placebo. Might not the experimenters, it was asked, perform a series of sham operations as a test? Then, Loyal Davis, distinguished neurosurgeon (and future father-in-law of President Ronald Reagan), angrily rose to announce that he had known about the operation from reports in the popular press. "I had hoped that the reports were grossly exaggerated," he began, but apparently not: Freeman and Watts were indeed wantonly destroying brain tissue. In clear derision of Freeman's nonmembership in the neurosurgical fraternity, Davis stated, "As a pathologist, he may not have much fear of looping out pieces of subcortical tissue," but his description "gives one's surgical conscience a slight twinge." Emptying a full quiver, he added, "The offhand manner in which this surgical procedure is described and discussed is no credit to the essayist as a surgeon, a pathologist or one who is searching for a scientific truth." What was needed instead were "the observance of all the strict conditions of a physiologic experiment." Others in the audience then joined the chorus of sarcasm and ridicule. Lewis Pollock, for example, simply stated, "First, this is not an operation but a mutilation." And not a harmless error, at that, for "many patients with recurrent depressions are highly competent and contribute largely to science, literature and art." He wondered, "What will be left of the musician or the artist when the frontal lobe is mutilated?"

Freeman later described his defensive reaction to the attack as being so emotional that "I almost bit the stem of my pipe off trying to regain control of myself." His response was to state that clinical work had shown that "a brain can stand a good deal of manhandling" and to repeat the point that "patients with these psychoses are in a serious condition and do not have much chance of recovery otherwise." In clarification of another misconception, he declared that they were *not* advocating its use for manic-depressives, involutional melancholics of less than a year's illness, or schizophrenics. "Is this operation justifiable?" he asked, rhetorically. "Most patients after operation," Freeman declared, "have been able to adjust better socially than before."[71]

In June 1937, Freeman and Watts presented their work at the annual convention of the AMA. Freeman, who continually apprised Moniz of the latest developments concerning leucotomy, wrote to him that newspaper coverage of the event had broadcast their results as far away as Paris and Shanghai. He reported that, although the work had been "roundly criticized" by many, it was given a warm reception "by those who in our opinion know something about the problem." More significantly, Wilder Penfield, director of the Montreal Neurological Institute who was pioneering the use of brain operations for the treatment of focal epilepsies, had astutely observed that the leucotome method left in place damaged brain tissue that might eventually lead to epileptic seizures. In response, Freeman informed Moniz, he and Watts were developing a new operative technique in which the corer would be replaced by a bistoury (a form of flat, dulled knife); the surgical approach would be from the side, not the top; and entry into the skull would be via a trephine rather than a burr, so as to minimize cortical damage. (The modified procedure would eventually become known as the "standard lobotomy.") The disciple had grown sufficiently confident to outstrip the mentor.[72]

In February 1938, Freeman and Watts, at the New York Neurological Society, described the significance of the operation for one particular class of neurotic patients, those known as "obsessive ruminatives." One patient, for example, was a young woman who had such a strong fear of contamination that she could not touch an object that previously had been touched by someone wearing shoes. Almost total social isolation resulted. After the operation, however, although she complained of a "lack of vivacity," she nevertheless was able to rejoin society. As proof, Freeman related that the patient had recently joined him and Dr. Brickner at the

Waldorf-Astoria for cocktails. By and large, though, the results were uncertain in this class of patient, they reported.

Brickner began the discussion with comments friendly to the two, saying that he had had the privilege of observing a number of their cases firsthand. It was true that the obsessions persisted and remained incapacitating, but "not to a degree comparable with that in the preoperative state." Results definitely were better in cases of agitated depression of long-standing duration. "There is little else to offer patients with such conditions," he stated, and continued, "That the procedure is radical is of little significance when one thinks of the years spent in institutions and of the possibility of suicide." The operation's effects, he argued, clearly were not due to suggestion, as the obsessions remained, but not with the same level of anxiety. Rather, Freeman and Watts had directly altered the "correlation between intellect and feeling tone in the brain," an effect unlike any other treatment. Brickner then added that not much actual cortex was destroyed in the operation, as the focal point of attack was the connections between it and the thalamus.

Kurt Goldstein, the leading expert on the psychological consequences of brain injuries, also rose to the speakers' defense. He opened with the statement, "Certainly every one was astonished, even shocked at first, on learning about operations of this type on persons with functional neuroses and psychoses." However, he wondered aloud, who has not seen the other treatments in use in psychiatry "without becoming frightened at first?" It followed, then, that "the heroic character of a method should not count against it." Goldstein had the opportunity of seeing some of these patients himself. Although his own observation was admittedly superficial, "what some of the patients told me about their condition before and after the operation was impressive." The affective attitude seemed to have changed completely, "and there was marked indifference to the obsessive ideas and hallucinations." Indeed, "the patients were not disturbed by their thoughts; they could be insensitive to them." "There is no doubt," he concluded, "that the main benefit of the operation lies in the diminution or loss of compulsive feelings, which the patients particularly appreciated."

The reception changed dramatically, however, when a succession of prominent, Freudian-oriented neurologists and neuropsychiatrists took the floor. Smith Ely Jelliffe redescribed the problem of obsessive neurosis in the Freudian terms of a brain region that had been overinvested with libido. Freeman and Watts's method of reducing this libido, he mused, reflected the questionable wisdom of "burning down the house to roast a pig." Theoretically, such an operation might be possible, he noted, if the specific region of the brain responsible for the pathology were localized.

He then criticized the two for failing to investigate the part of the brain involved in anal sensory perception, as it was well established in analytic theory that obsessions originate from anal sadistic urges; there was no need, therefore, to attack the whole frontal lobe. Jelliffe was even more dismissive of the core of Freeman and Watts's argument: that the operation was able to reduce tension of affect. "I doubt whether there *can* be any such reduction," he stated bluntly. For, in accordance with strict Freudian doctrine, "affect simply fails to be sublimated by higher degenitalized symbolizations and must find an outlet somewhere else." Jelliffe's attack did not stop at the meeting's door. Soon thereafter, a sarcastic review of Moniz's monograph appeared in the *Journal of Nervous and Mental Disease,* which Jelliffe edited. The review asked, "What has Moniz accomplished?" and replied, "No one knows, and I suspect least of all Moniz."[73]

Another analyst, Leland Hinsie, did not doubt that changes had occurred in the patients but insisted that the effects must be psychological in origin rather than physiological. For: "a psychoneurosis is 'hypochondriasis' of the mind. The laity believe that the mind and the brain are one. Hence, any medical or surgical procedure that aims to remove a disability in the head may afford relief." Not denying that Freeman and Watts had discovered a "useful investigative instrument," he doubted its relevance to psychoneurotic syndromes.

It remained for A. A. Brill, doyen of Freudian orthodoxy, to fire the hardest shot yet. He declared, "I cannot understand why such ideas are brought here, much less the fantastic conclusions drawn from them by some of the discussers." His answer: " I suppose all are so polite that anything may be ventured with impunity." Two of the patients under discussion, he noted, had been under his care, and in his opinion they were certainly doing much worse now. Like Jelliffe, he doubted that there was any reduction in affect of compulsions. How did Freeman and Watts measure such a thing? He ended his remarks on a note of ridicule, stating, "I believe that there is no reason that one should in any way be impressed by the seriousness of these presentations, in spite of the fact that I regard the authors highly." The material that had been presented "is no more conclusive of the validity of their claims than the putative cure of homosexuality by prostatic massage."

Freeman, in a curt response, denied that the operation was radical, as most of the frontal lobes was left intact. He was unperturbed that they had not localized the precise area; rather, this was a call for further research and work. That the positive results might be due to suggestion was rejected out of hand, for postoperative psychotherapy yielded minimal results. Brill, moreover, was simply mistaken about the identity of the patients. As to the condition of the patients following surgery, Freeman was simply stating that they were akin to paretic patients who had received malaria treatment, in that they might once again become usefully employed.[74]

At the end of the first year or so of Freeman and Watts's trials, the future of these brain operations in America remained uncertain. Their strongest support came from those who had firsthand contact with their patients; the problem persisted of how to convince the wider medical community of the procedure's rational basis. The most vocal criticism stemmed from those whose own professional turf had somehow been invaded, as when the pair presented a paper on the treatment of obsessive-compulsives before the New York psychoanalysts; these were precisely the kind of nonhospitalized patients who comprised the bread-and-butter practice of the analysts. From Freeman and Watts's perspective, they could afford to ignore detractors who summarily rejected their work as the latest "quack" remedy: the operations had too powerful an effect to be a mere illusion. Even so, although lobotomized patients were conspicuously changed from their preoperative state, it was difficult to articulate this difference in either lay or technical language. The ineffable nature of the operation's clinical effects thus prevented its supporters as well as its detractors from controlling the terms of the debate. Clinicians on both sides anxiously looked for an authoritative evaluation of the procedure's legitimacy from the perspective of laboratory science. Physiologist John Fulton was the one to provide that authoritative voice.

### Fulton's Perspective

In August of 1936, Freeman sent to Fulton his laudatory review of Moniz's initial publication on psychosurgery. Freeman and Fulton frequently corresponded about neurophysiological issues and, in the previous year or so, Freeman had been particularly inquisitive about the behaviors of Fulton's lobectomized chimpanzees. (Freeman and Watts were in possession of a typescript of Jacobsen's 1935 paper to the New York Neurological Society; Freeman also corresponded with Jacobsen.) Upon his return from Europe in mid-September, Fulton replied that he had acquired a reprint of Moniz's article in July and that he quite agreed that Moniz had taken an important step in the treatment of insanity. The deciding factor for Fulton was Jacobsen's observation that bilateral removal of the frontal association areas in chimpanzees permanently elimi-

nated experimental neuroses. He assured Freeman that Moniz had undoubtedly produced an equivalent effect with his surgery on human
beings. Freeman, in his later recollections of the factors that precipitated
his decision to pursue leucotomy, carefully noted Fulton's assurances. It
was "fortunate," he also recalled, that Watts had spent a year in Fulton's
laboratory.[75]

Fulton had not been informed, however, that Watts had already been
persuaded to make preparations for the first psychosurgery operation in
the United States and that the two Washington physicians had also obtained their first surgical prospect, A.H. Two days after Fulton replied to
Freeman's letter, the procedure was performed. Three weeks later (and a
few days after a second operation), Boston neurologist Henry Viets passed
through Washington and, on a chance visit to his former student, was
surprised to discover that Watts had taken up the Moniz procedure. Viets
forwarded to Fulton a diary entry of his trip, in which he had written that,
much to Watts's joy, the patient immediately became quiet and "normal"
following the operation. And although only a short time had elapsed, the
patient's family was already delighted with the improvement. Viets noted
that at first sight the operation did seem radical and foolish, but its remarkable results indicated good potential. He believed Watts to be a
cautious surgeon who was well aware that vehement opposition lay
ahead.[76]

Fulton replied that he already knew about Moniz's operation and that
he was strongly in favor of the procedure. Once again, Fulton turned to
his experience with the lobectomized chimpanzees: "As you probably
know, not one of our chimpanzees or monkeys with frontal association
areas out has ever had an experimental neurosis." "I have an idea," he
continued, "that when the last word has been said about catatonic demen-
tias and schizophrenia, we will find that the frontal association areas are
the parts of the brain principally involved, and when they get tied up in
knots, I can see no reason for not surgically untying them. . . . " Writing
to Watts the same day, Fulton repeated the above statements in almost the
identical words and concluded that Moniz's procedure appeared to be a
well-conceived physiological operation. He hoped that Watts would persevere and give it a fair clinical trial. Watts replied, "I cannot tell you how
much encouragement it [your letter] gave me."[77]

A weekly exchange of letters thus began between Fulton and his former
associate, in which Fulton offered greatly appreciated advice, reassurance,
and professional support. At one point, Watts noted that initially he had
been reluctant to risk such a procedure, as he had a reputation for being a
conservative neurosurgeon. But a review of the experimental and clinical

literature had convinced him of the merits of Moniz's operation. Watts wrote that his final decision to try the procedure was heavily influenced by Fulton's and Jacobsen's chimpanzee operations. By the time of this reply, Watts and Freeman had operated on three patients. Two of them, Watts reported, were kept out of institutions as a direct result. An additional case prompted Watts to inform Fulton that the procedure's results had exceeded his and Freeman's grandest expectations. Fulton congratulated Watts for his pioneering role and hoped that these experiences would embolden him to carry on, as he expected that in a year or so the procedure would constitute one of the "major phases" of neurosurgery.[78]

In early November, Freeman traveled to New Haven to discuss the physiological basis of the operation with Fulton; the following week, Fulton reciprocated with a personal inspection of Watts and Freeman's work in Washington. Fulton's diary entry captured the enthusiasm he felt after an examination of one of Watts's first patients. In Fulton's account, the woman had been for two years an "impossible" schizophrenic, requiring two nurses in daily attendance. After the operation, she was perfectly calm, rational, and entirely conscious of the beneficial change that the procedure had wrought in her psyche. "I felt somehow," he wrote, "that we were in the presence of one of the milestones of modern medicine." He continued, "I have seldom been more stirred and Henry Viets who came with me felt exactly as I had." Fulton returned to New Haven sufficiently confident about the new operation to mention to Watts the possibility of referring a young schizoid man from Minnesota who was the son of a family friend. Watts was thrilled by this compliment, all "puffed up" at the possibility of a patient traveling the long distance from Minnesota. Fulton then wrote to the mother of the patient to explain the new operation, once again alluding to the prevention of experimental neuroses in chimpanzees. Upon his return to Boston, Viets, an editor of the *New England Journal of Medicine,* fired off an unsigned editorial. After mentioning the six patients who had been operated upon, it stated, "Much more time is needed and many more cases should be reported before valuable conclusions can be drawn from this work." On the other hand, "The operation is based, however, on sound physiological observation and is a much more rational procedure than many that have been suggested in the past for the surgical relief of mental disease."[79]

Fulton's support for the procedure quickly went beyond the encouragement offered to his former pupil and extended into the general community, thus paving the way for the treatment's general acceptance. Beginning in November 1936, Fulton alerted an extensive family of correspondents – a group with whom over the preceding few years he had discussed problems

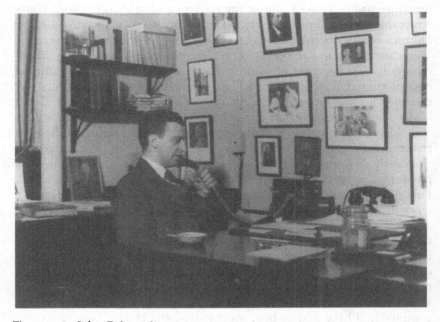

Figure 2.8. John Fulton dictating correspondence in his office. (Source: John Farquhar Fulton Papers, Yale University, Harvey Cushing/John Hay Whitney Medical Library)

of neurophysiology, neurosurgery, clinical neurology, and psychiatry – to the potential of the brain operations. In particular, Fulton had served as a private clearinghouse for discussions concerning frontal lobe function. Convinced now that lobotomy had a definite future, Fulton urged this network to consider the new procedure. The group included Henry Viets, Carlyle Jacobsen, Percival Bailey, Paul Bucy, Richard Brickner, R. Glen Spurling, Harry Solomon, Kenneth McKenzie, Spafford Ackerly, and John Lyerly. For example, Fulton asked Brickner whether he had been aware of Moniz's "impressive" new operation. "On the grounds of your observations and ours in chimps," he wrote, "it seems to me that the procedure is warranted and I hope we can stir up a few more courageous neurosurgeons to try it." In addition to broadening the operation's support, Fulton hoped to convince his favored investigators to seize a golden opportunity to "get in on the ground floor."[80]

Other prominent physicians, such as Harvard psychiatrist Harry Solomon, were intrigued by the new procedure but hesitated until researchers of Fulton's stature could provide a critical judgment "from the physiological standpoint." Fulton's correspondence with the neurosurgeon R. Glen Spurling illustrates how the Yale physiologist legitimated the new treatment. Interested in performing lobotomies himself, Spurling had contacted Freeman and Watts for surgical details but remained unconvinced that a neurophysiological rationale existed. Cognizant of Fulton's status as the leading authority on the overlap between neurophysiology and medicine, and hearing that Fulton had personally inspected the early cases, Spurling solicited Fulton's opinion.[81] Fulton replied in full and forwarded a copy of Moniz's monograph, admitting his own deep interest in the operation and then describing the significance of Jacobsen's studies. Before the operation, he wrote, the animals' behavioral disturbances had been "very real." For example, Jacobsen was forced to suspend experimentation for three to four months when an animal developed an experimental neurosis. But, Fulton emphasized, *"no animal with frontal association area out develops an experimental neurosis."* Fulton admitted that it was a long jump between case reports of experimental neuroses in cats and dogs to disturbances in man, but the gap had been narrowed by the chimpanzee investigations. And given the additional basis of Freeman and Watts's findings, he informed Spurling, test trials were indeed indicated. The letter was strong enough to sway Spurling, who replied that without it he would not have had the courage to attempt the operation. Spurling was not the only physician thus persuaded.[82]

Watts, in particular, was especially grateful for the many ways in which Fulton demonstrated active support. When the improvement upon Moniz's corer was being contemplated, for example, Watts duly consulted Fulton for advice. Fulton approved of the new procedure and "stood ready to help at any time." Direct professional aid had also been rendered by Fulton, who had revised the drafts of Watts's early lobotomy papers before both their delivery and their publication. But most of all, Watts was thankful for Fulton's role in stimulating others to look into the procedure and was relieved to learn from him that leading researchers and surgeons had also become convinced of the operation's neurophysiological basis and clinical future.[83] Fulton, quietly and assuredly, thus had laid the groundwork for the intellectual justification of the operation, fired up interest across a wide assortment of medical and scientific disciplines, and assisted its major proponents clear a number of minor hurdles. Soon, Fulton would also directly intervene and bail out Freeman and Watts when serious professional roadblocks threatened to put a halt to their activities. It had become common knowledge that Freeman and Watts enjoyed the full backing of Fulton's "powerful influence."[84]

## A Confession of Faith

Several rationales can account for Fulton's close involvement in the initial development of psychosurgery. As scientific justification for the procedure appeared to him to rest upon experimental findings that had originated within his own laboratory, Fulton naturally maintained a proprietary interest. He was also thrilled that the procedure had been introduced to America by a favored alumnus of his laboratory. Furthermore, he shared the excitement generated by a treatment that seemed to offer hope in a realm where fatalism was the rule.[85] Fulton's enthusiasm, however, extended beyond such considerations. To understand his full motivations – as well as identify the source of the larger community's enthusiasm for the experimental therapy – one must also appreciate what lobotomy as a research enterprise *symbolized* to Fulton, as well as to the group of neurologically oriented scientists and physicians whom he guided.

During his first decade as chairman of Yale's department of physiology, Fulton had to combat what he termed "static dead-house" neurology, a doctrine that in his opinion had pervaded the field in the United States. In 1933, Fulton outlined to Alan Gregg his blueprint for reforming neurology through the infusion of a new "dynamic neurology" into American medical education.[86] The ultimate goal of his program was to widen the scientific basis for future clinical advancements. Because the results of such work would have direct medical relevance to man, Fulton insisted on working with primates at a time when few went to the trouble. It was also this spirit that prompted him to dedicate his classic textbook, *The Physiology of the Nervous System,* to those who someday might "bridge the gap between the concepts of neurophysiology and the problems of clinical neurology." Fulton saw the young field of neurosurgery as the best available bet and invested his own time and energy accordingly. A close observer would later write that no one had ever done as much as Fulton had in bringing together a clinical specialty and its basic scientific counterpart; indeed, Fulton "made all neurosurgeons conscious of neurophysiology." In 1937, Sherrington told Fulton that his physiological laboratory would be the "sine qua non for the neurosurgeons of this generation."[87]

Fulton looked to a young group of research-oriented neurological surgeons to bring about neurology's transformation, an elite corps who banded together as the Harvey Cushing Society. Named after Fulton's mentor, the association consisted primarily of neurosurgeons such as Watts and Bucy who espoused Fulton's "dynamic attitude." Founded in 1932 by the first cohort of neurosurgeons to have trained under the pioneers (who had formed the Society of Neurological Surgeons in 1920), the new society demonstrated that the profession was in a restless growth phase.[88] In Fulton's opinion, 1932 was also the year when neurological surgery "came into its own," as demonstrated by its impressive showing at the First International Congress of Neurology. Until then, a neurosurgeon had been "virtually a carpenter who bored holes in patients' heads where the neurologists told him to go." Now, however, he had "emancipated himself to a degree that makes his position far stronger than that of the neurologist himself."[89]

The Harvey Cushing Society's potential as a source of professional reform greatly excited Fulton, who looked upon the members as a "vigourous, alert group identified with the new order of things," through whom "the importance of dynamic neurology could be taught to the coming generation of neurosurgeons." Elected as the society's second president, Fulton used the opportunity of his 1934 presidential address to sound the clarion call:

> I have the conviction that the future of neurology in this country lies very largely in your hands. I am devoting myself to the study of the nervous system because I confidently believe that within the next few years more light will be shed upon fundamental problems of clinical medicine from study of nervous function than from study of other systems of the body.

"This," Fulton concluded, "is a simple confession of faith."[90]

In particular, Fulton predicted gains in psychiatry, because "a few psychiatrists are now willing to allow that the psychoses may have something to do with the brain, rather than entirely with the heart as Aristotle thought." This reflected Fulton's long-held "earthy" attitude toward psychiatry. In 1932, for example, he wrote to one member that his inclination was to look upon every case of mental derangement as having an anatomical basis unless there was objective evidence to the contrary. The occasion for the letter was the colleague's statement that Fulton's own research promised to bring psychiatry into the domain of scientific medicine. Indeed, in Fulton's pantheon, Pavlov was a far greater scientist than Freud.[91]

Only a few years later, James Watts – encouraged by Fulton – presented before the Cushing Society his first paper on psychosurgery addressed to his neurosurgical peers. At the summation of the presentation, Brickner rose to state, "The facts as they now stand are important." It was clear that "these procedures should be tried." A consensus was reached that in the team of Watts and Freeman the procedure's evaluation was in excellent hands; the explorers were congratulated. At the dinner preceding the session, the group received an inspirational telegram from Ernest Sachs, the "dean" of American neurosurgery: "THE FUTURE OF AMERICAN NEUROLOGICAL SURGERY LIES IN YOUR HANDS. IT IS A GRAVE RESPONSIBILITY

BUT I CAN THINK OF NO FINER GROUP TO HANDLE THIS PROBLEM." A large number of the audience then present would indeed become influential leaders in the neurosurgical profession; along the way, these same physicians would pioneer the use of psychosurgery in America, seeing in it yet another demonstration of their field's rapid progress. (Of the Harvey Cushing membership in 1938, at least one-third would be directly involved in some psychosurgery project within ten years.) The great potential of the new brain operations to affect psychiatry as well as neurosurgery was not lost upon Fulton. If the operation did prove efficacious, the need for skilled neurosurgeons would sharply rise; as one correspondent suggested to Fulton, medical schools might have to "turn out neurosurgeons by the score." And, as early as October 1936, Fulton envisioned that psychosurgery programs would be incorporated into state mental hospitals, leading to significant reductions in overcrowding as well as social costs.[92]

Fulton thus saw in Watts's accomplishments a fulfillment of his "confession of faith." Just a few years later, Fulton would declare, on a lecture tour, that the lobotomy studies demonstrated the "close correlation which is now coming about between experimental physiology of the nervous system and clinical neurology."[93]

## Full Circle

Largely through the handiwork of Walter Jackson Freeman and John F. Fulton, many leading figures in the medical community came to regard Egas Moniz's startling claims as an attractive opportunity for research. Freeman, through his trademark blend of derring-do and calculated showmanship, focused clinical attention on the raw potential of the operations. Fulton, in linking Moniz's initial surgical forays to ideas implicit in the chimpanzee experiments conducted at Yale, drew attention to a putative scientific justification for lobotomy and convinced those who mattered that the controversial procedure should be allowed to prove itself, one way or the other.

It is not difficult to proffer reasons to account for why both Freeman and Fulton felt compelled to advance the cause of psychosurgery during its fledgling years. Freeman was under pressure to expand the base of his clinical practice and was also on the lookout for a brass ring that might earn for him the praise so richly enjoyed by his grandfather Keen, the dramatic presence whose protective shadow he never fully escaped. Fulton was loyally paving the way for the success of a cherished student and at the same time hoping to clothe his research empire in the mystique of a grand scientific accomplishment – an ambition that for him, too, remained elusive.

Although these kinds of explanations are quite useful in explaining Freeman's and Fulton's individual actions, nevertheless they leave unaddressed the larger issue of why the two were *successful* in promoting the Portuguese operation. Consciously or unconsciously, both men were riding waves of professional change that were dramatically reshaping medical research, education, and practice. As active leaders in the transformations then under way, though representing different parts of the infrastructure, both investigators saw in Moniz's report a catalyst that might hasten changes of a particular kind. For them, far more was at stake than the therapeutic relief of a handful of agitated depressives. Thanks to Freeman's and Fulton's savvy in linking the innovation to broader issues, leucotomy's development also assumed the symbolic importance of a cause, a timely call to arms that enlisted many others.

The brain operations for mental illness were not so much a technical breakthrough as they were an occasion to rearrange the existing social structure within a part of medicine. Moniz's leucotomy was in fact a simple surgical procedure and represented neither a neurophysiological nor a neuroanatomical advancement. Rather, his proposition implicitly involved a realignment in institutional and professional relations that had divided several disciplines. In essence, Moniz was suggesting that neurosurgery was applicable to an unlikely class of patients, the mentally ill, whose brain tissue was – to the chagrin of a generation of neuropathologists – seemingly healthy. Up to this time neurosurgeons rarely encountered a psychiatric patient, and psychiatrists or neuropsychiatrists would have had little reason to consult a neurosurgeon unless either tumors or focal epilepsy were suspected. In addition, for neurological researchers his idea was opening up new areas for explorations. As Moniz expressed in a letter to Freeman, "the human brain is not now closed to our investigations."[94]

For the particular neuropsychiatric community Freeman represented, Moniz's work represented the triumph of the "no-nonsense" organic approach to mental disease. In their perspective, progress in psychiatric therapy was mostly a matter of technological improvement, and thus the group kept a sharp lookout for promising innovations in drugs, medical machinery, or surgical interventions. (For Freeman and his fellow travelers, the various forms of psychotherapy were insufficiently medical and thus could be safely ignored.) As a bench research scientist, Fulton represented a somewhat different perspective: the belief that the motor driving therapeutic advance was not clinical trials but laboratory investigations that shed new light on the fundamental processes at play in the human organism. In particular, Fulton expected that progress in psychiatry awaited the time when neurophysiologists could map out the nervous system. Significantly, at that moment the two perspectives of Freeman and Fulton were converging, especially through the rise of the new field of neurosurgery.

The nascent specialty of neurosurgery brought together in a single practitioner a blend of bold surgical mastery, neurological acumen, and a passion for experimental physiology. Indeed, neurosurgery flourished in democratic America as in no other country, for nowhere else could the historically separate professions of the pragmatic surgeon combine so naturally with that of the learned neurologist and the laboratory physiologist.[95] The career path of Watts, who was extensively trained in all three disciplines, exactly typified the connections being formed between the separate worlds represented by Fulton and Freeman. Fulton saw in psychosurgery visible proof of the importance of this union. True to his vision, over the next decade the technique would indeed be pioneered by the young neurosurgeons who shared Fulton's vision of injecting a new, dynamic, and experimentally based neurology into American medical research and education.

Psychiatry's own historical moment offered a unique opportunity for the joining of neurology, psychiatry, neurosurgery, and neurophysiology. As discussed previously, psychiatry was under both internal and external pressures to adopt the methodology of modern science, whether the sophisticated overview of social scientists or the rigorous techniques of the laboratory experimentalist, or some combination thereof.[96] A large rift remained, however, between the academic laboratories and the isolated asylum. Fulton, in invoking Pavlov's model of experimental neurosis as the key explanatory basis of Moniz's operation, had hit upon the exact intellectual structure for bringing the psychiatric world within the purview of the laboratory. This framework allowed researchers to discuss and approach a topic that previously had been labeled "subjective" and hence off-limits to laboratory investigation.[97] Significantly, the neurosis of the Pavlovian model was not that of Freudian terminology but that of Meyerian maladaptation – the mental pathology that results when an animal is unable to cope with environmental stress. Mental illness, redefined by American psychiatrists in terms of maladjustment, referred to an individual's performance as a unit of the social organism. Thanks to Pavlov, this performance was yoked to laboratory research. It was all physiology.

Psychosurgery, thus packaged, became an object lesson of what the new, experimentally based psychiatry might yield. In 1944, Abraham Myerson, director of one of the few research institutes located in a state mental hospital, reviewed psychiatry's scientific status. The Russian physiologist Pavlov was the single most important figure in the history of psychiatry, Myerson wrote, as he pointed the way to the transformation of psychiatry into a genuine experimental science; his discovery of a method of analyzing pathological mental states in animals was a psychiatric "milestone." Myerson's essay concluded with a judgment on the new brain operations: "and whatever the value of psychosurgery will be, its advent will also be hailed as a boldly conceived attack upon the problems of psychiatry."[98]

There was no necessity that a connection would be made between the concept of experimental neurosis and the development of operations on the human frontal lobe. The association was first made by Jacobsen in an offhand remark meant only to add color when describing his otherwise dry behavioral protocols of experiments limited to nonhuman subjects. Jacobsen had had no intention of ever directly investigating the subject himself. Moniz, although often making reference to the results of Jacobsen's work, never once alluded to the experimental neurosis framework – it held no additional significance for him. Likewise, there is little evidence to indicate that Freeman or Watts had ever thought in terms of experimental neurosis before Fulton pointed out its significance: unlike Moniz, however, they immediately incorporated the explanation as their primary scientific justification.

There are specific historical reasons why such a connection was made at Yale, and in Fulton's laboratory. Moreover, the same factors that account for this moment of serendipity also illuminate why the "discovery" had such a significant impact upon the broader research community. Indeed, there existed only one primate laboratory in this country where such research was possible: there were particular circumstances why such unusual facilities were located at Yale. As mentioned earlier, the Yale Medical School, transformed by the Rockefeller Foundation in this period, exhibited a commitment to interdisciplinary research that would explore new laboratory-validated means of investigating and modifying human behavior. (Indeed, the celebration of Yale's IHR in 1929 corresponded with Pavlov's only visit to America, when the physiologist was shifting his own research focus onto psychiatric issues.)[99]

In short, although the development of psychosurgery in America was an unintended consequence of the overall Rockefeller mission, it was by no means an undesired one. Once Moniz's work became publicly known, it was immediately interpreted by Fulton and his group in light of the local meaning of the Yale program. Through Fulton's skilled promotional efforts, this local meaning was then translated into a professional significance far beyond what Moniz or even Freeman had anticipated. The reason why medical leaders here so readily accepted Moniz's proposition to link brain surgery to the challenge of insanity was due, in particular, to the broader professional currents that sought to extend the medical laboratory directly into the problems of society. Psychosurgery, which experimented with the very stuff of self, offered a dramatic opportunity to carry this enterprise forward.

The story of Becky and the rise of psychosurgery has now come full circle. On the one hand, the tale is an outright invention of Fulton's, a thinly veiled grab for a portion of the scientific limelight. On the other hand, there is another meaning embedded in the story. Although the famous account of the Yale experiment's direct effect on Moniz must now be seen as apocryphal, nevertheless the indirect role of Fulton's efforts to sustain the early development of the brain operations was indeed highly significant. Fulton's greater influence was not on Moniz, but on his later followers in the United States who were convinced by him that the innovation embodied a particular vision of medical progress. As suggestive as the results of Moniz and Freeman were, it is clear that it was Fulton's laboratory which provided the leverage point with which to displace professional attitudes from peremptory rejection to a cautious acceptance. That is the greater truth buried within Fulton's fable of Becky and the frontal lobes.

## Conclusion: Storied Success

How does this individual story of psychosurgery fit in with other stories of medical advance? From today's perspective, the parable of Becky and the frontal lobes can be easily dismissed as bad history formulated out of questionable science. Unlike science, though, bad history is not useless history. Quite the contrary: its utility is of a very calculated kind, although it is not immediately apparent. The truth lies hidden here – and in the usual accounts of scientific discovery – because of the special way in which scientists use history when telling the story of their innovations.

True concepts, we are taught, are timeless. The doctrine of uniformitarianism holds that the laws of Nature, revealed today, will also pertain tomorrow – it is on this basis that we can predict and thus master our fates. The doctrine also runs in the other direction, however, implying that today's revelations will also explain away yesterday's ignorance. It is a special feature of the scientist's worldview that as the present becomes clearer so too does the past. The sciences thus present themselves as the most *ahistorical* of knowledge enterprises: when it comes time to judge whether or not a particular theory or experiment is sound, the observer does so from a position that is shorn of any reference to location or time. Scientific facts exist outside of history.[100]

Belying this attitude, though, are the quiet and essential ways in which history is used to justify ongoing scientific missions. Indeed, there can be no sense of progress without first distinguishing current from past events. Typically, the introductory section of a comprehensive textbook – or even of a single research publication – begins with an encapsulation of the events that have led to the current state of knowledge, thus placing in high perspective the knowledge that is already known and that which is yet to be known. Newton's dictum "If I have seen further . . . it is by standing on the shoulders of giants," one of the more famous quotations in the history of science, nicely exemplifies the importance of a stable historical foundation to the ongoing research enterprise.[101]

Every story of scientific advance is thus but one link in the master narrative of how reason prevailed over ignorance, turning darkness into light and helplessness into mastery. The seductive power of Fulton's fable hence lies in its familiarity. This is a story that has been told many times before, though set in different locations and with different principals. A chance or serendipitous observation of an alert laboratory investigator precipitated the discovery of a practical therapeutic advance; Understanding and Utility once again marched on, hand-in-hand. This said, one might be tempted not to dwell any further on the matter, viewing these little stories of science as harmless forms of self-celebration – and not unjustified, at that. Except, of course, in Fulton's case.

Such stories are *not* so benign, however.[102] By shoring up the idealist model of scientific advance, they defend the scientific community from grave tensions, external as well as internal, that threaten its continuing ability to function. To begin with, these accounts preserve the public image of how medical science progresses, a process that as a whole is far more haphazard than it would be comfortable to admit. The core message of Fulton's story is the oft-sung refrain that laboratory advances prompted practical benefit, that workers in the field advanced no further than the guidelines provided by experimentally based knowledge. This is a carefully orchestrated illusion. As even Freeman admitted, Moniz's theoretical justification was thin at best.[103] (Moniz himself stated that the best justification for his bold experiment was found in the fact that it worked.)

The example of psychosurgery thus brings to light an unpalatable truth about how laboratory researchers and investigators in the field often come together. It is not uncommon for clinical investigators to move about from one approach to another, keeping an eye out for whatever yields an interesting result. And should something of promise appear, they quickly scramble around for a current theory with which to justify their original decision as having had a solid scientific foundation. The laboratory-based community of scientists, for its part, is all too eager to accommodate this ruse, thereby racking up yet another demonstration of how their research has paid off in practical fruits. For the whole enterprise to keep moving forward, the public has to maintain confidence in its belief that clinical investigators are not subjecting their patients to trial-and-error tactics, and that laboratory researchers are not pursuing idle phantasms.[104]

It is in the interests of all parties, then, to construct these kinds of historical fictions at the earliest opportunity. Indeed, on the very first page of Freeman and Watts's initial publication on psychosurgery, a description of the importance of Fulton's chimpanzees to psychosurgery can already be found – in spite of the fact that the reported operations had occurred *before* Fulton had brought to their attention the significance of experimental neurosis. As for Fulton, he shortly thereafter included a description of the connection in his landmark *Physiology of the Nervous System,* the first edition of which appeared in 1938. "Moniz," Fulton declared, "has applied Jacobsen's findings concerning experimental neuroses in chimpanzees to the surgical treatment of neuroses and of the major psychoses in man." Once implanted, the story was never challenged, and the importance of Becky only grew as the years passed. From that point forward, when others pursued the innovation, they too followed suit in citing the Yale research as the scientific rationale.[105] Indeed, in the years ahead Fulton's personal version of how Moniz had been influenced by Jacobsen's report on Becky became accepted as the official narrative, which has since remained unchallenged.[106]

Perhaps the best indication of what Fulton's parable was really accomplishing, in back-dating the moment when the laboratory and the field were joined, is provided by a retelling of the Becky parable that appeared in a 1954 issue of the *Mental Hygiene News:*

> In 1932 Dr. Fulton of Yale was given some chimpanzees and decided to test the validity of Starr and Burkhardt's work [nineteenth-century physicians who explored the use of brain surgery in mental illness]. First, he induced psychoses in the chimps using Pavlovian conditioning techniques. When they would respond to no other form of treatment, he operated on their frontal lobes with marked improvement in their condition.[107]

Every facet of this rendition was of course off the mark. The point of the story, however – that is, reinforcing the public's (erroneous) impression that the brain operations logically flowed from a deliberately focused set of experiments – was exactly on.

Another rhetorical function of the standard old chestnuts of scientific triumph is to obscure the rocky process by which consensus is reached within a scientific community. Through such accounts, scientists convince us – and themselves – that science advances logically and inexorably, driven forward by the intellectual methods of deduction and induction. Indeed, the capacity to demonstrate that research decisions are anchored to a long string of prior scientific discoveries is vital to the scientific community's ability to direct the flow of future research efforts.[108] In reality, scientists on the front lines are faced with uncertainty at every turn, having to choose among many competing research paths without ever knowing what really lies ahead. The basis upon which they decide to embark on this or that research avenue is a lot messier than is generally recognized. In addition to the intellectual factors, such calculations are dependent upon a broad range of personal motivations and social factors as well.

For a medical innovation to cross over from a status as an untested and daring venture to a more favorable posture as an experimental procedure worth pursuing, a select group of respectable physicians and scientists have to reach agreement that its potential benefits outweigh the possible risks. By some later commentators, the story of psychosurgery is seen as an example of what happens when scientists pay insufficient attention to the evidence at hand when making such calculations. One can make the case that the facts marshaled by psychosurgery's proponents, even from the perspective of the day's standards, were not so compelling as to force a neutral observer to agree that the procedure's advantages outweighed its deficits. To paraphrase Ludwik Fleck, however, in science – just as in art, politics, and life – *there are no neutral observers.*[109]

Because scientists work within institutional and professional confines that seem increasingly remote from the larger general culture, it has become that much harder to see their decisions as expressions of these broader currents. Even as the scientific community turned inward, though, it was substituting an *inner* culture that was no less influential in informing the actions of its members. When it comes time for scientists and physicians to gamble upon a particular line of investigation, the facts at hand go only so far – especially because such choices necessarily arise at the exact moment when the participants know the least about the new research paths. For guidance, they fall back upon other frameworks with which to manage the uncertainty. What they see ahead thus often comes to mirror the inner forces – professional, social, and cultural – that structure the community itself.

When considering whether to buy into a new research path, investigators ask two kinds of questions: were the initial findings illusory, and if not, what were their significance? The answers are not to be found in the original research papers, but elsewhere, in the personal circumstances of the participants. Fulton, it has been shown, was inclined to believe the claims of the early psychosurgeons for a variety of reasons. He knew the investigators personally and believed them to report honestly on what they saw. As to the matter of whether what they saw was spurious or real, Fulton had seen with his own eyes the dramatic emotional changes that followed bilateral frontal lobe damage in primates – Becky was by no means the only such example. In turn, the broader community of investigators trusted Fulton's judgment that the effects of the operation were not artificial but had scientific plausibility. No one knew better than he.

As to the findings' significance, Fulton had seen in the subject of psychosurgery the exact fulfillment of what his career had been about: the challenge of linking research on the brain to problems of vital human import. Situated as he was within a powerful institutional matrix then focused on precisely these kinds of crossover subjects, it was a natural extension for Fulton to view Moniz's report in this way. Fatefully, the particular intellectual framework Fulton used to communicate his favorable opinion of the Moniz operation happened to resonate strongly with currents converging across a wide range of disciplinary and professional interests. Fulton successfully articulated what was at stake in the claim that brain operations were a solution for mental disorder, and in leading others to see this potential as he had Fulton demonstrated his true role as a statesman of science.

Fulton's interpretation of what had happened to his chimpanzee Becky did not *prove* to the larger medical community that Moniz's brain operation was scientifically valid. Rather, it indicated to them that this type of medical venture was a likely place in which to fulfill their broader mission already under way. In his role as a respected authority in scientific medicine, Fulton was looked to by others precisely for his ability to articulate what this mission was, and where next to proceed. Defined by Fulton in these kind of terms, the brain operations now *made sense* to this group, and they took the next step.

In sum, the usual tales of medical innovation have lulled us, as well as the scientific community itself, into viewing the story of scientific advance in straightforward, unproblematic terms. A flash of insight solves a series of unexplained phenomena, which in turn prompts a useful innovation. The more we look at it this way, however, the less is understood of the broader historical processes at work in medical discovery: the real story is not *only* in the scientific apparatus. Traditional stories of science, camouflaged as innocuous forms of puffery, are in fact rhetorically powerful forms of displacement whose function is to turn our attention away from the inescapably human dimensions of medical science.

Thus, Fulton's own story of how his laboratory findings were the deciding factor in the origin of psychosurgery, an account that looks suspiciously like a vehicle for further self-aggrandizement, is actually an artful denial of Fulton's *social* role, his extensive personal intervention in constructing the later scientific consensus. Similarly, the longevity of Fulton's fable is not so much evidence of the essential gullibility of the scientific community as it is an expression of the vital need for all parties involved to gloss over the uncertainty inherent in medical advance, to shore up the fiction that therapeutic innovations always logically derive from prior laboratory gains. Finally, in holding to the model that an *idea* alone led to a specific application, Fulton's familiar story of scientific discovery denies the importance of the historical situation in which the participants lived and worked.

Fulton was well aware of the extent to which he had persuaded the larger medical community of psychosurgery's potential. Circumspect to a fault, he nicely expressed the delicate position in which he had placed himself. In a letter to one of the neurosurgeons he had so convinced, he remarked half-jokingly that, as everyone was proceeding on the basis of his opinion, if the operation eventually did not gain general acceptance, "I am afraid I shall have a good deal to answer for to St. Peter." This said, Fulton was willing to stand behind his exhortations. Although he had not yet formed a final opinion of the procedure, he concluded, "I do believe it is sufficiently promising to be given a trial."[110]

It is one thing to understand why the research-oriented community, guided by Fulton and what he represented, would invest their energy and reputations in an experimental trial of psychosurgery. A separate issue, though, is to elucidate why clinicians in the field would judge the new treatment to be of positive therapeutic benefit. In the final analysis, Fulton remained at the bench, far removed from the clinical scene; his perspective was not especially relevant in this other arena. The next step, then, is a closer examination of the early psychosurgeons and the contexts in which the procedure was viewed so favorably.

# 3

## Certain Benefit

### Initial Impressions of the Operation

Fulton's expectation that Freeman and Watts's work would lead to further clinical trials was quickly fulfilled. At the 1939 meeting of the AMA, Fulton prepared a multipanel poster exhibit that touted the significance of his research on the frontal lobes (see Figure 3.1). One panel contained a description of Moniz's innovation. "The results of his operation have aroused wide interest," it stated, "and the procedure is now being actively studied in various centers in the country including Washington, Jacksonville, and Boston." A combined total of nearly two hundred cases, the passersby learned, had resulted in good results and even "striking improvement." (To Fulton's great satisfaction, the exhibit was awarded a medal.)[1] As Fulton had hoped, the very first trials outside of Washington involved such notable neurosurgeons as James Lyerly, Francis Grant, and W. Jason Mixter – exactly the sort of group who might be trusted to proceed with caution and give the right attention to the considerations of neurophysiology. A closer look at these early years will illustrate why the findings of Watts and Freeman were initially confirmed and why Fulton would step back into the fray when their work was seriously threatened by professional censure and controversy.

The matter of psychosurgery, though, would not for long remain confined to the small professional world that was bounded by the intersection of neurological surgery and brain research. The procedure's fate also became wrapped up in the currents driving psychiatry. In the transition from its origins in the private office practice of Freeman and Watts to a broader location within the nation's system of mental hospitals, the technique acquired a luster that not even Freeman had anticipated, and with consequences for the relations between laboratory researchers and clinicians that not even Fulton had foreseen. In the years between 1937 and the end of World War II, a consensus emerged among many American physicians that psychosurgery was a treatment that indeed offered certain benefit. At the same time, those involved learned that the benefit was of only a certain kind. The challenge for these practitioners, it will be shown, lay in articulating precisely what these boundaries of advantage and disadvantage

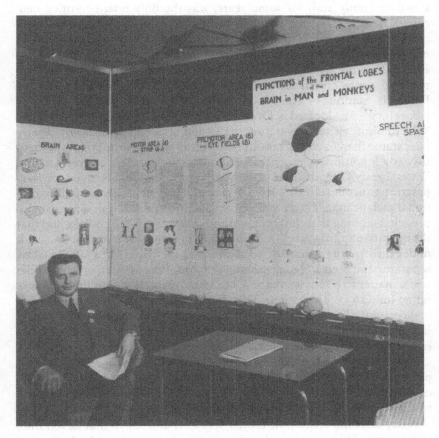

Figure 3.1. John Fulton and his medal-winning poster exhibit at the 1939 AMA Meeting. (Source: John Farquhar Fulton Papers, Manuscripts and Archives, Yale University Library)

were, a problem complicated by the very same factors that were at work in furthering the procedure's acceptance.

## James Lyerly

Soon after Freeman's and Watts's first cases, James Lyerly, a young neurosurgeon in Jacksonville, Florida, decided to try the operation. Educated exclusively in the South, Lyerly was a member of a distinguished North

Carolina family and, for some years, was the only board-certified neurological surgeon in his state. Although far from the centers of medical advance, he would remain in contact with recent developments in neurophysiology and neurosurgery through his active participation in the Harvey Cushing Society, of which he was a founding member, and through personal contact with leaders such as John Fulton. Yale's Anthropoid Research Station – Yerkes's primate colony that supplied Fulton's laboratory – was located in Orange Park, on the outskirts of Jacksonville. When Fulton visited the station, he would also visit with Lyerly. Lyerly later stated that his conversations with Fulton were of prime importance to his early lobotomy experiences.[2] Following the example of Freeman and Watts, Lyerly's first series of cases was comprised of middle-aged, private-practice patients suffering from severe agitated depressions and involutional melancholia. Lyerly was not satisfied with the Moniz-Freeman approach, believing that the corer was too destructive to the cortex and that the operative approach was a "blind" one, in which surgeons cut tissue not under direct vision. Instead, he abandoned the corer for a simple tissue separator and used a "brain speculum" to push the tissue apart so that the white matter to be cut was exposed to visual inspection. His first trial was on 19 June 1937. The patient, Theodore Trotter, was a white middle-aged male employed as a clerk. His depression started six months earlier when he began to worry about losing his job. Increasingly restless and fearful of ending up in prison, he eventually discussed suicide. He had been in a sanitarium since May, where he would spend his days wringing his hands, pacing the floor, and rubbing his head. At one point, an attempt at self-castration led to serious injury. Profoundly depressed, he had to be induced to eat. The diagnosis was involutional melancholia.[3]

A day after the operation, Trotter was alert and stated that he felt fine, but hungry. This was considered a significant change, as he had never previously spoken of hunger. He said that his fears in regard to work were unchanged, but now he was inclined to joke instead; there was no mention of suicide. Trotter was discharged within a month. At the end of August, he walked into Lyerly's office with a smile on his face, saying that he had no complaints, everything was fine. He was currently employed part-time in a grocery store. Nor did he show evidence of depression or any other emotional instability or cognitive abnormality. In November, however, a follow-up visit yielded signs of relapse; Trotter appeared nervous and depressed. After some discussion, these conditions were thought to have resulted from a noisy living environment; when he moved into a new home the symptoms disappeared. At the end of February 1938, Trotter came into the office looking bright, alert, and smiling. He stated that he never felt better in his life and that he had a steady job. Memory and concentration were as good as ever; he performed arithmetic without trouble. Perfectly relaxed, he declared to Lyerly that "he felt like his old self" again.

The second patient, Rosalyn Somers, was a middle-aged housewife who had been ill for over a year with involutional melancholia. Her worries were also centered on financial matters, as her husband was unemployed and her daughter about to marry. She became intensely restless, nervous, and greatly disturbed for a period of a month, after which she was discovered lying in a closed room with the gas turned on. Placed in a sanitarium, she refused to eat. When discharged, six months later, she weighed only eighty-two pounds. At home, she remained restless and agitated, and developed delusions that her daughter was trying to poison her. An operation was performed on 5 October 1937. Mrs. Somers was discharged from the hospital a fortnight later with her condition markedly changed. She was cheerful, laughing and joking. Upon examination a month later, she was found to have no impairment of memory or disorientation and responded intelligently to all questions. The sister of the patient described her as "an entirely changed person," one who "no longer worries about anything." The following March she returned for another examination and walked into the office smiling if not "radiant." Mrs. Somers declared that she felt happy and never better in her life. She enjoyed going places and attended the Women's Club frequently. She was doing all of her own housework and no longer felt nervous or tense as she had prior to the operation.

Emboldened by these examples, Lyerly soon operated upon a dozen more patients, half of them from private practice and the others drawn from a pool of similar patients at the Florida State Hospital in Chattahoochie. When he first reported on these cases at the May meeting of the Florida Medical Association in 1938, already four of these institutional patients had been discharged. No patients in the series had died; none had serious medical complications. The confusion following the operation was only transient. "In no case," Lyerly underscored, did the operation "appear to affect the patient's judgment, reasoning, or concentration, or his ability to do arithmetic." Lyerly's paper was well received. J. C. Davis, then president of the State Board of Medical Examiners, began his discussion by reiterating that each patient operated upon at the Florida State Hospital either had been released or was pending release. Such results, he declared, are "nothing less than miraculous." Noting that "words are inadequate to describe the mental torture that these patients with agitated depression experienced before operation," Davis concluded that "the value of the prefrontal lobotomy, estimated in terms of relief of human suffering, cannot be overrated." Similarly, P. L. Dodge, a psychiatrist in Miami, joined in the congratulations. From a psychiatric standpoint, Dodge declared, there was very little that could be done for involutional melancholia or agitated depression. Regardless of medical intervention, the condition advanced, with permanent institutionalization the inevitable result. Indeed, he noted, "there is nothing more depressing in all the field of nervous and mental diseases than is this particular type of patient." Such patients were "hopeless and helpless," and without such a treatment as lobotomy, they surely "will go on like such cases have gone for centuries past." Lyerly, in reply, cautioned that this was merely a preliminary report, and it was too early to know if the relief was permanent.[4]

By March of 1939, Lyerly's series had extended to twenty-six cases. His next communication elaborated upon his surgical innovation, which he claimed left undamaged the posterior portion of the frontal lobe and thus accounted for why "these patients do not have any serious mental deficit after the operation." To bolster this claim, Lyerly engaged the services of a psychometrician, who subjected the patients to a full battery of mental tests before and after operation. Lyerly then reported in detail on the third and fourth patient in his series, who also had results as good as in the first two cases. The last patient, for example, was a middle-aged druggist who had previously attempted suicide twice and had been institutionalized for a year and a half with severe depression. After a lobotomy, his condition improved so that forty days later he was sent home. His wife later wrote to Lyerly full of effusive thanks that her husband was himself again. Furthermore, she noted, his personality was an improvement upon what it had been before his illness.

Given his respected position, Lyerly's findings carried great weight, as when he reported his findings to the Harvey Cushing Society in 1938 and 1939. It was clear from the discussions, for example, that Watts himself was spurred on to improve Moniz's procedure by Lyerly's reports of lower deficits. Moreover, on a trip to the anthropoid station in March 1939, Fulton visited Lyerly and encouraged him to continue his work with lobotomies. (In 1940, Lyerly was also engaged in extensive three-way discussions with Carlyle Jacobsen and Fulton concerning the possible neuropsychological models that might account for lobotomy's success.) Other influential centers would also take up Lyerly's approach, such as those at the Mayo Clinic, Massachusetts General Hospital, and the Lahey Clinic.[5]

## Francis Grant

Watts's distinguished mentors, Francis Grant in Philadelphia, and W. Jason Mixter in Boston, were the next neurosurgeons in America to attempt the procedure, both beginning operations at the start of 1938. Grant, trained by Harvey Cushing and William Frazier, was at the top of the first generation of students to specialize in neurological surgery. Chief of the neurosurgical service at the Hospital of the University of Pennsylvania in 1935, he was highly influential in the instruction of young professionals. His neurosurgical colleagues would later eulogize him with the statement that "no one in his generation was held in more affectionate esteem by his colleagues."

Grant had been a consulting neurosurgeon at Delaware State Hospital, where Superintendent M. A. Tarumianz was attempting to build a treatment institution that might serve as a model for the rest of the nation. Through the meetings at the Philadelphia Neurological Society, Tarumianz had come in frequent contact with Grant, as well as with Walter Freeman and Jim Watts. In February 1938, Grant and Tarumianz together paid a visit to Washington to observe with their own eyes what Watts was up to with the Moniz procedure and to lay the foundation for implementing their own program at Delaware State. They watched as Watts operated upon patient "E.W.," and later Watts forwarded his operative notes to aid Grant in his future work. Next, both Freeman and Watts were invited to Tarumianz's institution, where they identified which patients were the best candidates for the operation.[6]

The first patient selected, Julia Koppendorf, was an unmarried elderly women. A high school graduate, Miss Koppendorf had worked for thirty years in the office of a large factory. She was considered an excellent housekeeper, taking pride in the neatness of her home. During menopause, she had suffered an intense attack of severe depression with agitation, becoming resistive and destructive; the attack lasted three months. In the summer of 1933 she became irritable, and eventually abandoned her housekeeping and employment. After developing delusions of persecution and hallucinations, she admitted herself to the Delaware State Hospital. In the hospital, she wandered about restlessly with a rosary in her hand, crying loudly, wringing her hands, full of condemnations of herself and others, and afraid that she was losing her mind. "I feel that my church has thrown me out and my people don't want me and my soul is lost," Julia would declare, "I want to go home to die. I've tried and tried, but I can't see Jesus." Over the years, she deteriorated further, occasionally having to be force-fed through tubes. She would frequently state that she had no soul and that she was nothing but a block of wood.[7]

The picture of agitated depression the patient exhibited was so striking that Freeman and Watts immediately chose her as the most likely surgical prospect. The family consented to the operation and so did the patient, who stated that anything should be done that might give relief, as death was preferable to her current misery. On 11 March 1938, Francis Grant performed Moniz's procedure. Two days later, the patient already was more cooperative and was enjoying her meals. When interviewed after a week, at times she rambled and was incoherent; on the other hand, she could not remember when she had felt so well. Psychometric examinations later revealed little change in intellectual performance. Upon her dismissal from the hospital at the end of the month, she was thought to have made a satisfactory adjustment. She lived with an ailing sister, greatly aiding in household work, and entered normally into the social life of her town. A year or so after the operation, the patient's nephew informed Grant that his aunt had been entirely restored to her normal condition.[8]

The published case report began with the statement, "Of all psychiatric conditions, agitated depression is doubtless the most distressing. The unremitting mental agony, unrest, apprehension, and the relentless pangs of remorse over minor or fancied misdeeds render the life of the victim little worth living." Without some means of radical intervention, "many of them can expect no relief from their misery until death intervenes." In the opinion of the physicians at Delaware State, the results of their first trial of the new procedure "were entirely those hoped for." Although part of the delusional content persisted, there was a complete disappearance of agitation and depression.[9]

Grant proceeded down the list of ten patients that Freeman and Watts had selected. Within a month, another two similar patients were operated upon; they too were soon discharged. Sarah Strawbridge, the sixth patient in the hospital series, had been admitted to Delaware State Hospital in 1936 after an agitated depression of five years' duration. Although her childhood was considered to have been generally normal and uneventful, Sarah had grown into someone who mixed poorly with her peers, lacked self-confidence, was at times stubborn and envious, and was – for lack of a better word – peculiar. Friends and family volunteered that she had few likable traits. Until her illness, Miss Strawbridge had been successfully employed as an office assistant. When her depression began, the patient became apathetic, ate poorly, and declared that she wanted to die. She told her relatives that she had developed strong affections for a married man who worked at a desk near her own and then tried to get them to arrange a tryst with him. The relatives stated that her sense of modesty and propriety had seriously eroded, and that it was not safe for her to go out alone, as she "might pick up any man." She became increasingly difficult to manage and was committed.[10]

Upon admission, Miss Strawbridge was cooperative and in touch with her surroundings, though apathetic. She adjusted poorly to ward routine, became reclusive and increasingly depressed, fearing that her job would not be held for her or that she might never recover from her illness. Feelings of self-condemnation erupted, particularly in regard to her attachment to the married man. In time, she complained of peculiar bodily sensations which developed into delusions that her heart and brain were dead and she no longer had control over her body. "Dear Susan," she wrote to a relative, "please don't allow anyone over here for I have no feelings only this thing beating in place of my heart. . . . I walk around and don't even feel it. All the insides of my head are gone and there isn't a chance of me ever getting home or having my body back again. To have to live like this is terrible yet I don't know how I could die for I don't have any heart of my own to die with."

A number of treatments were tried, each to no avail. These included the latest in experimental techniques such as hormone therapy and benzedrine sulphate. In July, a lobotomy was performed, after which Miss Strawbridge was found to progress rapidly. She showed far more interest in her environment, began to help other patients, and looked after her personal appearance. Three weeks later, she went for a short walk with her relatives, who were startled to find her talkative, demanding cigarettes and cocktails, and full of spontaneity. Tarumianz wrote to Grant that "There has been a remarkable change in this patient, which appears to affect even the basic personality." The hospital awaited further developments in this patient "with growing interest."

The next patient in the series was included only at Tarumianz's insistence. As Sally Gold was only in her early twenties and was reputed to be a brilliant student, Grant was quite reluctant to operate, but was persuaded by Tarumianz that her case was "entirely hopeless." Grant operated in October 1938. Apparently all went well enough; little more than a year later, Grant received an engraved invitation to attend Sally's wedding.

At the 1941 AMA meeting, Tarumianz reported on the lobotomy series at Delaware State. Of the ten cases that Freeman and Watts had chosen, seven had returned home within a few months of operation and had made good social and mental adjustments; two returned to active employment. One died, a result of operative error. With such results as this, Tarumianz concluded, "one cannot help but consider prefrontal lobotomy as an adequate type of approach in chronic cases after all other types of conservative as well as semidrastic methods have been tried."[11]

### Boston Conservatives

About the same time as Grant was operating in Delaware, Watts's other mentor, W. Jason Mixter, was attempting his first lobotomy in Boston at

Massachusetts General Hospital. He performed one operation in 1938 and one in 1939. Although the number of cases was small compared to those of Grant or Lyerly (and soon others), their significance should not be underestimated; for Boston and "Mass General" were at the center of modern medicine in the United States and had a reputation for conservatism. Mixter himself was the oldest neurosurgeon in Boston, a founding member of the Society of Neurological Surgeons (the most prestigious neurosurgical group in America) and chief of the influential neurological service at Massachusetts General.[12] His sober but favorable report on these cases published in 1941 was an important step in the legitimation of the procedure.

Mixter's direct involvement with these patients came through his association with Stanley Cobb, the director of Harvard's Department of Nervous and Mental Diseases and of the neuropsychiatric service at Mass General. In the middle 1930s, Cobb was groomed by the Rockefeller Foundation to run an ideal mental treatment center that might inspire changes nationwide. Part of Cobb's responsibilities in directing the Harvard program in psychiatry was to develop stronger programmatic ties to McLean Hospital, an elite private asylum that was opened in 1818 as an offshoot of Mass General.[13]

## The Case of Arthur

In October of 1938, Cobb had run out of treatment options when considering what to try next for Arthur Prescott III, a private patient of his who was then residing at McLean Hospital, for over a year, on his second admission.[14] Arthur Prescott III was born into an old New England family that was described as "prominent socially, efficient economically, and stable emotionally." His father, a successful businessman, presided over a large and harmonious family, in the middle of which was located Arthur. According to the other brothers, Arthur's childhood had differed markedly from their own. Sent to a military academy, he shied away from sports, fought his way out of difficult situations, and was expelled for uncooperativeness. Refusing to go to college, Arthur decided instead to make his own way in business. His father arranged a series of clerical jobs, all of which he detested. He began drinking "to escape his loneliness and unhappiness." Around 1910, in his early thirties, he borrowed approximately thirty-five thousand dollars to set up his own fashion business. The venture was remarkably successful, and Arthur quickly paid back the loans in full. Sufficient money rolled in to finance a flashy life-style. Arthur's sartorial habits and conspicuous displays of extravagance earned for him a reputation as one of Boston's colorful, eccentric dandies. To his brothers, this success had rendered him totally unapproachable, giving him an impenetrable air of "grand aloofness."

World War I shattered Arthur's life. He went overseas first as a noncombatant volunteer and then as a regular army private; he found it "mental torture to have to be in close physical and psychological contact with other unwashed people." Like so many others of his generation, on the battlefield Arthur suffered "shell shock" and was shipped home as a nervous invalid. Through his father's intervention, he was released from a psychopathic ward and awarded an honorable discharge. Arthur returned to business life only to find that the market for his product had collapsed and that his business associates were incompetent. Having scorned his family's earlier urgent advice to sell out, Arthur was now financially ruined. He first turned his hand to writing plays and short stories, but soon lapsed back into heavy drinking. His social life revolved around frequent dates with women whom his brothers described as either prostitutes or "semi-prostitutes." When Arthur's drinking bouts and sexual forays became too much for the family to tolerate, he was evicted to a separate apartment. On his sober days, Arthur went to work at a shabby downtown office, where he puttered around with petty business matters.

In the summer of 1927, Arthur's drinking had become so bad that the family implored him to enter Channing Sanitarium, a private facility, to dry out for a couple of weeks. Upon his discharge, the physician in charge assured the family that Arthur was not insane but simply had "an entirely warped outlook on life." Within a few years, however, Arthur became further depressed and was discovered unconscious in a bathtub with his throat and wrists slit by a razor. Much to his own disappointment, he recovered. He moved into a house in a small town outside Boston and arranged for a housekeeper to take care of him. When he realized that never again would he be productively employed, he returned to heavy drinking supplemented by large quantities of drugs. Over the next few years, his life continued to erode. When his housekeeper tried to protect him by hiding the drugs, he became suspicious of her. His brother defended the housekeeper, believing her to be an honest but "coarse" woman, even though he suspected that she had been having an affair with Arthur. Arthur began to believe that his family too was cheating him. In 1931, he drank intensely, remaining in bed for weeks at a time.

In January 1936, Arthur contacted his brother and asked him to take him to a hospital because he felt he was going insane. The brother advised him to consult the specialist Stanley Cobb, which he did. At Massachusetts General, however, Arthur left the ward against medical advice, claiming that it reminded him too much of the military hospitals in France. In February, the brother responded to another phone call and found Arthur naked and drunk. All of his treasured possessions were stuffed into his pillowcase in an attempt to keep his housekeeper from stealing them. It was clear to the brother that Arthur was deteriorating rapidly; something had to be done. He was persuaded to enter another facility. After three months there and little improvement, Cobb advised the family to commit him to McLean Hospital.

Arthur entered McLean in the summer, and over the next seven months he remained agitated, renewing his suicidal threats. Cobb noted that he was more quiet and reasonable since the previous year, but that he kept demanding to be released, and even threatened Cobb with physical violence when the conversation touched upon the subject of his relations with the housekeeper. To placate him, Cobb released Arthur to a retreat at a ranch in Vermont, convinced that it was only a matter of time before he would "wear out the better patients." Within a year, Arthur was back at McLean. The admitting notes describe him as in his late fifties, quite agitated, uncooperative, and concerned only with whether or not he could receive assurance that he would return home by Christmas. He was oriented, had no impairment of memory, and was in good physical condition, though underweight. Cobb wrote on the temporary care order (the document that legally committed him for observation) that, as the patient had been hospitalized for the last eighteen months, he had had no alcohol or bromides; although he was much improved physically, "sobering him up has uncovered a marked psychosis of the agitated depressive type."

Arthur was initially placed on a ward for patients who were only mildly disturbed. He expressed satisfaction with the room and was anxious to know whether his letters would be mailed. The next day, the attending physician signed an order allowing him to go for a walk with a nurse. On the walk, he attempted to escape and returned nervous and anxious. At the staff conference, the physicians discussed Arthur's case. Dr. Thomason stated that as "this thing has been going on for quite a long time" and the patient felt no great necessity to change, they could not expect to do much. Several other physicians then debated his diagnosis, wondering whether he was psychoneurotic or psychotic. In either instance, it was clear to all that the prognosis was poor and that he would be a great deal of trouble to care for. Dr. Jaffe related that the family complained that they had had "an awful time with him."[15]

Over the next few days, Arthur settled unsurely into the hospital routine. He had a habit of accosting everyone he came into contact with as to whether he would be out by Christmas. Arthur steadfastly denied that he was unhappy, saying that his only source of depression was his confinement. He appeared agitated and restless, spending much of his time writing letters, mostly to his housekeeper. For example, that first week he wrote to her, "MY WHOLE LIFE IS BOUND UP IN YOU AND WITH YOU LARGELY RESTS THE FATE OF OUR ENTIRE FUTURE LIFE!" He complained that he was being kept under lock and key and denied the privileges that he had been assured. "I love you passionately, tenderly and forever," he continued, and emphasized that "the point is to keep at them morning noon and night until they let me out of here." (He ended with the poignant biblical reference, "FADER, MEINFADER, HEIREST DU NICHT?") Apparently, the feeling was mutual. Toward the end of July, the housekeeper spoke with Arthur's staff physician and told him that she was disappointed in McLean's care. She added that she loved Arthur dearly and would marry him if he returned to normal.

Over the next few months, the clinical and nursing notes indicate that Arthur continued to spend his time writing letters, whining to all about his lack of privileges at McLean and complaining about the other patients. He denied that he had a mental problem. He was visibly agitated, constantly picking his fingers. His nonstop letter writing focused mainly on attempts to gain release. It was noted that the patient appeared content only if left alone to do as he pleased. In September, he wrote to his brother that he had been tricked into signing the commitment papers when he was still under the influence of drugs and pleaded for his freedom. He concluded the letter, "My suffering beggars description. BE MERCIFUL." To the staff physicians, Arthur presented the frustrating picture of a patient who was always on the verge of dramatic change and yet remained obstinately opposed to improved behavior.

In October 1938, Stanley Cobb returned for a consultation. He noted that Arthur's condition remained the same. Cobb was clearly exasperated. He wrote in the clinical chart that the "outlook is bad," and that therefore he was willing to "let the family try anything they wish," implying that he would consent to other arrangements should they insist. On the other hand, although Arthur's stay at McLean was as yet doing little clinical good, Cobb still advised further institutional care. He suggested yet another alternative, the "operation of 'frontal lobotomy' as practiced by Watts and Freeman." Cobb noted that Arthur "is just the kind of case that has been helped."[16] In December, Cobb returned for another consultation and found the patient somewhat less tense and more reasonable. He attributed the change to the new hope the patient found in the promise that the lobotomy might enable him to return home. In fact, Arthur demanded that Cobb sign an affidavit stating that, should the operation prove successful, he would be discharged within eighteen months. Cobb signed it. Permission for the operation was obtained from the brothers and the patient. During February, Arthur returned to his usual uncooperative, disagreeable self, content simply to lie on his bed and write his maudlin, often incoherent letters. Or he would follow the physicians around the ward, constantly badgering them as to whether he would be home by June 1939 and showing them Cobb's affidavit.

Arthur was transferred to Massachusetts General for a lobotomy on 24 March 1938. Mixter used Watts's and Freeman's new operation, without the corer. The operation itself was uneventful. Afterward, Arthur was found to be quieter and able to hold a more normal conversation. Upon his return to McLean, on 2 April, he was placed on Men's Belknap I, a minimal care ward, to encourage his socialization and to impress upon him that the doctors expected some change "as a result of the operation." Intelligence tests revealed little significant change, but it was wondered how reliable they were in regard to more complex functions. On 11 August, Arthur was prepared for discharge. The clinical summary stated that after the operation he was given full hospital privileges, was less agitated, could maintain a friendly attitude toward the doctors when interviewed, and in general was able to behave far more normally than before. The operation was judged to be a moderate success. Arthur was placed in the care of his family, who rented a beach home where he could be taken care of by his housekeeper. Four months later, Arthur's brother wrote, "He is perfectly well and his condition is better, if not the best that it has been in years." All the symptoms of depression, worry, and agitation had abated. It was noted that Arthur did lack the energy and drive that he had possessed when he was younger. On the other hand, he truly no longer had any desire for drugs or alcohol. Arthur read current literature, attended to his religious duties, and renewed his old acquaintances, with whom he got along quite normally. Most characteristically, Arthur could still "talk a good game."[17]

Two years after the operation, Arthur returned to Cobb's office for an examination to determine if he was sufficiently competent to remove the legal guardianship of his affairs. Cobb noted that when Arthur arrived, he appeared quiet, dignified, with a rather exaggerated exactness of speech and intonation – he was evidently on his best behavior. Arthur began the conversation by describing the poor health of his mother and his housekeeper but was not as upset or agitated as before. He did not drink. Cobb described Arthur's mood as calm and normal, and outwardly happy. His stream of talk was slow, measured, and with adequate expression, though pedantic. Speech was orderly and expressive. His memory for recent events was good. He remembered a French proverb and used it correctly. He subtracted sevens from one hundred as follows, "93, 86 . . . 9, 2, and from 2 not even you can do it," and then laughed. He showed some insight into his problems and stated that he hated all associations with his illness. He found his years in various institutions to have been "very sorrowful" but held no rancor. He had been so frightened by these experiences that he no longer had any desire to drink. Arthur summarized his current state as follows: "My soul is damaged but the head is all right." When the examination was over, Cobb asked Arthur why he was so interested in having the guardianship removed. His explanations were sound. Cobb then asked Arthur to dictate the letter he needed. He stated slowly and thoughtfully: "I have attended Mr. Prescott several times since February 1936 and am thoroughly conversant with his case. I definitely believe that he is capable of managing his personal affairs completely and I emphatically desire the termination of the terms of his guardianship at the earliest possible date."[18]

## The Case of Harry

A month before Arthur's discharge, Cobb found himself considering lobotomy in a second case. Harry Hartford was admitted to McLean Hospital during the Depression, a married businessman in his mid-fifties. The precipitating factor in the decline in Harry's life was the stock market crash of 1929, which shut down his office. He borrowed money to start again, but this effort yielded only further disaster. Worries led to long bouts of sleeplessness, anorexia, and an attempt at suicide with a knife. After his wound was sewn up (he remained a cripple), Harry then threw himself headfirst against a radiator at the hospital, inflicting further injuries. Subsequent attempts at suicide yielded other permanent damage.

At McLean, Harry's suicidal tendencies continued; he asked to be placed in a straitjacket, lest he tear his eyes out. During the following months his self-condemnations continued: he would recite homosexual limericks as proof of his vile nature. His physician noted that Harry believed that coitus was against biblical teachings, and that he had definite homosexual longings. "The homosexual trend," Dr. Hollingshead explained, "may be an expression of an unsatisfactory sexual life." On the other hand, he continued, "it may be part of his rather dramatic effort to prove himself the worst patient in the history of the hospital." Harry had little motivation to get better, having a poor home life and no business to return to. The hospital physicians found it difficult even to imagine that Harry might someday become whole again. It was feared that he might one day achieve some measure of adjustment, but just enough to commit suicide successfully.

In discussing this case, the other physicians noted that the problem was not with the patient's mode of thought, but with the extreme level of emotion; it was possible that if the emotion could be lowered, he might recover to a meaningful extent. The immediate difficulty was how to handle such an aggressive patient. It was noted that his nurse already had a black eye, and that he struck out at others in the hope that they would respond with sufficient force to kill him. The homosexual urges also added to the hospital burden. Dr. Rourke commented that Harry represented "a challenge to our medical and nursing supervision." The recommendation was to hold him on the maximum security ward and keep him in the therapeutic baths for as long as was necessary. It was clear to all that Harry "will be ill a long time."

As the years passed, the grim prognosis held. In addition to his continuous self-condemnations (he would describe himself as a bucket of garbage), Harry also developed a habit of smacking his lips noisily, which became permanent. He was informed that his favorite child had died, which deepened his depression and revived suicidal wishes. Eventually, he settled into a habit of muttering only in a jargon of words and it became impossible to hold a coherent conversation with him. The nurse's notes indicate that a typical day would find Harry noisy and active about the ward, shuffling and jabbering as he moved around. (Interestingly, his gait would return to normal if he believed no one was watching.) He also read a lot.

At the end of October, Cobb visited McLean to examine Harry, whom he diagnosed as an agitated depressive. He discovered no neurological abnormalities, but the physical exam was incomplete because Harry was uncooperative. The patient's ceaseless activity, muscular tensions, and flows of gibberish, in Cobb's opinion, were a form of psychological defense, but they also suggested something else. If one might "neurologize" about a psychiatric case, Cobb pondered aloud, this excessive cerebral activity might be meliorable through frontal lobotomy. The operation was further justified in Harry's case, Cobb argued, because of his advanced age and otherwise hopeless prognosis. Hallowell and Pauline Davis, pioneers at Harvard in the development of the new technique of electroencephalography, were brought in to examine Harry. They determined that Mr. Hartford did in fact have abnormal electrical activity throughout the cortex. Mixter also examined Harry and concluded that, as the underlying problem was attributable to increased activity of the frontal cortex, surgical treatment offered a reasonable chance of success. That the patient had not seriously deteriorated was in his favor; that he had shown no spontaneous improvement demonstrated there was little to be lost. Mixter was "glad to operate on him," but with less enthusiasm than in the previous case.

A staff conference was held the following week. Dr. Caufield began with a clinical summary which stated that the patient's condition had changed little in the past year. Harry continued to pace up and down the halls all day, or remained in his room muttering and smacking his lips. In his opinion, prognosis was poor, regardless of whether or not brain surgery was performed. In contrast, Dr. Boyle thought Harry was an excellent candidate for frontal lobotomy.[19] None of the doctors present could agree about the underlying pathology. Some suggested neurological conditions such as Parkinson's or a brain tumor, as indicated by the unusual EEG. Others attributed his mannerisms to psychological defenses. Dr. Rourke noted that Harry had been doing fine in life until "things crowded in on him." Dr. Hollingshead captured this frustration by stating that trying to diagnose Harry was akin to interpreting art in a museum: you see only what you are already interested in. A further diagnostic procedure was called for that uncovered some atrophy in the left part of Harry's brain; this was attributed to a presenile condition. As a result of this finding, Walter Freeman was consulted for advice. Freeman recommended surgery, and permission was obtained from the family.

On 2 February, Harry Hartford was transferred to Massachusetts General for a lobotomy. Immediately following the operation, he began to talk rationally, although for only a few hours. A week later, with the patient still hospitalized, the clinical notes stated that he was much improved, "in the way that we hoped he might be." In particular, his agitation, motor restlessness, jaw-champing movements, and continuous gibberish had all greatly diminished. He was returned to McLean, where the next few weeks were not stellar. The nurses noted that Harry was talkative, though in his usual peculiar jargon. He was uncooperative when getting out of bed and struck the nurses twice. In March, however, Harry began to show slow signs of improvement. He was described as carrying out the ward routine very quietly and cooperatively, and had even gone out for a drive with friends. April was even better. Harry went to town to see a movie and did not mumble in his jargon during the outing. Later in the month, he was talking to everyone in a sensible manner. He visited home one day and wrote a letter to his wife without difficulty. Moreover, Harry showed considerable mirth and humor in his conversations, laughing and joking with patients on the ward.

Harry's startling transformation impressed even Dr. Caufield, who earlier had expressed doubts that a lobotomy might achieve anything beneficial. In his clinical note of 13 May, Dr. Caufield wrote that the "patient has markedly improved, now being able to carry out most of the activities quite naturally and taking an obvious interest in everything." Harry spent a lot of time reading and participating in sports, and had gone out for frequent rides with friends and family. He conversed with the other patients and was cooperative and friendly toward the physicians. In addition, he walked in a more normal manner and had "entirely given up his peculiar manneristic talk." In June, Harry was transferred to a better ward. The nurses' notes indicate that he "behaved well at all times" in the unrestricted environment. In the first week of August, he went on a vacation trip with his daughter and returned a week later. Upon his return, the nurses described Harry as doing very well, becoming more talkative with the nurses, often laughing with them. A few weeks later, he was placed "on visit," pending discharge.

In the year after his return home, Harry's nephew informed the hospital that their former patient was continuing to make improvements. He was apparently happy and living in a small apartment with his wife, and his activities were increasing. The nephew found it highly significant that Harry's sense of humor had definitely returned; he told a joke and the patient laughed heartily. A few years later, the hospital phoned the household and learned from a sister that Harry was getting along very well. He had appointed himself money collector for the building, soliciting on behalf of the Red Cross, the Salvation Army, and the like. His sister described him as entirely recovered. The physician then spoke to Harry himself and found him to be "absolutely normal."[20]

Mixter, along with Tillotson and Wies, published a report on these two cases in the journal *Psychosomatic Medicine* in 1941. (Cobb's direct role in selecting these patients was played down in the report, but the significance of the article's appearance in this journal – the house organ devoted to Cobb's own clinical orientation – was clear.)[21] The article began with the disclaimer that "We have been slow to use frontal lobotomy as we have felt that a destructive operation without demonstrable brain lesions was a radical procedure." They set out criteria for consideration, including well-established agitated depression, lack of mental deterioration, a chronic condition with no chance of improvement, and severe states that require constant institutional care. The two patients, chosen over three years, met all these criteria. The results generally matched Freeman's and Watts's description of how the operation both relieved some symptoms and produced another set. On the negative side, patients lost spontaneity, initiative, and thoughtfulness about the future. General knowledge and memory remained undisturbed, however. On the positive side, the operation reduced the energy content of ideas and emotions that had previously resulted in grossly psychotic behavior. Extreme agitation, negativism, and poor appetite all disappeared. In both patients, suspiciousness, odd mannerisms, agitation, and irritability vanished; and anxiety and nervous tension diminished, replaced by a partial return of a sense of humor. One, in addition, gave up drugs and alcohol. They concluded that, through lobotomy, the psychosis is not "cured" but some sort of permanent "desensitization" takes place. And although the frontal lobes definitely figure in higher intelligence, "this destructive operation has not destroyed the ability to reorganize the elements of the personality to a considerable functional level." Frontal lobotomy, then, was definitely indicated for those patients who met the right selection criteria.

## Other Early Trials

The work of Lyerly, Grant, and Mixter soon inspired others in the United States to experiment with Watts's and Freeman's new procedure (in these early years, Watts just as often, if not more, was cited as the leader, as it was a neurosurgical innovation). Case reports began to appear from around the nation, focusing on either the new Freeman-Watts procedure or the Lyerly approach. Patients targeted for the operation remained mostly cases of severe agitated depressions or involutional melancholias. A new trend was developing, however, as patients selected for the procedure increasingly came from institutional as opposed to office-practice populations.

In Seattle, Washington, a young man who worked at Boeing was operated upon according to the Lyerly method in 1941, with good results. "It is probable that we will have a normal, responsible member of society," his physicians declared, "one who is able to take his place in the world and do his work properly." In Wichita, Kansas, a fifty-year-old woman with severe anxiety neurosis who had attempted suicide was becoming worse; following a lobotomy, she laughed out loud for the first time in four years. Eventually, she resumed all of her social obligations and assumed responsibility for running the household. Her husband stated that she had been restored to her former self. Other early locations of operations included Hartford, New York City, Rochester, and Toronto.[22]

Ten patients, beginning in 1941, were operated upon at the Medical College of Virginia. Most of the "miserable, unhappy, restless individuals who paced the floor wringing their hands, moaning, groaning, sometimes yelling and screaming," it was reported, "were transformed into "quiet, placid, uncomplaining persons who showed little concern about their troubles." The "striking fact" was that almost all of the patients showed some degree of improvement, with the large majority "capable of living and adjusting in their home environment," which was "in sharp contrast to their preoperative behavior." Thus, "many hopeless, chronically mentally ill individuals who appear to be destined for an institutional existence the rest of their lives," as a result of this procedure, "make a social recovery and most of them are able to live in peace and quietude in their own homes."[23]

Perhaps the best example of how Watts and Freeman, Fulton, and Lyerly set the psychosurgery programs in motion was the example provided by the neurosurgeons at the famous Mayo Clinic in Rochester, Minnesota. The 1939 meeting of the Harvey Cushing Society, at which Lyerly described his improvement on the psychosurgical technique, took place at the Mayo Clinic. Staff neurosurgeon J. G. Love was so impressed by the demonstration that he made a trip to Jacksonville to learn directly from Lyerly. Love performed his first operation on 28 February 1940 – only a few short weeks after Fulton himself had lectured to the clinic on the neurophysiological significance of lobotomy.[24]

In the published series of staff proceedings, it was stated that the clinic had been skeptical when the first results of such an operation were published. The demands of the patients' families had forced them to reconsider, however, prompting investigations by Love and others. Eventually, a series of forty-two patients were operated on by 1943, mostly agitated depressives who were brought over from the local state hospital. "Needless to say," Love reflected, "I am very happy to have had some part in the care of these unfortunate individuals." He described the horrendous conditions of institutional life as something that every physician should be forced to witness. To see these suffering patients improved by lobotomy was indeed "a pleasant part of medical experience."[25]

## New Pastures

A second wave of interest in the surgical relief of mental illness began when Edward Strecker, clinical director of the Institute of Pennsylvania Hospital, asked Grant if he might perform some lobotomies on his patients. Between October 1938 and May 1941, twenty-two of the institute's clients were given lobotomies. What distinguished Strecker's series from previous work was the use of brain surgery in cases of chronic schizophrenia, the most serious form of mental illness. Moniz as well as Freeman and Watts had argued that lobotomy would be of little use for such intractable cases. In September 1940, the University of Pennsylvania celebrated its bicentennial with a series of distinguished addresses by faculty members. Strecker used his address to publicize the achievements of the

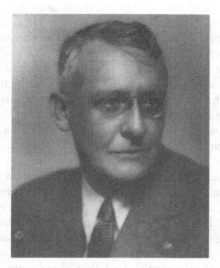

Figure 3.2. Edward Strecker. (Source: Archives of the American Psychiatric Association)

new somatic treatments in psychiatry and to announce the successful application of brain surgery to the problem of schizophrenia. The results of the lobotomies, Strecker stated, were "truly amazing." Although the original speech discussed the brain operations only briefly, a press release was prepared that described in further detail the dramatic transformations. *Time* magazine, for example, related how Edward "Streck" Strecker, "psychiatric bigwig," had arranged for a lobotomy on a young woman whose psychosis led her to rip her clothes off and to fly into rages; she was so violent that she required tube-feeding. After the operation, however, she was calm enough to play bridge and sculpt.[26]

At the next meeting of the American Psychiatric Association, held in Richmond, Virginia, in May 1941, Strecker and his associates reported on their innovative use of lobotomy. In contrast to the prevailing guidelines, their patients were not the melancholias of late middle age, who were generally well preserved, but young adults with severe schizophrenias of long standing, usually described as mentally dilapidated or deteriorated. Their conclusions were based on the first five patients, all of whom had been observed postoperatively for at least one year. The first case was a schizophrenic woman in her middle twenties who had been under Strecker's care for over five years. She had a long history of stormy misadventures, including suicide attempts in which she set fire to her clothes and slit her wrists. She had been paranoid, delusional, and hallucinating. A lobotomy yielded no immediate relief. A year later, however, she had improved to the point where she was employed as a hostess at a resort and performed satisfactorily. She learned to play golf and even played in highly competitive tournaments. A similar patient had a violent fear of being kidnapped, would smash all the furniture in the house, and attack her nurses. After the operation, she became talkative, pleasant, and cooperative, and took an active interest in her environment. Her mother wrote to the doctors, "I want you to know how very much I appreciate all that you have done," for the operation "undoubtedly benefited her to a certain extent."[27]

By January 1940, Strecker was sufficiently confident in the procedure to recommend it in the case of Eileen, the sister of a personal friend, who had suffered from schizophrenia for over ten years. He explained that "a friend of mine, Dr. Francis Grant (I am sure you know him socially) is one of the outstanding neurosurgeons in the world and, in addition, is one of the few neurosurgeons thoroughly familiar with the technique of this operation." He strongly emphasized that there were no assurances it would prove beneficial. Nonetheless, it was his opinion that a lobotomy might offer "a fairly good prospect for improvement." The operation was performed on 16 January 1940. On 6 March, the sister wrote to Grant that she recently lunched with Eileen and the visit was a great success. Eileen showed interest in everything and behaved normally and with considerable poise. She showed no signs of nervousness or tension, initiated considerable conversation, and joked. "I feel that Eileen's progress is a very precious and thrilling thing," she reported, "and I hope with all my heart it can be maintained if not increased."

Over the next few months, it became clear that, although the patient had substantially improved, she would still require some form of institutional care. At the end of October, the sister again wrote to Grant, using the salutation "Dear Chubby," which was his nickname. She described how Eileen was still improving, although she did at times laugh inappropriately and make odd noises. Eileen had taken up some arts and crafts, and had accompanied her twice to the World's Fair in New York City. "I am delighted with the results of the operation," she concluded, "irrespective of whether or not she recovers completely (I know she won't) because of the absence of the unbelievable and desperate suffering she endured for years." She was now "content about her" and deeply grateful to him and Dr. Strecker.

In analyzing their results, Strecker and his associates forthrightly stated that with prefrontal lobotomy "recovery must not be expected," and that they were "frank to admit that surgery seems a potentially dangerous and definitely brutal method to use in the treatment of mental dysfunction."[28] Indeed, two of the other reported cases seemed much more ambiguous in their results. Nevertheless, it was clear to them that all of the patients did improve somewhat, even after one discounted the difficulties always inherent in the measurement of psychiatric gains. (Psychometric tests revealed little change in intelligence.) Talents in arts and crafts or athletics, long dormant as a result of psychosis, reappeared. In the overall picture, a fundamental change in the emotional structure of the patients was effected, for the better. True, sophisticated pursuits of the prepsychotic personality were replaced by a tendency to derive pleasure from the simpler things in life, such as an ice cream cone, a dog, or a movie. Yet, contrary to widespread professional belief, destruction of the frontal lobe did not lead to an inevitable release of inhibitions. Some of the patients regained a measure of self-control and maturity that was startling. One such patient regained sufficient resourcefulness and common sense to rescue a friend who was seriously injured when they were out horseback riding.

Institute staff members learned that the best indications for lobotomy were not diagnostic criteria, but an appropriate constellation of symptoms revolving around a patient's level of agitation, destructiveness, mental distress, and overactivity. Their experience had also led them to maintain a narrow, strict set of guidelines for selecting operative candidates. It was their heartfelt opinion that psychosurgery was not a "standard method of treatment applicable to any large section of psychiatric practice." Irreversible mutilation was irreversible mutilation, period. When all was said and done, however, "there is no denying the fact that surgery is sometimes effective and must be considered."[29]

That Strecker's group pioneered the application of psychosurgery to the "forgotten patients on the back wards" was not pure happenstance.[30] To begin with, it was highly unlikely that any new intensive medical therapy might make its first appearance within the nation's vast system of public institutions, in spite of the fact that close to 85 percent of all hospitalized patients resided in state hospitals. There simply existed too many barriers – geographical, financial, and professional – between state hospitals and the other major centers of medical advance. Such barriers were less common in Europe; it is therefore not surprising to find that whereas Moniz began his operations in Portugal's national psychiatric hospital, when the procedure was transplanted to America it initially took root in the private practices of Walter Freeman and Jim Lyerly. Only after the new procedure had been somewhat established did it shift to those state hospitals willing to invest their scarce resources in an unproved treatment. Even then, patients selected for the operation were basically similar in pathology to the original private-practice patients, differing only in the degree and duration of their conditions. To regard chronic schizophrenics – the bedrock core of the isolated institutional population – as suitable for a new medical treatment required the crossing of several barriers. (Moniz's reported failures with schizophrenics also dampened enthusiasm.)

In the previous generation, some states had committed themselves to establishing special research centers that did offer occasions for experimental ventures. However, these kinds of facilities – various freestanding psychopathic institutes and neuropsychiatric wards in teaching hospitals – dealt primarily with the less serious psychoneuroses or psychotic episodes of short duration. Once a patient's stay extended beyond the state's statutory limit for temporary commitment pending observation, he or she would be transferred to a state hospital. Almost by default, then, one would expect that any connection made between Moniz's procedure and the severer problems of mental disorder would occur at an elite private hospital such as Strecker's Institute. There, the clientele could afford the added costs involved and the physicians would have access to the latest techniques.

In practice, however, barriers prevailed in this domain as well. As evidenced by the case history of Arthur Prescott III above, few of these facilities were equipped to care for long-term, seriously disturbed individuals. In addition, private asylums tended to be just as isolated from centers of medical progress as were the public ones. Indeed, only a few such institutions existed that offered both long-term care for deteriorated psychotics and an opportunity for first-rate medical research. A list would include the McLean Hospital in Belmont, Massachusetts; the Institute of Living in Hartford, Connecticut (which was closely allied with Yale Medical School); and the Institute of Pennsylvania Hospital in Philadelphia. Each of these sites, as it happens, would eventually develop extensive programs of psychosurgery that focused on its uses for schizophrenias of long standing.

The Institute of the Pennsylvania Hospital, however, was doubly special. There was no hospital that better demonstrated, simultaneously, Adolf Meyer's clinical philosophy of psychobiology, Thomas Salmon's professional vision of a unified neuropsychiatry, and Alan Gregg's ideal of a center for psychosomatic research and teaching. It was precisely for this reason that the institute was singled out by the Rockefeller Foundation as being a key site for the reinvigoration of American psychiatry. (The Pennsylvania Institute was one of the first psychiatric facilities to offer a full three-year residency qualification program, and by World War II it claimed to have trained more leading psychiatrists than any other location.) The foundation was sold on the special meaning of the Institute, which was advertised to them as the "the only situation in which are found chronic and acute psychoses, neuroses, and what can be described only as nervous symptoms in gifted and ordinary people."[31] In a single site, close to a major university medical school (Strecker was also chairman of the University of Pennsylvania's psychiatry department), researchers, clinicians, instructors, and students could focus on any kind of mental disorder, from the minor to the severe. The unusual mission of the Institute of the Pennsylvania Hospital was to link fast-breaking medical advances to the problem of the long-care institutionalized population. Psychosurgery was a natural extension of this mission.

Strecker's findings on psychosurgery had a decisive professional impact for several reasons. First, the Pennsylvania Institute's avowed commitment to an eclectic treatment program, in which somatic therapies were considered as valid as psychotherapeutics, lent further credibility to its medical reports. Second, at the time Strecker held a position of unusual esteem in both the public and the professional arenas. Two years after the report on psychosurgery was published, Strecker would assume the presidency of the APA during its symbolically significant centennial year and would preside over the commemorative meetings in his own city of Philadelphia. To the public, Strecker was lauded by *The Saturday Evening Post* as one of the top five psychiatrists in America. He alone, however, was publicized as "the man who made psychiatry respectable."[32]

## Early Converts

It was not long before others were inspired to follow Strecker's lead. Tarumianz, for example, was greatly impressed, and in August 1941 Grant was asked to try his hand on two schizophrenics at Delaware State. The first patient had been constantly combative and homicidal but in just a few days after the operation was serene enough to request newspapers and magazines. Results of the procedure on the other patient were no less remarkable. A catatonic who had been mute for nine years in the hospital, she sat up after the operation and asked for the beautician to come and give her a manicure.[33] And at Nebraska State, results consistent with the "encouraging" report of Strecker's were found in a small series of chronic schizophrenics, in a program guided by noted neuropsychiatrist A. E. Bennett.[34]

A team at Elgin State Hospital in Illinois set out to duplicate Strecker's work, convinced by his portrayal of "miraculous results." It was no mystery to them why Strecker's report had set off a firestorm of interest in the brain operations. Over the previous decade, the shock therapies had quickly gained the "paramount position in the armamentarium against the affective and schizophrenic disorders." The most disappointing aspect of this otherwise bright story, however, was that none of these treatments had proved useful once the mental illness passed the acute phase. It was not surprising, then, that "recent reports of improvement or even recoveries in chronic schizophrenics following bilateral prefrontal lobotomy were received with enthusiasm." (Their own trial at Elgin, however, ended badly; their report would constitute the only negative result published in the next decade.)[35]

Significantly, Walter Freeman himself identified the lobotomy program at the Institute of the Pennsylvania Hospital as having constituted a crucial turning point. Strecker's display of therapeutic "courage," Freeman felt, had reawakened the possibility of psychosurgery for a population that even he had abandoned as "unfruitful."[36] Moreover, the potential of what Strecker had accomplished was not lost on the general public. In a 1941 article in *Harper's Magazine* on psychiatric progress, filed by science writer William Gray, the story of psychosurgery was used to conclude the section on the new somatic treatments. It began with a brief description of the Moniz and Freeman-Watts operations, but the majority of the section was a narration of Strecker's triumphs. Noting that previous attempts had been restricted to the emotional disorders of middle age, the account focused on Strecker's innovation of using lobotomy on chronic schizophrenics. Gray retold the saga of the young woman tortured by voices whose existence was an endless hell; lobotomy restored her fully to life. "It is doubtful if in all the annals of mental disorder," Gray breathlessly declared, "a more dramatic 'improvement' can be found."[37]

As the emphasis shifted to the chronic schizophrenics in state or city hospitals, the pace of the operations quickened. Two of the largest early programs were at the Willmar State Hospital in Minnesota and the St. Louis City Hospital (later St. Louis State Hospital) in Missouri. At Willmar, neurosurgeon Harold Buchstein performed forty-six operations on mostly schizophrenic patients between January 1941 and May 1942. Of the twenty-nine operated upon in 1941, six had already returned home by the time of his report's publication in 1943. Four others were making satisfactory social adjustments; in no case was the psychosis aggravated. "While these results are not spectacular," Buchstein reported with Superintendent Magnus Petersen, "it must be remembered that . . . [the subjects] were formed from clay rejected by the potters." Because spontaneous remission rarely occurred in these kinds of long-standing cases, they argued, the operation alone must be credited for the positive changes.

Petersen and Buchstein, obviously moved, wrote that psychosurgery thus "kindles hope in a realm of psychiatry where despondency reigns." Between June 1941 and April 1944, 101 patients were given lobotomies at the St. Louis City Hospital, two-thirds of whom were chronic schizophrenics. None of the patients were reported to be worse after the operation. Although the outlook for all of these patients was "nil," after surgery thirty were discharged; fourteen of these were regularly employed and reported as essentially normal. In the opinion of the hospital staff, "prefrontal lobotomy is slowly but steadily proving its value."[38]

In both of these sites, the emergence of psychosurgery programs can be traced to the long reach of Fulton's laboratory. Buchstein, the Minneapolis-based consulting neurosurgeon to Willmar State Hospital, had recently returned from a postgraduate year under Fulton's supervision in 1939. His own interests in the procedure focused on the opportunity it offered for further research into the neurophysiological relations between the frontal lobe and the autonomic nervous system – a typical Yale project.[39] The tie to St. Louis was even stronger. Fulton inadvertently drummed up local interest in the Moniz procedure with his exhibit on the frontal lobes at the 1939 meeting of the American Medical Association, which was held in St. Louis (Fulton's visit was reinforced by a lecture on the subject given by Walter Freeman some months later). Furthermore, when Washington University in St. Louis started up a department of neuropsychiatry in 1941, they hired for their first medical psychologist Fulton's former colleague (and collaborator on the Becky experiment) Carlyle Jacobsen. Jacobsen had not abandoned his research interest in the frontal lobes, and he turned his attention now to the physiological underpinnings of psychosurgery. Leopold Hofstatter, the staff physician at the City Hospital who was first author on its psychosurgery publications, later attributed the emergence of the lobotomy program largely to Jacobsen's arrival. Once the program was under way, Jacobsen personally conducted the psychometric examinations before and after the operations.[40]

It can be argued that the St. Louis City program was in fact the first major trial of psychosurgery at a public institution in that it involved teams of first-rate neurosurgeons, an active university department of psychiatry, and experimental psychologists. A distinguishing feature of the St. Louis series was the sophisticated neurophysiological input into the design of the lobotomy program. (The team claimed that intellectual deficits were far fewer than those seen in other lobotomy trials, and attributed this to their own improved operative technique, which was based on a comprehensive reexamination of neurophysiological function.)[41] For this kind of interdisciplinary, state-of-the-art medical program to take root in the back wards of a publicly funded mental facility, an unprecedented level of cooperation would first have to occur between otherwise separate institutions and professions.

These kinds of disciplinary rearrangements that resulted in the appearance of an elaborate program of brain surgery in a public mental hospital did not happen by themselves. Here, too, is evident the handiwork of the Rockefeller Foundation's calculated patronage, which saw in St. Louis a unique opportunity to bring about its vision of a laboratory-based psychiatry. For some time, Washington University had been a favored recipient of Rockefeller money, ever since an earlier endowment of seven million dollars had established it as the premier medical center in the region. Beginning in the early 1930s, the foundation targeted the university as one of its primary sites for the development of clinically oriented neurophysiology. Here, basic research into nerve physiology was to be closely integrated with strong programs of neurology as well as neurosurgery. Under the direction of Ernest Sachs, for example, the St. Louis neurosurgical unit was growing into the nation's largest such training program, which is how the City Hospital came to have four visiting neurosurgeons on staff, at a time when even one would have been a rare achievement.[42] Moreover, beginning in 1938, the foundation began to supply an additional fifty thousand dollars a year to create a wholly new department of neuropsychiatry, whose mission it was to demonstrate how psychiatry might be reintegrated into general medicine through university-based laboratory research (Karl Menninger, for example, protested that the St. Louis grants were diverting psychiatry away from its proper focus in clinical work). Thanks to the aggressive funding of the Rockefeller Foundation, researchers across a broad array of disciplines were thus focusing anew on the problem of mental disorder and reached out to nearby mental institutions for a supply of suitable material. In the wards full of chronic psychotics at City Hospital, this unique group of motivated, interdisciplinary investigators found a natural place to connect brain research to mental pathology – in the form of psychosurgery.[43]

### Freeman and Watts

Freeman and Watts did not sit idly by as others began to file reports on their results with psychosurgery. Between 1938 and 1941, they quickened the pace with which they performed lobotomies and invested an even greater percentage of their professional energies in assuring a future for the procedure. In Freeman's case, psychosurgery became a dominant feature of his career. Looking to the distant future, Watts did not want to concentrate his neurosurgical practice on any one technique, and thus he made a conscious effort not to commit himself as fully as did Freeman. What was discussed among the profession first as the Watts and Freeman procedure soon was referred to as the Freeman and Watts technique.

Both men clearly were motivated by the excitement that comes from being in the forefront of medical innovation. In psychosurgery, the pair had found a career-making challenge that engaged all of their intellectual, technical, and clinical skills. Moreover, neither Freeman nor Watts was financially well-off at the time, and the monetary rewards that lay ahead were quite compelling. The patients who might qualify for such a procedure were in almost limitless supply and in desperate need of something; the procedure itself was relatively simple, with low mortality. Working within the American medical custom of charging whatever the market could bear, such operations yielded anywhere between a low of twenty-five dollars and a high of fifteen hundred, depending upon individual circumstances. Fees often reached five hundred dollars – a tidy sum for an afternoon's work.[44]

Freeman positioned himself at the center of the storm he knew was brewing within the profession and rode it out to a position of high visibility. Egas Moniz, recently incapacitated by a homicidal patient and nearing retirement, faded from the scene. Freeman dutifully kept Moniz up to date about the psychosurgical developments in the United States, describing the setbacks as well as the successes in individual cases, and deferentially requested advice. It was clear to both parties, though, that the procedure's fate had passed from Moniz's hands to Freeman's.[45]

In short order, Freeman discovered that his unique position as lead examiner for the specialty Board of Psychiatry and Neurology offered a perfect vantage point from which to seed a new therapy. The extensive travel to centers of neuropsychiatry around the country, where the professions' best and brightest stood up to prove themselves the equals of their mentors, ensured that the rising generation of experts would familiarize themselves with whatever Freeman was up to. Moreover, in preparation for these trips, Freeman would arrange for a demonstration of psychosurgery at nearby mental institutions whose administrators were all too eager to collaborate with a physician of Freeman's stature. Such an opportunity might not come again for some time – or at least until Freeman's follow-up visit. Indeed, within the course of a few years, Freeman had added to his professional correspondence an elaborate network of hospital superintendents and clinical directors who were scattered about the national landscape. Perhaps no other medical leader in America was in as close contact with this isolated medical constituency.

On a trip to Milwaukee, for example, Freeman interviewed patients lined up by the local sanitarium's director and then selected a group that, in his opinion, should have lobotomies. On the institution's behalf, Freeman would then personally relate his decision to the relatives, explaining his reasoning. He informed the husband of one patient, for example, that his wife "would be strikingly benefited by the operation," for she showed "so clearly the emotional distress and preoccupation that are more or less specifically relieved by [it]." Saying this, he then described a range of complications that might ensue. Freeman did not recommend the operation for everyone. To another patient's sister, he wrote, "On the whole, I think the chances are against it, and I would not recommend it," in spite of the fact that "I am naturally optimistic and a taker of chances." To the husband of a different candidate, he wrote regretfully that the chances of his wife being benefited by the operation were "too slender to warrant it." She would "manifest certain tendencies towards irritability and aggressiveness that would render nursing or even institutional care still necessary continuously." Freeman closed the letter with a philosophical musing: "The only thing that I can say is that next year maybe something else will turn up that will throw prefrontal lobotomy into the discard. I certainly hope so."[46]

Freeman also pursued a more public means of furthering the development of lobotomy. He and Watts kept up a hectic pace of presentations at professional societies and publication in the leading journals. Freeman sensed that what was needed was a no-holds-barred campaign, and went to work. At poster sessions of scientific meetings, for example, he would stand in front of his table snapping a clicker like a barker at a state fair; before he delivered a paper at a local medical meeting, he might arrange for a newspaper reporter to attend, promising a juicy story. Stories of how surgeons could cut out worry and mental illness struck a receptive chord among a public clamoring for the next triumph of medicine.[47]

John Fulton himself had occasion to experience just how hot the topic of psychosurgery had become. In 1940, he was invited by the national chapter of Sigma Xi to lecture to audiences around the country about recent scientific accomplishments (the tour included sixteen cities in three weeks.) Fulton drew up a list of several possible topics, and to his surprise – and dismay – all twelve of the local chapters wanted to hear the same thing: an explanation of the importance of the frontal lobes. Even though his talk referred to a broad range of developments in neurophysiology, what the audience latched onto was the new operation of lobotomy. Even *Science Service,* when covering his speech to the Mayo Clinic, entitled it "Brain Operations, Removing Parts of Frontal Lobes, Found to Aid Some Types of Hopeless Mental Patients." For Fulton, the trip resulted in his own education as to the level of desperation that mental patients and their families felt. As each of the lectures was closely reported upon by the local press, Fulton would return home only to find a stack of letters from strangers pleading with him to arrange a lobotomy. He sardonically referred to these letters as his "fan mail" and forwarded more than a few to neurosurgeons for whom he could vouch.[48] Fulton would soon find himself drawn back into the professional fray as well.

### Backlash

It was not long before Freeman and Watts found themselves caught up in a strong backlash. In particular, the more public aspects of the lobotomy campaign generated considerable antagonism within the medical profession and left the pair vulnerable to serious charges. In 1940, science journalist Waldermar Kaempffert observed a lobotomy operation performed by Freeman and Watts. Greatly impressed, he considered writing a feature article on psychosurgery, the first to appear in a national publication. When he queried the New York Academy of Medicine on the topic, he was surprised to discover bitter opposition there – such words as "crime" and "criminals" were mentioned. Kaempffert turned to Fulton for advice, who responded by describing the academy's opinion on the operations as "all wet." This proved to be sufficient incentive for Kaempffert to follow through on his article. Kaempffert then obtained from Fulton appropriate background references on the subject, as well as some editorial assistance.[49] The article was eventually published in *The Saturday Evening Post* in 1941 and produced a scandal that prompted more than one medical society to pursue the censure of both Freeman and Watts. Unknown to Fulton beforehand, the printed version of the article contained several photographs in which Freeman and Watts were identified by name. At the time, this was regarded as a form of medical advertisement – a serious breach of medical ethics. Once again, Fulton rose to the occasion. He declared to those proposing censure that, if necessary, he would stand behind Freeman and Watts "to the last ditch." At the American Neurological Assocation he was able to quash the censure motion in executive session.[50]

The controversy that always surrounded psychosurgery was beginning to boil over. Whereas previously it had been confined to discussions conducted in private corridors or in the semiprivate context of discussions that followed papers at professional meetings, condemnations of Freeman and Watts began to appear in regular editorials and other communications. In May 1940, for example, the lead editorial in *The Medical Record* was titled "The Lobotomy Delusion." Unsigned, it began by asserting that in recent years a new type of "meddlesome surgery" had been introduced into this country, "frontal lobotomy by name." It derided the attempts to "to pluck from the brain a hidden sorrow" as both dangerous and wrongheaded; such fundamental aspects of personality were a product of the whole organism, not localizable to any particular region of the brain. The "mutilating surgeons" who would venture forward on this path were admonished to reread the Hippocratic oath.[51]

In 1941, Gregory Zilboorg's history of medical psychology chastised psychosurgery as a form of medical sadism. Attacks by such psychoanalytically oriented practitioners, however, were not unexpected. More worrisome for Freeman and Watts's venture were the issues raised by Stanley Cobb in his comprehensive 1940 review of neuropsychiatry published in the *Archives of Internal Medicine*. Although it was through Cobb's initiative that lobotomy was introduced at McLean, his public thoughts on the subject reflected a deeper ambivalence. He supported its use for patients of older ages who had no chance of recovery. Even then, however, he was troubled by the operation's total effects. "Is the surgeon justified," he wondered aloud, "in depriving a patient of the most important part of his intellect in order to relieve him of emotional troubles?" Cobb left the question unanswered, content to table the issue until more was known scientifically. He voiced bitter skepticism, however, that Freeman and his supporters were the ones to accomplish this research. Freeman's phrase "pre-frontal lobotomy" he ridiculed as an anatomical misnomer; the current studies on frontal-lobe function were dismissed out of hand as lacking valid controls. Cobb complained that even though scores of patients had been subjected to the operation, there existed not a single report that was "convincing as scientific evidence."[52]

In reaction to the growing interest and controversy spawned by the various forms of psychosurgery, in June 1941 the AMA's Section on Nervous and Mental Diseases took the unprecedented step of hosting a "roundtable" forum of experts on both sides of the issue. Moderated by Paul Bucy (a favorite ex-associate of Fulton's), the panel consisted of presentations of late-breaking findings by Freeman, Lyerly, Tarumianz, and Strecker. Roy Grinker, a Chicago-based neurologist and Freudian sympathizer, set the tone for the debates that followed. (A somewhat sanitized transcript of the discussants' comments was published in *JAMA*.) Grinker prefaced his comments by stating that "he was no angel," and that he had been invited to criticize the procedure as best he could. The interest in lobotomy, he thought, originated in the hopes of those who wanted to swing the therapeutic pendulum in psychiatry away from psychotherapeutics toward more physical methods. "It is not a far cry from psychochemistry to psychosurgery," he sneered, in an oblique attack on Walter Freeman (who some years earlier had published a minor paper with this title). He reflected that a great deal of emotion existed on both sides, a situation not unlike the debate in religious circles on abortion and contraception.

After a few more biting remarks on the poor judgments of those espousing lobotomy, Grinker took the opportunity to underscore that although ordinary intelligence tests were unable to pin down what was lost in the operation, "I think all of the members of the panel are agreed that there is some defect." There was a great danger that lobotomy resulted in only a "spurious kind of normality," thus permitting the patient to return to situations of responsibility "with disastrous results." Extreme caution must be applied when advocating the procedure, for "once one cuts, there is no return." Diminished anxiety, Grinker continued, is not necessarily a good thing; anxiety is what drives man's adaptive mental mechanisms. The only "rational" treatment, in his opinion, was "psychologic therapy." There might exist a very narrow grouping of people, Grinker allowed, for whom psychosurgery was indicated. The greater danger, however, was that the operation would expand beyond tight guidelines. In particular, Grinker was extremely anxious about "the general group of people floating around this country with psychoses and psychoneuroses who will, if we are not very careful, be mutilated by this operation."

Grinker's comments, as expected, sparked intense discussion. Freeman attacked Grinker for basing his harsh assessment on the reports of lobectomies performed for cancer and epilepsy, not on the actual lobotomy literature. In Freeman's view, moreover, Grinker's call for highly elaborate, technical intelligence assays, was simply off target. Such tests were inapproprate, for what mattered was not a patient's performance in an artificial context but how he or she did in life. Patients would undoubtedly fail some of Grinker's tests, Freeman conceded. "These patients are, however," Freeman countered, "able to carry on the normal details of their everyday existence in a rather satisfactory manner." Freeman also attacked Grinker's comment that a patient's anxiety could be construed as beneficial: this was sheer wishful thinking on the part of psychoanalysts.

Palmer and Tarumianz entered the debate, taking issue with Grinker's insinuation that the lobotomy patients had been denied the fruits of psychotherapy. Not true, they asserted. The lobotomy patients all had had long-term counseling and, in some cases, psychoanalysis. Palmer discovered a point of vulnerability in Grinker's otherwise formidable attack. As Grinker complained that the hospitalized schizophrenics and melancholiacs had not had sufficient psychotherapy, Palmer asked him point-blank to state what percentages of success he expected such treatment to achieve with this class of patient. Grinker was forced into strategic retreat, unable to hazard even a guess, explaining that in psychotherapy success depended upon too many complex factors. His unsatisfactory response confirmed the suspicion of those supporting the brain operations that the strident attacks of the psychoanalysts could be comfortably shrugged aside. Let them tend first to their own glass houses.[53]

For the general medical community, the result of the debate was a cautious wait-and-see attitude. An editorial in *JAMA*, written by Morris Fishbein, accompanied the publication of the roundtable discussion. Tempering the enthusiasm of its proponents, Fishbein noted that it was inconceivable that any such procedure might completely restore a human being and that its detrimental effects were at present only partially understood. Nevertheless, "an emotional attitude of violent unreasoning opposition to this form of treatment would be inexcusable." Yes, he continued, it was a mutilating procedure, but this was a characteristic of many surgical procedures and in itself did not rule against it. Until such time as more scientific evidence could be produced, "no doctor can yet assert that this is or is not a truly worthwhile procedure." Although the editorial did not certify the procedure as being of proven therapeutic benefit, it did imply that lobotomy was of sufficient value for current clinical trials to continue. The roundtable's positive result for Freeman and Watts was not so much Fishbein's tacit benediction but the evidence that they no longer were alone in their crusade. Lobotomy was now being explored by a growing number of prominent researchers and clinicians who represented a broad spectrum of the neuropsychiatric domain, from private practice to the state hospitals.

## Psychosurgery, the Monograph

The real turning point for the pair came in 1942 with the publication of their *Psychosurgery*, the first comprehensive guidebook to appear on the subject. The route to publication had been rocky and by no means assured. In July and October 1940, Freeman and Watts submitted their manuscript first to Macmillan and then to W. B. Saunders, two important medical publishers. Their manuscript was declined as either too controversial or too expensive. Undaunted, they tried C. C. Thomas, known for his well-produced volumes devoted to neurological subjects. During the summer of 1941, Thomas agonized over the decision to publish, wary of the storm that Freeman and Watts seemed to invite. He consulted Fulton, who for many years had been a valued source of confidential editorial opinion and an important author for Thomas's firm. Fulton lobbied hard on behalf of Freeman and Watts. In response, Thomas wrote that he had received many letters "blasting Freeman and Watts all over the lot" but, as Fulton's opinion was always the most reliable, he would accept the manuscript. Watts thanked Fulton for this support, convinced that without it Thomas would never have signed a contract.[54]

The landmark text was the culmination of everything toward which Freeman and Watts had worked. In a single volume the reader found an exhaustive overview of the scientific literature, richly detailed case histories, summaries of clinical findings, and a snapshot of the operation's national as well as international use. It began with a historical account of surgical attempts to cure insanity, from the ancient Incas up to the modern era. This preamble was followed by comprehensive chapters on frontal-lobe physiology, normal as well as pathological. The reader then was walked through the latest surgical techniques for bilateral prefrontal lobotomy and given a thorough, practical guide as to what to expect postoperatively and how to respond. In the final set of chapters, the authors analyzed the effectiveness of the operation by diagnostic category and propounded a new theory of frontal-lobe function. Included in the book was a supplementary set of analyses by psychologist Thelma Hunt that compared postoperative and preoperative results.

For Freeman and Watts, the theoretical basis of the operation had now stabilized. Moniz's original model of a neuronal basis for "fixed ideas" was superseded by the American model of maladjustment that emphasized an individual's capacity for survival in a social environment. Evidence indicated that the frontal lobes were essential to "satisfactory social adaptation." Some individuals, however, had a "perverted activity in these areas" and might function better in life if the frontal lobes were "partially inactivated," the authors asserted. After the operation, although fixed ideas and compulsions often persist, the " 'sting' of the disorder, is drawn," for the disabling fears that accompanied these pathologies were banished. Almost all of the lobotomy patients, they declared, "find existence more pleasurable, and they can adjust better in their environment" (Freeman and Watts, *Psychosurgery*, [1942], 294).

The current state of the technique was presented in strongly positive though qualified terms. "Prefrontal lobotomy is being tried out here and there in tentative fashion," Freeman and Watts wrote, with "some excellent results and a good many failures" (18). As to their own results, by April 1941 (the date of the volume's final revisions) the pair were able to report upon seventy-four patients. The results were presented to the readers in the form of both easily readable tallies and detailed case histories. One table counted the symptoms reduced by the operation while another listed the new problems produced. In this manner, readers were left to make up their own minds as to whether the operation seemed worthwhile. For example, it was reported that nervous tension had been

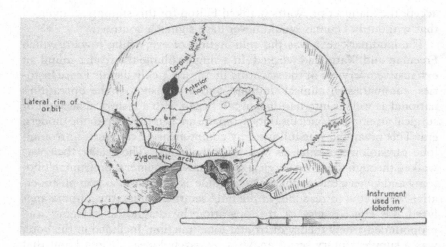

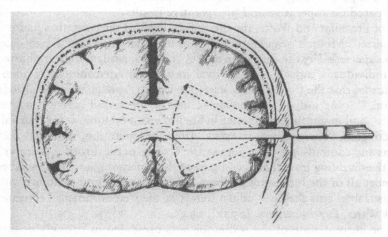

Figure 3.3 a, b. Diagram of a Freeman and Watts standard lobotomy. (Source: Walter Freeman and James Watts, *Psychosurgery,* 1942. Courtesy of Charles C. Thomas, Publisher, Springfield, Illinois.)

present in seventy-two of the patients; after lobotomy, persistent relief was obtained for fifty-seven of these. Fifty-four patients had previously demonstrated suicidal desires; lobotomy reduced this to three. The symptoms produced were just as thoroughly documented. The reader learned that thirty patients developed a persistent lack of initiative. Tactlessness

appeared and remained in forty-three, laziness in twenty-nine, and euphoria in twenty-two. A simple inspection of the two sets of tables, the authors argued, revealed that "the balance would seem favorable to prefrontal lobotomy" (294).

The pair were careful not to oversell their subject. Readers were warned
that the method was not to be used indiscriminately, but only on those
patients facing disability or suicide who had proved refractory to other
treatments. There were no guarantees of a successful result, either. For, as
Freeman noted (with one of his trademark flourishes of the macabre), in
some instances the operation "succeeds too well." If anything, they tried
to present a realistic picture of what might happen. "Our bad results have
been emphasized," it was explained, "in part from a desire to instill
caution" (vii). Thirteen patients, the authors indicated, did so poorly that
a second, deeper operation was attempted. Three of these ended up in
"mental dullness." The reader thus learned of the occasional fatal hemorrhage and of the fact that in many patients the imagination was severely
infringed. The two even went so far as to include the poignant testimony
of the son of one patient, who stated, "Frankly, Dr. Freeman, I don't know
of any way that I might suggest to anyone to more effectively cause the
deterioration of an entire family than that operation" (292). The final
impression was that the technique was by no means perfected, but that
improvement was expected at some point in the future.

*Psychosurgery* broke new ground not just because of its unusual subject
matter but for the mode of its presentation. The dry statistical tables had
been accompanied by lengthy case histories scattered throughout the
book, a stratagem that constantly focused the reader's attention on the
human dimension of psychosurgery. But these were not ordinary medical
case presentations, either. Each formed a novella in its own right, written
in a frank and often lurid format. Freeman had a flair for pulp nonfiction,
a talent honed over the years in the lecture halls of the medical schools
where he took great pride in simultaneously engrossing and appalling his
audience with the rawness of medical reality. (His classes developed something of a cult reputation, as medical students would invite their girl-
friends along to experience the thrill – or, alternatively, watch in satisfaction as their dates passed out.) In a literary equivalent to cinema vérité,
readers of *Psychosurgery* would follow the progression of an individual
patient as he or she moved from a hellish existence on the ward (described
in all its gritty detail) to selection as a candidate for surgery. Such stories of
torment and suffering were told through the patients' own voices and
those of their families, friends, and hospital staff.

The dramatic moment then came when the subject was brought into the operating room – perhaps kicking and screaming, and tearing off his/her clothes in a desperate attempt to escape. The operating room setup was described, and Freeman and Watts would get to work, talking to the patient, who was under only local anesthesia. The story picked up there, as the readers listened in on the actual conversation, recorded in transcript. ("QUESTION: What's going through your mind? PATIENT: A knife" [109]). The main drama over, a new narrative of gradual recovery and self-growth began, starting with such basic matters as regaining sphincter control and learning how to hold a spoon, and ending with resumption of housework or even a job. Many would make the uncertain passage, others not. Contact with these stories was maintained through extensive use of photographs of the patients taken before, during, and after the operation – often quite haunting.

At the same time that it played to the morbid fears and fascination of the public, the book nonetheless also worked at a highly technical level, supplying all the expected medical imagery of x-rays, neurophysiological diagrams, histological analysis of brain cells, and photographs of the actual clinical charts. Freeman's genius lay in his unprecedented integration of the two genres, interweaving the trappings of laboratory science with the fabric of everyday life. The book worked something like contemporary anatomical teaching aids that were composed of multiple layers of colored cellophane. Indeed, as the reader turned the pages of *Psychosurgery*, he or she would find pictures that began with exterior views of the head and, as layer by layer was peeled off the skin and then the skull, ended up with the deepest reaches of the brain exposed. Unlike typical medical texts, though, the layers were not confined to the body. Freeman also superimposed colorful verbal sketches of the patients' personal hygiene, domestic relations, job skills, and the like. In effect, the composition of the book itself demonstrated the exact claim that was at the core of the psychosurgery enterprise: brain physiology and human life were now connected, in a way that was understandable to laboratory science and open to practical intervention by trained physicians.

The unusual power of *Psychosurgery* in projecting this message to the average reader was noted at the time. The superintendent of a state hospital in South Carolina, for example, wrote to Freeman that his seventeen-year-old daughter had read it and told him: "Daddy, this is the most interesting medical book that I have ever seen. Even I can read it and understand what I am reading about."[55] Science journalist Waldemar Kaempffert reported in the *New York Times* that, after having read extensively in the literature on brain studies, he felt it was safe to say that "there is no book" like *Psychosurgery*. "*Psychosurgery* is not too technical even for laymen," he explained. Moreover, "this department found it more exciting than most novels. And why not? Probing into the brain, breaking up fixed pathways and compelling the thalamus and the prefrontal lobes to find new ones, watching uncontrolled minds slowly return to more normal ways of thinking – no novelist ever had a more thrilling subject." And even if psychosurgery did not have scores of successes to its credit, "This book is bound to be read by every progressive psychiatrist, neurologist, and psychologist," for "its approach is practical and realistic."[56]

Within the medical profession, the book was indeed an instant classic: the letters poured in from around the country to congratulate Freeman and Watts on their achievement. Tarumianz, for example, called it a "masterpiece." Their publisher, Charles C. Thomas, was thrilled to report that by all accounts the book was "No. 1" in quality. He was particularly impressed by the comment of the prominent neurosurgeon Max Peet, who said that before reading the book he had been leery of the procedure but was now convinced. From Toronto, psychiatrist Kenneth McKenzie informed them that it was "the only book on psychiatry that I have been able to understand." As another example, Wilder Penfield, head of the influential Montreal Neurological Institute, sent a card to Freeman: "It is beautifully and thoughtfully done. It will prove to be a building stone in a structure of therapy in a field where little therapy has stood the test of time." Perhaps the best tribute came from John Fulton himself when he requested that the original typescript be sent to Yale University for inclusion in its history of medicine collection.[57]

## Certain Benefit

From the time of the monograph's publication in 1942 to the end of the Second World War, the use of the operations grew steadily but not dramatically. A review of published and unpublished studies, conducted by Lloyd Ziegler in 1943 for the *American Journal of Psychiatry*, enumerated 618 lobotomies as having been performed in eighteen centers in the United States and Canada, with the large majority performed since 1939. Of these 618, twelve patients had died as a result of the operation and two had committed suicide; eight had been made worse. Summary results indicated that 194 had improved, 214 had recovered, and 277 were still in the hospital. A remarkable 251 were outside of the hospital, working full- or part-time. Three patients were serving in the military. "Intellectual impairment, which was feared most," Ziegler reported, "has been found to be much less than expected." Modern medicine, he observed, has taught us that we can survive with one less lung, or kidney, and now

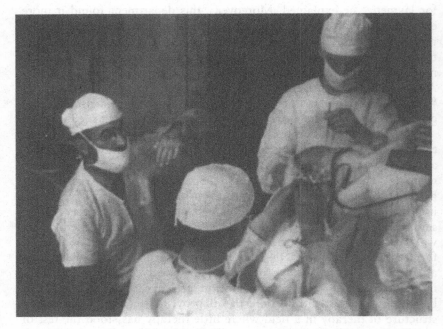

Figure 3.4. Scene from a film of Walter Freeman and James W. Watts performing a lobotomy, 1942. (Source: *Prefrontal Lobotomy in the Treatment of Mental Disorders,* film produced by Walter Freeman and James Watts. Courtesy of the National Library of Medicine.)

perhaps we can live with less frontal lobe as well. He concluded his review by stating that "this interesting therapeutic endeavor deserves a good trial over the next five to ten years." Ziegler's tabulations were supplemented in 1944 by the neurosurgeon A. Earl Walker, in the first comprehensive review article to appear on the topic of psychosurgery. The review revealed that 107 articles and monographs had already been published and were appearing at a rising rate.[58]

The increasing number of lobotomies did not indicate that the controversy or doubts surrounding the procedure had been dispelled. Walker noted the growing concern as the lobotomy tallies climbed into the hundreds of cases, with many patients having "paid a high price for their freedom from fear, worry, and anxiety." Some critics of the operation, he noted, characterized lobotomy as producing a "new disease" in the patient which was "no less severe than the original affliction." Analogies were made to "the placid, slow-moving life of the Lotos-Eaters far from the Utopian existence."⁵⁹ Walker's doubts, like Cobb's, were reminders that, for many prominent figures within the scientific and medical communities, the jury was still out as to the procedure's ultimate value. However, these kinds of reservations, although strongly voiced, did not halt the lobotomy programs under way.

From the perspective of those on the front lines in the mental hospitals, it was clear also that the procedure was not well understood scientifically. Nor had it been subjected to "the acid test of time that will determine its value." Nonetheless, all indications were that the method had "sufficient merit to justify further trial." Institutional psychiatrists around the country began to pay closer attention to the possibility of offering psychosurgery to their own patients. By 1944, two psychiatrists at a southern hospital defended their decision to begin a lobotomy program by simply stating that the method of Freeman and Watts "has become an accepted practice and is now being used more extensively."⁶⁰

Freeman, too, saw definite signs that a sea change had occurred in the overall attitude toward psychosurgery. Perhaps the strongest evidence that the tide had turned in its favor was the introduction of psychosurgery onto the wards of St. Elizabeth's, the federal facility where Freeman's own career had begun. In 1937, when he first broached the possibility of performing lobotomies on its patients, Superintendent William A. White made little attempt to conceal his hostility. "It will be a hell of a long while before I'll let you operate on any of my patients!" he told Freeman.⁶¹ By 1943, after White's retirement, the first brain operations were performed – a turn of events that even years later Freeman would retell with some relish.

Toward the end of the war, Freeman resumed his correspondence with Moniz, now retired. In April 1944, Freeman proudly informed Moniz that he and Watts had performed 230 lobotomies, and that more than half of these patients were usefully occupied. He was also happy to report the results of Ziegler's survey and that, by his own reckoning, psychosurgery had been attempted in as many as twenty-five to thirty centers in North America. "Psychosurgery," Freeman observed, "is being adopted more liberally throughout the country now." And in 1946, Freeman reported, "the resistance in this country to the concepts of prefontal lobotomy is gradually disappearing." He boasted that even the great neurosurgeon Walter Dandy, at "conservative" Johns Hopkins, performed one.⁶² The brain operations had survived their baptismal trials.

For those physicians who had witnessed the effects of psychosurgery, there was little mystery why the procedure had advanced beyond its status as an experimental method of questionable merit and limited availability to the next phase, that of tentative acceptance and broad clinical trials. As Lyerly expressed to Fulton in 1940, "I am sure a good procedure which obtains excellent results to the satisfaction of the patient and the family should not be allowed to die and that the work will continue to progress under its own merits." The issue boiled down to a simple set of questions. As George Kisker asked in his review article, "Does it get results?" and "Is it a useful addition to the psychiatric armamentarium?"[63] From what the investigators had seen with their own eyes, the answer was strongly affirmative. In the brain operations, psychiatry had discovered a medical resource of uncommon strength. Over and over again, hospital psychiatrists watched in disbelief as their most intractable and wretched patients were visibly transformed.

For example, Harry Solomon, director of the prestigious Boston Psychopathic Hospital, noted that until his own facility began its lobotomy program in 1943, he had shared the skepticism of others concerning the claims of Freeman and Watts. He too assumed that "next to Ananias, they were the best story tellers and the best liars the world had heard of." Solomon, however, in "a moment of irresponsibility," agreed to try it out on a series of twenty-three chronic, "hopeless, unquestionably schizophrenic patients." The results were not something for which he was prepared. That such patients were given "a new lease on life and [have] become reasonable persons again," Solomon reported, "has rather shaken my stability." At Boston Psychopathic, one of the largest psychosurgery programs in the world was soon launched. "Like all converts," Solomon observed, "I should like to do a little evangelical work."[64]

Freeman and Watts must be included among those convinced by the raw power of the operations. However cynical one might be about the motivations for the pair committing so much of their professional energies to developing the new treatment – in Freeman's case, with a level of drive that surely bordered on the pathologically obsessive – it would be wrong to downplay their faith that, in the cause of psychosurgery, they had found a true means of rescuing innumerable persons from otherwise hellish fates. As the years progressed, Freeman kept in touch (through phone calls, correspondence, and personal visits) with literally thousands of his lobotomy patients, and what he learned from them and their families only deepened the pair's belief in the essential good they had accomplished. Hanging on a wall in Watts's office was a poem, decorated with hand calligraphy, written by a patient who had been the recipient of Watts's sixty-eighth lobotomy:

> Gentle, clever your surgeon's hands
> God marks for you many golden bands

They cut so sure they serve so well
They save our souls from Eternal Hell
An artist's hands, a musician's too
Give us beauty of color and tune so true
But yours are far the most beautiful to me
They saved my mind and set my spirit free.[65]

To Freeman and Watts, the carping of their colleagues in the laboratories – and of psychoanalysts in posh consulting rooms – was unlikely to divert them from their course, for the proof of what they had accomplished was found, not in a microscope slide or a published dream interpretation, but in the unfiltered statements of those whose lives they had touched.

## New Complications

Freeman and Watts introduced psychosurgery into America only to discover that once the procedure had broken free of its initial hurdles the expanding number of operations engendered a new set of complications. With every additional report documenting yet another instance of remarkable gains, clinicians in the field were that much more convinced that "prefrontal lobotomy seems to offer something of importance in the handling of the intractable neuroses and psychoses."[66] That the operation yielded significant benefit they were certain. But it was also increasingly clear that the benefit was of only a certain kind, and limited to a particular form of suffering or behavior. The harder the practitioners attempted to pin down the procedure's advantages and disadvantages, and the indications of when to use it, the more the existing methods of assessment were revealed as inadequate to the task. This was a case of familiarity breeding not contempt but confusion.

Paradoxically, the confusion was produced by exactly the same set of factors that were fueling the procedure's dissemination. It is the common destiny of most medical innovations to be tried out, even if only halfheartedly, on a range of conditions and disorders far different from those which their innovators had originally anticipated. In the case of psychosurgery, this clinical drift was especially significant. Following the well-publicized reports of Strecker and his associates at the Institute of the Pennsylvania Hospital, the use of psychosurgery crossed over into the long-term, deteriorated institutional population – the kinds of patients who were filling up the nation's vast system of state hospitals. As early as 1943, observers tied the increasing rate of lobotomy to Strecker's discovery that psychosurgery was useful for these institutionalized psychotics.[67]

Strecker's further observation that the best guidelines for selecting operative candidates were based, not on specific categories of disorder but on severity and type of symptom, in effect eroded Freeman's and Watts's original protocols that did restrict the procedure to a well-specified type of patient. Moreover, it was not long before Freeman and others began to argue that the certain benefits offered by lobotomy implied that patients should not be left to languish in mental institutions where they might deteriorate past the point of reclamation. It was through this logic that Grant, for example, had been persuaded to operate upon schizophrenic women in their early twenties. The perceived utility of the operation grew in direct proportion to the expansion of the diagnostic categories considered appropriate for the procedure, resulting in a broad mix of indications for the operation. It was this same heterogeneity, however, that hobbled attempts to define in precise terms the operation's advantages and disadvantages.

Whereas the operation had previously been applied to only one type of well-defined clinical condition, now it was used for a wide assortment of clinical problems, each with its own problematic package of possible outcomes. The cases were not commensurate, however. After lobotomy, a young schizophrenic's hallucinations might cease, but her delusions continue; although a businessman's depression might lift, he was no longer employable; and a catatonic mute for ten years might speak again, but when reunited with family be unable to establish satisfactory relationships. Freeman and Watts could point with pride to the growing number of publications that, due to the size of their lobotomy programs, had to report their results in summary tables rather than individual case histories. Even as these tallies grew from tens into hundreds and then even into thousands of cases – objective evidence that a lot of psychosurgery was indeed occurring – such reports were revealing less and less about *what* was happening. As the self-appointed head of the psychosurgery campaign, Freeman found himself obliged to make sense out of an avalanche of material that in the years to come was getting ever harder to synthesize and manage.

In truth, the fate of psychosurgery had become linked to factors that extended well beyond Freeman's, Fulton's, or any one person's control. Once the method had gained a reputation as a useful treatment for patients with chronic mental illness, the usual professional mechanisms that were assumed to check the growth of innovative procedures no longer applied.

New medical treatments historically appear first in America, not on populations at the bottom of the socioeconomic ladder, but on those at the top. Only the well-to-do have access to physicians at the forefront of medical advance. (In a private aside to Fulton, Wilder Penfield saluted his clientele, who not only offered themselves up as experimental guinea pigs but also paid him handsomely for the opportunity.) In the clubby world of the elite physicians, the limits of acceptable risk were patrolled by unwritten but often closely watched gentlemen's agreements.[68] The very first cases of psychosurgery were no different, as Freeman found himself second-guessed and monitored by the "conservative" physicians in Boston and Philadelphia, and even by Menninger in Topeka.

In a sort of "trickle-down" process, it is only when a procedure has been found to have some general value that it enters the rest of the medical system (and then only after a constituency comes forward to push for its inclusion). As the example of psychosurgery demonstrates, however, the shift from the private offices of the neuropsychiatrists and their elite clientele to the state mental hospital system carried with it some important consequences.[69] No longer were discussions about the procedure limited to the private correspondence of elite physicians. They had become a matter for open discussion with governmental bureaucracies that were beholden to trustees, legislatures, and public opinion. Moreover, the kinds of evaluations made as to whether psychosurgery worked would be very different in the institutional context than it was in the private-practice environment. The dramatic success of psychosurgery – as well as other somatic treatments appearing at the time – thus opened up the deep professional rifts that still existed within the field of American psychiatry, despite claims of unification. Each of the many subgroups of psychiatry had its own inner culture, its ways of seeing and doing things, as well as its own set of local challenges. The future of psychosurgery was no longer simply in the hands of the elite neuropsychiatrists or neurosurgeons (which included Freeman), but became caught up in broader historical currents.

Furthermore, once psychosurgery was identified by the profession and the public as a treatment of possibly vast potential, the idea was shattered that any orderly connection might still exist between the laboratory researchers who were supposed to regulate new discoveries and the clinicians in the field. The scientists closest to the scene, such as John Fulton and Stanley Cobb, had expected that psychosurgery would follow a classical model of technological diffusion, in which the laboratory spins off innovations of great utility in the extramural world. Until such time as the proper scientific tests were conducted, these new treatments were to be designated as "experimental," and thus considered off-limits to the average working physician. The assumption was made that those in the laboratory and the field would work in tandem. From the outset of his involvement with the story of psychosurgery, Fulton was well aware of the considerable potential that Moniz's procedure might have for psychiatry as well as neurosurgery. As early as October 1936, for example, Fulton predicted that the treatment might ease the overcrowding then prevalent in the nation's mental hospitals, at the same time greatly lowering the costs of caring for the severely mentally ill. Although he was solidly in favor of the medical community proceeding with the operations, he remained undecided in regard to its actual validity: final proof had not been obtained. Fulton's support of the procedure had been predicated on the idea that a series of small, carefully designed clinical trials in elite academic institutions would ensure a deliberate, responsible evaluation of the procedure's merits.[70]

Such conditions proved to be extremely problematic, however. For example, Fulton knew that Freeman and Watts, confined by the demands of private practice and by limited access to research facilities, would themselves be unable to take the neurophysiological lead. The task of bringing together the academic centers (which contained the trained researchers) with the remote state hospitals (which housed the vast clinical material to be studied) was more difficult than first supposed; the profession might not wait until such time as these realignments could be effected. In 1944, researchers Stanley Porteus and Richard Kepner published a pioneering psychological monograph on psychosurgery in which they detected just such a breach. They appealed to the wider psychiatric community to abstain from further lobotomy programs until the conclusion of the necessary scientific studies. From what they had already seen of families demanding this treatment for their loved ones, they were not optimistic. "There is a great danger," they warned, "that lobotomy may become too popular." Looking back in 1950, Cobb confirmed their worst fears. Psychosurgery, in his view, had indeed "moved away too rapidly from its physiological basis and was somewhat prematurely applied to patients." By way of explanation, Cobb simply stated that "the need was great."[71] Even to him, it was not clear how, in light of psychiatry's circumstances, the tale might have been otherwise.

The story of psychosurgery thus demands that we turn to a consideration of the factors outside of the laboratory and the office clinic for a deeper understanding of just what this desperate "need" was. Psychosurgery, it seems, gained additional momentum not just because of what it was expected to do for particular cases of mental illness but for what it might accomplish for all of psychiatry in America.

# 4

## Active Treatment
### Somatic Therapy and State Hospital Reform

One may question whether shock treatments do any good to the patients, but there can be no doubt that they have done an enormous amount of good to psychiatry.

Louis Casamajor (1943)

In the half-decade following the end of World War II, brain operations for the relief of mental illness soared dramatically. Whereas in 1945 approximately 240 lobotomies had been performed in America, they more than doubled annually until 1949, when at least 5,000 patients were operated upon (see Figure 4.1). Between 1936 and 1951, close to 20,000 patients received some form of psychosurgery in America. The primary site of the procedure was in the nation's vast network of state mental hospitals, which accounted for 85 percent of the psychiatric beds in the United States; at least 63 percent of all state facilities had used psychosurgery. Yet it would be wrong to assume that the story of psychosurgery transpired only inside the walls of state hospitals. During their heyday, the brain operations were in fact employed throughout the institutional geography of American psychiatry, which included private asylums, general hospitals, university medical centers, psychiatric research institutes, and veterans hospitals. Indeed, the last three on this list had a higher rate of participation than did the state hospitals. For example, 80 percent of all psychiatric research institutes in America used psychosurgery at some point, and so did *all* thirty-seven of the new (and then well-regarded) VA hospitals.[1]

The issue no longer seemed to be whether to operate but how to refine clinical indications and surgical techniques. Psychosurgery's legitimacy was further reinforced by the convening of the First International Congress of Psychosurgery in 1948 and by the awarding of the Nobel Prize in Medicine to Egas Moniz in 1949. An influential neurologist noted in 1951 that, although lobotomy initially had been viewed as a "desperate experiment," within just fifteen years it had become "an accepted routine, a useful procedure widely employed." Its *nonemployment* in any hospital,

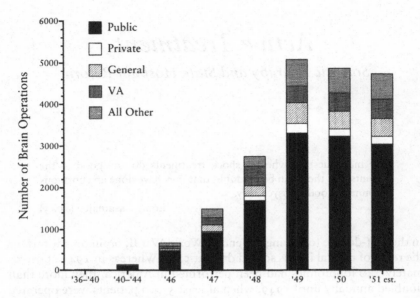

Figure 4.1. Psychosurgery in American mental institutions, 1936–1951. (Source: Chart prepared from data in *Proceedings of the Third Research Conference on Psychosurgery,* 1954)

another prominent psychiatrist declared, would "require an explanation."[2]

To explain this turn of events, the story moves away from the individual psychosurgeons and their patients who have dominated the narrative thus far and shifts to an overview of the special challenges then facing both the mental hospital system and the psychiatric profession as a whole. The "great need" that Cobb cited as having fueled the procedure's diffusion was in fact not one problem but an amalgam of problems. Psychosurgery rose from its status as yet another promising therapy to that of a fundamental part of contemporary psychiatry because it appeared to address a wide range of timely issues. In the right combination of circumstances therapeutic innovations become valorized as "active treatments," celebrated for their social and political utility as well as for their clinical potential.

### The Shame of the States

In 1946 Americans awoke to the massive social problem posed by its mental hospitals. Readers of the May issue of *Life* magazine were scan-

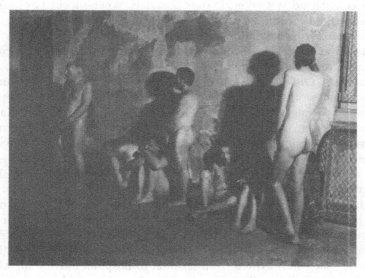

Figure 4.2. Incontinent ward, Byberry State Hospital, from Albert Deutsch, *The Shame of the States* (New York: Harcourt, Brace, 1948). (Source: Archives of the American Psychiatric Association)

dalized to learn from Albert Maisel's pictorial essay that the nation's state mental hospitals had degenerated into "little more than concentration camps on the Belsen pattern." This was not idle hyperbole. The graphic photographs that accompanied the piece demonstrated brutal neglect and dire conditions. At Philadelphia State Hospital and Cleveland State Hospital, for example, wards were shown in which patients were abandoned, provided little or no clothing, and left in physical restraints. Overcrowding was so severe that floors in some wards were not visible due to the closeness of the patients' beds. Thousands of inmates spent their days in physical restraints. Others, isolated in dungeons, lay in their own excrement. Long hidden from public discussion, here was the shameful story of "the abused, the beaten, the drugged, the starved and the neglected" (see Figure 4.2). This essay was not the first such exposé in the postwar years. The *Life* magazine report, however, had a powerful effect in mobilizing both journalists and public opinion. What once had been taboo for public discussion became fodder for journalistic sensationalism, and superintendents nationwide found their own institutions propelled into the public spotlight when local newspapers produced a flood of similar reports.[3]

Maisel's article was based primarily upon the experiences of conscientious objectors, mostly Mennonites and Quakers, who had served their enlistment period as workers in state hospitals. When shocked by hospital conditions, this group did not shy away from controversy. In 1947, a far more extensive presentation of the conscientious objectors' story was published as an abridged collation of some two thousand confidential, firsthand reports that originated from hospitals in twenty states. The compilation, *Out of Sight, Out of Mind,* stunned readers with a picture of a grim, cruel world that might have been scripted partly from the pages of Dostoevsky's tales of daily life in Siberian prisons, the rest from Kafka. Inmates lived a routinized life devoid of dignity, being herded through traumatic five-minute meals and fortnightly mass bathings and shavings. A heartless bureaucracy demanded the requisition of every necessity; yet little arrived, no matter how vital. Ten pairs of shorts and seven shirts might be the sole allotment of clothing for several hundred patients. The few doctors available were besieged by paperwork, unable to spend more than half their time in direct patient care. Patient contact for the most part was provided instead by attendants on the lowest rung of the staff ladder, workers drawn from a pool of uneducated transients. Known as "bug-housers," such staff drifted from hospital to hospital, moving on when-ever their alcoholism, idleness, or brutality became too blatant to ignore or hide. Training of the attendants might consist solely of a demonstration of how to sign out a set of keys. Readers encountered frank portrayals of rape, sodomy, and even death at the hands of sadistic attendants and incompetent doctors, whose prescriptions for nightly sedatives occasion-ally proved fatal. Attendants offered no excuses; doctors salved their con-sciences with the grim sentiment that such patients were luckier than the survivors. Skilled editing had woven this collection of personal testi-monies into a tapestry of systematic dehumanization.[4]

The muckraking campaign intensified when Albert Deutsch published *The Shame of the States* the following year. Based on a year and a half of journalistic investigations and his photo essays in *PM,* a left-leaning New York newspaper, the book took the reader on a detailed tour of state hospitals around the country, some remote, others well known. In addi-tion, Deutsch presented statistical data revealing serious defects in every aspect of the mental health care system. Recognized as an authority on the history of the mental hospital, he helped to awaken public as well as professional awareness of the enormity of the problem.[5]

Were state hospitals, for the typical patient, really a bottomless "snake-pit"? Historian Gerald Grob points out that sensationalist accounts of institutional life, which have appeared at almost predictable intervals over the past century, often mistake occasional brutalities and excesses as being representative of the everyday quality of life. Rather, conditions varied greatly between hospitals, and even within a particular hospital or ward.[6] The asylum was a fragmented environment composed of many sub-worlds, whose features hinged upon such localized variables as proximity to a workable bathroom or the kindness of the individual attendant or head nurse. Generalizations must be applied with caution.

A broad survey of the institutions' annual reports from this period does indicate, though, that the mental health care system was in serious trouble. As a rule, these publications combined statistical tables of patients admitted and discharged, with an inventory of repairs and improvements needed in the upcoming fiscal year, one part testimony of services rendered balanced against pleas to the legislature for further appropriations. In these pages, the superintendents expounded upon the erosion in physical plant and the decline in the purchasing power caused by inflation. They offered running commentaries on the pressing need for new sinks, toilets, sewers, shingles, and kitchen facilities, and on the rising prices of pork, coal, and muslin. Morale of the hospital corps, too, they reported, was ever plummeting. As these reports were written by superintendents and their medical directors as proof of taxpayer monies being well spent, it is safe to assume that actual conditions were in fact worse than reported. Read together, such materials present a medley of lament, the keening of large bureaucracies overwhelmed by rapidly deteriorating circumstances. The nation's entire system of mental health care was in dramatic decline, unable to cope with existing responsibilities at a time when demand for its services was rapidly increasing.[7]

The primary concern was overcrowding. It was not uncommon for a hospital whose maximum capacity was set at twenty-three hundred patients to hold as many as thirty-two hundred. At one Ohio institution, for example, a ward whose capacity was rated at twenty-five beds was filled with over a hundred cots placed side by side. To get to one of the ward's three toilets, even the elderly patients had to climb over one another.[8] Lack of personnel was another perennial complaint. Contemporary surveys indicated that in over one-third of the state hospitals, the ratio of patients to physicians exceeded 250 to 1. Superintendents admitted that institutions offered prospective employees a long work week, an emotionally taxing job, low pay, little recreation, and substandard housing. Turnover was appallingly high. During the 1948 fiscal year at Pennsylvania's Norristown State Hospital, for example, six hundred staff members were appointed but three hundred and fifty resigned, and almost two hundred were fired. It was not uncommon for states to resort to commandeering attendants from local jail cells. Chronic shortfalls in operating expenses also placed mental institutions in perpetual crisis. Unlike other state agencies, which could defer acquisitions until better years, state departments of mental hygiene could not put off purchasing food, fuel, and clothing for the patients. In 1947, the West Virginia hospital system was unable to afford the small luxury of publishing annual reports in which to complain about its lack of money.[9]

It was the common feeling among superintendents that hospital conditions were "at a low ebb." One director stated that his physicians were working "beyond the limits of their physical endurance." The 1948 annual report of Topeka State Hospital in Kansas incorporated distressing observations of one state inspector. As the official walked from ward to ward, eyeing in disbelief straitjackets, patients bound to bedposts, and overcrowded wards in buildings long since condemned, he commented upon the "air of utter hopelessness." "You know it is probably sinful and contrary to your knowledge of medical science," he concluded, "but you find yourself thinking that most of these people would be better off dead." The prevailing mood of the profession was perhaps best encapsulated in an aside by a psychiatrist that appeared in the *Psychiatric Quarterly*, a professional journal devoted to the concerns of state hospital physicians. Hospitalization, the physician noted, was "identical with doom."[10]

## A Formula for Disaster

In little over a century, what had begun as a series of small asylums averaging no more than several hundred in residence had, by the middle of the twentieth century, expanded into a sprawling network of large and often immense institutions, some containing as many as ten thousand patients.[11] Patient populations had risen at an alarming pace, even when the figures were corrected for rate of population growth. Nationally, the total daily census of the state hospitals increased from 159,000 in 1909 to 480,000 in 1940, a figure roughly equal to the number of beds in all nonpsychiatric hospitals combined. The hospital population's rate of growth had been almost twice that in the general population (see Figure 4.3).[12]

The fate of the state mental hospitals was governed by a three-legged mathematical relation: the number of patients admitted, the speed with which they were discharged, and the availability of beds to house them. All three variables were changing for the worse. First, a dramatic rise occurred in both the number and the rate of admissions. In New York, for example, new admissions rose from fifty-six hundred persons in 1920 to thirteen thousand in 1940, which amounted to an increase from 65 to 101 admissions per hundred thousand population. Psychiatric leaders, hoping

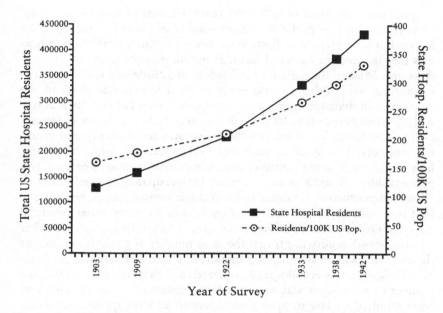

Figure 4.3. U.S. state hospital population, 1903–1942. (Source: Chart prepared from data published by the United States Bureau of the Census, 1904–1946)

to forestall fatalistic perceptions that the precipitous increases were due to an epidemic of mental illness, ascribed the higher institutionalization rate to such factors as a greater public acceptance of hospitalization, decreasing size of family housing, and the longer-lived population that placed more persons at risk for senility and cerebral arteriosclerosis. In addition, the Great Depression had exacerbated tensions of living and strained families' abilities to nurse troubled members.[13]

Second, retention rates stayed high. With discharges lagging ever further behind admissions, contemporary observers decried the lack of therapeutic progress that exacerbated the developing crisis. In New York, for example, the rate of recoveries per hundred admissions declined from 22.5 in 1910 to 19.0 in 1940. Especially distressing was the rapid drop-off in the recovery pattern of mental patients. A growing weight of evidence indicated that of the patients who were institutionalized for longer than two years all but a few would remain in the hospital until death intervened.[14]

The true significance of such statistics has been hidden by the tendency of contemporary observers (as well as later commentators) to measure hospital usage in terms of either the yearly number of admissions or the bed census that reported the average number of patients residing in the institution on a given day. Both measures were static, time-blind indicators that ignored the essential fact that not all patients were equally burdensome. Most of the patients admitted spent as little as a few days in the institution, while others would never leave. It is better to think of the institution in dynamic terms, as a vessel into which patients flow at one end, then out at the other. Its beds, thus conceptualized, may be construed as kinds of turnstiles, some of which turn over more slowly and others more rapidly. This dynamic analysis reveals a fatalistic logic. No matter how swiftly most of the turnstiles spin, some small portion of patients will prove stubbornly resistant to treatment. The occupancy of a bed by one of these semipermanent residents leads to tragic consequences, however, in that it eliminates one of the turnstiles for use by many other potential patients. Over time, even a low retention rate will retire enough beds that an institution's ability to process the large number of patients pressing at the entrance will be significantly impaired. This tragic but seemingly inevitable sequence was colloquially referred to as "silting up." Limiting the number of admissions was not an option, however, for state institutions were required by law to open their doors to all who applied. Such dire circumstances were not lost on contemporary observers. In his presidential address to the APA in 1939, Richard Hutchings noted that "our institutions promise to become in time vast infirmaries with relatively small departments for younger patients and curable disorders."[15]

The last variable was the aggregate bed capacity of the state hospitals. Crisis would be avoided so long as the net resident population grew at a rate consistent with construction of new hospital facilities. For every turnstile immobilized by a chronically ill resident, a new one had to be installed. Unfortunately, hospital openings had peaked in the expansion of the 1880s and 1890s, with no upswing appearing again until the 1940s, too little and too late (see Figure 4.4). Similarly, the funds spent on hospital maintenance and expansion did not keep pace, a problem severely complicated by the Depression. Here, too, Hutchings expressed the foreboding felt by all in the profession. Inadequate expansion, he stated, has "given rise to apprehension for the future."[16]

Two damning aspects of social reality in the 1930s and 1940s had prevented hospital psychiatry from building the social consensus necessary for a forceful political lobby. First, because a fearsome social taboo still surrounded mental illness, the afflicted and their families were unlikely to

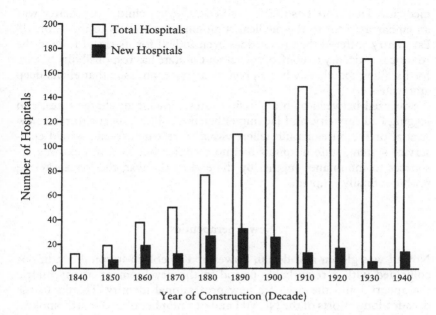

Figure 4.4. Construction of state hospitals in the United States, by decade. (Source: Chart prepared from data in J. K. Hall, ed., *One Hundred Years of American Psychiatry,* 1944)

take bold steps to gain recognition as a constituency, an exercise in self-identification. Even the location of the institutions, which typically were located in isolated areas, reflected the social ostracism of the mentally ill. Second, those who advocated any form of public support of health care typically were met with withering political hostility. Albert Deutsch, in his contribution to the APA's 1944 Centennial Meeting, described the peculiar abyss into which the psychiatric profession had fallen. He pointed to the telling yet rarely emphasized fact that one of the world's largest systems of publicly supported and managed health care had existed in the United States for over a century and was then expanding at a dramatic rate. It was called psychiatry. "It is insufficiently realized in the heat of partisan debate over state medicine," Deutsch argued, "that nearly one-half the hospitalized patients of all types in this country are already maintained under state care."[17] This was no debate over semantics but an issue that struck at the core of the profession's dilemma. Psychiatry was dependent precisely upon the state funding denied so vigorously to general medicine. Denigrated as the state's needy "foster-child," psychiatry was an embarrassment to the medical community as well as to the public.[18] Psychiatry suffered then (as it does even today) for its sin of forcing the American citizenry to confront whether the state has responsibility to care for its ailing members who happen to be poor, an issue that elicits deep ambivalence.

Squeezed between high admission rates, slowing discharge rates, and lagging bed capacity, and lacking either the political means to raise new capital or the bureaucratic wherewithal to restructure an ossified civil-service system, state hospitals had no recourse but to strain existing resources to inhumane lengths. By the end of the war, the long-festering problem finally erupted.

## New Therapeutics

Not all was gloom and doom, however. The ebb in hospital conditions coincided with a remarkable period in the development of psychiatric therapeutics and the rise of a new professional identity. Thanks to the decades-long efforts of the NCMH and of a number of psychiatric spokesmen, the public had become convinced that modern psychiatry offered a service that was of use to more than just the institutionalized insane. As described previously, Adolf Meyer had outlined an expansive vision for reconstituting the field, in which the modern psychiatrist focused instead on the problem of maladjustment – broadly defined – and its melioriation through psychotherapy and resocialization. Indeed, as he lived until well after the war, Meyer had the privilege of seeing his vision become reality (though only partially), as growing numbers of psychiatrists shifted their work to urban private-practice settings and took up residence in schools, factories, community clinics, and even policy circles.

As impressive as were the professional gains engendered by the new model of psychiatry, the historical base of the medical specialty was not as clearly transformed. Although the extramural basis of the profession was rapidly expanding due to the emerging psychodynamic framework, psychiatry was still mostly a matter of state hospital practice, an environment which virtually ruled out individualized treatment. Even avid supporters of psychoanalysis ruefully admitted that the method could not handle "mental patients in the mass."[19] Intensive psychotherapy of *any* kind was rarely an option, for the delivery of such labor-intensive services was far beyond the resources of the state hospitals. Moreover, the majority of mental hospital patients were severely psychotic, a condition that even Freud admitted was unsuitable for analysis. One of the lasting ironies of this period, as historian Gerald Grob has highlighted, was the fact that the much ballyhooed professional agenda of the NCMH had passed by the mental hospitals.

## Shock Therapies

The rise of the new model of psychiatry did not come without professional resistance, as debates erupted over the scientific validity of the various forms of psychotherapy, especially psychoanalysis. (The intraprofessional battles are discussed at length in Chapter 8.) However, to the majority of the psychiatric profession who still labored in the state hospitals such squabbling was irrelevant. Institutional physicians were not necessarily hostile to psychotherapy. In fact, many supported it as the psychiatric ideal – laudable, but as yet unattainable. As a matter of practical reality, these doctors looked instead to a series of therapeutic innovations that had developed alongside the psychodynamic movement.

The introduction in the late 1920s of Wagner von Juaregg's fever treatment for general paresis raised hopes that other physiologically oriented cures for psychiatric conditions were within reach. Beginning in the mid-1930s, wave after wave of somatic therapies were introduced into America, revolutionizing institutional practice. (As a rule, all of these began overseas.) The most important were the various forms of "shock" treatments that triggered convulsions and states of unconsciousness in the patient, either through injection of metrazol (a form of camphor), insulin-induced hypoglycemia, or direct applications of high voltages to the head. Until shock treatments, hospital psychiatrists had very little in the way of drugs or medical procedures by which to treat specifically the symptoms of mental illness. Asylum physicians, to be sure, always resorted to this or that potion to calm the "furors" of their clients or, alternatively, a tonic to stimulate them, if needed. In the second half of the nineteenth century, more potent drugs were developed, such as the various barbiturates and bromides, as well as the infamous chloral hydrate (knockout drops). Although useful in the management of difficult patients, such chemicals often proved dangerous to handle and actually did very little to change the underlying mental or emotional dynamics.[20]

With the arrival of the shock therapies, a profession that had been known for its therapeutic "nihilism" became giddily engaged in developing an extensive array of specialized treatments. In 1938, statistician Benjamin Malzberg reported encouraging evidence for the effectiveness of insulin therapy based on an analysis of a thousand patients treated with it in New York state hospitals. A national survey in 1942 revealed that between 1935 and 1941 seventy-five thousand patients in the United

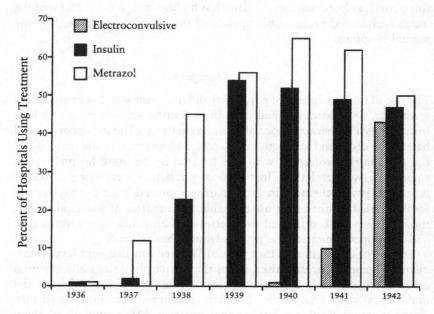

Figure 4.5. Shock therapy in American mental institutions, 1936–1942. (Source: Chart prepared from data in Lawrence Kolb and V. Vogel, "The Use of Shock Therapy in 305 Mental Hospitals," 1942)

States had received some form of shock, and that the new treatments were rapidly spreading throughout the institutional system (see Figure 4.5).[21]

The shock therapies were by no means ideal treatments, being often dangerous as well as difficult to administer. Insulin shock, for example, consisted of inducing hypoglycemic comas six days a week, up to ten weeks in a row. Patients were terrified by the daily entrance into states of near death, while the inherent risks of the procedure necessitated constant monitoring of the patients by trained nurses. Even large hospitals were rarely able to maintain more than fifty beds for insulin treatment. Metrazol offered the advantages of avoiding deep comas and greatly reduced cost, but its simulated epileptic seizures and spasms were so intense that fractures occurred routinely in the spine and other bones. Electroshock – the cheapest and simplest procedure – was also risky because of the number of bones fractured. Although greatly admired for their clinical effectiveness, the new therapies thus had their drawbacks. Shock therapy had "thrust its none-too-pretty form" into the psychiatric field, observed Har-

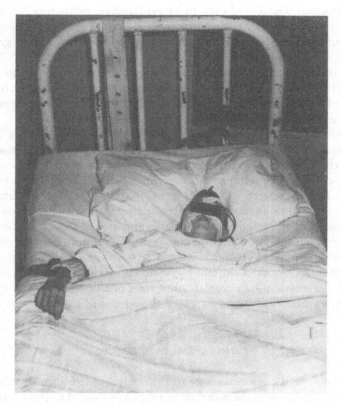

Figure 4.6. Patient receiving insulin shock. (Source: Archives of the American Psychiatric Association)

vard psychiatrist Harry Solomon. And whatever the method of producing shock, he added, the process itself was "distasteful."[22] Some physicians argued that the successes of the procedures were directly proportional to the fear induced; the mere threat of further treatments would quickly spur patients back onto the path of right living.

Nonetheless, institutional psychiatry was strongly affected by this revived "cult of curability." Special commissions, numerous journal articles, and state hospital annual reports indicated cure rates approaching a remarkable 85 percent, depending on type and duration of mental disorder. Public interest in psychiatry's new treatments was generated by featured stories in magazines and newspapers.[23] But even this newly formed positive image, hospital physicians were disappointed to discover, was double-edged. Pessimism withered only to be replaced by premature optimism. Families of patients, as well as patients themselves, began pressuring hospitals and state departments of mental hygiene to perform ever greater miracles, to use the new therapies even in inappropriate cases.[24] Social prestige thus rested, not upon the profession's ability to provide an absolute number of cures, but upon the ratio of its actual rate of success to that expected by the public. Ironically, the success of the new therapies engendered even further public dissatisfaction.

It would take a Dickens to describe adequately the contradictory world of the state mental hospital in the 1930s. The emergence of the wave of somatic therapies occurred at the very moment of the heightening crisis in hospital conditions, juxtaposing a curious blend of opposite circumstances. The expansive optimism generated by the new treatments' capacity to reclaim significant numbers of patients was tempered by a realization that whole groups of patients threatened to slip beyond the reaches of even the latest therapeutic advances. Brutal custodial neglect and deteriorated living conditions coexisted with the arrival of new medical treatments, creating a situation in which hospital psychiatrists looked to a new age of scientific psychiatry but were unable to finance or implement it fully. Such paradoxes hastened the advent of psychosurgery.

### Neurosurgeons by the Score

Within the overall clinical ecology of the mental institutions, psychosurgery's own particular niche was thus more or less limited to those patients who, because of unsuitable diagnosis, duration of institutionalization, or history of relapse, were believed unlikely to benefit from any other available treatment. Lobotomy rose to such prominence, nonetheless, precisely for the reason that over the years this residuum (which consisted mostly of chronic schizophrenics) had accumulated into something quite substantial. That psychosurgery was the first – and for a time the only – treatment believed even remotely effective in the management of chronic mental illness is a consideration whose effect on clinical decision making would be hard to overestimate.

Perhaps the strongest confirmation of this ecological influence is revealed by the specific pattern of the operation's use. Although the brain operation was initially targeted on cases of agitated depression and involutional melancholia, Strecker's report on its applicability to chronic schizophrenia led others immediately to follow suit (see Chapter 3). This clinical crossover, by the end of the war, was almost complete. Clearly, the vast expansion in the use of lobotomy was due to the penetration of the procedure into a huge area as yet unoccupied by competition from other viable therapies. That the original purpose was so quickly superseded in importance is especially remarkable, for even the most fervent promoters of lobotomy never back-pedaled from the supposition that its clinical effectiveness in schizophrenia was poor when compared to its results in cases of agitated depression, involutional melancholia, and certain kinds of obsessive-compulsions (a ranking that has remained unchallenged even through the later "waves" of psychosurgery in the 1960s and 1970s).

Although the expenditure of several hundred dollars on a single medical procedure was a considerable outlay for the financially strapped hospitals, the economics implied that the nation could not afford *not* to pursue vigorous programs of psychosurgery. Suddenly, a lot appeared to be at stake. Policy analysts in this period stated that, as institutional psychiatric care was essentially a government-subsidized service, new treatments for chronic mental illness offered savings to society not only in "human misery" but also in public expenditure, in amounts that would "stagger the imagination." At the 1941 AMA roundtable forum, at which claims were first made for the broad applicability of the operations in the institutional context, M. A. Tarumianz of Delaware State put exact figures on the amount of public money involved. He calculated the effects of a full program of lobotomy within his own institution of 1,250 patients, where 180 suitable candidates could be found. Including the expenditure of $250 in surgical fees for each operation, over ten years the hospital would have saved more than $350,000. "These figures being for the small state of Delaware," he commented, "you can visualize what this could mean in larger states and in the country as a whole."[25]

Lobotomy thus appeared to be an attractive technological solution for a problem that was both an intractable clinical challenge and an immense social burden. In 1948, the New York Neurological Society heard a report on the latest in a series of new psychosurgery techniques. "At the current stage of psychiatric therapy," one discussant excitedly responded, the new form of lobotomy would prove to be "a boon to the large number of the chronic and serious mentally sick patients, that large group which have been neglected as described by Albert Deutsch in his recent book, *The Shame of the States*."[26]

## A Larger Agenda

Even its most optimistic supporters knew, however, that psychosurgery by itself was "not the answer."[27] The need to deploy effective treatments for the severest cases of chronic mental illness was extremely important, to be sure, from the perspective of both patients and hospital. But the severe challenges then confronting American psychiatry were broader and deeper than that posed by the existing backlog of intractable cases, notwithstanding that for those who worked on the wards such cases certainly were urgent and compelling. Rather, the critical problems were structural in nature. The current sad conditions were in fact surface phenomena, dramatic evidence that the massive, complex social constructions governing the system at its most basic levels had become outdated and unworkable. If substantial and lasting changes were to occur, it was clear to all observers, immediate attention had to be given to overhauling the mental hospital both in its image and its reality; to relegitimating the profession within the wider medical community; and to rebuilding the public's faith in mental health services. At every level, psychiatry required reconfiguration. Hospital administrators, lay reformers, and psychiatric leaders together fought for this activist agenda. The fate of the somatic therapies – and psychosurgery in particular – was caught up in these ongoing currents.

The first priority was a rebirth of the mental hospitals. In 1937, C. C. Burlingame, flamboyant director of the elite Institute of Living in Hartford, Connecticut, depicted psychiatry's hoped-for destiny. "I can envisage a time," he declared, "when we in the field of Psychiatry will entirely forsake our ancestry, forgetting that we had our beginnings in the poorhouse, the workhouse and the jail. . . . I can envisage a time when we will be doctors, think as doctors, and run our psychiatric institutions in much the same way and with much the same relationships as obtain in the best medical and surgical institutions. . . ."[28] In this speech, Burlingame was expressing the heartfelt beliefs of hospital administrators and psychiatrists nationwide that, under current circumstances, mental institutions were hospitals "in name only," and that psychiatry was considered a medical specialty more by historical association than by what its current practices suggested. Or, as one superintendent explained, so long as the people as a whole fail to recognize that "a mental hospital is not an institution for the poor, nor is it a welfare institution, but that it is a hospital," policy recommendations "will continue to be nothing more than futile gestures and serve no useful purpose."[29]

As revealed by their annual reports, state mental hospitals in the 1930s and 1940s appear indeed to have been custodial institutions whose primary concern was sheltering, housing, feeding, clothing, and maintaining the physical health of its residents rather than being "real treatment hospitals." Even a hospital considered progressive by contemporary standards in 1939 would spend, per capita, sixty-two dollars for food and nineteen on clothing, while medical and surgical supplies cost a little more than a dollar. Space devoted to psychiatric therapies in these reports was scant. Contributions appearing under the heading of "Medical Department" or "Psychiatric Treatment" might amount to a solitary paragraph in a thirty-page document. In the *Annual Reports* of the Connecticut State Hospital, for example, the installation of linoleum received more attention than the year's psychiatric program. Routine health care, such as tallies of dental work, was given more notice than psychiatric therapies. Such accounts indicate that little effort was made to distinguish psychiatric treatment from attempts simply to provide general medical care. The reports also disclose that state hospital physicians were compelled to devote a majority of their time to administrative and bureaucratic tasks, with few hours actually available for clinical contact with patients. Psychiatrists, obliged to supervise ward personnel, wasted as many as three to four hours filling out the forms necessary to hire a single attendant.[30]

If state mental institutions preserved the characteristics of poorhouses, contemporary psychiatrists noted, they also reflected their ties to the jail-house, as they were still suffused with a "penal atmosphere." In almost every phase of institutional life patients were governed by correctional procedures. For example, they were routinely transported to hospitals, not in ambulances, but handcuffed, in squad cars. And if immediate entrance to a local institution was delayed by overcrowding, such patients were placed in county jails until vacancies arose. The admission process itself resembled incarceration. Even in New York, considered a progressive state, three-fourths of the hospitalized patients underwent court commitment. Patients were arraigned before a judge, a procedure that "smack[ed] of criminal proceedings rather than medical treatment."[31]

As in prison environments, once individuals entered the state hospitals they were stripped of personal identity through the institution's harsh regimentation of clothing, feeding, bathing, and shaving. Privacy was nonexistent, every moment being supervised and dictated according to explicit rules. Patients were subjected to the same erosion of citizenship rights as were criminals. Their mail was censored, their personal belongings vulnerable to random seizures, and their voting rights removed. Unsavory aspects of prison life also prevailed, including rape by inmates or attendants; maintenance of discipline through coercion, humiliation, and information obtained from "stoolies"; and thriving black markets. Even exiting the hospital occurred through penal rituals. Once or twice a year a patient was brought before an institution's "Parole Board," which decided whether to place the patient on "probation" or to allow release to the custody of a guardian.[32]

Weighed down by their negative legacy of custodial and disciplinary functions, state hospitals were further weakened by their conspicuous inability to resemble bona fide medical facilities. In 1944, the APA's Committee on Psychiatric Standards and Policies admitted that the psychiatric services in state hospitals had never matched the services of other branches of medicine found in general hospitals. "How then," the committee wondered, "do psychiatrists expect the medical profession as well as the public to recognize mental institutions as true hospitals?"[33] The disparity between psychiatry and the rest of medicine had widened by the 1940s as the standards of what constituted hospital medicine had appreciably risen in the public's estimation. Thanks to such celebrated advances as the new sulfa drugs and penicillin, and improvements in surgical technique and anesthesia, general hospitals in mid-twentieth-century America had become temples to the new scientific medicine, a far cry from their earlier image.

First, to those workers attempting to advance the cause of mental health care, the broadening gap between the idealized image of good medicine and the unpleasant realities of psychiatric practice was a cause of intense frustration. This predicament was depicted in a novel by Ellen Philtine, the pseudonymous author of *They Walk in Darkness* (1944), which was based on her real life experiences as the wife of a staff psychiatrist at Pilgrim State in New York. In the story, a forward-looking senior physician, Dr. Goldschmidt, exclaims to Peter Carson, an assistant psychiatrist:

> "Treatment!" ejaculated Goldschmidt. "Ach, you like to work and you are idealistic. You are green yet in such places. It is verboten to do anything for your patients here!" he shouted. "This is a hospital? Better call it a prison! You think you have come here to learn psychiatry? . . . This is work for doctors? . . . You worry, how will you make your attendants understand a medical viewpoint. Have they a vocation? You are right, they regard themselves as jailers! . . . Anybody cares here for patients?

Goldschmidt concludes his tirade, "There is no treatment here – there is only discipline!"[34]

Second, psychiatry's troubles extended beyond the present concerns of the state hospitals and touched every component of the mental health care profession. Addressing the centennial meeting of the APA in 1944, Alan Gregg declared contemporary psychiatry to be the "most isolated of medical specialties." He was attempting to spur the membership into action the way S. Weir Mitchell did in his famous address at the association's fiftieth anniversary.[35] Gregg outlined the manifold problems facing the profession in its research, education, lack of psychiatric facilities in general hospitals, and the distance between mental hospitals and the rest of the medical system. The audience was unlikely to take offense, for Gregg's address was merely the latest in a series of pleas for serious reform that had been broadcast by the profession's own leadership.

Support for psychiatric research was felt by psychiatrists to be unconscionably low in proportion to the prevalence of mental illness. In 1946, Senator Claude Pepper testified to Congress that the combined private and public expenditures on mental health research was less than twenty-five cents per case of mental illness in the United States, compared to a hundred dollars per case of polio. (In 1947, a total of less than three million dollars was spent on psychiatric research nationwide.) As the great majority of experimental investigations were supported solely by the limited discretionary funds of the state hospitals, it was clear that American psychiatry had failed to develop reliable sources of research support. Compounding these budgetary restraints, the historical prominence of the state hospital in American psychiatry was seen to cripple research in other ways. Only a small number of hospital psychiatrists had been adequately trained in scientific methods, and the few qualified personnel available were hamstrung by hospital job descriptions unsympathetic to the demands on time required by rigorous experimental work.[36] Moreover, the status of research as an activity worthy of public monies was never fully established; the eliteness of the task seemed far removed from the gritty world of the state hospital. Elgin State Hospital, for example, one of the few institutions with an endowment for maintaining a comprehensive research program, printed on the title page of its in-house publications the disclaimer, "NOT FROM TAX MONEY."[37]

Several states had attempted to develop programs of research in mental illness by establishing specialized facilities, originally called psychopathic institutes and later either psychiatric or neuropsychiatric institutes.[38] Typically located near prestigious medical schools, the institutes were small in size and amply staffed with comparatively well-educated researchers. Although started with high hopes in the first two decades of the century, their actual success was limited, as they were overwhelmed by the intractability of the psychiatric problem and slowly but surely co-opted by the demands of their service role. Instead they became diagnostic centers for the intake and distribution of patients into the rest of the mental health care system. The large numbers of patients to be examined and the rapid turnover prevented any realization of in-depth clinical studies.[39] Support for research in psychiatry – as was the case in many other areas of medicine and science – was left to the private philanthropies such as the Rockefeller and Commonwealth Foundations.

Medical education was another area of grave concern for the profession. Contemporaries complained that most medical schools gave psychiatric education short shrift, the few hours devoted to the study of mental disorders amounting to little more than textbook instruction, with little direct clinical contact. Equally worrisome, the numbers of students planning to enter the psychiatric profession were woefully inadequate to meet current needs – let alone the mushrooming demand. The training that young physicians did receive in the mental hospitals was described by the APA as "desultory." In his speech, Gregg stated that such a situation, in which future medical specialists entered a profession untrained, unsupervised, and assumed competent, was "unthinkable" in any other area of medicine. Such practices, he noted, would disgrace a surgical ward.[40]

To measure the degree of psychiatry's isolation from general medicine, an observer would have to look no further than to the nearest general hospital. As late as 1940, only a minor fraction of the nation's 4,300 general hospitals contained psychiatric wards. A large percentage would not admit psychiatric patients for any medical complaint – including emergency health care.[41] It was unlikely that many medical students would have acquired much experience with psychiatric patients during their hospital residencies. Mainstream medical practice was, in effect, virtually insulated from contact with patients exhibiting recognized mental disturbances.

Lastly, reformers knew that their campaign was not simply a matter of infusing sufficient funds into the state hospitals or of incorporating the mental health care system into the existing medical infrastructure. The existing practical limitations of modern psychiatry were familiar enough, but the *perceptions* of its inherent limitations were held to be just as damaging. The battle for psychiatry's future thus was also fought on a spiritual front, one that consisted of the public as well as professional attitudes toward psychiatry. Psychiatry's new age would happen only if people believed in it enough. The task was clearly an uphill push, for popular opinion still regarded most of psychiatry as somehow unlike "real" medicine.

One set of negative evaluations centered around the current practices and institutional realities. In the words of Alfred Bay, a mental health official in Illinois, the public believed that mental patients were simply "put away" until they "snapped out of it." Another set of perceptual barriers were linked to the public's understanding as to what constituted mental pathology. An official bulletin of the American Hospital Association, for example, stated that the treatment of mental illness could not advance until such time as "old ideas of 'insanity' were dissipated by the demonstration that its patients can be studied as objectively, efficiently and scientifically as those in any other branch of medicine." Psychiatry would have to connote, in every aspect visible to the public, the image of a genuine medical enterprise. Some even argued that progress in revising the public's attitude about psychiatry would have a direct impact on clinical efficacy. As stated in the *Mental Hygiene News,* "the attitude of acceptance" of mental illness as a disease like any other, and of psychiatry as part of the medical system, had in itself "a great therapeutic value."[42]

## Strategies of Reform

The tide eroding mental health care in America was plainly visible to working professionals and external observers alike. How to reverse this process was not as clear-cut. Various and at times conflicting strategies were pursued by a diverse set of interest groups. As described earlier, for example, the Rockefeller Foundation invested heavily in a scenario where the future of psychiatry was to be located in university programs of research and training, such as Harvard's Department of Nervous and Mental Diseases as led by Stanley Cobb. Other philanthropies, such as the Commonwealth and Russell Sage Foundations, placed more stock on shifting the service role of the psychiatrist away from a base in the mental hospital, with its traditional emphasis on severe mental diseases, to the community clinic (located in the school, factory, or urban center), which stressed instead the psychopathologies of everyday life. And, as also previously mentioned, some elite private institutions such as Strecker's Institute of the Pennsylvania Hospital sought to combine these two approaches.

These particular currents were largely peripheral to the problem at its core, however, for the bulk of the profession was still married to the state institutions and the psychoses that were unreachable through office- or clinic-based psychotherapy. In recognition of this hard reality, other leaders of American psychiatry mapped out a plan that pinned its future on reworking the mental health care system from the inside out. Rather than abandoning the mental hospitals, the aim here was to reinvigorate them as the basis of a newly medicalized psychiatry, one that might reclaim the confidence of both the larger medical community and the public.

Believing that the postwar period would be "one of the most crucial in our history," the APA Committee on Psychiatric Standards and Policies began work in 1944 on a series of proposals to guide the reconstruction of the profession. The natural focus of such efforts, they stressed, was the system of state mental hospitals, still "the very foundation of psychiatry."[43] If psychiatry were to achieve adequate recognition, institutional standards would have to be raised; it was from here that "all medical services emanate." Or, in the phrasing of later reports, "Mental hospitals should lead the way."[44] In essence, the committee was drafting the blueprints for the fulfillment of Burlingame's vision of American psychiatry, where a future psychiatrist could claim to be as "medical" as any other physician and the public would receive a level of service in mental institutions akin to what they might find in general hospitals.

In particular, the committee argued for a new integration of state mental hospitals with general hospitals and medical schools. This might involve appointing university faculty to the hospitals' rosters of visiting and consulting medical staff, establishing residencies and internships in nonpsychiatric specialties such as surgery, and working state hospitals into the clinical rotations of medical and nursing students. It was hoped that such measures might free the institutions' staffs from the labor of general medical tasks – work for which it was acknowledged they were poorly trained – thus allowing psychiatrists to concentrate upon purely psychiatric duties. In return, the mainstream medical world would gain access to a wide body of clinical material, but, more importantly, extramural physicians would become cognizant of the special problem of mental illness, and perhaps even bring a fresh interdisciplinary approach to its resolution. Other important measures advocated were the establishment of specific acute-care medical units in the mental hospitals, setting higher standards for psychiatric residencies, and promotion of research within each institution.[45]

The avalanche of negative publicity caused by Maisel's 1946 exposé redoubled the profession's reform efforts. APA President Samuel Hamilton, for example, sent a letter to alert each member of the association to the need for immediate action. In the face of the hardships imposed by war shortages, he wrote, hospital psychiatrists tended to absolve themselves of blame that might be sloughed off on the indifferent legislatures; others outside the APA reinforced this do-nothing attitude by fingering an apathetic public as the source of the hospitals' difficulties. "This will not do!" thundered Hamilton, as the time had come for the entire association itself to "present forcefully to the public and to their legislatures all the shortcomings and deficiencies in the hospitals and to demand the backing necessary." Hamilton included an addendum from the latest report of the Committee on Psychiatric Standards and Policies, which stated that as long as mental patients were treated in institutions funded at a daily rate between sixty-five cents and two dollars per capita, "the American public will not consider psychiatry as a legitimate scientific branch of medicine."[46] The committee also noted that if the public were educated to accept psychiatry on the same level as it had recognized other branches of medicine, it would be possible to raise the standards of mental hospitals to those of general hospitals "within the next ten to fifteen years."[47] Positive public perceptions were a cause – not just a consequence – of progress. It was the duty of psychiatrists to alter these perceptions.

Hamilton's call to arms was echoed by a composite army of lay advocates, organizational leaders, hospital psychiatrists, and state officials, who campaigned together to rescue psychiatry by reversing the decline in hospital conditions. An awkward dilemma arose. At the same time that the public was being asked to place greater confidence in mental hospitals, the same audience was to be shamed into underwriting a massive infusion of funds on the grounds that the state hospitals "were a shameful disgrace, unfit for human occupancy, that they all stank." An expedient solution was to emphasize the need to deliver more psychiatric treatments into the state hospitals, thus attributing current failure to a lack of adequate resources but at the same time establishing that better care was indeed within reach. As Alfred Bay later noted, it was precisely the lack of such "bottle goods" that had been responsible for the public's negative perception of psychiatry. The measure of the reform campaign's progress, it seemed, would be the hospitals' ability to distribute all currently available treatments to every patient who might benefit from them, as well as to encourage and provide for the aggressive development of additional therapeutic measures. The California Department of Mental Hygiene, for example, proclaimed that "we are coming closer and closer to the day when we can truthfully say that California's share of the 'shame of the states' has vanished," by "doing everything for the victim of mental ills that medical science can do."[48]

## Active Treatment

The primary goal of this broad-based campaign to reform the mental health care system was thus to transform the isolated state hospitals into truly modern hospitals, a process envisioned as the first step in remaking the entire profession. The key strategy in this campaign was to establish what were termed "active treatment centers" that might repudiate the custodial legacy. By "active," contemporaries were referring to those medical advances that dramatically improved patients for the better, providing visible proof of the power of scientific medicine to affect the individual organism. At the same, time, however, they were also consciously referring to the significant *indirect* benefits, the power that such public displays have to mobilize the social body. Medical advances, it was rediscovered, can be "active" politically as well as clinically.[49]

All of the somatic therapies were found by the profession to be especially "active" treatments, in both meanings of the term. The new treatments appeared as concrete examples of what a science-based, medical psychiatry could accomplish, and reinforced psychiatrists' claims to being providers of bona fide medical care. Hospital psychiatrists and administrators – at least those who considered themselves to be progressive – strove to introduce such therapies into the state hospitals both for their direct clinical effects and for their secondary benefits as rallying points that might convince the public to support necessary reforms. Apparently the lessons were cumulative. The new therapies were thus developed in successive waves, as facilities created for the application of insulin shock treatments were redeployed for metrazol and then electric shock. Lobotomy programs, which completed the new somatic armamentarium, rode the wave of interest in revitalizing hospital psychiatry through the implementation of "practical scientific progress."[50] As lobotomy was understood to project the most medical image of the somatic therapies, programs of psychosurgery, in turn, became especially valued showpieces by which state hospitals further sought to proselytize the new medical psychiatry – a rhetorical means of reversing the damage caused by longstanding "regressive" attitudes. An instructive example of this association is provided by the story of the development of psychosurgery within New York, a state that boasted the largest – and arguably the most influential – mental health care system in the nation.

## The Empire State

New York State's long history of support for progressive mental health care and research was often cited by reformers, such as Albert Deutsch, in their accounts of how forward-looking policy decisions could have far-reaching, positive consequences. Deutsch in his history *The Mentally Ill in America,* which was published in 1937 as a guidebook for reform, singled out New York's State Care Act of 1890 as having begun "a new epoch" in the care and treatment of the mentally ill. As he described it, this law shifted responsibility for care of the insane poor, who had been housed in county almshouses, entirely to the state mental institutions. These institutions were also provided capital for needed expansions and were upgraded in image by such tactics as replacing the term *asylum* by that of *hospital.* Deutsch credited New York's example as inspiring other states to pursue similarly enlightened legislation.

In 1895, the Empire State founded the Pathological Institute of the New York State Hospitals, the country's first organized psychiatric research center. Over the next three decades the center (eventually renamed the

New York State Psychiatric Institute) evolved into one of the world's largest and most eminent such institutes.[51] Perhaps owing to its generous support of the institutions and its aggressive efforts on behalf of mental health care, New York found itself with both the most mental patients in absolute numbers of any state and among the highest rates of admissions per 100,000 population. Between 1920 and 1947, the number of patients on the books in its state hospitals rose from 38,300 to 84,500. In 1947, New York State contained 9.9 percent of America's residents yet 17.7 percent of all state hospital inmates.[52]

By the end of World War II, it was clear that the system's once proud reputation was severely tarnished. Energetic efforts were made to rebuild and reorganize the system through spending initiatives and reform legislation. Between 1943 and 1950, the New York State Department of Mental Hygiene (hereafter NYSDMH or Department) grew into the largest agency of the state, consuming one-third of New York's operating budget and employing an equal proportion of all state workers, reaching in excess of 24,000 employees. The total population in residence at the mental institutions in 1951 amounted to a staggering 104,800. The reform momentum gained crucial support from Governor Thomas Dewey's personal commitment.[53]

The first turning point was a 1944 report of the Commission to Investigate the Management and Affairs of the Department of Mental Hygiene, a panel established after an embarrassing outbreak of amoebic dysentery at Creedmoor State Hospital. Dewey charged the commission to recommend sweeping changes in the organization of the Department and called for a halt in the hospitals' deterioration, a reorientation of treatment, and a blueprint for future growth. After a detailed inspection tour of each facility, the commission concluded that the primary deficiency of the state's mental institutions was their status as "principally custodial institutions" rather than hospitals "in the true sense of the word." Progress in these institutions, they continued, simply had not kept up with the pace set by general hospitals; more emphasis had to be placed on psychiatric therapy.[54]

New York State officials wanted to recapture the Department's status as the premier mental health care system in the country. In this quest the delivery of adequate psychiatric treatment was given the highest priority. Hospitals were strongly encouraged to intensify their therapeutic efforts, a challenge that often extended beyond the issue of insufficient resources. The commission report noted that some institutions used the new shock therapies while others did not, and the variability correlated neither with the numbers of patients and personnel nor with financial means. Rather, some hospitals simply allowed "inertia" to set policy, in contrast to those "alert" institutions that seized the initiative by implementing the latest treatments.[55]

The early years of the development of the shock therapies in America demonstrated the readiness of institutions in several states, and in particular those in New York, to expand into new therapeutic ground. The use of insulin, metrazol, and electric shock in the United States was often pioneered in New York mental hospitals. For example, Manfred Sakel himself, the developer of insulin shock, was brought several times to the United States by the NYSDMH to supervise personally the use of the procedure. At Harlem Valley State Hospital, Sakel taught six-week clinics in 1936 and 1937 to representatives of hospitals statewide, and to others who traveled there from around the country. New York State also led the way in evaluating the new therapies through its unprecedented Temporary Commission to Evaluate Shock Therapy, which analyzed with some sophistication the results of studies at Brooklyn State Hospital.[56] The shock therapies thus rippled through the state hospital system, pushed onward by an emerging cadre of hospital administrators, psychiatrists, and NYSDMH officers who were committed to broadening the range and availability of psychiatric treatments. This vanguard at the same time was campaigning to overhaul the mental health care system, recasting it in the image of modern medicine. Psychosurgery, the latest development in the onrush of somatic therapies, was also swept up in the reform momentum. In the state that claimed the nation's largest, most progressive psychiatric program, psychosurgery became a featured part of reform activities.

### "Pilgrim's Progress"

The first psychosurgery operations in New York were performed on an outpatient basis or arranged by the family. The exact numbers are unknown, as few reports of these cases were ever published. Official use of psychosurgery in New York's state hospitals did not begin until after the war, when Pilgrim State Hospital initiated a pilot series in 1945. Binghamton and Brooklyn State Hospitals followed in 1946. At its peak in 1950, almost all of New York's twenty facilities were employing the procedure, with a total of more than eight hundred such operations performed that year alone.[57] The single largest program was at Pilgrim State Hospital, which operated on 350 patients in 1951 and over 1,300 in the span of five years.

The lobotomy trial at Pilgrim began in March of 1945, when a resident physician with neurosurgical training was sent to Washington to observe Freeman and Watts's technique and returned to perform four lobotomies.[58] The resident soon left the hospital, thereby terminating the first series. It was not long, however, before the hospital resumed the operations under the sustained interest of the hospital's director, Harry Worthing, clinical director, Henry Brill, and a local neurosurgeon, Henry Widgerson. During the late 1940s and early 1950s Pilgrim State had grown into the largest mental institution in the world. True to form, its venture into the use of lobotomy resulted in the most elaborate program in the nation.

When Pilgrim opened in 1932, one of the newest institutions in the state, it was envisioned as New York's flagship mental hospital. In the late 1920s, the NYSDMH had responded to an anticipated need for additional hospital beds to serve the New York metropolitan area by planning the construction of a mental health facility of unprecedented size. Given a choice between building two five-thousand-bed hospitals at a cost of fifteen million dollars each and the option of building one ten-thousand-bed hospital for twenty million dollars, the Department opted for economy. The result was a vast complex whose size and scope boggled the mind. The new hospital was placed on central Long Island farmland, sufficiently distant from Manhattan to provide cheap acreage but close enough to be accessible by the Long Island Railroad, to which the hospital would build its own spur. Over the course of two decades an entire city was built from scratch on two thousand acres of "dreary, burnt-over waste of stunted pine and oak." Pilgrim State Hospital grew to approximately one hundred buildings, connected by nine miles of underground tunnels. According to contemporary newspaper accounts, the contract was the largest single brickwork project of its day. Opening with two thousand patients in 1932, by 1950 Pilgrim housed more than eleven thousand patients and employed twenty-five hundred personnel, including forty-four physicians.[59]

The hospital was named for Charles Pilgrim, a retired state hospital superintendent who had been commemorated for his trenchant efforts to promote progressive psychiatry throughout the state hospital system. The symbolism was intentional. From its outset, the new hospital was committed to a policy of providing the latest in psychiatric treatment and set itself up as an exemplar of enlightened medical administration, a standard for other state mental hospitals to follow. The hospital staff was indeed quick to introduce every major therapeutic development, starting with malaria therapy in 1932, Pilgrim's first year of operation. In 1936, the hospital sent a doctor to study under Sakel at the Harlem Valley clinic; metrazol was introduced in 1938; and in 1940 Lothar Kalinowsky, the American pioneer of electroshock therapy, personally started the hospital's own such program. "Treatment continues to be stressed as the primary function of the hospital," the hospital's *Annual Report* proclaimed in 1944.[60]

Impressed by the results of the first lobotomy series, the hospital began a second series in March of 1947. Sixty-six operations were performed the first year. Initial results of the operations spoke for themselves: restraint, seclusion, and sedation had all become largely unnecessary. Expansion of the program was recommended. "We have found," investigators declared, "that chronic behavior disorders of very varied patterns have proved more amenable to prefrontal lobotomy than to any procedure hitherto known to us." The Board of Visitors concluded from its 1948 inspection that Pilgrim "has not only used the older and proven therapies but has been constantly on the alert to use the newer methods." By way of example, they cited the appointment of Henry Widgerson, a neurosurgeon, to the visiting staff and his commencement of a substantial lobotomy program. The Medical Services Department noted that its greatest expansion was in the surgical division; of 265 major operations performed that fiscal year, 205 were lobotomies. In just its second year, the lobotomy program was treating twice as many patients as was the insulin program. The Board of Visitors commented upon the impressive results of the hospital's psychosurgical efforts, stating that they followed its development "with interest."[61]

The next few years showed heightened interest and satisfaction. In 1950, the Board of Visitors noted "with pride" the "active treatment program" and with some self-satisfaction cited the results of the 350 lobotomy cases that had recently been published in the *Psychiatric Quarterly*. The program itself had expanded to nearly three hundred patients in a single year, with operations scheduled two days a week for a monthly total of between twenty-five and thirty lobotomies. The following year, the board stated that "the hospital looks with favor on the use of prefrontal lobotomy" – a thousand patients were already under study. Widgerson appeared on the staff roster as "Lobotomy-Neurosurgery." Pilgrim's prefrontal lobotomy program had become its clinical showpiece.[62]

When exploring each of the new physical therapies, the staff at Pilgrim refrained from experimenting with physiological manipulations, such as dosage strengths, new chemical means of terminating comas, or special combinations of therapies. Rather, their attention was focused on the special problems of deploying medical innovations within an institutional context, with particular emphasis placed on economies of scale and organization. For example, in a standard shock-therapy unit, patients would have to be transported to and from various hospital wards for treatment and subsequently returned, a serious strain on hospital personnel. In addition, this movement severed clinical contact between patients and their supervising physicians. Pilgrim advanced the principle of establishing an independent psychiatric treatment unit that retained patients for the duration of the shock-therapy process, a period of possibly several months, lasting even through resocialization and retraining. Such a unit was established in the medical-surgical building that also doubled as the admitting center, where new patients were held for observation, given a course of treatment, and if necessary eventually parceled out to the back wards. Over time, the treatment center became the clinical focus of the hospital. Pilgrim had thus set up a context for the aggressive treatment of recently admitted patients. If one therapy proved unsuccessful, it was soon followed up by the next treatment in an attempt to keep the patients from entering or returning to the back wards.[63]

Pilgrim's efforts in psychosurgery were a natural extension of the existing shock-therapy program and indeed in some ways its fulfillment. The clinical director of the institution noted that "The experience and organization developed in connection with these methods [shock therapies] were now ready for trial of any new technic which seemed to offer hope to the residuum of cases which had been resistant to known modalities. . . . It was at this point that psychosurgery began to receive extensive trial."[64] The lobotomy program was established in Building 28, the same facility set aside for the development of the shock therapies. As the psychosurgery program enlarged, it drew increasingly upon the special orientation and advantages of the shock unit. To monitor the patients' critical first postoperative week, the lobotomy unit made use of this building's centralized nursing and medical care. Pilgrim's psychiatrists had published an extensive account of how centralized, efficient organization was a key component of a shock-therapy unit's success; the lessons were transferred to its administration of the brain operations.[65]

As the number of successful cases mounted, the hospital reapplied its earlier strategy of institutional rehabilitation that had proven so effective with the shock therapies. Lobotomized patients were not returned to their original wards but remained in specially graded resocialization wards (in Building 28) until such time as they were sufficiently improved to enter less restricted wards or, if recovery went even better, into convalescent care. If the latter event occurred, patients were incorporated into the hospital's after-care clinic, located in the facilities of the New York State Psychiatric Institute on 168th Street in Manhattan. At the clinic, two days a week were reserved for electroshock and lobotomy patients.[66]

In short, Pilgrim's lobotomy program was a direct expression of the hospital's explicit mission to explore the possibilities of the latest psychiatric treatments in a large hospital setting.[67] Psychosurgery had become a visible part of the hospital's active treatment program and a symbol of its commitment to further psychiatric progress.

## New York's Ray of Light

Pilgrim's favorable experience with psychosurgery was not unlike that of other state hospitals in New York. Of eighteen hospitals and two research institutes in the state, the annual reports of sixteen cited some use of psychosurgery, with only one institution reporting unsatisfactory results.[68] The rest described positive results similar to those cited by Pilgrim. Superintendents declared that their psychosurgical programs yielded "highly gratifying results," and that the procedure had become an "integral" part of hospital treatment programs.[69] Henry Snow, Binghamton State Hospital's clinical director, published the accomplishments of the hospital's initial lobotomy trial. "It is remarkable," he enthused, "that out of a group of 27 deteriorated, destructive and assaultive patients operated upon, patients for whom everyone had lost hope, we should find eight now at home and the ninth on her way home." Such results, he added, were "beyond anyone's expectations." Binghamtom went so far as to boast, in 1950, that six players on its successful patient softball team had had lobotomies. The director declared that the institution would employ the procedure so long as the results continued to justify its use; the program in fact was to continue longer than a decade. Some hospitals were able to build upon their existing shock-therapy facilities and personnel to provide the necessary components for an on-site lobotomy capability. Others, such as Middletown, Harlem Valley, and St. Lawrence State Hospitals, transported their psychosurgery candidates to nearby hospitals that did offer lobotomy. Alternatively, patients were temporarily released into the custody of their families, who then brought the patients to general hospitals for the operation.[70]

Although within the New York hospitals the lobotomy programs varied greatly in size, organization, and duration, these institutions shared a common set of expectations as to what psychosurgery might accomplish both clinically and politically. Psychosurgery was incorporated into their treatment programs at the precise moment when the NYSDMH was stressing the importance of increased therapeutic efforts. For example, in 1945 and 1946, Binghamtom State Hospital's Board of Visitors praised the institution for its accomplishment of raising the level of treatment activity and keeping current with modern, scientific treatment methods. A few years later, when the Board of Visitors summarized the gains made by the hospital, it complimented the institution and medical staff for their "active therapeutic program," singling out for commendation the consulting neurosurgeon who performed the lobotomies. And Binghamton's achievement in inaugurating the state's first continuing program of psychosurgery was broadcast in *Mental Hygiene News,* the official organ of the NYSDMH. (In addition, a picture of a lobotomy being performed at Binghamton was included in the 1947 *Annual Report* of the NYSDMH, in its section on therapeutic advances.) Boards of Visitors at several other institutions likewise praised their own psychosurgery programs as proof that "modern treatment techniques" were being implemented. At Brooklyn State Hospital, the psychosurgery program was insuring that its "active and vigorous treatment schedule" would reach "a larger number of patients than ever before."[71]

Psychosurgery programs were also cited by the New York hospitals for their important role in the campaign to bring modern medicine into the state institutions, in that they bolstered connections to university medical schools, enhanced resident training programs, and introduced modern neurosurgery into the institutions.[72] Given special regard was the importance of lobotomy for stimulating efforts in psychiatric research, models of what science might accomplish within the special circumstances of the state hospital context. For example, the *Annual Reports* of Rochester State Hospital reveal that a five-year follow-up study of its lobotomy patients was the most technical research ever accomplished at the hospital. The hospital proudly noted that a color film made of psychosurgery operations and subsequent patient rehabilitation won the Biological Photographic Assocation medal for medical photography. Lobotomy investigations at Pilgrim and Binghamton also resulted in these institutions' most ambitious research endeavors and noted publications.[73]

Indeed, not only did New York state boast the largest psychosurgery program, it could also lay claim to having established an experimental investigation of unprecedented scope, more complex than any other project ever before attempted in American psychiatry. Scores of investigators from Columbia University, the Neurological Institute, the New York State Psychiatric Institute, and other disparate institutions, representing a diverse assortment of fields, joined together in a sophisticated psychosurgery study that was the single most ambitious project of the day in terms of scientific protocols, depth of patient evaluation, and funds committed. Known first as the Columbia-Greystone Project, then as the New York State Brain Research Project, its cost was underwritten in three successive special appropriations of the state legislature that totaled approximately

$250,000 – at the time an extraordinary research expenditure. Governor Dewey himself appears to have been the catalyst for the development of the larger Brain Research Project.

This celebrated investigation gave high visibility to New York State as a leading site for medical research in psychiatry. In an editorial in the *Psychiatric Quarterly,* Newton Bigelow, the State's Commissioner of Mental Hygiene, went so far as to describe this project as one of the most promising psychiatric investigations then under way.[74] New York's importance as a center of research in psychosurgery – and by extension all psychiatry – was further enhanced when the fledgling National Institute of Mental Health sponsored three annual conferences on psychosurgery, the era's only significant, in-depth national discussion of a psychiatric therapy. The conferences were held in New York City, under the auspices of the directors of the Columbia-Greystone experiments. The editor of the First Psychosurgery Conference was none other than Commissioner Bigelow.

Through psychosurgery, the state hospitals in New York were proving that they were exactly the kind of "alert" institutions the NYSDMH was trying to foster, that is, "in the vanguard of progress."[75] Governor Dewey claimed in 1949 that, within two years, New York State would be doing more for mental hygiene than the rest of the country combined and would boast the finest psychiatric system in the world. "We needed desperately the vision," he stated, "to start curing instead of just caring for the patients." By way of illustration, Dewey then cited the results from a lobotomy program in a single New York state hospital, where 164 procedures had been performed in the previous two years. Twenty-seven percent of these patients, the governor noted, had made a good adjustment at home.[76]

When the two years had passed, Dewey delivered a retrospective on the rehabilitation of the NYSDMH that had occurred since he had initiated his commitment to its reform:

> After nearly 10 years of persistent effort our work in the field of mental hygiene is beginning to take on the pattern long developed in the field of public health. In spite of difficulties in getting people to the difficult, often discouraging, work in our mental hospitals, in spite of doubled costs and seemingly everlasting shortages of building materials, custodial institutions are becoming hospitals, and research is destroying the former complacent assumption that thousands of our people must irrevocably be committed to end their lives in institutions. . . . Within the last nine years shock therapy, group therapy, occupational therapy and psychosurgery have taken a major place in the programs of our state institutions. In the last year alone 800 brain operations were performed on severely disturbed patients. Marked

improvement has been shown in many cases previously thought
hopeless.[77]

True, the numbers of patients undergoing lobotomy appeared small in
comparison to procedures as widespread as electroshock, which might
have been used on upwards of 20 percent or more of the total hospital
population. Nevertheless, the implementation of the lobotomy programs
held great symbolic power. Here was tangible proof that the Department
was at last on the path to enlightened mental health care, a route pioneered by the NYSDMH for other states to emulate.

The decades preceding the introduction of the somatic therapies had been
characterized as a period steeped in "darkness." By the early 1950s, however, a new optimism was emerging. In 1950, the editor of the *Mental
Hygiene News* wrote a short piece in the twentieth anniversary edition of
the publication in which she reflected upon the accomplishments of both
the Department and all of psychiatry. The editorial, titled "Two Shining
Decades," described how it had been "the brightest era in psychiatric
therapy"; for in this period psychiatry had come into its own as a medical
specialty: the new treatments – psychosurgery included – illustrated the
newly found clinical efficacy. Similar articles on clinical progress in the
state never failed to include psychosurgery as evidence of the new "light"
that had been shed. (About this time, the *Mental Hygiene News* adopted
as its masthead a dramatic picture of a darkened landscape pierced by the
light of Liberty's torch.) The magazine also published an article on the
history of the Department, with a section on gains in medical treatment
due to recent scientific progress; the only photograph accompanying this
section depicted a lobotomy operation.[78]

The connection between the reform efforts and psychosurgery was not
lost on contemporary observers. In 1948, the *New York Times* responded
to popular concern about conditions in the mental health care system by
conducting its own investigation. The *Times* concluded, in a display of
cautious optimism, that New York's institutions were slowly shifting their
emphasis from "mere custodial care" to treatment and research, though
due to bureaucratic inertia many hospitals were slow to increase the levels
of therapy. Brooklyn State Hospital, it was discovered, shone in contrast
to these other laggards. Its director, Clarence Bellinger, was quoted as
explaining that "we are a hospital, not an asylum." In confirmation, the
*Times*'s own inspection reported that "Brooklyn is a treatment institution," for "in the medical-surgical unit, two or three lobotomies are performed weekly. . ." (Deutsch himself had lauded Brooklyn State, which
previously had pioneered the use of insulin in the state hospital context,

for putting in place the nation's most active shock-therapy program.) When a psychiatric journal published a biographical note on its clinical director, Christopher Terrence, it first described his contribution to this innovation and then noted the "active part" played by him in the application of lobotomy, personally assisting at more than three hundred such operations.[79] The implication was one of a continued commitment to progress.

Also in 1948, a representative from the famous York Retreat in England visited Pilgrim State for the purpose of awarding the hospital its prestigious Tuke Medal, heaping praise on Worthing for his success as a psychiatric administrator. The representative stated that had he not seen the evidence with his own eyes, he would not have believed that a large institution could be so excellent. The award was cited in *Mental Hygiene News* in a notice of recent events at Pilgrim, a column that also mentioned the return of the hospital's clinical director from a trip to Washington, D.C., where he was instructed in the latest method of lobotomy. In the eyes of contemporaries, these surely were not unrelated events. A few years later, the Association for the Improvement of Mental Hospitals, Inc. – a mental health lobby – bestowed its Adolf Meyer Award upon Harry Worthing, Superintendent of Pilgrim State Hospital. The award, presented at a radio broadcast ceremony attended by mental health care officials, read: for his "Successful Inauguration of Enlightened Psycho-Surgical Treatment and Rehabilitation Programs for Patients Formerly Considered Incurable."[80]

## A Measure of Progress

Not just in New York but in states throughout the country, psychosurgery programs arose out of efforts by departments of mental hygiene and individual hospitals to infuse medical standards and practices into otherwise custodial environments, a campaign that had begun with the introduction of the shock therapies in the late 1930s. The experience and resources that were garnered from the introduction of insulin, metrazol, and electric-shock treatments – for example, how to establish acute-care facilities, train nurses and doctors to work together in intensive patient therapy, and raise funds for special medical efforts – were in turn applied to the development of lobotomy programs. The practice of psychosurgery thus captured some of the momentum that had advanced the rapid development of the shock treatments. In November 1948, radio commentator Carl Downing devoted a show to the introduction of lobotomy into his home state of Washington. His invited guests included Don Sergeant, supervisor of the mental institutions. "Can you tell us, Don," he asked, "how psychosurgery is affecting the mission of our state hospitals?" Thanks to the brain operations (and other physical treatments), Sergeant declared, "our hospitals are now centers of treatment rather than custodial institutions."[81]

In line with the pattern seen in the example of New York, those institutions and personnel that had played significant roles in introducing the various shock therapies – often with the additional purpose of establishing a "real treatment hospital" – were usually the same ones that brought into existence programs of psychosurgery. For example, Longview State Hospital in Ohio, one of the few institutions in the 1930s that supported a more than token research enterprise, would later boast that it was the first state facility to use electroshock; psychosurgery here was begun as early as 1942. In California, the first state hospital to employ lobotomy was at Stockton, the same institution that initiated the state's first use of insulin shock. The first state hospital to employ psychosurgery on a mass scale was State Hospital #4 in Farmington, Missouri. Its superintendent, Emmett Hochter, was something of a local hero for his progressive psychiatric reforms. And so on. To contemporaries, the moral was clear: progress begat further progress.[82]

Perhaps the best example of this link between hospital reform and the development of psychosurgery was that provided by the efforts of Mesrup Tarumianz, director of the Delaware State Hospital. As noted previously, in 1938 Tarumianz orchestrated the first formal uses of psychosurgery on state hospital patients in America. At the time, he was praised in the *American Journal of Psychiatry* as the visionary leader of an institution "dedicated to the principles of medical treatment of the mentally ill"; the hospital itself was rated as one of the best financed and supported institutions in the country, testimony to what an enlightened legislature might accomplish. Two psychiatric observers from the prestigious Pennsylvania Hospital went so far as to comment that, as Delaware State "has taken the lead among state hospitals" in adopting lobotomy, they were very proud "to feel, as it were, that we are in the same community with th[is] progressive hospital." Tarumianz's influence in the profession would continue to grow; in the mid-1940s, as chairman of the APA Committee on Psychiatric Standards and Policies, he drafted the association's policies for hospital reform.[83]

Nationwide, psychosurgery programs thus came to be regarded as another "measure of progress" for hospital psychiatry, indicators that pointed out which hospitals were trying to "keep up with the modern trend in the care of patients." At the simplest level of explanation, when state hospitals each year dutifully reported the numbers of lobotomies performed on their patients, they were merely following the bureaucratic mania for counting that had carried over from the nineteenth century, in which large numbers were thought to reflect a high level of governmental service. In Buffalo State Hospital's *Annual Report,* for example, the Occupational Therapy Department reported that the patients had made 2,604 scratchpads and rebound 341 books in the previous fiscal year, in the same way that the electricians stated they filled 1,840 repair orders and fixed 1,660 pieces of furniture. For these purposes, the specific types of therapy were less relevant than were the total number of treatments. They served as a gross record of the hospital's psychiatric activity, just as the number of hot meals delivered was a sign of its humane care and the number of cavities filled an indication of competent health care. At one hospital, for example, applications of the various treatments were listed as if part of an accounting tally, so many wet packs wrapped and electroshocks given, and then all of the treatments lumped into a single grand total. Although this chart was absurd from a clinical standpoint, it made good sense at another level, registering the point that the hospital delivered a respectable level of publicly paid-for services.[84]

The somatic therapies fit well into this tradition. Easily enumerated medical events, the new treatments provided an opportunity for hospitals to provide quantitative, documentable proof of the delivery of psychiatric services. Indeed, during the war and into the immediate postwar years – the period of the severest strain on hospital life – hospitals proudly pointed to their tables of psychiatric treatments delivered as testimony that, in spite of the prevailing difficulties, the institution's treatment program was if anything *expanding.* The superintendent of one state hospital, for example, after discussing at length the many problems bedeviling his institution, supplemented his commentary with the bright note that the figures on clinical services "definitely indicate that there has been no tendency to neglect the important psychiatric procedures . . . insulin, electric shock, electronarcosis and lobotomies." Here was a ready index by which the institutions could be compared against one another and rated as to the vigor with which they were pursuing the new psychiatry.[85]

Psychosurgery programs nationwide were also instrumental in the wider efforts to reduce the gap that separated the state hospitals from mainstream medicine. In 1950, an influential survey of the conditions of the nation's mental health care system was sponsored by the Council of State Government. The council report stressed the importance of research projects to the mission of the state hospital. Psychiatric investigations, declared the council, "break the isolation of the hospital" by "forging a bridge" between the mental hospital and the university medical center. This was especially true of psychosurgery projects, of which most were cooperative endeavors, establishing significant ties between state hospitals and local neurosurgeons, psychologists, general hospitals, university medical schools, and research institutes. In the survey, several states singled out their lobotomy programs as proof of the progress achieved in remedicalizing their mental health care systems.[86] The council also credited research programs with indirectly raising the quality of patient care through attracting better doctors, as these projects were one of the signs by which a "young alert physician contemplating training in psychiatry identifies the hospital in which he would like to serve his residency." The most prevalent such sign of a progressive hospital was, in fact, lobotomy. The council's survey of current research identified almost two hundred ongoing investigations in state hospitals; forty-nine (25 percent) were psychosurgery studies – more than any other category of research.[87]

As cited earlier, Pilgrim State Hospital in 1944 declared that "treatment continues to be stressed as the primary function of the hospital."[88] Today, this plank of progressive medicine is so commonplace as to be hardly worth noticing. But in the 1940s the importance of becoming a "real treatment hospital" was the critical issue upon which the profession was staking its future.

## New Attitudes

Psychosurgery was also useful to the psychiatrists who were waging an ideological campaign to convince the public, the general medical community, and themselves that psychiatry indeed had medical treatments, deployable in medical settings, that functioned according to medically understandable precepts. As Karl Bowman noted in his 1946 presidential address to the APA, the vital problem confronting the profession was how to dispel the long-standing negative connotations attached to psychiatry and the treatment of mental illness. In particular, Bowman insisted that "Mental illness is a form of disease. Psychiatry is a branch of medicine. We must keep this relationship constantly before the public."[89] The point was just as important to establish with the health care professions as it was with the general public.

The development of the shock therapies gave reformers the exact ammunition they needed to thwart what were termed "regressive" attitudes toward psychiatry. In the words of New York State's *Mental Hygiene News*:

> The physical therapies have emphasized the essential unity of mind and body. The fact that mental illnesses are in a degree amenable to procedures easily comprehended by all as "treatment" goes far to establish the attitude that these are really illnesses like all others, and not incomprehensible reactions which split the victim away from

the rest of mankind and from ordinary concepts of sickness and treatment.[90]

Moreover, as a consequence of shock-therapy programs, mental hospitals found themselves actively incorporating medical practices. Due to their involvement with the new somatic treatments, for example, psychiatric nurses felt buoyed by a chance to act for once as "real" nurses. Pilgrim State Hospital explained that, as a result of its shock-therapy unit, relations between the mental hospital and the medical public had improved, for in contrast to the previous "hospital regimes" the new procedures were "comprehensible on medical grounds." An article in *The New England Journal of Medicine* declared that the shock treatments would "bring the field of psychiatry a little closer to that of general medicine."[91]

The psychosurgery programs were easily incorporated into this campaign. The director and clinical director of New Jersey State Hospital at Trenton, for example, explained how the lobotomy program they had instituted at the hospital would "mark another step" in the long road toward demonstrating that mental illness was in the same category as medical and surgical conditions, and toward convincing the public "to regard mental patients as individuals suffering from treatable disorders, rather than as candidates for custodial care." The Council of State Government's 1950 report noted that the new brain operations, along with the rest of the recently introduced somatic therapies, had already increased psychiatry's status as a medical specialty.[92]

Indeed, for those involved in institutional work the preparation for a lobotomy operation was clearly the single most medical event in the hospital's repertoire. Patient records and published reports reveal that workups for an inmate undergoing psychosurgery were quite elaborate, running the gamut from blood tests to urinalyses, metabolic recordings, and EEGs, not to mention a battery of psychological tests, if available. Rarely, however, did such data ever bear any relation to the operation itself or to the path of postoperative treatment. Rather, the hospital was orchestrating an extensive show of medical care in which lobotomy patients played featured roles in the institution's central drama. (The effect that such displays alone had on clinical outcome was well appreciated – so much so that the early reports of the operation's success were often derided as being not physiological in origin but psychological.) Its dramatic impact on the entire institutional staff, in important ways, was equally intense. In addition, such displays were deliberately used to strengthen professional relations within the general medical community. For example, at the Second Mental Hospitals Institute, the director of a state hospital in Iowa described an occasion on which, in the interests of fostering ties between hospital psychiatry and general medicine, he had invited the local medical society into his institution to witness a psychosurgery demonstration.[93]

The surgical imagery of the brain operations had a powerful effect on perceptions of mental illness. Scores of feature articles in magazines and newspapers across the country tracked each psychosurgical development; writers seemed fascinated by the apparent simplicity with which a surgeon could "cut out" the "worry center" of the mentally ill. An editorial in the *New York Times*, for example, stated that "surgeons now think no more of operations on the brain than they do of removing an appendix," as "it is just a big organ . . . no more sacred than the liver."[94] Modern psychiatry, it seemed, had advanced at last to the point where the treatment of mental illness was now as mundane as when surgeons repair other malfunctioning body parts. The demonstrated success of lobotomy also was seen as effective in undermining the dualistic model of mind and body, the widespread belief that mental functions could not be understood in physiological terms – a philosophy that many professionals thought was a hindrance to further progress. When a new lobotomy procedure was presented before the New York Academy of Medicine in 1949, one discussant noted that the paper's most noteworthy contribution was that the researchers were looking for something of "material" importance and had attributed mental illness to a brain disturbance. Another participant commented that the mind had, in the past, been treated too much by "verbalism" as if it were an isolated entity – a thinly disguised attack on systems of psychotherapeutics. Yet another was enthralled by how the project demonstrated that "personality itself can be influenced by attack upon precise areas wherein lie the organic pathology of man's behavior and conduct."[95]

Not a small portion of psychosurgery's effectiveness in proselytizing for a newly medicalized psychiatry derived from its much publicized pedigree as a product of laboratory science. More so than any other psychiatric therapy then available, the other somatic treatments included, lobotomy was heralded as proof positive of what rational scientific investigation might accomplish. The origin of the brain operations, after all, was conspicuously laid at the doorstep of John Fulton's Yale laboratory, an establishment with an impeccable scientific reputation. And almost daily, it seemed, scientists were reporting advances in neurophysiology that elucidated the brain's centers of emotion. In contrast, even the strongest supporters of the various shock therapies freely admitted their "empirical" (i.e., haphazard) derivations and lamented the continuing lack of physiological understanding as to their modes of cure. The culminating moment of psychosurgery's appeal as an emblem of scientific psychiatry arrived in 1949, of course, when Egas Moniz was awarded the Nobel Prize.

## Psychosurgery and the Management of Despair

One of the most important (if intangible) benefits of the psychosurgery programs was their ability to inspire hope at the very moment when the profession was at an ebb in morale. The problem, as Deutsch described in 1944, was that "the relatively low recovery rate in mental disease, together with a combination of many other factors, has tended to build up an atmosphere of defeatism in many state hospitals." As a result, the "better doctors, intensely interested in active treatment and clinical research, often leave state hospital posts for more hopeful fields of work." Worse yet, Deutsch argued, psychiatry would not move forward as a medical specialty unless talented and dedicated medical students could be convinced to enter the field – hardly a likely event unless the profession could offer the possibility of rewarding medical work.[96] In effect, the precipitous decline in psychiatry's image had developed a momentum of its own, which led only to further professional deterioration. Psychosurgery, in particular, was looked to as a resource for breaking the vicious cycle.

Although the shock therapies helped promote new optimism in psychiatry, they did have distinct limits. Worthing, for example, stated what most experienced users of the new therapies knew all too well: in no instance should shocks be employed on patients who had been hospitalized for more than a year. "Failure to observe this rule," he remarked, would result "in fruitless work which only serves to reactivate the therapeutic nihilism which is even yet a silent partner in a our state hospital practice." Bernard Moore, a psychiatrist at Yale and director of the Connecticut Lobotomy Study, remarked that, despite intensive efforts, the state hospitals contained large numbers of patients under restraint in locked wards. To the psychiatrist, Moore added, "their presence is a frustrating reminder of his relative therapeutic impotence." Worthing, on another occasion, reflected that "only one who has lived in close contact with the regressed and disturbed wards can appreciate . . . the vague sense of blame that is involved in therapeutic failure."[97] Mental hospitals stood as painful testimony to the helplessness of psychiatrists.

Psychosurgery, in providing a timely attack on the final barrier dividing curable from incurable, sparked new optimism within the profession. Harry Solomon, director of the Boston Psychopathic Hospital, credited the procedure with having improved the overall attitude toward the chronic psychotic; in his opinion, psychosurgery brought about no less than a worldwide "awakening of hope for the recoverability of patients ill for many years." In the combination of shock therapy and psychosurgery, others underscored, the profession had discovered "a magnificent stimulus to psychiatric treatment and research."[98] Hospital psychiatrists and administrators echoed that psychosurgery led to noticeable gains in hospital morale beyond what even the most energetic shock programs could accomplish. Programs of psychosurgery allowed institutional physicians to bask in the all too rare experience of watching their clinical handiwork have some visible impact in an otherwise unrewarding area. The 1948 *Annual Report* of Middletown State Hospital in Connecticut began with the familiar litany of depressing hospital conditions, but some rays of optimism provided counterpoint. "There have been brighter sides to the picture during the biennium" and of these, the hospital staff declared, "most notable has been the introduction of the operational procedures known as prefrontal lobotomy."[99]

With the growing proof of the efficacy of the new armamentarium, reformers considered public apathy toward psychiatry no longer excusable, for where "there is help, there is hope."[100] Presented as a complete system of treatment, the new somatic therapies reassured the public. Based on a logic of increments, in which each shock therapy, if unsuccessful, was followed by the next therapy or combination of therapies, the system constituted a formidable attack.

For example, it was the experience of some hospital psychiatrists that through electroshock therapy 40 percent of a group of recent admissions might be restored; unsuccessful cases were then treated with a program of insulin shock therapy, reclaiming another 40 percent of the remainder, or an additional 24 percent of the original total; and lastly, metrazol might be deployed, or some combination of all three, returning another group of patients to their homes. With such a progression of treatments, up to 70 percent or so of newly arrived patients could be successfully treated, it was asserted. Psychosurgery completed the system, offering a final intervention for the residuum of patients who were still resistant to treatment. For at least 72 percent of such patients, advocates claimed, brain operations could at least "do something." Harry Solomon argued that if a progressive hospital incorporated lobotomy into its treatment program, 95 percent of those admitted could eventually return home.[101]

The hope and reassurance generated by the new system of therapy should not be undervalued, for these emotions were vital to the maintenance of the social relations that existed between psychiatric professionals and the public. Mental disorders were and remain terrifying, baffling events for the families of those afflicted as well as for the patients themselves, the suffering further compounded by the amalgam of shame and guilt caused by stigmatization. More than those of most other medical specialties, psychiatry's disease entities are unpredictable as to course and duration, vague in nosology, and mysterious in etiology. Relatives were crushed in spirit as they watched their loved ones temporarily improve only to slip back once again into the depths of mental disorder. When families reached the limit of their tolerance and financial resources, their only recourse was to entrust the patients to the care of the state mental hospitals. Understandably, the families of mental patients looked to psychiatrists and their mental institutions to provide a structured, medical context in which the fate of their loved ones could finally be resolved.

Thus, the social function of the state hospital was the management of despair. It is no exaggeration to claim that one of the most important tools employed by psychiatrists in the fulfillment of their tasks was the inducement of hope in patients, families, and the wider community. In the world of mental health care, optimism was not merely a consequence of progress, it was integral to the forward movement. "Hope," declared the caption of a Pennsylvania Department of Mental Hygiene bulletin, was "a lodestar."[102] Psychiatrists discovered soon enough that the development of the new somatic treatments provided procedures and techniques which, in addition to their direct therapeutic value, reassured families that "something" and "everything" possible would be done for the patients. Due to a psychosurgery program at Greystone Park State Hospital in New Jersey, hospital administrators received "uniformly favorable" reactions from relatives who appreciated that "an effort was being made to do something for patients who otherwise, presumably, would have very little expectation of ever leaving the institution."[103] Another superintendent explained: "Emphasis is placed on treatment and remedial measures, and advantage is taken of all new therapies and discoveries. . . . Our favorable discharge and recovery rates are results of these efforts. With our first contact with the patient and the patient's family, attempts are made to direct a feeling toward hope of recovery."[104] As long as any sort of treatment was still possible, the family could cling to the slimmest of chances that the patient was not permanently lost.

Here, then, was the special message of psychosurgery as put forward by state hospitals: now there was no point at which the family would have to rule out hope. The Brooklyn State Hospital's *Annual Report* of 1951 revealed lobotomy's true role in the overall treatment program when the hospital staff boasted that it "always maintains a hopeful attitude so far as prognosis is concerned." Those cases "which do not respond to psychotherapy or shock therapy, and who remain here for more than three years," it elaborated, "are selected as suitable cases for surgical intervention." Although from a philosophical perspective the profession was often fragmented into warring therapeutic camps, within the workaday world of the state hospital all treatments were considered better than no treatment, and institutional psychiatrists thus tended to work toward the implementation of a unified therapeutic system. New York State's Department of Mental Hygiene took credit for an "increasing emphasis on treatment" by publicizing its "substantial advances in psychosurgery and group therapy" – a seemingly unlikely pair. Although he was an avid supporter of psychoanalysis, even Deutsch, in his description of an ideal state hospital treatment program, included psychosurgery as a desideratum. In sum, if psychotherapy was hailed by many psychiatrists as the "cornerstone" of the new age of modern psychiatry, psychosurgery served as its *capstone*.[105]

## Conclusion: Civilized and Humane Science

In the years immediately following World War II, psychosurgery achieved a coveted status as one of the core therapies in the arsenal of modern psychiatry. To contemporary observers, the dramatic rise in the use of lobotomy was no mystery – it was perceived as an answer to a series of grave, overlapping problems. Although psychiatry in America was expanding its base through the growth of office practices, employment in community clinics and industries, and university appointments, the bedrock of the profession remained the nation's vast system of state institutions that housed more patients than all nonpsychiatric hospitals combined. Within these mental hospitals the single most pressing problem was what to do with patients suffering from chronic psychosis, a condition for which no good treatment options were available, the new shock therapies included. At the same time, the institutions had been placed under tremendous pressure to find new ways to return these patients home. Commitment rates had recently soared even as budgets and infrastructure shrank; decades of neglect had rendered the system unable to handle the rising demand.

When Strecker and his associates announced that psychosurgery was useful for long-term schizophrenias, the procedure was eagerly seized upon as a partial solution to the present crisis. Although these types of patients were not thought to be the "best" candidates for the procedure – other diagnostic categories were considered by all involved to yield more favorable and reliable results – it apparently worked well enough. It can be

argued that, from an ecological perspective, the treatment rapidly penetrated into a niche of almost limitless size that as yet had no competitors.
Its viability was assured for the foreseeable future. Moreover, implicit in
the social contract that ensured the continued (albeit minimal) survival of
the state hospitals was the expectation that the psychiatric community
would exhaust all means possible to restore a mentally disturbed individual to society and family – never giving up hope, no matter how desperate
or dim the situation. Lobotomy's special value, as a treatment of last
resort in a realm where none before had been available, was its considerable extension of this contract.

Programs of lobotomy, it has been shown, also became swept up in a
broader reform movement in American psychiatry that sought to remake
the state mental hospitals into genuine medical facilities and thus secure
the viability of the profession as a whole. The first step in this campaign
was to demonstrate to the public, to the general medical community, and
to themselves, that psychiatry was just as "medical" as any other specialty,
able to cure specific illnesses with specific treatments; overturning the
long legacy of regressive attitudes and doubts would be a hard-fought
battle. Psychosurgery, arguably the most medical of the new psychiatric
treatments – it alone boasted a laboratory pedigree and involved high-tech
procedures such as neurosurgery – was thus discovered to have great
*symbolic* value in proselytizing for the new image of psychiatry, as well as
for convincing the public to reinvest in, not abandon, the nation's mental
hospitals, to do the right thing and wipe away the "shame of the states."

Appealing to both institutional needs and progressive ideals, psychosurgery thus gained considerable impetus from the state mental hospital's
unique, Janus-like historical position. In this period, state mental hospitals
still faced backward, using organizational structures, facilities, and attitudes that lay in their origins in the poorhouse, the prison, and the era of
administrative psychiatry. At the same time, however, they faced in an
opposite direction, looking yearningly toward the future, where psychiatric treatments might hold to laboratory standards. The combination of
historical circumstances that defined the procedure as an invaluable hospital therapy, both for its ability to better conditions within the institution
and for its lure as a progressive scientific enterprise, led to a paradoxical
utilization pattern. Hospitals in opposite situations, those which suffered
from the worst deterioration and stress and those which claimed to provide state-of-the-art treatment and research, found psychosurgery to be
equally compelling – though for different reasons. Ambitious programs of
lobotomy were thus created in remote Texas state hospitals as well as in
the nation's newly revamped system of Veterans Administration neuropsychiatric facilities, whose high staffing levels, revolutionary combina-

tion of teaching, research, and treatment, and placement within general hospital facilities embodied the dreams of state hospital reformers.[106]

In sum, the special appeal of psychosurgery arose from the particular circumstances of the day, in which the huge clinical problem it addressed represented at the same time an immense burden on society, a problem which the public had recently been sensitized about and had demanded action on. Because society as well as the profession looked especially favorably on those solutions which were associated with scientific medicine, the procedure gained an additional source of impetus. Contemporary psychiatrists were on the lookout for precisely the kinds of medical innovations that might be as useful in the political and social arena as they were in the clinical domain. In psychosurgery they discovered just such a combination, exactly the kind of "active treatment" that was needed.

At the time, although psychosurgery was by no means considered a perfect fulfillment of the new psychiatry, it nonetheless represented the attitudes and approaches that were held to constitute steps in the right direction. As Bigelow remarked in the *Psychiatric Quarterly* with respect to the Columbia-Greystone lobotomy research, here was "the most promising means presented in many years for casting light on many of psychiatry's dark places." Hospital psychiatrists might have harbored strong reservations – as many did – concerning lobotomy's clinical effects, but they approved wholeheartedly of what lobotomy programs did for the development of institutional psychiatry. "One may question whether shock treatments do any good to the patients," one psychiatric reformer stated in 1943, "but there can be no doubt that they have done an enormous amount of good to psychiatry." Such physicians felt assured that when patients in the future benefited from some substantially improved form of treatment, the patients would owe them thanks for doing what had to be done to guarantee that medical progress in psychiatry would continue to thrive. "Despite the justifiable protests against the empiricism, the brutality, and the hazards of the various drastic techniques," declared *Harper's Magazine,* the encouragement provided by even a handful of successes will "open the way to the expanded research that is so greatly needed, attracting both the gifted men and the necessary dollars to finance their studies."[107]

In 1948, the superintendent of Western State Hospital in Washington was so taken with the results of a recent trial of lobotomy at his own institution that he wrote to his counterpart at Oregon State to convince him to invest in a similar program. In closing the letter, Dr. Keller congratulated his correspondent for having at last obtained funding for several new buildings. "In this state mental hospital work," Keller noted, "it behooves us to march together along the most progressive lines." "Never has the public or the profession taken such great interest in psychiatry," Keller explained, ". . . and this is the great opportunity for mental health." Several months later, Keller's hospital was awarded a large grant for the construction of a research building. Credit for this turn of events was attributed to the lobotomy program. As one hospital psychiatrist explained in a private letter to Walter Freeman, "Dr. Keller was certainly aware of the value of having something active underway such as the trans-orbital [lobotomy] series" when the matter was under consideration in the legislature.[108]

Today, it is hard to imagine that lobotomies – or shock treatments, for that matter – could ever have been tethered to progressive platforms for social change. Contemporary psychiatrists and mental health care reformers faced no such contradictions, however. In the interests of presenting a coherent, clean line of attack, such advocates projected an oversimplistic yet politically effective conception of psychiatry, one constructed in black and white with few intervening shades of gray. In highlighting what had been achieved and what remained to be accomplished, the reformers placed treatment-oriented psychiatry in stark opposition to a past of purely custodial care in the hospitals. The representations found in the professional literature and the public exposés merged into a collective morality play, set in the state hospitals, where the forces of Past and Future were locked in mortal combat. In this polarized view, the emphasis on treatment programs, on transforming the mental institutions into "true" hospitals, took on a special significance. This was the critical arena in which the stranglehold of the past would finally be broken.

Hospital psychiatrists and lay advocates of mental health reform thus seemed to face a simple binary choice: there was old, bad psychiatry and there was new, good psychiatry. Each image included a constellation of intertwined, associated features. Old psychiatry was a mixture of custodial care, therapeutic nihilism, restraints and beatings, unscientific methodology, geographic and professional isolation, and dualistic conceptions that separated mind from body. In contrast, in the new psychiatry, mental institutions would be akin to general hospitals in levels of facilities, staffing, and partnership with medical schools; patients would be treated with respect and dignity; and the public would accept mental illness as exactly equivalent to any other physical ailment. To stand in favor of the new reforms was to assume a posture against the past punishment, stigmatization, and inhumane neglect of society's outcasts and to argue for their replacement by enlightened medical attitudes. Reformers such as Deutsch dedicated their efforts to the realization of "civilized, humane, and scientific treatment."[109] The components were not separable.

One might still reasonably wonder if, in the rush to implement programs of psychosurgery, the patients' well-being might have been subordinated to the interests of institutional expediency. For example, not the weakest reason Strecker's report achieved the response it did was its statement that lobotomized patients, even if not cured, make better hospital residents. Here too, however, contemporary psychiatrists saw no contradiction between progressive medical ideals and practical professional realities. In order to understand how they arrived at this conclusion, a closer examination must be made of the historical context in which the psychiatrists formed their therapeutic judgments.

# 5

## *Human Salvage*
### *Why Psychosurgery Worked in 1949*
### *(and Not Now)*

The Commonwealth can foot the bill
For the "poor-sad-folk" who are mentally ill.
Free eats for those who can't pay taxes;
The violent ward for indigestion.
                    Patient B.B., Ward A, Boston Psychopathic Hospital (1950)[1]

For American psychiatry in the 1940s, the only solution to the present crisis was to repudiate its past, to reach out to the promise offered by the scientific medicine of the future – a challenge that came at the precise moment when it was least possible to finance or implement this vision. Programs of lobotomy, as shown previously, were one of the favored strategies whereby state departments of mental hygiene demonstrated their commitment to the new medical ideal. For the procedure to develop beyond the initial few research institutes or flagship mental hospitals, however, and become a treatment that sustained interest throughout the mental health care system, it first would have to earn a reputation as a method of proven practical and not just symbolic value.

Showpieces are sold on the basis of their technical sizzle and dramatic appeal as illustrated by a handful of ideal-case scenarios. Administrators at a typical mental hospital were more concerned, though, with the less flashy matter of what a therapy might accomplish for the *average* patient it was used upon, and whether favorable results were possible for a large number of patients. Apparently, medical directors at well over half of the nation's state mental hospitals were sufficiently convinced, to the extent that they incorporated lobotomy into their own treatment programs in some manner. And within those facilities that did not offer the procedure, medical authorities explained this omission as due only to an immediate lack of financial, staffing, or institutional resources. Indeed, interest in the new therapy was no mere flash in the pan – lobotomy programs in a single hospital might last ten years or longer.

Judged solely on the basis of frequency of use, psychosurgery thus had passed through its experimental phase and out of the restrictive realm of clinical trials as well. Remarkably, a hospital's decision to opt for lobotomy was no longer considered remarkable. The cause of psychosurgery's success was obvious to contemporary psychiatrists. In the words of one, "the main reason for doing the operation is that it usually works; it brings results sufficiently successful to make it worthwhile."[2]

What was considered obvious in the 1940s and 1950s, though, may jar the sensibilities of more recent observers. Given what has later become known about the delicacies of brain function and the complexities of psychiatric illness, it strains credulity that such a crude procedure as the original lobotomies might truly have yielded therapeutic benefits for a great many patients. Here, one stumbles into the paradox that forms whenever a medical therapy widely favored by the profession at one point in time becomes mired in disrepute at another. A great disparity exists, to be sure, between the little that Walter Freeman and his followers knew in 1940 about the neurophysiological implications of an injury to the forebrain and all that is understood by current neurobiologists. One would be perverse, however, to declare that the underlying physiological reality had also changed in the interim. All other conditions being equal, a frontal-lobe cut observed today should yield results no different than those reported upon in the literature forty years ago. If it really cured then, it should still cure now. How is it possible that something that worked so well two generations ago no longer appears to?

Typically, such a paradox is disposed of by undermining the validity of the original clinical reports that had claimed success with the treatment. One or both of two strategies is usually employed in this effort. The first strategy identifies where such physicians badly erred in their practice of medicine. A doctor's responsibility as a clinician is to pick and choose from the universe of possible medical interventions the best match for a patient's particular illness and condition. Medical decision making of this kind, although based on difficult technical issues, appears nonetheless as a straightforward affair, a fundamentally rational process of first limiting the search to treatments of proven effectiveness for the clinical problem at hand, and then ranking them in reverse order of likelihood of severe side effects.

This deliberative process, it is believed, is at the core of what it means to be a physician. Thus, when the question arises as to whether a doctor (or group of doctors) acted appropriately in deciding to use a treatment like lobotomy, what is really demanded is a reconstruction of this clinical deliberation, a sort of medical audit in which we refigure the clinician's original tally of perceived benefits and deficits for the treatment in question, to find out where the calculation went askew. This recalculation is not expected to be especially arduous: in the present example, take the published record of the psychosurgeons' clinical deliberations and subject it to the acid test of today's knowledge of brain function.

Thus, our ability to sit here in historical judgment is predicated precisely on the assumed invariability of natural phenomena, a stability that defies time and place. In the early nineteenth century, physicians treated their syphilitic clients with large doses of mercury. Is this proof that in the prescientific era patients were subjected to torture for no good reason? Or the contrary, that the doctors of yesteryear had sufficient clinical skills to identify a potent means of cure? No problem. Conduct a series of controlled experiments to ascertain the true pharmacological properties of mercury in regard to syphilis. It either works or it doesn't.

In the case of lobotomy, a similar urge beckons us to peer into the past through the window offered by current laboratory medicine, whereby we will no doubt verify that, as such sweeping brain operations do not work today, consequently they never did. It would follow, then, that the psychosurgeons failed to exercise an appropriate level of medical prudence and were overcome by some combination of hastiness, self-delusion, and other defects of judgment. Consciously or unconsciously, they must have misrepresented the procedure's true clinical effectiveness and downplayed or overlooked its obvious hazards. The judgment of history seems inescapable: although the advocates of psychosurgery might not necessarily have been bad persons, perhaps even well-meaning in intention, nonetheless they were flawed physicians who victimized their clients.

The second line of argument stresses a different test of what constitutes good medicine, one that deemphasizes the issue of whether or not a treatment is clinically effective and focuses instead on the purposes of its use. In this view, that the operations were useful in some regard is stipulated without contention. If anything, the procedure is considered to have been *too* effective. The more important issue, it appears, is that a powerful technology was being applied to the wrong targets – and for the wrong reasons. This particular concern underlies what has been portrayed as perhaps the most frightening and damning aspect of the whole psychosurgery story. Lobotomies, it has been alleged, were performed upon patients not for a putative cure of some grave ailment but simply to render society's troublesome individuals more complacent and compliant. Medicine had found an all-too-easy way to reshape society's square pegs to fit into round holes; it was only a matter of time before a tool with such potential for abuse would be put into play by authoritarian and repressive forces. A distinction is thus drawn between those physicians who acted solely on the basis of their clients' true medical interests and those who capitulated to the dehumanizing pressures of bureaucratic and social expediency – or to simple greed.

Whereas the first approach leads critics to condemn the psychosurgeons as good men who made bad doctors, the latter one suggests that they were effective doctors but malevolent persons. Framed in this manner, a historical assessment of the psychosurgeons reverberates between the unsavory images of ineptitude and immorality. In either instance, the original success of the treatment as a bona fide medical therapy is forgotten. The story of psychosurgery, thus revised, no longer remains bound up in paradoxes but serves as yet another object lesson that truth can be denied for only so long. Ironically, this kind of moral has been kept in circulation by apologists as well as critics of psychiatry.[3]

But is it accurate? In those instances in which a controversial new treatment is deployed by only a small cadre of physicians with marginal reputations, such a judgment might seem warranted. However, when the example under study is distinguished by its widespread diffusion, this explanation engenders more problems than it solves. Such is the case with psychosurgery, the promoters of which represented a substantial and respected segment of the medical profession. Are we to believe that *all* of these physicians were incompetent or irresponsible, or worse?

The problem lies in the commonly held assumptions about what influences and structures medical decision making. One belief in particular, shared by professionals and the lay public alike, has significantly shaped the narrative of modern medicine and has led to the conundrums mentioned above. The medical evaluation of a therapy, it is assumed, concerns only such data as are derivable from laboratory printouts and objective clinical signs and that speak only to the physiological efficacy of the treatment under consideration; a reconstruction of how any one therapy was evaluated by physicians thus may proceed without reference to the immediate historical context in which they acted.

To the contrary, when physicians consider the appropriate therapeutic response to a case at hand they do not think merely of one treatment at a time but map out whole campaigns with fallback strategies already in place: they work within entire systems of care. Moreover, the process by which clinicians deliberate over the suitability of a particular medical treatment – what might be termed the "therapeutic calculus" – draws upon a wide range of variables, some of which are restricted to the confines of physiology and diagnostics, and others of which reflect wider realities. Every step along the way, including the original description of the presenting problem, the perceived urgency of medical intervention, the

structure of the treatment plan, and even the medical evaluation of success
or failure, are all informed by broad social, professional, and cultural
currents. Medicine is more than a matter of curing disease. Rather, its true
work lies in solving the *problems* that are thought to originate in disease.
This function is more wrapped up in human, time-dependent concerns
than is generally admitted.

If these lessons are applied to the example of psychosurgery, another
way will be found around the historical dilemmas. Such an approach will
help to clarify why some well-meaning and capable doctors in postwar
America could reasonably arrive at the conclusion that a lobotomy was
both beneficial and necessary. It will also account for why so many of
them did precisely that.

It is the contention here that the decision to use lobotomy had become a
natural – and in some ways inevitable – extension of the overall treatment
plan within which psychiatrists functioned in the 1940s. Psychosurgery
rose to prominence in this period because countless thousands of patients
fell into the category of "last resort," and at a point in time when such a
label indicated that desperate action was required. The historical challenge, then, is to explain both the expansion of this category and its
heightened fatalism.

One might wonder how a treatment with such grave drawbacks could
ever have been viewed as a useful therapy. Lobotomy, however, never was
advertised as a form of medical cure, but as a kind of partial *salvage,* an
attempt to make the best of a tragic set of conditions existing at a particular moment. When figured according to the day's concerns and measured
against the available therapeutic options, for many physicians psychosurgery did in fact appear to be both humane and medically prudent. It
made clinical sense – at the time.

And if there was a high road to lobotomy, there was a low road too: it
was not just the patients who were in desperate circumstances in the
1940s but the institutions as well. It is certainly true that psychosurgery
also worked from the standpoint of hospital administration, and that this
consideration alone factored heavily in the selection of many patients for
the operation. The question remains why the physicians at the time saw
no inherent conflict between their clinical perspective and that of the
institutions in which they served. Once again, the answer is to be found in
the historical context, in the continuing institutional legacy that dominated every aspect of mental health care. No contradiction was seen between them because psychiatry during this era was construed as the medical specialty formed at the junction of private and public health; a person's
restoration to productive citizenship was in fact the operational standard
of mental well-being. Ironically, the high estimation of psychosurgery was

the logical conclusion of the reform platform around which the new medical specialty of psychiatry was constructed in America in the decades between the world wars.

## Last Resort

The story of why physicians resorted to the use of psychosurgery cannot be told without reference to the then prevailing system of psychiatric therapy, to the overall treatment plan and the logic of its unfolding – clinical decision making is not reducible into a string of isolated events. To begin with, the attractiveness of a new therapy is dependent upon the known effectiveness of its competitors. One might say that the therapy which is selected is not the *right* treatment so much as it is the *best available* one. In the case of psychosurgery, if other treatments had been on hand that offered even a remote chance of success in cases of chronic mental illness, Moniz's article on lobotomy might have received an altogether different response. Clinicians looked eagerly to lobotomy precisely for the reason that this was the only treatment which offered, with at least partial substantiation, a regular hope of success in such cases. By simple reason of default it won a prominent place in the therapeutic armamentarium. Indeed, as many as twenty years would elapse before a competing treatment (namely, the major tranquilizers) was introduced.

Also, there is a subtle but powerful influence often at work within the overall system of therapeutics. Such was the case with American psychiatry in the 1940s when the general treatment plan was well understood and articulated, newly reshaped by the conspicuous success of the somatic therapies. In brief, if a patient did not respond to the lower levels of treatment, the next, more severe tools of the armamentarium were automatically applied. Psychiatrists began with those therapies considered least intrusive, such as hydrotherapy, physiotherapy, and light sedatives, or, if resources permitted, group or individual psychotherapy. These were followed in turn by the various shock therapies – electroshock, metrazol, and insulin – employed at first individually and then in combination.[4] Psychosurgery fit well within this schema and, in important ways, was its natural extension.

What matters here is the inexorable logic of a system that was built upon the slow ratcheting up of ever more powerful weaponry, a process that gained momentum as it proceeded forward. Those working within such a system did not even have to be conscious of its effects to be pulled along by the current. Once the precedent had been set, a "slippery slope" was constructed in which new patients started at the top and – unless they exited at an earlier stage – inevitably slid into candidacy for the institution's psychosurgery program. Just as a person reading in a room with afternoon light might later not realize that the sun has set, so the same gradualness of the treatment plan created a context in which an otherwise very dramatic decision, such as an order for a lobotomy, might be glossed over as a natural and nonextraordinary event. It may even be argued that once psychosurgery had developed a clinical reputation, the decision to operate was in large measure already preordained by the prior one to intervene medically.

The source of what influenced physicians to use psychosurgery on a widespread basis thus originated at a slightly earlier historical turning point, when the profession first adopted the regimen of the shock treatments and launched what even contemporaries referred to as the modern era of "heroic therapy." Indeed, it was the prior experience with insulin and metrazol shock that had eroded whatever psychological barriers remained against subjecting mental patients to drastic medical interventions. One observer remarked as early as 1938 that the medical community certainly was astonished when the brain operations were first announced. But, he noted, "we have become accustomed to such heroic methods." Who has not, he wondered, seen the exceedingly dangerous condition of patients undergoing metrazol and insulin therapy without being frightened? In just a few years, however, such procedures were accepted without misgivings. No doubt, he presciently implied, the same will soon be said of lobotomy.[5]

In raising the standards of what psychiatrists were expected to accomplish, the success of the shock therapies paved the way for the introduction of even more drastic treatments. With their failures that much less likely to be tolerated, psychiatrists were prodded into ever more aggressive modes of intervention. In an individual case in which all of the usual treatments had been exhausted, the psychiatrist's declaration that "nothing more could be done" was thought to crush any remaining hopes of the patient as well as his or her family – a development that in itself was expected to have grave consequences for the patient's future well-being. Psychiatrists thus faced an unforgiving choice: give up the treatment plan after so long a journey, or continue forward, however uncertainly. And, as mentioned previously, the psychiatric system as a whole contained something of an imperative to maintain the therapeutic momentum, to stay with a program of "active treatment." As psychosurgery represented the first real treatment for chronic mental illness, it provided the essential capstone to the treatment plan that was otherwise still missing. Now, no patient would ever be so sick as to escape the therapeutic reach of modern psychiatry. A large measure of lobotomy's success thus lay in its defense of the overall treatment record of the profession at a time when therapeutic failure was growing politically embarrassing. Like other such weapons of last resort, psychosurgery did not need to be deployed often to convey a message of reassurance; its mere presence in the background was sufficient to sway public sentiment.

But used it was in great numbers, a circumstance that still begs explanation. For so many individuals, why was it believed that nothing *less* severe than a lobotomy might work? Curiously enough, it was the recent success of the shock therapies that also stigmatized these patients as even more intractable than was previously thought; the issue here was not just the failure of the profession or of the procedure, but that of the patient as well. The newly discovered ability of modern medicine to send home a large number of recently admitted patients within an average time of six months had the unanticipated effect of drawing increased attention to those patients who remained uncured. A study at Pilgrim State Hospital, for example, examined the fate of a hundred successive patients who had not shown signs of recovery after a course of shock therapy. A year later, only eight of these were discharged; after four more years, this total had expanded to only thirteen.[6] Such lessons had important ramifications for how the profession regarded long-term mental illness.

The evaluation of a specific treatment occurs in the context of an interlocking web of clinical interpretations that exist at a particular moment. When the shock therapies were celebrated for their success, this was not an isolated event but necessarily reverberated throughout the psychiatric system. Raising optimism for one group of patients thus had the equal and opposite effect of lowering it for those who remained outside the treatment pool of eligible candidates. The situation of these chronic patients seemed more dire than ever before, inviting the further attention of medical science to find a cure for them too, a newly constituted problem in search of a scientific answer. In the 1930s, when a patient was diagnosed with severe schizophrenia, hospital authorities might shake their heads sadly and leave his or her fate to the natural course of the disease and the usual ward routines.[7] By the late 1940s, however, professional circumstances had produced a new kind of urgency.

In addition, there is a direct relationship between the perception of a particular therapy's efficacy and the perceived status of an individual patient's clinical condition. When a patient did not respond well to a treatment like insulin shock (which was assumed to work in a majority of cases) the lack of success was blamed, not upon the treatment's shortcomings, but was shifted back onto the patient. The patient's condition was thus reassessed as being more serious than previously believed. In this manner, patients became labeled in the literature and clinical records as "shock resistant," or even "shock-fast," now proven to be so gravely ill that nothing less severe than the next-higher assault therapy was indicated. The therapeutic armamentarium, once begun, became an internally propelled juggernaut, with each thrust forward self-justified by the results of the previous step.

It seems ironic, if not perplexing, that patients who received no treatment were somehow held to be clinically better off than those who were given the benefit of therapy but demonstrated little response. (In illustration, a patient hospitalized for only six months but who had failed a course of rigorous treatment might thus be perceived as more hopeless than a patient who had been hospitalized longer than two years with only custodial care.) The confusion stems from an assumption that, when physicians examine patients, the clinical assessment occurs in the decontextualized environment of a clinic or laboratory. All that matters, it is believed, is the bag of bones, nerves, and fluids present for the doctors' direct inspection. (Much of the image of the timeless nature of medical practice stems from this belief.) On the contrary, every patient is enshrouded by thick layers of personal history, much of which is directly relevant to the clinician's success in reaching a proper diagnosis, prognosis, and treatment plan. This is especially true in psychiatry, where the record of a patient's prior difficulties often constitutes the most important medical facts of the case. Some physicians – such as emergency-room triage teams, perhaps – confront a nameless and decontextualized body in their work. The large majority, however, must deal not just with organisms as they are when they walk in the door but with time-bound persons whose medical "careers" stretch well into the past and into the projected future as well.[8]

The usual response on the part of medicine to contain this messy historicity is to treat it like any other empirical problem. Thus, medical students are ingrained with rigorous methods of how to "take a history." The more rigorously such a task is performed, it is thought, the more physicians will base their judgments on hard facts. The reality is not so positive. Establishing the medical history is a notoriously tricky and uncertain art, to be sure, even when the patient is rational, articulate, willing to cooperate, and of the same ethnic or class background as the interviewer. Psychiatrists, worse yet, must rely mostly on the doubtful testimony of family members and friends (ruefully dubbed "informants"), who have their own willful or unconscious reasons for hiding or distorting the record of events.

The problem of identifying the true medical history of the patient goes even deeper than this, however, for the simple reason that doctors themselves distort the historical record they are trying to study so detachedly. In a phrase, there are no unspoiled or virgin patients in the modern world; there is no convenient way for physicians to step outside the historical process even for a momentary reflection on an individual case. As the case of the shock therapies exemplified so well, doctors do not simply establish a diagnosis and then choose a series of remedies, as if the two were somehow wholly distinct. A corollary to the classic adage that one cannot step in the same river twice is the proposition that once someone steps in a river he or she is no longer considered to be the same person. The simple fact is this: a patient who has received this or that treatment will no longer be regarded, clinically, in quite the same way as someone who has not. Every additional step along the way, each further contact with the medical system, has the subtle effect of reshaping interpretations as to what was the original presenting problem. A consequence of this dialectic is the situation that medicine, at some fundamental level, responds to conditions it itself has at least partly produced.

For many conditions, the perceived recoverability of an individual patient is thus not so much measured by the medical instruments as it is *created* by the accumulated history of prior clinical efforts. When contemporary psychiatrists explained that psychosurgery was only for cases of last resort – that is, for the "residue on the filter paper" – they unknowingly indicated this truth.[9] If mental hospitals were filled with what Walter Freeman described as "failures in life," a sort of undifferentiated sludge of humanity, then the new scientific psychiatry was believed to distill out any nuggets that still lay buried in the muck. The cast-aside byproduct of this distillation was necessarily even baser stuff. Already established as failures by society, and now proven by science to be unusually intractable cases, the patients who fell into the category of last resort were truly twice damned. It is for these reasons that psychosurgery appeared, in the 1940s, to be the last chance such patients had to leave the institution.

Although physicians might declare that a patient's condition was not expected to respond favorably to any of the usual modes of intervention, the decision to try a treatment of "last resort" in such cases was by no means automatic. There always remained the choice of simply not doing anything, letting nature take its course. Given the particular conditions of American psychiatry in the 1940s, however, the option of standing pat was considered a poor alternative. This urgency stemmed from the combination of two perceptions: the low chance of improvement should no further aggressive psychiatric treatment be attempted, and the assessment of the patients' quality of life given the reality of the existing hospital conditions.

Recent statistics had come to light that reinforced the professional wisdom that if any significant change were to occur spontaneously in a patient's condition it would happen in the first two years or so after onset. The Pilgrim study, for example, analyzed the typical fate of those admitted to a mental hospital. One thousand consecutive hospital discharges were tallied by year of patient admission. Over 90 percent of the discharged patients, it was determined, had been hospitalized for less than two years. Only eighty-six – less than 9 percent – had resided there for two years or longer. The situation was even more striking when discharges for the existing hospital population were tabulated. Although at least 45 percent of Pilgrim's residents had lived there for five years or longer, only a negligible fraction of this group – less than 1 percent – had been discharged during the sixteen months of the study. The implications of these and similar findings were clear: without some sort of dramatic intervention, the vast majority of chronically ill patients would be "doomed utterly to spend their lives in a mental hospital."[10]

Moreover, as mentioned in the previous chapter, getting patients out of the mental hospitals was an imperative in the 1940s. Epidemiological reports verified that mental hospitals were extremely unhealthy environments. Dysentery, tuberculosis, broken hips, pneumonia, and typhoid were common events. Each day spent in an institution exposed a patient to grave risks of increased morbidity and mortality. The prospect of permanently consigning a stricken individual to the confines of an asylum is hard enough, in any decade, even if the receiving facility were an exemplary model of benevolent care and lavish resources. Given the day's harshness of life within America's state hospital system, whose worst examples were soberly likened to concentration camps, such a prospect was to be avoided at all costs. Under such circumstances, a long life in an institution was not thought necessarily preferable to a short one.

Such was the situation when the cascade of reports on the use of lobotomy in the nation's state hospitals first appeared. Large-scale programs revealed that discharge rates hovered between 10 and 30 percent, even if the procedure was used on the most hopeless and intractable cases. It is understandable, then, that psychiatrists would see the treatment as a new means of deliverance, discovered none too soon. For Herman Snow, clinical director at Binghamton State Hospital, it was psychosurgery's net *humanitarian* benefits that swayed him, with its ability to save "a moderate percentage from the camisole, restraint sheet or seclusion room." J. L. Pool, a noted neurosurgeon and lobotomist, spoke for many of his colleagues in arguing that, when facing a choice between leaving a patient "behind bars in an institution" and performing an operation which might return the patient home, the decision was obvious, even when there was a risk of personality change.[11]

## A Salvage Operation

Lobotomy was rarely advertised as a procedure with only positive attributes, even by its most fervent supporters. "It seems quite certain," Freeman and Watts stated in the second edition of *Psychosurgery,* that someone seeking mental relief "has to pay a certain price." From the outset, observers scrutinized whether the price paid was worth it. "Is the surgeon justified," Stanley Cobb wondered aloud in 1940, "in depriving a patient of the most important part of his intellect in order to relieve him of emotional troubles?" "In each case we must ask ourselves the following question," stated a Yale psychiatrist during a 1948 radio interview, "whether it is justified to expose the patient to an operation which may remove some of his very human qualities in order to alleviate his symptoms of mental illness."[12] The decision to perform or not perform the operation was not an easy one.

The results of the operation were necessarily a mixed bag. On the plus side was the immediate and almost palpable reduction in torment exhibited by the patients, as described in earlier chapters. The touted ability of the procedure to save patients from the "misery of mental illness," an effect whose emotional draw should not be underestimated, appeared reason enough for many psychiatrists to order the operation. Other positive attributes, it was believed, included a reduction in obsessive behavior and excess emotional energy, a renewed interest in social activity and the environment, a receptivity to resocialization, and an indifference to pathological mental events that would otherwise paralyze the individual. Mortality rates generally ranged between 1 and 3 percent, a figure considered quite acceptable. On the minus side, however, it became generally recognized that psychosurgery patients were likely to suffer such ill-effects as loss of creativity, inability to react appropriately to environmental challenges, enuresis, torpidity, and epilepsy (scar tissue from the operation produced convulsions in as many as 10 percent or more of cases, a complication that did cause considerable concern). Even Freeman argued that in a patient given a standard lobotomy a naturally occurring disease had been replaced by an artificially induced one. He, and others following his lead, referred to this resultant state as the "lobotomy syndrome."[13]

The equivocal performance of lobotomy was further assured by the fact that the majority of the patients selected for the procedure during its heyday were not the "ideal" obsessive-compulsives or agitated depressives but the "low-grade" chronic schizophrenics languishing in the state hospitals. For most of them, whatever benefits followed the operation were less than what had been hoped. The important consideration here, however, is that, given the special circumstances of the day, the prospect of even slight gains was magnified in importance and likely to be viewed as an occasion for prompt action.

The therapeutic calculus is often erroneously thought of in terms of an absolute standard that measures a treatment's effectiveness in regard to a particular pathological condition. Rather, when physicians balance the positive against the negative, the process results in the *relative* judgment that the scales tip more toward the use of particular therapy as opposed to not. Such a process does not always indicate by how much one side of the ledger outweighs the other: the slimmest of margins may suffice. Indeed, the goal of lobotomy was not cure but *salvage*. It was to reclaim – if just partially – souls that otherwise would be forever consigned to the darkness of the nation's asylums. "The human salvage resulting from the operation," stated one New York hospital superintendent, "has been one of the most heartening developments of the last few years."[14] The economic metaphor is particularly apt, for the question of whether a salvage operation is worth the effort is conditional upon precisely these kinds of equations of marginal value, which in turn are dependent upon a range of shifting market conditions. There was no question that lobotomy patients were profoundly different in personality and behavior after their operation; whether this change was considered a net plus was contingent upon the special circumstances that existed in 1940s America.

To begin with, given the abysmal conditions of the state hospital, any treatment that offered any reasonable chance of exiting the institution with some semblance of humanity intact was considered of sufficient value to sway the therapeutic calculus on its use toward the "profit side of the ledger." As suggested above, the option of simply not doing anything had its own considerable dangers and unpleasantness. In the case of lobotomy, its potential downside was further mitigated by the certainty with which physicians held that the chronic patients would never change for the better without drastic intervention. Even critics of the operation, such as neurosurgeon Eric Oldberg, nevertheless agreed that it should be used for hopeless patients who "had nothing to lose."[15] At the time, to do nothing would merely allow a patient to drift toward an early death or to remain trapped in a nightmarish limbo of constant suffering. Under such circumstances, the scales were balanced in favor of the operation even before the weighing began.

From the perspective of the families, too, the overall risks often seemed preferable to simply watching their loved one continue on as before, a situation which often became unbearable. In 1940, Francis Grant vainly tried to stop a hemorrhage that occurred during an operation upon an elderly woman. She died shortly afterward. The husband's reaction, Grant found, only confirmed his original decision. "Although the outcome we had hoped for did not materialize," the husband began his poignant letter, "I realized the dangers attendant upon such an operation, and I am satisfied that you did all within your power in a difficult situation." "While no one could foretell the extent of the mental improvement had she lived," he continued, "I feel that it is providential that she should be taken as she was rather than, without the chance of an operation, that she should continue year after year to suffer that mental agony which for so long had been her lot."[16]

That the particular behavioral changes produced by lobotomy were interpreted as in themselves beneficial was also a matter of historical circumstance, the culmination of a century-long legacy in which insanity became defined in institutional terms. Physicians at Delaware State Hospital reported that, thanks to lobotomy, "many of these miserable, unhappy, restless individuals who paced the floor wringing their hands, moaning, groaning, sometimes yelling and screaming . . . were transformed into quiet, placid, uncomplaining persons who showed little concern about their troubles." From today's perspective, what is to be made of this particular trade-off? At one level, the immediate reduction in human suffering seems indeed a blessing, the kind of uncontested good that is associated with other great medical triumphs. At another level, though, one might cringe at the price paid by the individual patient – as well as at the sangfroid of the psychiatrists. Freeman, as usual, cut right to the heart of the matter in explaining how he weighed the scales. A lobotomy patient might suffer a reduction in "personal dignity," he stated, but this was more than balanced by a gain of sufficient "social adaptability" to reenter the work force. "Even if a patient is no longer able to paint pictures, write poetry, or compose music," Freeman bluntly noted, "he is, on the other hand, no longer ashamed to fetch and carry, to wait on table or make beds or empty cans."[17] Is this not prima facie proof that the patient's mental well-being was improperly gauged?

It would be wrong, though, to judge these sentiments from the standpoint of current sensibilities, even if the events in question were fairly recent. Participants saw the world in different ways, even then. Such evaluations of the brain operation were in fact consonant with the medical as well as the public understanding of what mental illness was all about. In the 1940s, a time when the great majority of patients were still declared legally insane prior to commitment, insanity was thought of in institutional terms; the majority of contact with psychiatrists still occurred within hospital settings. As far as the collective memory held, it had always been this way. Someone might be nervous, eccentric, or distracted, to be sure, but this was not the same as designating him or her *insane*. Insanity had acquired a special, additional connotation, reserved mostly for those citizens who were so severely disturbed as to require constant care. With the matter of sanity and asylum care thus intertwined over the course of the previous century, this particular social recourse had come to define the boundaries of mental health. Although psychiatric diagnosis appeared vague, confusing, and tentative, with the nosological labels changing faster than the subsequent generation of medical students could acquire them, the judicially rendered verdict of sane or insane remained a social fact of palpable constancy.

Furthermore, as much as medical personnel in the asylums grumbled about working in a domain in which their tools and even conceptual building blocks were so tightly controlled by extraprofessional factors, they too inevitably bowed to the situation. Confinement in a mental institution, a social fact, thus also became reified into a clinical fact, the defining moment in a mental patient's medical history. Admission to a mental hospital was taken as visible proof that a citizen had failed in life, lacking the strength of character or mind to continue as before. The converse held true. Living once again outside the institution was considered the best indication that a patient had "recovered" – though of course still tainted by stigma.[18] Few thought about serious mental illness in such terms as self-actualization, realization of human potential, inner harmony, and empowerment – all vocabulary and concerns of a later time.

Contemporary psychiatrists were not insensitive to the issue that something more was involved in the definition of mental illness than such simple operational definitions – they were certainly uneasy about equating discharge statistics with cure rates. But more sophisticated methods of clinical assessment did not yet exist, and the average clinician had little else to apply other than such summary judgments. One report on psychosurgery argued that the issue was easily resolved:

> If we are willing to carry out a therapy whose purpose is the practical one of returning the patient again to the community in a state of comfort and usefulness to himself and to others, then figures of successful releases are a useful measure. The patient, his family and the community are likely to consider such a release as a highly desirable achievement. At worst it permits the patient to spend a larger proportion of his life in remission and a smaller proportion in the hospital.[19]

Whatever psychosurgery did to the patients, it had changed them in such a way that, according to the standards of society and the medical profession, they were better off than if no such operation had been performed.

## Taxeaters into Taxpayers

The equation of insanity with institutionalization had always been a source of great ambivalence for the psychiatric community. In a sense, psychiatrists had become trapped by their own success, having built up their medical specialty on its location inside the asylums. In the late nineteenth century, the agenda was to reestablish the medical definition of mental health by transforming the image of the asylums into that of genuine hospitals. The concept of insanity, however, was not so easily reworked. The profession remained caught within a dual reality defined both by their roles as medical specialists and by their responsibilities as hospital administrators; the problem of mental illness remained wrapped up in institutional concerns as well as clinical reality. When a new treatment was introduced onto the wards, it was almost inevitable that the issue of clinical efficacy would be evaluated in hospital terms as well as medical ones.

Lobotomy programs were thought to be successful because they met both sets of standards. From the perspective of those concerned with workaday conditions in the state hospitals, psychosurgery appeared a godsend, an instrument whose considerable utility could not be ignored. State hospital psychiatrists and administrators saw a vital need to free up beds claimed by the chronic mentally ill, a population that required a disproportionate level of hospital services and prevented the institutions from treating newly hospitalized patients – individuals for whom modern psychiatric medicine had proved regularly successful. A multiplier effect was involved. In the span of a year, a single bed released might be used to treat several acutely ill patients, thus lowering the future number of patients developing chronic conditions. As described previously, the best way to assess mental hospital statistics is by a dynamic model, where each bed is viewed as a kind of turnstile. Some turnstiles rotated fast, others slowly, through which patients flowed in and out of the institution. The immediate problem was that too many of the turnstiles were stuck. Psychosurgery was the only tool found effective in reclaiming such turnstiles for their optimal use: curing patients who still were curable. Some lobotomists thus justified the operation on the utilitarian grounds that, even though they posed some risk to the individual patient, the programs were necessary from the standpoint of the greater good.[20]

In the years after the war, as both the number and size of the lobotomy programs were steadily growing, the results seemed to match or exceed expectations. For example, a Duke University team, operating on 284 patients drawn from Raleigh and Butler State Hospitals in North Carolina, reported a 14 percent discharge rate. The Connecticut Cooperative

Lobotomy Group proclaimed that as many as 36 percent of 294 patients went home. Physicians at Rochester State Hospital wrote: "all patients selected for this operation are long standing cases of schizophrenia and have shown no response to the usual modes of therapy – yet, over one-third have shown sufficient improvement to leave the hospital and adjust well enough to be cared for in the community." Similarly, at Marlboro State Hospital in New Jersey operations upon two hundred patients, of whom practically all had been confined to small seclusion rooms for up to twenty years, led to the hospital's release of twenty-six. In retrospect, physicians at St. Louis State Hospital in Missouri boasted in 1953 that – thanks to its lobotomy program – almost one hundred patients had been discharged.[21]

The fiscal implications were especially compelling. Tarumianz's earlier prediction that significant sums would be saved by ambitious lobotomy programs seemed to have been borne out. In 1952, a report from the Trenton State Hospital in New Jersey claimed that operations on its worst class of patients had resulted in seventy-nine discharges, representing a yearly savings of $91,695.30. And for those who did not return to active employment, benefits still accrued to the hospitals. Many previously intractable patients, following a brain operation, were assigned to occupational therapy and became productive members of the hospital's own work force. Hospital labor performed by psychosurgery patients, one institution noted with surprised satisfaction, actually exceeded the cost of their maintenance.[22]

Lobotomy might return patients to their homes, but did this represent a true saving or simply a transfer of the costs of medical care to patients' families? On the contrary, Tarumianz had argued, patients were restored to socially useful functions, either to housekeeping or to former jobs. Perhaps the strongest positive claim made on behalf of psychosurgery was its potential to reach into the back wards of mental institutions and reclaim a fair percentage of their intractable patients for society. The significance was not lost on its advocates. In their monograph *Psychosurgery,* Freeman and Watts had reported an astonishing fact: at time of publication, approximately two-thirds of their lobotomized patients were usefully employed, earning at least a partial living or keeping house. Freeman advanced this claim with confirming photographs and case histories. One such "after" photograph was captioned "employed and going to night school." Another, "he worried because he couldn't find a job and couldn't find a job because he worried so much." Lobotomy, the reader learned, ended this vicious circle by allowing the patient to find "both a job and peace of mind." Most suggestive were those case histories that illustrated lobotomy's peak potential. A soldier reentered active duty and eventually won a service medal; a businessman returned to his office; and an inventor institutionalized for several years patented an innovative lathe.[23]

Freeman and Watts's claims were reinforced by testimony from hospitals across the country. The psychosurgical literature swelled with such stories of remarkable transformations. A lobotomized patient at Weston State Hospital in West Virginia was hired as a station agent by the C. & O. Railroad. A woman hospitalized for ten years at Norristown State Hospital in Pennsylvania resumed her former position as a public school teacher; another, after several years of severe mental illness, became a regular member of a nationally known orchestra. The large-scale psychosurgery programs buttressed such individual accounts with impressive aggregate figures, showing that a consistent percentage of patients were returned to regular employment.[24]

Rarely did skilled workers return to their original occupation. As the hospital population was comprised mostly of unskilled laborers and non-professionals, this limitation did not dampen overall enthusiasm for the procedure, however. Freeman, true to form, best articulated the operation's raw economic allure to society and its administrative agents. Applied to the right patient, Freeman boasted, lobotomy alone could make the difference between a "taxeater and a taxpayer."[25]

## Administrative Cures

The popularity of psychosurgery in the mental hospitals involved more than just the possibility of discharging patients home. Even its most ardent supporters reported that at best only one-third of lobotomized patients might eventually leave the institution. Inevitably, hospital staffs and administrators would judge programs of lobotomy on how well the typical postoperative patient fared *within* the institution. Although spectacular results were achieved only infrequently, such reports stated, the large majority of psychosurgery patients were nevertheless greatly improved – at least from the standpoint of hospital psychiatry. After a lobotomy, patients who once had posed the worst behavioral and nursing problems now constituted significantly less of a management burden. In effect, the goal of lobotomy had become codified as two-tiered. Psychiatrists at Logansport State Hospital in Indiana described how "the improvement which is sought and which lobotomy may accomplish may be of two varieties." First, they explained, "some are improved so much that they can be discharged to the care of relatives." The others, however, "remain as institutional cases but are more cooperative."[26]

Strecker, in his landmark report on lobotomy for chronic schizophrenics, provided the first succinct description of this second feature of psychosurgery. Patients selected for lobotomy operations had been "disruptive of hospital morale" and "impregnable to management or even approach." Yet after an operation a very large reduction had occurred in the patients' "destructive and dangerous clashes with the environment." What Strecker termed the procedure's "outstanding clinical result" became psychosurgery's most visible selling point. Its ability to transform violent and destructive patients into "rather pleasant, harmless persons" was extolled by research publications, clinical surveys, annual reports of state mental hospitals, and literature supplied by state departments of mental hygiene. "In many cases," the director of Pilgrim State Hospital contended, "we have found ourselves able to discard for the first time in years, the use of restraint, seclusion and chronic sedation where previous attempts to relax precautions have resulted only in difficult or dangerous situations." Through its psychosurgery program, noted the California Department of Mental Hygiene in 1948, "many old chronic cases, who are noisy, intractable, uncooperative and assaultive, quiet down and become reasonably well-behaved patients." Freeman boasted that lobotomy patients became "quiet, orderly," even exhibiting "cheerful compliance with the ward routine."27

Individual case histories could be quite dramatic, as when Hohman and his colleagues presented the story of a fifty-nine-year-old, violent schizophrenic patient who had been hospitalized for twenty-five years. This destructive patient caused several thousand dollars of damage each year, necessitating two seclusion rooms. (The second room was used to contain him while the first was being restored.) Miraculously, after lobotomy he was able to live placidly and comfortably inside the hospital. Another patient had grown resistant to normal methods of sedation, spending her time in seclusion rooms, screaming incessantly. Postoperatively, she entered occupational therapy and was ready to be transferred to work in the laundry. The reports from the large-scale trials sometimes included short vignettes of individual patients alongside the summary tables. One inmate, for example, was said to have been changed "from a seriously assaultive and destructive problem" into someone who "is neat and tidy and works in the kitchen."28

Psychosurgery was hailed as being of enormous benefit to the beleaguered state hospitals for these and other contributions to ward life. Lobotomy patients, it was found, created fewer incidents of destruction of sheets and clothing, bed-wetting, soiling, and refusing food. An article from Marlboro State Hospital in New Jersey stated that it was nearly impossible to overemphasize the conservation of hospital personnel resulting from its lobotomy program; approximately seven-tenths of the patients required much less supervision, with no case proving more difficult to manage than before surgery.[29] In Massachusetts, a survey of the institutions that participated in its centralized program of psychosurgery found uniform agreement upon the overall reduction in overactivity, aggressiveness, and belligerency on the halls. One superintendent stated that by simply observing the level of agitation on a ward he could tell whether psychosurgery had been used. The director of Pilgrim remarked that one of psychosurgery's "unmeasurable gains" was its auxiliary effects. By quieting a single chronically noisy and provocative patient – someone who had kept the rest "stirred up" – just one operation might significantly ease the burden of caring for an entire ward. Figures and statistics alone, such superintendents emphasized, could not reveal the levels of institutional improvement that stemmed from an active use of lobotomy.[30]

The discovery that the typical lobotomy patient became well adapted to institutional life was at the outset viewed as a fortuitous side-benefit. However, it was not long before the operation's collateral effects – pacification and increased manageability – were established in their own right as guidelines for the selection of lobotomy candidates. Psychiatrists at Binghamton State Hospital in New York provided an example of this shift when they described psychosurgery's use in cases where care "is extremely difficult because of antisocial behavior, including assaultiveness, biting, hair pulling and other dangerous tendencies." Further,

> every hospital worker will remember certain vicious and extremely dangerous patients who have created great problems in nursing care and it is our hope that this operative procedure will eventually reduce to a minimum that type of behavior on wards of mental hospitals. Many a nurse or attendant has been slapped, bitten, has had her hair pulled and her uniform stripped off, by this type of actively aggressive patient. This method of treatment promises to be a real boon to all engaged in psychiatric nursing on disturbed wards.

This behavioral concern was candidly expressed by Freeman when he wrote that a patient might as well be excluded from consideration for lobotomy when a nurse's notes read "gives no trouble on the ward." Psychosurgery's popularity in state hospitals was directly related to its growing reputation for alleviating "troublesome problems of management to hospital administrators."[31]

The use of a psychiatric therapy for the express purpose of maintaining hospital order was of course not original to psychosurgery; this tendency originated from the time institutions were first opened. The new wave of somatic therapies, however, had intensified this legacy. Even as these treatments were revolutionizing medical care of the mentally ill in the 1930s and 1940s, they were also transforming the management of troublesome patients. Before, hospital staffs had only minimal tools available for controlling such difficult patients as the chronically disturbed or those who broke suddenly into an acute psychotic episode. Traditional resources included a variety of physical restraints, such as cuffs, camisoles, chains, and thongs; isolation, in the form of seclusion rooms, dark rooms and cells, into which patients were segregated for periods ranging from hours to days or perhaps longer; and heavy sedation through drugs such as chloral hydrate, paraldehyde, and barbiturates, though these were limited in effectiveness due to problems of toxicity and tolerance.

The vigorous extension of asylum hydrotherapy in the first third of the twentieth century illustrated the high interest in discovering techniques of patient management that were based on physiological interventions. Hydrotherapy, already in use for centuries, had been recast in a newly scientized form. Psychiatric hydrotherapy consisted of applying water in various external ways to affect body temperature and circulation, a putative means of indirectly toning up the psyche. The most common forms of this treatment were continuous tubs that kept a patient immersed in a bath of running water of constant temperature; wet-sheet packs, in which a patient was "mummified" in wet bedsheets and placed in a darkened room; and water sprays of varying temperature, spread, and duration. Here was a complete system with which to regulate psychiatric conditions. For lethargic patients, stimulating sprays were indicated; at the other extreme, for manic patients, tubs and wet packs were proven pacifiers. During the 1930s, elaborate hydrotherapy rooms and suites were incorporated into mental hospital construction, evoking a style of brass-age asylum architecture one might attribute to Jules Verne.[32]

In addition to its purely clinical purposes, hydrotherapy soon developed a covert reputation as a disciplinary tool. For example, in Ellen Philtine's fictionalized account of Pilgrim State Hospital (the novel *They Walk In Darkness*), a senior psychiatrist winks at his young acolyte when lecturing that the use of hydrotherapy is proscribed if used for other than purely medical reasons. His own example taught otherwise. When dictating the clinical notes on a garrulous patient, the psychiatrist reports that the individual had "called examiner s-of-a-b as well as other epithets." His answer was to shout to the staff, "Into the tub!"[33] The novel is set at the end of the 1930s, a crucial period when optimism generated by the introduction of the somatic therapies collided with the brutal realities of the impending crisis in hospital conditions. The hard-pressed staff discovered soon enough that the new somatic therapies yielded the unexpected benefit of additional, much appreciated behavioral tools, and were effective forms of sedation and behavioral control. Hospital workers scrambled for

new ways to use the shock therapies to alleviate particularly distressing
behavioral episodes, or virtually any problem that might arise in a typical
workday. In this manner the new treatments became self-consciously used
for administrative and not just "curative" purposes.

In the early 1940s, the compromise of accepting that chronic patients, if
not curable, could at least be controlled became known and implemented
nationwide as "maintenance therapy." Insulin, for example, when used in
lower doses not producing a coma, was found to have a useful sedating
effect. Because the subcoma technique did not require constant nursing
attention as in the case of full treatment, its use was practicable at a
distance away from the medical facilities in the acute ward, thus allowing
penetration into the back wards.[34] Metrazol shock, a popular substitute
for insulin, was also used for "administrative problems" associated with
disturbed psychotics. The maintenance therapy of choice, though, was
electroshock. Its simplicity, portability, cheapness, and relative safety allowed hospitals to employ it both as a planned system of treatment
throughout the hospital and as a means of responding to acute crises as
they arose. When used in female chronic wards at Harrisburg State Hospital in Pennsylvania, for example, patients were found to be "quieter, more
cooperative, less destructive and less untidy." The technique, termed
"symptomatic shock" by psychiatrists at Pilgrim, could control "serious
feeding problems and serious behavior disorders."[35]

For especially difficult cases, hospital psychiatrists found that the frequency of such treatments might be increased as the situation demanded.
The repeated use of electroshock, it was reported at a New York State
Interhospital Conference, would lead to hospital improvement in the form
of "control of destructive and assaultive tendencies of the patients" and a
change "in the atmosphere of the ward and the environment." (One patient received as many as eight hundred total shocks.) The much respected
superintendent of Norristown State Hospital in Pennsylvania, Nolan D.
C. Lewis, discounted criticism that maintenance electroshock was perhaps utilized beyond "conservative discretion." He argued instead that
one hesitated to restrict its use given the lack of personnel needed to
operate continuous baths or to employ alternative sedative measures. The
recommended treatment for those patients who had already failed to respond to maintenance therapy, stated one article in the *Psychiatric Quarterly*, was to shock them twice a day two days in a row, until control was
regained. The method was called the "BEST" treatment, an acronym for
"Blitz Electro-Shock Therapy." Testimonials on behalf of this strategy, the
authors noted, came from "exhausted and pessimistic" employees who

had labored for years with such patients. Similarly, psychiatrists at Kings Park in New York found that an article of theirs on "regressive shock" drew worldwide attention.[36]

In short, the use of the somatic therapies for the specific purpose of upgrading the ward behavior of chronic patients, and not out of any particular hope of cure, was stumbled upon accidentally and then refined during the successive application of metrazol, insulin, and electric shock. Psychosurgery became a natural extension of this tactic and quickly established a reputation as the most effective – read permanent – means of behavioral control. With the continued use of psychosurgery, the dual purposes of psychiatric treatment became so clearly differentiated that psychiatrists split their own terminology when describing the procedure's effects. In addition to "clinical recovery" and "cure rates," psychiatrists in the psychosurgical literature referred to patients in terms of their "institutional improvement" or "hospital recovery." One researcher went so far as to suggest dividing the evaluation of lobotomized patients into two categories, that of "curative improvement" and "administrative improvement." William A. White, in his 1925 presidential address to the APA, noted that in the dehumanized state hospitals the patient relinquishes "control over his body and even his life itself to this gigantic piece of medical machinery."[37] In some sense, the fate of the patient and that of the institution had since become even further intertwined. Disturbances in normal hospital operations, occasioned by a patient's obstreperous behavior, were seen as having a solution in common with the new medical technologies that could tame a patient's inner conflicts. Psychosurgery truly offered an administrative cure.

## Apologia

One can make the argument that institutional psychiatrists, in deciding to use the brain operations on their patients for administrative cures, were simply doing the best they could under trying circumstances: the staff were guilty, but with an explanation. In her novel, Philtine sensitively portrayed how a commitment to the curative ideal inevitably becomes subordinated to the more pressing matter of managing difficult patients. The reader follows along as the protagonist, assistant physician Peter Carson, agonizes over the shift in his own standards during the course of his professional seasoning. At the beginning of the story, a senior physician instructs Carson that a state hospital doctor's entire arsenal is "restraint, hydrotherapy and sedatives – that's all."[38] The irrepressible Carson will not let it rest there. The young idealist pours out his heart to Dr.

Goldschmidt, a German émigré, who alone on the staff believes in such progressive ideas as Freudianism:

> Soberly he began outlining his problems: the lack of nurses, the scarcity of attendants, the absence of the most essential equipment. And how could doctors so overburdened with routine find time to treat their patients? What was the program for the treatment of chronic cases? . . . "Oh, I know on reception service the new patients get shock-treatments. But down here in these chronic buildings, so far as I can make out, all the emphasis is on keeping 'em quiet. Well, hell, any dumb attendant could learn to give sedatives and stick violent psychotics in the tubs! There must be more to it than that, or why would they need doctors at all? . . . So I keep asking myself: what in hell do you do for these chronic patients? Isn't there some plan for cure, some special treatment that will eventually get them out of here?" (p. 83)

Peter's ambition leads him to experiment with a new drug that had proved efficacious in short-term trials and to extend its use to more difficult chronic cases. He sketches his goal to the Superintendent:

> when I take some of those patients out of restraint, it doesn't seem long before I have to put them back. The routine drugs we use here don't seem to quiet 'em, unless you keep on giving the drug, and then the patient may become toxic. Well, it means I've got to find a drug that will quiet 'em and keep 'em quiet, without toxicity. (p. 139)

Peter invests his hopes in a (fictional) drug called "sodium octathal," believing that somehow its toxicity could be nullified. Another doctor cautions him not to be too enthusiastic about the new drug:

> I think it wise to warn you – ah, most other investigators have since agreed with me – not to expect any mental changes. Physical improvement and more co-operative behavior. But that is all. Also the danger of toxicity –
>
> [Peter] I don't care, sir! I've seen too much around here to hold out for absolute cures. I think it'll be important just to quiet 'em down, so I can cut out restraints! (p. 279)

Thus, under the numbing demands of state hospital life, Peter's passionate drive to discover a cure for the masses suffering in the chronic wards was soon downgraded into an anxious scramble for a treatment that would at least establish some sort of order – even if it involved a substantial risk to the patient.[39]

An awareness of the pressures that hospital psychiatrists faced of course does not dissipate our concern that the clinical interests of the patients were so overshadowed as to shift the blame from that of the individuals who worked in the hospitals to the wider social dynamics that led to the poor conditions. This kind of apologia is misleading, however. To frame the issue in terms of the dilemma faced by psychiatrists, in having to choose between their roles as managers and as healers when evaluating the somatic treatments, is an anachronism. Although psychiatrists at the time clearly made distinctions between the administrative and curative effects of their medicaments, it would be wrong to assume that in discussing these functions they regarded them as incommensurate realms. If anything, the exact opposite was held to be true. In this period, the goals of therapy and behavioral readjustment were seen not as antithetical but as linked and consistent. To more recent observers, such a blatant conflation appears as yet another indictment of the psychiatrists, further proof of the kind of deliberate or malicious disregard for their patients' welfare that led to such episodes as psychosurgery. A reexamination of what it meant to be a psychiatrist in the 1940s, however, will help to account for why these physicians saw little conflict between their dual responsibilities and thus embraced *all* of the somatic treatments' functions as valid medicine.

This will become clearer with a closer look at the inner structure and functioning of the mental hospital system. Psychosurgery, along with the rest of the new somatic therapies, was grafted onto a model of psychiatric therapy still heavily rooted in its administrative locus. A patient's clinical status, the pattern of treatment use, and even the criteria for assessing mental well-being were defined in institutional terms. In such a world, psychosurgery appeared to offer a viable path along which patients might return to improved health, not just better behavior.

### The Structure and Function of the Modern Asylum

Although state mental hospitals varied greatly in size, condition, and other such structural features, as a rule they followed the same general administrative and clinical organization. Mental institutions actually were a collection of many separate facilities that were divided into wards segregated by sex and occasionally age, and further differentiated by degree of discipline and supervision needed to maintain order and hygienic conditions. The spectrum of ward types began with loosely supervised "open" wards in which patients were entitled to come and go as they pleased. In the middle were "day" wards, locked only at night. These were followed by "chronic" or "deteriorated" wards, which housed patients who required the most nursing care. At the far end were "disturbed" wards, which contained the most violent and disruptive patients.

In essence, state mental hospitals were a continuum of varying security and nursing environments, ranging from minimum supervision to maximum, and from those that provided little nursing attention to others that offered continual caretaking. If the mental hygiene department was situated in a populous state and consisted of multiple institutions, then the system as a whole may have been similarly differentiated, with particular hospitals devoted to the separate functions. Receiving hospitals, for example, corresponded to acute wards where incoming patients were observed, diagnosed, and after initial treatment transferred to an appropriate ward. Some states also supported specialized outpatient clinics, hospitals dedicated to the care of the chronic mentally ill, and isolated facilities for the criminally insane.

The mental hospital experience, from the patient's perspective, was a journey of indefinite length that led from ward to ward and from hospital to hospital. Transferred through a variety of facilities, the patient discovered in each new destination a confusing environment that was inhabited by unfamiliar residents and authority figures, with varying sets of daily routines that required the adoption of different strategies for survival. An informative map of the world traveled by the inmate would not be based on its physical geography, in which different residences were known generically as "Ward 23" or "Building C" – or perhaps benignly called the Adolf Meyer Pavilion. More accurately, it would be categorized into behavioral zones that established when a patient's conduct, if unsatisfactory, required deportation to a harsher environment or, if satisfactory, provided a visa to one less restricted. Unless death intervened, the trek ended when the patient either had traveled through ever better, more civilized wards, ultimately surfacing to be reunited with family and friends or, alternatively, had sunk lower and lower, ultimately reaching the "snakepit" from which few were reclaimed.

Surprisingly, such a map would hold little meaning for those seeking to navigate on the basis of clinical reality as codified in medical textbooks. To begin with, mental hospital organization did not reflect the contemporary classification of mental disease. Psychiatrists frequently noted that any given ward was a seemingly random blend of psychoneurosis, schizophrenia, manic-depression, paresis, alcoholism, and paranoia. It was not diagnostic considerations that determined how patients were distributed throughout state hospitals but specific behavioral features. "In the everyday management of a state hospital we don't put our patients, for instance, on a disturbed ward because they have schizophrenia," declared the clinical director of Worcester State Hospital in Massachusetts. "Similarly," he continued, "we do not remove them to the quiet ward because they have ceased having schizophrenia and now have a psychoneurosis, and we don't send them home on that basis."[40] Psychiatrists lamented the lack of medical staffing and facilities that prevented a clinically rational segregation of patients. The functional unit of the hospital was not the patient, but the ward. A psychiatrist's primary responsibility was to insure viability of ward life, a duty that was part personnel officer and part quartermaster. Psychiatrists were assigned to buildings, not patients.[41]

What was true for patient diagnosis held for therapeutics. Meagre resources did not allow for a careful matching of specific conditions with a particular treatment, or for careful follow-ups sorted by category of mental disease. The hospitals simply were not organized in that way. Patients drifted between wards and buildings, precluding any semblance of clinical continuity. Therapies were thus implemented and evaluated in terms of their applicability at the ward level. The medical treatment of choice would prove to be not a "magic bullet" that might cure patients stricken with a specific mental illness, but a trusty shotgun that could be used without regard to diagnostic labels. One of the most difficult jobs confronting hospital psychiatrists, an observer remarked, was the daily evaluation of scores of patients with regard to their management and treatment. Given state institution realities, he noted further, the two were "practically inseparable."[42]

From this perspective, the distinction between psychiatric therapies as medical treatment and as a form of behavioral control began to dissolve. In psychiatry, the natural history of a patient's disorder was tracked in terms of his or her path through the institution (or institutions). In a general hospital, the course of a disease was monitored on patients' charts through measurements of body temperature and of blood cell count, and changes in tissue structure and heart rhythms. But in mental institutions the patients' current and past mental status was indicated by the types of wards in which they resided and the success of their adaptation to them. (In the nurses' notes of McLean Hospital, for example, when a patient was transferred to a different ward the event was recorded in red pen.) Prognoses and clinical progress were logged in institutional terms; institutional history and clinical history were indistinguishable. Such behavioral maps in the world of mental health were in fact the primary guides to clinical decisions.[43]

## Socializing Medicine

It was thus no secret that the mental hospital, stripped to its barest essentials, was fundamentally a hierarchy of living environments differentiated mostly by degree of regulatory control. One would be mistaken to conclude, however, that when contemporary psychiatrists acknowledged this point they were at the same time admitting that their professional world was therapeutically bankrupt, inherently *non*-medical in outlook and action. To the contrary, it was precisely this behavioral apparatus that psychiatrists at the time seized upon as their core treatment method for restoring a patient to mental health.

As previously described, in the first third of the twentieth century state hospital psychiatrists lacked both effective somatic treatments and psychotherapeutic tools for dealing with severe mental illness. Whereas the nation's general hospitals were proudly displaying the latest gifts of scientific medicine, the mental institutions had received little such benefits. Frustrated by the prospects of an unfulfilled future, psychiatrists reached backward to a usable past, rediscovering the rich nineteenth-century legacy of "moral therapy" in which hospital routines formed the basis for reconstructing a patient's character. In so doing, these physicians perceived in the ward hierarchy a therapeutic gradient that paralleled the various stages of mental deterioration exhibited by patients.[44] The hospitals' varying ward environments, originally formulated out of administrative and bureaucratic necessities, were thus reenvisioned as vital elements of a rational, coherent system of therapeutic intervention through which patients might gradually be retrained to cope with the stresses of everyday life.

Each ward level defined the extent of the psychiatric challenge as well as the appropriate therapeutic response. The specific contribution of hospital psychiatry, also known as administrative psychiatry, was thought to be the skillful application of hospital routines and personal guidance that would bring to bear just the right level of remedial training and resocialization. Such combinations were labeled variously as Habit Training, Recreational Therapy, Dance Therapy, Occupational Therapy, and Industrial Therapy. Hospital therapies were to be applied in correspondence with the patient's level of contact with reality and ability to behave appropriately. In Habit Training, severely regressed patients were retoilet-trained and taught everyday skills such as eating with utensils. Recreational Therapy referred to light diversions such as movies, plays, and dances that might draw patients back into closer touch with their social world. Occupational Therapy was reserved for those who had some social awareness and usually consisted of arts and crafts and simple hospital tasks. In Industrial Therapy (called Occupational Therapy in some places) those patients who had improved the most were integrated into the hospital's labor force. It was common for wards to be designated by the types of hospital therapy employed.

In short, prior to the introduction of the new somatic therapies there existed a coherent system of care believed to be effective in its own right. The move to declare the mental hospital as not just the primary site of psychiatric healing but the major mode of therapy as well was nicely captured in William Russell's 1932 presidential address to the APA. Russell told his brethren what they already knew: that the most important therapeutic resource available to psychiatrists was the social structure of the hospital itself. The *medical* practice of the mental hospitals, he underscored, was "social treatment." It was only after the advent of the new physical therapies that the "hospital regimen," or "allied" therapy, was differentiated into a separate category of lesser medical status. Before, it was simply psychiatry.[45]

Ironically, it was the rise of Meyerian concepts of mental disorder and its emphasis on the noninstitutional basis of modern psychiatry that had paved the way for the remedicalization of the asylum along social precepts. As previously described, in place of legal insanity or mental disease as the defining concept of psychiatry, Meyer promoted a radical standard of maladjustment or maladaptation as the index of mental pathology. The target was not to heal a sick body or set a broken mind so much as to restore an individual to proper functioning within the larger body politic. Psychiatrists no longer had to concern themselves with hunting for the precise physiological defect that had disabled the individual or, alternatively, to investigate the error of thought that led to character disarray. Instead, what mattered was simply to promote a better functional relationship between the individual and the environmental challenges posed by family, employer, and society.

The rank and file in the mental hospitals found much to like in the Meyer reform platform, even though the primary thrust of the campaign – especially in the hands of the NCMH and Thomas Salmon – did not target the institutions as a major beneficiary. (Historian Gerald Grob has described how the vision of these reformers fatefully turned psychiatry *away* from the institutions, with disastrous consequences that erupted decades later.) In particular, they discovered within the maladjustment model an opportunity to repackage the traditional hospital programs in a way that would cast a newfound *medical* cachet upon their work. In the Meyerian worldview, White's observation that a mental hospital was a "gigantic piece of medical machinery" was meant literally.

In the new framework, patients in the institutions were not healed in a strictly physiological sense but refurbished through its powerful social apparatus. By working their way through the series of graded behavioral environments, inmates gradually retraced the process of growing into responsible adults; if successful, they emerged in a form that was perhaps not as adequate as their premorbid personality, but one nonetheless sufficiently adaptable to handle the stresses of everyday life. The measure of psychiatric success was based on a relative standard of social performance, not an ideal standard of physical health. Only one criterion mattered: was the patient more able to cope than before?

Thanks to the success of the adjustment model of mental disorder, the mental hospital had been reconceptualized as a microcosm of external society in which physicians might oversee the process whereby patients relearned the habits of good citizenship. Psychiatry in the modern world was to have no walls separating the asylum and society. In this framework, the hospital's emphasis would be on reeducating a fragile individual to survive in a society fraught with complex environmental challenges. The goal was adaptability and survival; the most important indicator was that of adjustment – a measure of the soundness of the fit between an organism's capabilities and the demands of its immediate environment. In the new psychiatry, concerns about the inner mental life of patients – such qualities as their range of emotional coloration, depth of capacity for interpersonal attachments, or self-actualization of talents – were largely irrelevant to the healing process. This was no Freudian paradise. In 1942, a special New York State Commission to Investigate the Care of the Mentally Ill summarized the institutions' arduous task as promoting "a proper adjustment to life," to be achieved through furnishing the patient "with a course of activity which will develop his self-reliance and diminish his introspection."[46]

Moreover, it was the public health framework of the new psychiatry that led these physicians to see the disturbances of their patients on the wards in distinctly medical terms. Although Meyer's doctrine of psychobiology claimed a monist's view of mind and body, the psychiatry that he and Thomas Salmon built around it was inescapably bivalent in professional responsibility. From one perspective, the goal was to satisfy the needs of the mentally disordered; from the other, the goal was to repair the breach in the social fabric. The mentally ill were not just the disturbed but those who were disturbing; the mission of the new psychiatrist was to intervene whenever a maladjusted person threatened the social order.

Professional ideology aside, the tension between the two roles of course never did go away. On a daily basis, however, such problems tended to be swept aside by a corollary set of assumptions within the maladjustment model that equated mental health with social contentedness.[47] The fact that someone was unhappy with his or her life situation, and expressed this anger through hostile words or actions, was itself interpreted as further evidence of psychiatric morbidity; that psychosurgery calmed the troublemakers and restored peace on the wards was thus considered, within this framework, as final proof of lobotomy's *clinical* effect. This

## PREFRONTAL LOBOTOMY SUMMARY

Name _Case 121_ Sex _F_ SMWD _D_ Age at first operation _31_
Education _Highschool_ Occupation _Housewife_
Diagnosis _Dementia precox. hebephrenic_ Date of onset _1934_ Disabled since _1935_
Hospitalized _Oct 1935, 3 mo.; since Aug. 1938_ Shock therapy _Metrazol_
Date of lobotomy _March 24, 1942_ Reoperations _____ First contact _8/25/41_

| FOLLOW-UP | V—visit | | R—report | | L—letter | | P—photograph | | |
|---|---|---|---|---|---|---|---|---|---|
| YEAR | 1942 | 1943 | 1944 | 1945 | 1946 | 1947 | 1948 | 1949 | |
| Jan. | | Keeping house | Employed | Employed | Employed | Partly employed | Partly employed | Partly employed | |
| Feb. | | | | | | | | | |
| Mar. | LOBO-TOMY | Employed | L | L | | | | | |
| Apr. | R Home | | | L | | | | | |
| May | R | | | | | | | | |
| June | V P | | | | V P Home | | R | | |
| July | | | | | | | | | |
| Aug. | | L P | | | L | R | L V | | |
| Sept. | Keeping house | | | | | | | | |
| Oct. | L | | | | Partly employed | | R | | |
| Nov. | | | R L | | | V P | | | |
| Dec. | R | | | | V | L | | | |

Figure 5.1. Card used to rate progress in a lobotomy patient. (Source: Walter Freeman and James Watts, *Psychosurgery*, 2d ed., 1950. Courtesy of Charles C. Thomas, Publisher, Springfield, Illinois.)

perspective echoes through patient records from this period, whenever physicians would justify the decision to operate on the basis of the need to make patients "more comfortable" – for themselves, their family, and the hospital staff. Indeed, whatever it was psychiatrists hoped to communicate to friends and family that they had accomplished by the operation, this particular expression was something that got across. For example, the person who signed the permission form for the operation on Helaine Strauss, a patient at an elite private hospital, wrote to the staff, "I fully realize that this operation will have little effect on her mental condition but am willing to have it done in the hope that she will be more comfortable and easier to care for."[48]

And should a patient actively resist a course of treatment recommended by the psychiatrist – even one so terrifying as insulin shock or brain surgery – this defiance itself was objectified as being an irrational fear to be cured, not placated. Indeed, as psychosurgery was thought to work best on "agitated" patients, the more a patient complained about being subjected to such a procedure, the better the prognosis. The best type of lobotomy patient, Freeman noted, was the one who had to be dragged into treatment kicking and screaming (see Figure 5.2).

In the experience of the hospital physicians, the single most potent tool in the therapeutic armamentarium for relieving patients trapped in a world of unending misery was psychosurgery. That it also rendered the unmanageable patients more manageable, and made hospital life more bearable for all, was thus additional evidence of lobotomy's clinical powers. Matters of private health and public health had converged. When Paul Howard, a psychiatrist at McLean Hospital, reported on the results of a comprehensive study of lobotomy in England, he paraphrased its findings as follows: 11 patients became worse, 244 were unchanged, 295 became milder, 166 were now "cooperatives," and 242 had become "citizens."[49]

In sum, according to the maladjustment model, a patient's manageability inside the hospital became a direct indication of his or her capacity to survive in the external social world. In this way, the very practical problem, faced by institutional physicians, of maintaining order was transformed into a medical issue, not just a penal one; from their perspective they were always doctors, never wardens. Manageability and improved mental health were now the same thing.

### New Wine in Old Bottles

The introduction of the somatic therapies, therefore, did not signify a revolutionary break with existing treatment philosophies but in important ways were interpreted as their fulfillment. As in all medical science, when new treatments are introduced they do not at once sweep aside the conceptual frameworks attached to the previously dominant therapies. Indeed, the opposite often holds true: the new therapies are seen to work in much the same way as the previous ones, only more so. The somatic treatments, and lobotomy in particular, yielded patients who looked and acted differently; the reason such changes were interpreted as signs that the patients were now *healthier* lies in the direct continuity between prior models of health and the new treatments. Such treatments made sense to the participants because they fulfilled traditional ideas about how patients were restored to well-being.

In the example of psychosurgery, the most conspicuous such carryover was the great attention paid to mental patients' physical weight. Inmates in the institutions were notoriously underfed, sometimes by circumstance and sometimes by choice: refusal of food was one of the most frequent ways in which patients expressed their "negativistic impulses" or paranoid delusions. Forced feedings, usually performed through rubber tubes inserted through the nasal passages, were one of the more unpleasant aspects of hospital life, for all involved; the threat of such an ordeal was a common punitive tool. The matter of weight was not inconsequential, as frail patients were more apt to succumb to hospital diseases and stresses. Hospitals also saw their share of anorexia, a poorly understood condition in which young women wasted away to an inevitable death. In the medical records, the patient's weight was one of the few measures the hospitals had to assess the general health of the patient; some state hospitals, in their annual reports, even published summary tables on the weight gains of their patients.

As it happens, one of the more frequent side effects of the brain operations was an almost total loss of appetite regulation. Following lobotomy, patients reported a constant urge to eat and rapidly put on great amounts of weight; gains of fifty to a hundred pounds were not unusual. The physicians who reported on the results of lobotomy made direct correlations between the weight gains and a return to happier, sturdier living. In the second edition of *Psychosurgery,* Freeman and Watts included a before-and-after picture of a woman who had weighed only 85 pounds at the time of operation, and three years later 210. The text reported that twelve years later the patient "is still obese and perpetually hungry but runs her sister's household and enjoys life."[50] When compared to their former gaunt selves, the fat lobotomy patients were the very picture of good health.

It was not just these frameworks of *physical* health that were used to measure a patient's well-being. It might be expected that the overtly physiological aspects of the somatic treatments would undercut the traditional model of how patients were restored, such as the hospital social programs of basket weaving and mattress sewing. In fact, the story runs in the other direction. Due to the Meyerian model of maladjustment, such hospital activities were considered by psychiatrists as their most potent *medical* tools, and the effects of the physical treatments were subsumed within this preexisting paradigm. This continuity was an important factor in why psychiatrists at the time interpreted the primary behavioral effect of the operations – their capacity to transform unmanageable patients into tolerable hospital residents – as direct evidence of a clinical and not just an administrative gain.

Indeed, the new somatic therapies were incorporated into state hospitals as direct supplements to the ongoing regimen of retraining and resocialization. Spokesmen from the California Department of Mental Health argued that hospital routines were, strictly speaking, the only true therapies. Most psychiatric techniques, they suggested, were really "experiences in helpful living," as "the serving of attractive and palatable meals, the right kind of recreation, music, reading material, hobbies, and work, all combine to form the recovery pattern." The more "technical" methods such as psychotherapy, electroshock, and psychosurgery, it explained, were "essentially functions through which the more simple techniques can reach the patient." New York State's *Mental Hygiene News* reported that "the physical therapies have been carried on as an integral part of the basic hospital program," being all the "various modalities that go to make up the complex structure of a modern mental hospital," such as occupational and recreational therapy. The latest additions to the therapeutic armamentarium, it elaborated, "neither reduced in importance nor replaced the older methods." Rather, they "lent them new effectiveness."[51]

Patients after psychosurgery were especially dependent upon the strength of an institution's resocialization programs. Although published investigations on lobotomy widely differed on such fundamental matters as particular mental disease targeted, patient demographics, and choice of operative technique, there existed a general consensus as to proper aftercare. Such reports cautioned that if the operations were to result in any meaningful, lasting level of restoration, postlobotomy patients must be incorporated into hospital therapies, beginning with habit training and ending with intensive occupational therapy. Psychosurgery patients tended to lack a certain amount of self-initiative, it was conceded, but remarkable gains were thought possible with proper attention and guidance. Programs of lobotomy were thus coordinated, heightened applications of the existing hospital regimen. Indeed, as no special outlays or reorganization was needed, "Any description of post-lobotomy care," wrote the administrators at Pilgrim State, "becomes a dissertation on ordinary state hospital procedure."[52] Some institutions, such as the Institute of Living in Connecticut, did go so far as to retool their retraining and resocialization program toward the particular needs of lobotomy patients, transforming the services into showpieces of what hospital therapeutics might become if given sufficient resources.

The goal in psychosurgery, as in all the other therapies, was reeducation of patients so that "previous undesirable habits could now be replaced by more acceptable behavior."[53] This framework extended into the domain of neurophysiology, molding the scientific explanations for the brain operation's effects. Although individual explanatory models were as varied as the methods of surgical attack, nevertheless a single theme was common to all, one that resonated well with the program of resocialization. The psychosurgical literature rested upon a model of brain and behavior, held by lay as well as professional audiences at least since the nineteenth-century writings of William James, in which it was believed that neuronal pathways underlying a person's habits would, over time, become rigid and fixed; as described previously, Meyer's model of mental disorder itself was built upon the concept of habit training.[54] Such beliefs helped to imbue chronic mental illness with a neurologically justified pessimism. Patients who remained in institutions for many years, in an unvarying environment that led to stereotyped behaviors, were doomed to a neuronally fixed, irreversible "institutional psychosis."

Lobotomy's unique power, within this framework, was its ability to break up the neuronal pathways that had become fixed, thus opening the possibility of reprogramming. One prominent supporter of psychosurgery, for example, described how it produced "a new malleability," thereby enabling "the restoration of a patient into useful society." A Missouri legislative report on the state's treatment of mental patients explained lobotomy's effects as caused by a disorganization of neural pathways. Two weeks after an operation, patients' confusions subsided and they were able to "relearn normal habits of living." Postlobotomy patients were often described as "immature" personalities and were likened to persons abruptly regressed to the earliest levels of life. Walter Freeman put it most aptly when he stated that psychosurgery works by effecting a "surgically induced childhood." An article for psychiatric nurses stated that the goal of lobotomy retraining programs was to develop "these emotional children into lovable grownups."[55] Used upon patients whose current antisocial or withdrawn behavior otherwise precluded any chance of ever being incorporated into programs of hospital therapy, psychosurgery was seen to offer a chance for redemption otherwise nonexistent. If the state hospital could be viewed as a proving ground for personal re-growth, then psychosurgery in effect offered a sort of neurophysiological shortcut. Patients who had slipped to the far end were, after the operation, reinstated at the beginning and ready to start the challenge anew. Through lobotomy, the staff at Pilgrim State Hospital declared, the patient is "ren-dered more amenable than before to the hospital regimen." Thanks to the brain operations, "now the basic hospital process of upgrading of the patient can begin."[56]

The maladaptation model of mental health also shaped the medical evaluation of those patients who were not released. A simple inspection of published lobotomy reports reveals a pattern of patient evaluation monot-onously uniform in its emphasis on the use of simple behavioral scales. Although the results were tallied under such basic clinical headings as "much improved," "improved," "slightly improved," or "no change," these categories represented administrative shorthand for the level of be-havioral change. "Much improved," for example, signified that a patient was "restored to being a . . . cooperative and agreeable individual, engag-ing in ward work, dressing and undressing without help, . . . and with complete freedom from all assaultive tendencies."[57]

Although contemporary psychiatrists did speak in separate terms of "curative improvement" and "administrative improvement," they saw little underlying conflict between the two goals. Rather, it was universally assumed that the difference between "recovered" and the other categories was one of degree, not kind – it was the same axis, only at a lower level. This is clearly evident in a lobotomy investigation done at Winnebago State Hospital in Wisconsin, which devised a "Winnebago Scale" that ranged from zero to four:

0. No change.
1. Slight improvement: loss of some drive, no longer requiring protective restraint but can't devote much time to productive activity or hospital activities.
2. Improved sufficient to adjust on a quieter productive ward. Can spend some time daily in occupational therapy.
3. Improved enough to adjust at a county hospital level. Can devote some time to productive activity. . . .
4. Improved enough to return home.[58]

Hospital psychiatrists thus judged a patient's mental health status against a continuum that stretched from total dependency in the back wards to self-sufficiency extramurally. It is within this overall model that lobotomy programs were fitted. "I have never selected a case for psychosurgery . . .

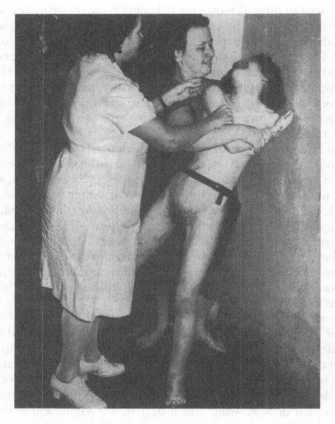

Figure 5.2. Resistance in a patient chosen for lobotomy. Caption states, "Other patients have to be held." (Source: Walter Freeman and James Watts, *Psychosurgery,* 2d ed., 1950. Courtesy of Charles C. Thomas, Publisher, Springfield, Illinois.)

on the basis of diagnosis alone," declared Malamud, "but on the basis of . . . the patient's ability to adjust to his setting."[59] Other examples of this continuum can be found even in the language used by psychiatrists when recommending the operation to the family of a patient. Psychosurgery, explained one psychiatrist, "may be recommended as the procedure most likely to give the patient a chance to adjust better in the hospital or even to adjust outside the hospital."[60]

In short, when psychiatrists reported that a patient who had not been fully restored by lobotomy was nevertheless living at a "higher hospital level," or had become a better "hospital citizen," they thought they were

stating that a measurable clinical gain had in fact occurred. To characterize the motivation behind the large-scale programs of psychosurgery as
arising solely from the desire to upgrade the behavior of society's deviates
(whether in the hospital or outside) is thus an oversimplification and a
distortion. It is a telling fact that during the heyday of psychosurgery,
supporters of the procedure typically recommended *against* its use on
patients with severe conduct disorders. Henry Brill noted, for example,
that "primary homosexuality, psychopathic behavior of the primary type,
alcoholism, and various fringe antisocial tendencies are not benefitted."
As another example, when the Veterans Administration established
centralized guidelines for its large psychosurgery program, such personality traits were listed as specific indications that the procedure was *not* to
be used.[61]

Such constraints were consistent with the general theory of lobotomy.
Surgery alone, it was believed, could not reconstitute the patient's underlying personality. A hardened criminal before the operation would remain
a criminal (though perhaps a less effective or motivated one).[62] Pycho-
surgery, as mentioned above, was believed to work by enabling resocialization to begin, through bringing out the patient's premorbid capabilities
for positive growth. As social deviates were considered to have lacked any
faculty for self-regulation even in childhood, it was concluded that the
procedure would be unable to build upon what was not there and, if
anything, would probably deinhibit even further destructive tendencies.

### Conclusion: A Measure of Desperation

From today's perspective, the assertion by psychiatrists in the 1940s that
lobotomy profoundly altered the behavior and personality of their patients is easily believed. The additional claim of theirs that these changes
were a great *medical* benefit is less apparent. If anything, the early testimonials in support of the procedure are often used to impugn the medical
credentials of those who espoused them. It just does not seem possible that
a treatment with such a poor reputation today could have worked so well
fifty years ago. Framed in this manner, the story of psychosurgery seems to
force us to make a choice between the perspectives of physicians then and
now, with unfortunate consequences for the former.

In the final analysis, however, health is determined not on an absolute
scale but a relative one, a matter of perceptions. A figure that looks light
against a given background looks dark if shifted before a lighter one. It is a
matter of contrast – and so too in medicine. Thus, the perceived urgency
of medical response depends both upon the backdrop of how intractable a

case looks and the consensus as to what will befall the patient should nothing further be done. Similarly, the perceived benefits and deficits of the intervention are judged against an appraisal of what the patient has left to lose. In addition, the results of any one treatment are judged within the preexisting paradigms of what a patient who is on the mend looks like. In short, as the therapeutic calculus reports only the direction of the pointer, not the magnitude, the slimmest of margins might suffice: small changes in such perceptions thus can have significant effects on clinical decision making. All of these background conditions or perceptions, moreover, are themselves direct products of historical circumstance, and are thus open to change. The efficacy of a treatment is not so stable, after all.

Psychiatrists interpreted the effects of lobotomy as a therapeutic boon because in the context of the 1940s its relative merits stood out in stark contrast and its drawbacks were muted. As has been shown, several circumstances had led to the creation of a large class of patients perceived as in desperate need of a heroic cure. The recent success of the shock therapies for acute patients had drawn attention to the chronic ones who remained untreated and thus uncured; in addition, the failure to improve of many patients who had received a course of active treatment had led to their reclassification as cases of exceptional obdurateness – for them, nothing less drastic was expected to work. In effect, the psychiatric system as a whole had sent patients down a path of increasingly grave action. Psychosurgery's success as a treatment of last resort was thus contingent upon the perception – caused by the newly raised expectations – that for so many patients modern psychiatry had become a failure. Thanks to the appearance of recent statistical surveys, psychiatrists were also convinced that in cases of long-term mental illness the rate of spontaneous improvement was negligible. The patients were not going home on their own. Compounding this overall perception of therapeutic fatalism was the palpable danger of leaving patients on the wards, whose everyday conditions were as dangerous as they were unpleasant. The option of simply leaving patients to their own fate was no longer tenable.

Psychiatrists at the time thus felt a need to do something, at virtually any cost. When Freeman described lobotomy as a "measure of desperation," his statement simultaneously undercut and promoted its use: it both acknowledged the procedure's limited clinical justification and accentuated the widespread need it addressed.[63] In effect, the therapeutic calculus was already set to report favorably upon any treatment that offered even a modest chance of discharge from the institution, even before Strecker popularized the use of lobotomy on hospitalized schizo-phrenics. If clinicians were convinced that a class of patients had "nothing left to lose," it would not take much for a new therapy to attract their notice.

When the physicians looked beyond the discharge statistics and scru-tinized in closer detail what psychosurgery actually did to their patients, they approved of what they saw for several reasons. First, the power to transform a person who had been hounded by unending mental torment into a cheery and unperturbable state was something unique to lobotomy. In today's post-tranquilizer era, it is hard to imagine how highly this attribute was valued, and why it would outweigh even considerable haz-ards and side effects. To John Fulton, who personally witnessed the first American trials of penicillin (which he had brokered and described to Howard Florey in Britain), psychosurgery was just as dramatic in its effects in the mental realm. Moreover, in returning some portion of the patients home, the therapeutic value of lobotomy was further magnified by psychiatry's institutional legacy. In the public's as well as the profes-sion's perspective, the definition of insanity was closely associated with a person's location; to be living at home was considered the most reliable index of mental health. In a private report to Fulton, the director of the Connecticut Cooperative Lobotomy Committee concluded that, if the "primary purpose" of mental hospitals was "to relieve human suffering and to restore patients to happy and productive lives in their homes and communities," then psychosurgery was well suited to the task and de-served the support of all psychiatrists.[64] In fulfilling the exact mission of modern psychiatry, psychosurgery was thus proclaimed a resounding medical success.

These kinds of results, however, held only for those conditions that were considered most favorable for the operation. The great majority of the operations were performed upon chronic schizophrenics, a class of patient that led to more equivocal results. Thanks again to the perception that they had nothing to lose, even small or ambiguous gains were con-sidered valuable – or at least valuable enough to proceed. Indeed, given the prevailing perceptions, it was hard for psychiatrists to imagine how such patients could be any worse off than they already were. (The possibility of a few more holes in an already sinking ship was not considered of much consequence.) The price paid in the alterations of personality and intelli-gence was not considered especially worrisome, for the reason that the state hospitals were filled mostly with men and women of the working class; their livelihoods and social position were not seen as being depen-dent on the higher virtues. The trade-off was acceptable because nobody expected much from this class of person, anyway. Thus, the background against which the side effects of the operation would be judged was already so dark as to cover a multitude of drawbacks. Furthermore, the threshold of tolerance for all kinds of drastic procedures had recently been raised by the wave of shock therapies.

As has also been shown, it was the perceived utility of the operation on those patients who would remain institutionalized that was perhaps the procedure's most successful selling point to those who worked within the harried mental hospitals. In declaring that lobotomy offered a small but nonetheless significant chance of returning chronic schizophrenics home, Strecker ensured a durable place for the procedure within the profession's repertoire. This niche was vastly enlarged, however, by his further claim that physicians might profitably use the procedure for the explicit purpose of transforming noisy, destructive patients into uncomplaining and complacent individuals. Psychiatrists nationwide soon began to sing the praises of lobotomy for its ability to effect "administrative" improvements on the wards.

At first glance, this two-tiered evaluation of the operations would appear to affirm the harshest portrayals of the psychosurgery story, in which the state hospital physicians are thought to have willfully subordinated their responsibilities as physicians to their duties as institutional bureaucrats. It was not therapy that lobotomy delivered, but a powerful means of social control. As argued here, however, this reading is anachronistic and unfair to the participants, who saw little conflict between the two roles. To begin with, the long tradition of psychiatry's institutional legacy had created an environment in which mental illness was necessarily viewed through the lens of hospital administration. Moreover, Adolf Meyer's model of mental disorder had created a framework that was used to remedicalize the wards along sociological lines; the resocialization of patients became the highest road to mental well-being. Lobotomy in particular was viewed as the only treatment able to change the severely mentally ill in such a way that they might rejoin the normal hospital programs. Now even the most deteriorated patients had a chance (however modest) of becoming better hospital citizens, the first step toward reclaimed mental health. Thus, even in the more typical and less ideal cases, the procedure appeared to hospital physicians to transform patients into a condition that approximated, both physically and behaviorally, what someone looked like who was on the road to mental recovery. The results of lobotomy thus made sense within the preexisting system of how mental patients were restored. In sum, from the perspective of psychiatrists in the 1940s, the medical interests of the patient, the hospital, and society at large, had all found a felicitous convergence.

Here, then, is the answer to the opening riddle. Any one of the factors outlined above might have been of sufficient import to sway the consideration of performing a lobotomy in an individual case. At this particular time, in fact, all indications generally pointed in the same direction, collectively providing a powerful argument that programs of psychosurgery were therapeutically useful. However, each of these prevailing perceptions and conditions, against which the effects of lobotomy were measured, was in turn dependent upon specific historical circumstances that might change at any time. Why psychiatrists in the 1940s declared lobotomy an effective treatment yet physicians today strongly disagree is not because either group is necessarily wrong. Rather, the world itself has changed in the interim.

As an "active treatment," psychosurgery was valued in the mental health care systems for its indirect political benefits. And given the conditions of the time, the psychiatric profession saw in the procedure a worthwhile addition to the therapeutic armamentarium. An altogether different issue, however, is not how the *typical* patient came to be operated upon, but a *specific* one. What kinds of factors were brought to bear that would impel a particular physician to recommend an operation on the patient in his office? A closer examination of individual case histories will reveal that such decisions are sited in a specific historical place as well as time; it will also prompt us to rethink the challenges all physicians face when they are engaged in the medical arts.

# 6

## Localizing Decisions
### Psychosurgery and the Art of Medicine

To an ethnographer, sorting through the machinery of distant ideas, the shapes of knowledge are always ineluctably local, indivisible from their instruments and their encasements.

Clifford Geertz (1983)

How did psychiatrists arrive at the conclusion that one of their *own* patients might benefit from a lobotomy? The previous two chapters were concerned primarily with the development of psychosurgery programs within the nation's extensive system of mental hospitals, and with the formation of a consensus among a number of professionals that such a drastic procedure did produce clinical results worth the risks and side effects. Lobotomy worked – at least according to the general standards of mental health and psychiatric practice of the 1940s. This kind of story was told in overview form, as its featured players included scores of psychiatrists, twenty thousand or so lobotomy patients, and almost a half-million other inmates, all scattered among several hundred different institutions throughout the country. Thus far, the analysis has boiled down to sociological conceptions such as the forces of professionalization, institutional pressures, shared ideas of mental health, and the like. Easily lost along the way, however, are the lessons to be learned from the opposite perspective, a close-up examination of events in fine detail. We may have identified what were the characteristics of the average patient selected for the operation, and what was thought to be the usual postoperative course. This is not the same, though, as re-creating why a Mrs. Smith did or did not receive psychosurgery, and what befell her.

At stake in the question is the regard we have for the individual psychosurgeons as practicing physicians. The everyday work of a doctor involves, fundamentally, the process of reasoning which of the available therapies is medically most appropriate for the patient waiting in the consulting room. In the case of those physicians who recommended lobotomy, was there any rigorous method to their attack on madness?

Some of the offhand remarks of the participants are not reassuring on this point. At a 1946 professional meeting in Boston, for example, a group of local physicians just starting up their own psychosurgery programs queried Walter Freeman about what specific kinds of patients were suitable for the operation. Freeman would not be pinned down. "The more this procedure is being used," he noted, "the more indications there are for it." The private conversations among the psychiatrists, as they debated what next to try, could appear even more cavalier, even at the best medical facilities. In 1948 at McLean Hospital, one of the nation's premier private facilities, the possibility of a lobotomy for a female patient with obsessive compulsions was raised in a staff conference. The physician who suggested the procedure was prodded by an associate to explain the medical justification. "Any and all," was his response, a remark that was only partly facetious.[1]

It would be wrong, however, to consider such weak rationales as proof that these doctors were indifferent to the standards of good medical practice. To a large extent, the reluctance of the participants to state in precise clinical terms who would and who would not benefit from a lobotomy stemmed from the psychiatric profession's distrust of its own diagnostic system, a nosology that suffered from widespread inaccuracy and variance. As mentioned earlier, what mattered more to the physicians on the wards than this or that diagnostic label were the particular behavioral and emotional features of their individual patients.

Offhand comments notwithstanding, the devotees of lobotomy clearly were targeting something as they walked the asylum halls. Moreover, the lack of a well-defined, explicit set of protocols for the selection of patients should not be cited as evidence that the psychiatrists themselves held serious doubts about their ability to distinguish likely prospects from poor ones. If anything, as time progressed, some of the physicians who were experienced with the operation grew even more confident in such decisions. To be sure, positive self-perceptions can be misleading, too. The simple fact that the participants may have had a high opinion of their ability to discern the need for a lobotomy in a particular case is not, of course, sufficient reason for observers today to arrive at an equally sanguine assessment.

Ultimately, the only way to arrive at such judgments is through historical case studies. What is needed is a close scrutiny of a selected group of physicians and their patients, re-creating both the contours of this profile that was used to identify particular lobotomy candidates and the logic of its application. Perhaps then it will be clearer how Mrs. Smith's doctor arrived at the conclusion that this procedure might work for her.

The records of the McLean Hospital in Massachusetts provide an exceptional opportunity for just such an intensive study. First, the institution had an active psychosurgery program that lasted more than a decade, and second, it diligently preserved its files in one of the finest archival programs of any mental health facility in the nation. Moreover, the individual patient records at McLean are unusually rich resources, filled with detailed nursing notes, frequent clinical assessments by the medical staff, long and meticulous family histories, correspondence between patients and those on the outside, and even transcriptions of important staff meetings.[2] From these and other materials, it is possible to replicate life on the wards, shadow the nurses as they observe the inmates, react to the hopes and fears expressed by the patients and their families, and overhear the discussions of the hospital psychiatrists as they debated what next to do. One can thus piece together a narrative that traces the overall development of the hospital's program of psychosurgery and, at the same time, reconstruct in some detail how at McLean one patient rather than another came to be selected for lobotomy.

Admittedly, McLean Hospital was a well-financed private hospital, a far cry from the back wards of the state hospitals. What happened within its walls is nevertheless instructive. Whereas the poorest of state hospitals present a scenario of psychiatry at its worst, a milieu in which lobotomies might have been ordered for explicitly nonmedical and hence the wrong reasons, McLean provides a contrary example of medicine at its best, an opportunity to examine the circumstances under which patients were lobotomized for more medical – and thus putatively the right – kinds of justifications. Furthermore, psychiatrists at the state hospitals felt a strong connection to their cousins in the private facilities. If the harsh reality of the wide gap in institutional resources separated the two domains, the ideal of what a practicing psychiatrist should be joined them. The McLean physicians were what the less fortunate psychiatrists aspired to be someday. In this sense, what happened within the walls of McLean resonated throughout the profession.

The chapter opens with an account of how the overall pattern of treatments employed by the McLean physicians was formed in the intersection of several historical currents: the specific nature of the hospital's clientele and the kinds of clinical problems they presented; the long legacy of the institution's commitment to state-of-the-art therapeutics and research; and the distinctive medical orientations of its administrators and staff. As a consequence of these circumstances, at McLean in the 1940s it was more likely than not that some sort of trials of the new brain operations would occur.

The sustained use of lobotomy, though, depended upon whether the staff developed a firm conviction that the procedure had something to offer their own clients. Indeed, at McLean, as at so many other hospitals in the postwar years, the growing satisfaction with the procedure's results led to a rapid increase in the number of operations performed. Here, too, as a description of the hospital's own published and unpublished tallies will indicate, lobotomy's status was soon upgraded from experimental technique to a featured part of the regular treatment program. This kind of summary account simply gauges the extent of the procedure's changing fortune, however. It does not provide much insight into the reasons underlying the physicians' assessments.

To confront this issue the chapter next turns to an examination of the individual patient files at McLean, and a case-by-case reconstruction of what the hospital physicians encountered when evaluating the results of lobotomy. As these materials will demonstrate, it was immediately evident to the staff that the reported power of psychosurgery was no illusion. The dramatic changes in emotional constitution, personality, and behavior were unlike anything they had witnessed before in the treatment of chronically ill mental patients. In the majority of cases, they learned, the effects of the operation were certainly not all beneficial, but a mixture of good and bad. For some patients, the results were unfortunate – even tragic. Most significant of all to the McLean staff, however, were the handful of cases in which the operation had produced a remarkable turn-around, the kinds of "miraculous" results that the advocates of psycho-surgery had bragged about but no one else believed. These examples convinced the staff that, given the presumed hopelessness of the patients under consideration for such a drastic treatment, psychosurgery was worth its risks and detriments.

Once the staff had been persuaded of psychosurgery's potential merit, the next priority was to devise rational guidelines for its use. The third section of this chapter concerns the evolution of these guidelines, the shifting amalgam of clinical indicators that comprised the rules of inclusion and exclusion. Which kind of schizophrenia did best? How old was too old? What was the right length of prior hospitalization? As revealed by the animated discussions in the case conferences, the staff's first attempts to construct a protocol for lobotomy were halting and unsure, and exhibited a heavy reliance upon the work of others to guide their way. As the staff's experience with the procedure grew, so did their self-assurance. Eventually, they came to recognize a good lobotomy candidate when they saw one – or so they said.

Ironically, the reality of what kind of knowledge base the staff had generated for the selection of psychosurgery patients fell far short of the scientific ideal as expressed in the staff conferences. Instead of pointing to well-defined diagnostic criteria – or any other desiderata of medical science – the McLean physicians defended their decisions on the basis of individual clinical judgment. In their considered opinion, the patient simply had what the lobotomy would cure.

What can be inferred about the quality of medicine practiced at this venerable institution from the manner in which the McLean physicians sorted out who should receive a lobotomy? The question hinges, of course, upon the standard against which the practitioners are to be judged. Sometime in the recent past, it is generally assumed, medicine was transformed from an unreliable art into a more trustworthy science. With the essential core of medical practice now generally likened to the work of an applied scientist, the decision to use a particular treatment in an individual case is held roughly equivalent to the process of choosing which solvent to add next in a complex chemical synthesis. From this viewpoint, the story of lobotomy at McLean is useful mostly as a means of dating just how archaic were the practices of 1940s psychiatry, a profession at the time clearly far more art than science.

There is an alternative way of approaching this story, one that calls into question the assumed dichotomy between art and science in medical practice. From this perspective, the story of the McLean physicians is doubly revealing. In addition to the insight it provides about the process by which psychiatrists in this period selected lobotomy, it also occasions a reexamination of our assumptions concerning what it is that physicians actually do – even in the supposedly advanced present.

The kinds of guidelines physicians use are not equivalent to those which aid scientists. In the place of exact formulas that are universally true across time and place, physicians fashion together rough but coherent sets of working rules and guidelines – what may be termed clinical frames – to sort out which modes of action might yield the most reliable results for *their* patients.[3] Such frames are formed in a dialectic inherent to all clinical practice: the dual obligation to work within the profession's standardized norms of therapy and yet, at the same time, abide by the idiosyncratic lessons derived from personal experience. As a matter of practical reality, then, physicians must continually balance the conclusions presented in medical textbooks and journal articles, which are based on thousands of unnamed patients distributed around the globe, against what they personally observe when a handful of local patients, whom they know quite well, undergo similar procedures or medications. What results, then, is a form of knowledge that is neither universal nor absolute but is limited to place as well as era, localized for a given set of problems and conditions. Indeed, it is this continuing tension between the limits of generalized knowledge and the need to respond to the difficulties of particular human beings, I suggest, that renders medicine fundamentally *both* an art and a science: the two aspects are inextricably woven together.

The remainder of the chapter focuses upon the complex way in which such frames are constructed and the consequent constraints within which individual physicians must work. To begin with, even though the eighty lobotomies at McLean did require eighty separate decisions, they were not entirely unrelated events. Through the use of retrospective statistics – that is, comparing the pool of patients selected for the operation to those who were not – it is possible to recapture some of the selection criteria that, consciously or unconsciously, were in the minds of the physicians as they walked along the corridors. A stable clinical frame had emerged.

First, the guidelines did not conform to the kinds of formulas that appear in textbooks. What will emerge from the analysis is a story not of one frame in use but of multiple ones. Psychosurgery was tried on a broad variety of patients for widely varying and even opposite reasons, even when the operations were performed within the same institution and were ordered by the same physicians. At McLean, as at other institutions, the issue of which treatment was given to whom was as much a matter of local clinical geography as it was one of adherence to a preexisting slate of diagnostic indicators that had been set by the profession at large.

Second, as illustrated in the case records, the attempts by the McLean psychiatrists to use psychosurgery in the most effective manner demonstrates another truth about medical practice: namely, the kinds of factors that go into the clinical frame are much broader than those in laboratory science. Indeed, the evaluation of a patient's clinical status involves far more than what transpires in the world beneath the skin. In the psychiatrists' experience, the success of an operation often hinges upon such nonphysiological factors as the attitude of the family, the patient's livelihood (and need for it), and marital status. Cultural and clinical geography are superimposed on the same map.

Third, medical decision making is a less than pristine process, necessarily involving the consideration of factors that are not usually regarded as central to the business of being a good doctor. The psychiatrists at McLean Hospital wore multiple hats. In addition to their role as clinicians, they also acted as administrators, researchers, and social workers. Each of these activities imposed a distinctive perspective as to what was the central problem with the patient and what might be done about it, and thus the task of choosing the most appropriate route of treatment was often compounded by separate and often conflicting value systems.

The answer, then, to why Mrs. Smith's doctor determined that a lobotomy would work for *her* is not to be found in any textbook of the time. There was no good formula available for identifying lobotomy candi-

dates, for the reason that physicians constructed and used their tools in a
manner very different from that of applied scientists. Rather, Mrs. Smith
was judged by her physician to be roughly analogous in psychiatric
makeup and life circumstances to others who had successfully been
treated – by him and his colleagues. Unlike textbook medicine, the clinical
frame had been forged in the intersection of scientific knowledge and the
personal experience of the physician, and included a range of considerations not usually describable in the language of laboratory science.

The previous two chapters have explored how the perceived value of a
drug or procedure is not something derived from its inherent physiological attributes alone, but is generated by the specific context of the time.
Thus it was without contradiction that lobotomy could work at one point
in time but not another. From a closer look at the way in which individual
physicians select a treatment for a given patient, it will become evident
that the clinical frames used for this winnowing process are also bound by
the qualities of the place and circumstances in which they are generated.
Lobotomy might thus might work here but not there; medicine can have
local styles. Finally, as will become evident in the case of psychosurgery at
McLean Hospital, the human dimensions of medical decision making are
not a fault that can be eradicated by additional progress in science but
remain an integral component of what it means to be a physician.

## The Hospital on a Hill

The story of lobotomy at McLean hospital properly begins with the hospital's prior history, its distinctive legacy of providing long-term care for the
most gravely disturbed mental patients and, at the same time, of employing the most advanced therapies regardless of their disciplinary or theoretical origins. The news of Moniz's operation was thus looked upon in
the same pragmatic light as any other therapeutic innovation: as soon as it
was no longer considered to be an experimental risk, it would be introduced onto the wards. The intent was to be neither the first nor the last,
but the best.

If it had been your fate to go insane in mid-twentieth century America,
there was likely no better place to end up than at McLean Hospital in
Waverly, Massachusetts. Not the least important reason was what it said
about who you were. Because it was one of the most elite such facilities in
the nation, if not the world, admittance to McLean meant that your
family was willing and able to spend considerable sums on your behalf,

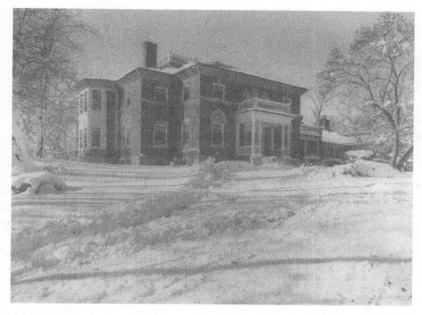

Figure 6.1. McLean Hospital in winter. (Source: McLean Hospital Archives)

perhaps indefinitely. And as McLean was a modestly sized hospital, limited to approximately two hundred beds of which only a portion became available each year, admittance was also contingent upon the personal approval of its staff. Perhaps your father had made the acquaintance of Franklin W. Wood, McLean's director, at a recent charity ball, or maybe your brother-in-law was distantly related to Dr. Stanley Cobb of the Harvard Medical School, who was a neurological consultant on the staff roster. Money wasn't everything.[4]

Then again, deep pockets did make for gracious living. As appealing as were its elite competitors – for instance, the Institute of the Pennsylvania Hospital, Chestnut Lodge, the Austen Fox Riggs Foundation, the Institute of Living, or the Menninger Foundation – none of these matched the sheer pastoral splendor of the McLean environs. In 1895, McLean Hospital was relocated from its prior site in the Somerville section of Boston, which had become an urban slum, to Waverly, a rural suburb seven miles from Cambridge. The new facility was spread out on a hillside of sprawling trees, open meadows, and tasteful gardens, at a site hand-picked by Frederick Law Olmsted, the celebrated landscape designer.[5] In its architecture, the

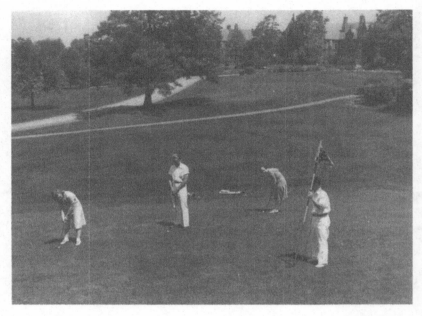

Figure 6.2. McLean Hospital recreation. (Source: McLean Hospital Archives)

reborn institution was a statement against the prevailing fashion of asylum design that followed the "Kirkbride" plan, in which segregated wards radiated outward from centralized facilities. Instead, the trustees looked overseas, to the British mid-century style of scattered cottages. Construction materials included red brick, colored marble, and limestone, with each building individually designed. It would have been difficult for an observer at a distance to discern that this assortment of buildings, which looked like nothing more than a random accumulation of "gentleman's country residences," was in fact a mental hospital. Closer inspection would have revealed such refinements as oak paneling, handsome stairwells, and well-stocked libraries, further confusing matters, as well as a separate Episcopal chapel on the grounds. The necessary administrative offices were confined to a building distinguished by its yellow brick and large circular driveway; the usual institutional infrastructure of steampipes and plumbing, as well as the pathways for the movement of food carts, bedding supplies, and disturbed patients, were all discreetly provided for in a warren of below-ground tunnels. To the trustees, the goal was to construct an environment where "a class of educated people of means" might feel entirely at home, gathered together as "a large family living in different houses."[6]

For those who still maintained – or had recovered – sufficient presence of mind to take full advantage of what McLean had to offer, the days might drift painlessly by, filled with genteel pleasures. Mornings might be spent on workouts at the gymnasium, strolls in the garden, sculpture, or croquet. After a hearty lunch, there were the afternoon teas, piano recitals, billiards, tennis, golf on McLean's own course, and a chance to sunbathe outside or catch up on one's reading. Regular outings with family members, perhaps going shopping or for a drive in the country, were strongly encouraged. Evening entertainment included movies, knitting circles, and listening to opera on the radio. Before retiring, there were milk and cookies.

Lest residents might feel that they were missing any of the small necessities of life, a fully stocked canteen billed them for such sundries as stockings, cigarettes, lipstick, powder puffs, and cocoa butter, and for such services as taxis, music lessons, and the occasional permanent wave. Patients were allowed to maintain extensive personal wardrobes, which they would expand to keep up with their social activities within the hospital or alter to reflect the dictates of current fashion; a housecoat, silk blouse, tweed suit, the right color shoes, a mink stole, and even a kimono might all be within easy reach.[7] Maintenance of proper decorum was a high priority. The better mental institutions liked to idealize themselves as microcosms of the democratic society outside their walls; McLean's inner social reality, though, reflected an even smaller microcosm. To observers on the scene, the true test of whether or not a suffering dowager had fully recovered might boil down to the finesse with which she hosted teas or wrote polite thank-you notes when attending such events sponsored by others.

The nineteenth-century vision of an asylum as a large family endured at McLean as in few other institutions. Believing in the importance of an active family role in the rehabilitation of the patients, the administration expended considerable staff resources in maintaining close contact with the relatives, keeping them up-to-date with significant clinical changes and planning for their next visit. Moreover, as many of the patients entered with conservatorships and trust funds, the hospital was enmeshed in the everyday details of managing the patients' affairs, a responsibility that often did not end with their official discharge.[8] The medical staff, too, was small enough to re-create the kind of professional culture that had existed in an earlier era. Often living on the grounds, the physicians would meet every night for a formal dinner under the patriarchal eye of the director, Franklin W. Wood. Perhaps most significant of all was the lack of a clear boundary between the two cultures. The original asylums were predicated on the assumption that the physicians and patients shared a similar culture, a circumstance that changed radically when the state institutions expanded in the late nineteenth century to include the immigrant poor.[9] At McLean however, with its wards filled by judges, priests, socialites, university professors, businessmen, and artists – and their families – the doctors and the clients often came from the same social strata. The boundaries were further blurred by occasions when the staff at McLean would admit their own relatives. (For years, the wife of one staff physician was a conspicuous such example.)

In stark contrast to the conditions that existed for the hundreds of thousands of citizens who fell into the nation's system of state mental hospitals, patients at McLean suffered no comparable loss of individuality.[10] Here, in some buildings, every patient occupied his or her own room. Social status was not stripped away, but reinforced in comforting ways. Nurses and attendants were instructed to refer to patients by their proper names, exhibiting as much deference as possible, while physicians approached them "as equals and companions." If anything, McLean prided itself on its ability to cater to the individual wishes and whims of its clients, within reason. "If the patient did not like the lamb we served for dinner and asked for lobster," remembered a former steward, "we gave lobster." The hospital was able to provide service like "the Ritz Carlton," he added, for the simple reason that the patients could afford it.[11]

Such an idyllic picture was of course just a surface reality. The hotel-like atmosphere pervaded only a portion of the total environment at McLean. Indeed, many sanitaria at the time excelled McLean in the sumptuousness of their facilities, suggesting even closer approximations of country club resorts. Channing, Ring, Wiswall, and Valley Head, for example, all were within traveling distance from Boston and were filled with an equally illustrious clientele. The difference between them and McLean, however, was not a matter of economics, but of morbidity. These other institutions were the first line of defense for individuals with acute or relatively minor complaints or disturbances. Grandmamma was having one of her fits, mother was tired and needed a summer off, William Jr. was suspected of sleeping with the wrong kind of person, Uncle George had gone on a bender again – the indiscretions and problems of the well-to-do were thus quietly and tactfully swept out of view.[12] Whole families would cycle through the same institution, one generation dutifully following the other; its solicitous superintendent would assume the role of a concerned godfather who was armed by his extensive foreknowledge of the family's hidden skeletons. Once admitted, clients who manifested serious mental or behavioral disturbances tended to scare off the rest of the guests, however. When this happened, the superintendent would regretfully inform the family that the sanitarium no longer could be responsible for the care of their loved one, and would offer to place the call for them to McLean Hospital.

What set McLean apart from the other sanitaria was its willingness to accept and care for, on an open-ended basis, patients suffering from severe or chronic mental illnesses.[13] On any given day, its clientele thus exhibited the same kinds of clinical problems on display at any state hospital. Similar to the large mental institutions, McLean was comprised of a series of graded behavioral environments that ranged from the "open" or "higher" wards like Appleton House and Belknap for women to the "lower" and hence "worse" wards of Codman Hall, East House, and, lowest of all, the "locked" ward of Wyman. Within each building the floors were also rated, from I to III ("I" being lowest), further differentiating the levels of disturbance.[14]

Unlike the state hospitals, as much as 50 percent of McLean's admissions were voluntary, which accounted for its better wards being filled with patients who might sustain the illusion of a country club atmosphere. The pleasant veneer merely concealed the darker aspects of life in a mental hospital, however. Even though some individuals might live quite nicely on a good ward for months if not years, they did so in the uneasy knowledge that they were surrounded by trapdoors to harsher environments, which in turn had their own trapdoors to even worse places. (As in the hallucinatory world in which Lewis Carroll deposited his suffering Alice, at McLean Hospital people suddenly came and went, and in the strangest of ways.) A tour of the rest of the wards at McLean thus would reveal a clinical terrain not unlike that found in the largest of mental institutions. Here, too, catatonics, involutionals, agitated depressives, and the senile might be observed to denude themselves, bang their heads on the furniture, smear feces on the walls, sit in puddles of urine, scream through the night, and stare off into space for months at a time. McLean Hospital was visible proof of the psychiatric adage that the privileges of race, class, and wealth provide no sure defense against the ravages of mental illness. Fine trappings notwithstanding, the possibility of total mental dissolution was always there, in the shadows.

What McLean was able to offer, for those whose minds did come apart, was a level of around-the-clock care that was truly second to none. State hospital administrators could only fantasize about both the extent and quality of nursing that was a reality at McLean. During the first few months of a patient's stay at McLean, the monitoring was nonstop; a day nurse as well as a night nurse might enter daily a full page of detailed notes into the patient's chart. Such reports reveal the close attention paid to the patients' social interactions, mood swings, deviation from normal routines, and standards of personal grooming and hygiene, as well as such physical matters as dietary intake, frequency of elimination, coughs, and headaches. The nurses were always at the ready with soothing words, assistance in getting dressed and eating, a sponge bath, an ace bandage, or castor oil. At the same time, McLean was also distinguished by its high level of medical care, general as well as psychiatric. Thanks to the corporate ties between McLean and Massachusetts General, as well as the Harvard University Medical School, the patients could expect that their physical ailments would receive the finest medical attention. (Patient records were filled with the same kinds of specialist reports and laboratory findings that might appear in the leading university hospitals.) As for the caliber of its psychiatric staff, McLean was successful in attracting men and women of the highest standards, who represented a broad range of training and interests, from psychoanalysis to metabolic research. When a patient was consigned to the care of McLean, his or her family knew that, if it was within the power of medicine to reclaim their loved one, they need look nowhere else. They could take comfort from the knowledge that whether custodial care or the latest in medical intervention was required, everything possible would be done.

## Clinical Orientation

By the 1940s, McLean boasted a rich legacy in the care of the mentally ill. Founded in 1811, one of the first asylums to be organized in America, its initial string of directors were at the forefront of institutional treatment of the insane. And when Edward J. Cowles assumed control in 1879, he set the institution on a path that would assure it a preeminent place in psychiatry well into the next century. Cowles's energies were devoted mostly to the relocation of the hospital, an arduous undertaking that was hampered by fluctuating financial conditions. In addition, however, Cowles championed a new vision of psychiatry in which the medical care of insane patients would derive from advances in psychology and physiology. The depth of his commitment was evidenced by his decision to spend a sabbatical year – an unusual decision at the time – with G. Stanley Hall at Johns Hopkins, studying the new experimental psychology.

He began by organizing in 1882 the nation's first training school for nurses involved in the care of mental patients, a move that would insure a supply of an educated and professional staff in the decades to come. Next, in 1890, much to the displeasure of the trustees, Cowles hired a young researcher, William Noyes, committing the institution to financing one of the only such laboratories in the nation. (Noyes's research successors would shortly include such future notables as psychiatrist August Hoch, psychologists Shephard Ivory Franz and F. Lyman Wells, and biochemist Otto Folin.) Also under Cowles's stewardship, McLean invested in a medical library, transformed record keeping from ward books to individual folders, and began a tradition of regular scientific meetings – all forward-looking innovations.[15]

In the 1930s, McLean again revamped. From 1932 until 1948, the administrative functions were controlled by Director Wood, and the clinical responsibilities were supervised by Kenneth J. Tillotson, Psychiatrist-in-Chief. Tillotson had come to the hospital with a strong vision of where he believed the future of psychiatry lay, a vision that was steeped in Adolf Meyer's eclectic doctrine of psychobiology. "In speaking of psychiatry I am using the term in its broad sense," Tillotson told the Boston Society of Psychiatry and Neurology in 1932, "and with the connotation that it should have." Such a heading, he argued, should include "all that is concerned with mental disorder," problems that "range from the simplest maladaptations to situations and environment to the most intricate psychotic conditions where manifold factors of body and mind take their part." As to particular clinical orientation, McLean's philosophy was to follow the teachings of Meyer, who counseled the need to view the patient as a whole, thus avoiding "a strict adherence to any particular school." "On our hospital staff," Tillotson stated, "we have attempted to get personnel with a wide range of experience and a diversification of opinion." Organicists and functionalists, biochemists and psychologists, Kraepelinians and Freudians, he claimed, were all hard at work at McLean. (Tillotson's own career included some analytic training, a penchant for arcane sociological theory, and laboratory-based physiological research.) The common goal of all these diverse approaches, he stated, was exactly the Meyerian standard of "restoring those who have failed to make satisfactory adjustments to life." True medical advances in psychiatry, Tillotson also expounded, would only come about when the modern mental hospital reflected the same combination of treatment, training, and research found in other specialties.[16]

Over the next decade or so, Tillotson set about transforming McLean into this vision of the modern mental hospital. (The vision was by no means unique to McLean, as the Meyerian model dominated professional ideology; few places, however, had the resources to realize it as fully.) Clinical ward rounds were established, entailing staff conference presentations on individual patients. The resident training program was expanded, and the ties to Harvard Medical School were strengthened, with medical students rotating through on a regular basis. The commitment to

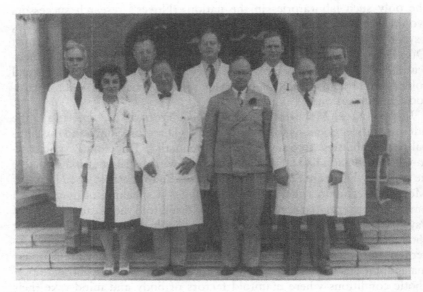

Figure 6.3. McLean Hospital staff, 1948. The staff present are: *back row,* Howard, Carter, Hallenbeck, Perry, and Jossman; *front row,* Lorenz, Tillotson, Director Wood, and Tompkins. (Source: McLean Hospital Archives)

basic science was extended with the work of John C. Whitehorn (then current chairman of the APA's Committee on Research), which was followed by the opening of a freestanding research division headed by Jordi Folchi-Pi, a future pioneer in neurochemistry. Links between the laboratory and the wards were established with the recruitment of Mark Altschule, an early advocate of clinical physiology in psychiatry.[17] Treatment and care were changing as well. In his speech, Tillotson noted that admissions patterns were shifting, with important consequences for clinical policy. Larger numbers of acute psychotic and psychoneurotic patients were showing up at their doors, exactly the kinds of patients who might benefit from medical advances. Staff and personnel had to be increased, along with significant additions to the occupational therapy department, laboratory facilities, and hydrotherapy equipment, all with the explicit objective of curing or restoring the recently admitted patient.[18]

Everywhere he looked in the 1930s, Tillotson observed that the hospital was reawakening to the challenge of modern mental health care. In addition to the rejuvenated hospital programs, new specialized modes of psychiatric care were introduced in rapid succession. Beginning in the middle of the decade, formal psychoanalysis had been initiated in a small number of patients. Although McLean was by no means a Freudian outpost, several members of its staff made use of the opportunity provided by the hospital to take analytic training in Boston. Rather, McLean vigorously promoted the importance of psychological contact between patients and physicians, a mode of intervention that fit well with the institution's ideology of individually based treatment and resocialization. "The various types of psychotherapy," stated the *Annual Report*, ". . . always claim first place of importance in any psychiatric hospital such as ours."[19]

At the same time that McLean was moving toward this psychotherapeutic goal, the new somatically oriented treatments also were introduced, though with an initial reluctance. Priding itself as "conservative" in the use of any kind of medication (for example, at McLean the preferred means of calming agitated patients was hydrotherapy and other labor-intensive responses rather than heavy sedation), the hospital was not one of the first facilities to try out shock treatments. At the end of 1937, however, Tillotson noted that the hospital was proceeding forward with shock therapy, due to "the demand for its use by professional colleagues as well as by the relatives of patients." It so happened that in 1938, Manfred Sakel, the European inventor of insulin shock treatment, was on an extended tour of the United States; characteristically, McLean engaged him to oversee personally the procedure's introduction in Waverly. The hospital was not, however, especially thrilled with either insulin or metrazol shock, which were also tried; the arduousness and hazards of such procedures did not sit well with what its clientele had come to expect in the way of treatment. Moreover, McLean was still primarily a facility housing chronic mental invalids, the kinds of patients for whom shock treatments yielded what were judged to be only temporary improvements.[20] The hospital appeared to be more immediately impressed by the results of its experimental trial with psychosurgery, which was first performed on a male agitated depressive in March 1938, and then on another in February 1939.[21]

What Tillotson – and, by extension, the clinical staff – were *really* excited about were the results of a new program of treatment known as "Total Push," in which the patient's body and mind together were reinvigorated. As Tillotson described it, Total Push was based on "principles of activating, retraining and re-educating the inactive, apathetic, dilapidated and deteriorated patients," through implementation of an "active program of physiotherapy, exercise, games and occupational and diversional therapy"; this was used in conjunction with vitamins, ultraviolet, and special diets.[22]

By the beginning of the Second World War, the cumulative effect of all the above developments had resulted in a sense that psychiatry at McLean had dramatically quickened and intensified. The combination of shorter hospitalizations and the incorporation of the "more active types of therapy," Tillotson wrote in the *Annual Report*, "has tended to activate the psychiatric work," so that the hospital had developed "an intensive therapeutic program for every patient admitted" – a theme reiterated over the next few years. Moreover, with the additions to the research staff, nursing services, roster of medical residents, specialist consultants, and the department of psychology, McLean was moving forward once again. There was even some suggestion that psychiatry no longer would rest content with reaching the right diagnosis or obtaining insight into a psychopathology. The new goal, Tillotson noted, was to find "some means of eradicating the morbid condition."[23]

The war years, however, soon forced McLean to alter course. Extreme shortages in personnel led the institution to take such steps as shutting down some wards and limiting admissions. In treatment, the first casualties were the Total Push program and the wide availability of psychotherapy. In their place, McLean redoubled the somatic interventions of electric shock, subcoma insulin, and prefrontal lobotomy, which required far less hospital labor. (In 1941, the introduction of electric shocks supplanted the use of insulin shock.) Setting the stage for a dramatic upswing in the use of such treatments, the *Annual Report* in 1945 noted that, although these "drastic therapies" were in fact being used "empirically," nevertheless they "unquestionably produce profound alterations in the internal biological milieu."[24] The use of electric shock would peak in 1948, when one hundred and fourteen patients received it, while ambulatory insulin crested in 1947, with one hundred patients.[25] Neither treatment was perceived to make all that much difference for the severely mentally ill, however. For them, the hospital turned to psychosurgery.

### Frontal Assault

The hospital's first series of lobotomy patients ended in 1941, after three male and two female agitated depressives were sent to Massachusetts General Hospital for a lobotomy by W. Jason Mixter, the renowned neurosurgeon. In 1945, a second wave was commenced when lobotomies were given to nine women of varying diagnoses, who had a median length of hospitalization of over seven and a half years. The *Annual Report* for that year noted that the procedure "has proven highly beneficial to certain patients whose behavior and aggressive psychotic symptoms rendered them incapable and unresponsive to all forms of treatment and constructive nursing and medical care." Such good results, it added, were leading them to consider it for patients of shorter-term hospitalization.[26]

McLean's expanding program of psychosurgery generally reflected national as well as local patterns. As a result of the publicity surrounding Strecker's use of lobotomy on chronic schizophrenics, the procedure had taken on a special allure for facilities such as McLean Hospital. Massachusetts, in particular, was quick to begin the use of psychosurgery on the long-term institutionalized insane; special committees were set up by the Department of Mental Hygiene in the early 1940s to investigate its potential. Beginning in October 1943, the Boston Psychopathic Hospital started an ambitious psychosurgery program, drawing patients from around the state hospital system, who were shipped there specifically for the treatment and then sent back. Under Harry Solomon, the program grew into one of the largest in the nation. In the small neuropsychiatric community of Boston, personnel often overlapped in the various institutions, however, and it was not long before professional currents that appeared at one location showed up at another. (Harry Solomon, for example, was also an active member of McLean's consulting staff, and recommended a lobotomy on a patient there as early as September 1945.)[27]

The first public discussion of McLean's second wave of lobotomy came at the January 1946 meeting of the Boston Society of Psychiatry and Neurology, when Tillotson and Frederick Wyatt (McLean's psychologist) met with Jason Mixter and Harry Solomon to discuss a paper presented by Walter Freeman. Tillotson used the occasion to describe McLean's positive results with eleven chronic schizophrenics, and how the success was due largely to the intensive Total Push program of reeducation. Significantly, Tillotson also broached the possibility that, if the physicians were sure of their diagnosis, "why should not prefrontal lobotomy be done early?"[28] Indeed, from this point on, McLean's program was no longer limited to cases of very long-term institutionalization, a shift that would account for much of its rapid expansion during the next few years.

Another nine patients were operated upon in 1946, three of them men. The *Annual Report* found it remarkable that about 50 percent of the lobotomy recipients, who otherwise "would become continuous treatment and chronic hospital patients," were now able to leave the hospital, requiring only minimal supervision. Some of them were even now able to "resume active and useful vocations." Thanks to an upgraded surgical facility on the premises, patients selected for lobotomy no longer had to be transported under guard to Massachusetts General, a difficult undertaking. (Mixter now traveled to McLean; with surgical fees running as high as $600 an operation, psychosurgery had become a lucrative side-specialty.) In the following year, the *Annual Report* somewhat obliquely remarked that "we have been conservative in the selection of our patients" for psychosurgery, and then announced that an additional seventeen operations had been performed. (The fourteen operations performed during the calendar year of 1947 would in fact be the peak period of lobotomy's use at McLean.) Again, the hospital authorities were impressed by the "remarkable results."[29]

In 1948, J. Butler Tompkins, the psychiatrist who had been chief of the Women's Division during the initiation of the second wave, published a report in the *American Journal of Psychiatry* on the hospital's experience with thirty-six patients. The brief account indicated that all but two had been benefited by the procedure, and that half were able to live fairly normal lives at home. Tompkins attributed the good results to "the individualized postoperative hospital care" available at McLean. After summarizing Tompkins's findings, the 1948 *Annual Report* stated that intensive study of the psychosurgery patients by the hospital's psychologist, Frederick Wyatt, failed to determine any major intellectual or emotional deficits caused by the procedure.[30] During this year, another twelve lobotomies were performed, all on female patients.

The year 1948 also saw changes in hospital staffing, which among other consequences had a potential for greatly reducing the interest in the psychosurgery program. Tompkins, Dorr Hallenbeck, and Frederick Wyatt, all physicians who were closely involved with the psychosurgery patients, had tendered their resignations. More significant, however, was the sudden resignation of Tillotson, which placed Paul Howard in the post of acting chief psychiatrist (a position he would fill for the next seven years). Howard was even more psychodynamically oriented than was his predecessor, and the *Annual Report* soon reflected this emphasis. Whereas Tillotson would write of the value of psychotherapy within a psychiatric institution, Howard simply defined McLean as a "psychotherapeutic hospital." Nevertheless, this did not mean that McLean would beat a quick retreat from the shock treatments and lobotomies. As elsewhere, the priority in this period was still that of using any available "active treatment" that worked; the supposed deep antagonism between somatic interventions and psychotherapy was often more rhetoric than reality. (It is interesting to note that one of Tompkins's prior publications, which appeared in *The Psychoanalytic Review,* was a description of a case of penis envy.) At McLean, the one was in fact interpreted as a route to the other. "One of the more cheerful aspects of hospital psychiatry today," Howard explained in the 1949 *Annual Report,* was that the "newer physiological influences have softened rigid psychotic symptoms or persistent anxiety," leading to a greater accessibility to psychotherapy. For beyond the "dramatic alterations in the course of psychosis and neurosis brought about by physiological, medical, and nutritional treatment, or by electric shock, insulin, and lobotomy – lie the personality needs of each maladjusted person."[31]

After another ten lobotomies were performed in 1949, Howard took it upon himself to prepare an internal report on the hospital's experience with psychosurgery, which to date had amounted to a series of over sixty patients. In the mostly favorable paper, which was delivered at a McLean staff conference, Howard noted that 45 percent of these patients were living outside of the hospital, and of those discharged, one-third lived without supervision, one-third with only mild supervision, and the rest required considerable care. Of the patients remaining in the hospital, most showed a moderate degree of improvement, "perhaps moving up a ward," with only a few cases showing no or little improvement. "Almost all observers agree," Howard emphasized, "that the patients become more contented individuals and have a more satisfactory existence than before the operation." He described how one patient was given a lobotomy "because she would almost certainly have killed herself if she had not been operated upon." After lobotomy, the patient "was still the same person and could feel the same tensions, but they no longer piled up on her." Now, "she reads, takes college courses, got herself a job, and has expanded her social life." The audience was invited to listen in on a psychiatric interview with the patient, as Howard had brought along a phonographic recording of the session. "I think the few brief sentences that I will play," Howard suggested, "will show her intellectual preservation, her social and personal sensitiveness and the relief of the misery which she formerly suffered."[32]

One gathers from the talk itself that, in Howard's opinion, lobotomy was still poorly understood, and in the individual case a definite gamble, but nonetheless justly occupied a prominent role in the therapeutic armamentarium. There was a pressing need, Howard noted, to do something about the chronic invalids who were a drain on the nation's resources; one could not ignore the operation's indisputable ability to relieve suffering. In short, the hospital staff had responded to the news about psychosurgery with the same mixture of caution and then deliberate action with which it had investigated the potential of any other new therapy on the scene. They consulted with the relevant medical experts and then introduced the procedure into McLean with the assistance of the finest technicians available. Before making any final commitments to an expanded program, however, the hospital staff waited until they could examine the results themselves. They would make up their own minds. Once convinced, the method would be assigned a consistent role within the rest of the hospital program.

At McLean, the obligations that went along with the nineteenth-century concept of elite stewardship were very much alive. The self-conscious goal of the staff at Waverly was to be neither too eager nor too hesitant to commit to a new mode of therapy; their duty was to school themselves in any procedure or intervention as soon as it had established itself as offering a reasonable chance of benefit. Duly appreciative of their unique position within the profession, the physicians at McLean felt obliged to add to the store of practical knowledge surrounding psychiatric treatment; they could investigate new techniques to a depth not available to others. And so too with psychosurgery. Thus, Howard introduced his report with the statement that lobotomy was "one of the therapeutic approaches which is being worked out at the present time." The contribution of these approaches at McLean would be not one of surgical mechanics or physiological understanding but one of refinement in use. The staff ventured into such matters sure in the knowledge that what was learned locally, in their own carefully tended garden of psychopathology, would eventually trickle down to influence others throughout the profession. Compared to their peers at such places as the Menninger Foundation or the Institute of the Pennsylvania Hospital, who often publicly campaigned before lay as well as professional audiences on various psychiatric issues, the staff at McLean were more reticent and subdued. Sometimes a soft-spoken, measured voice holds greater authority.

## The Good, the Bad, and the Mixed

Although the program of psychosurgery at McLean might have originated in the institution's long-standing interests and particular approach to psychiatry, the continued use of the procedure was dependent on what the staff encountered on a case-by-case basis. To the hospital's psychiatrists, the results that mattered most were not those that occurred in distant institutions and were described in the medical literature, but the ones witnessed with their own eyes.

If the physicians at McLean were pressed to explain why they supported the use of psychosurgery, they might point to any of a number of patients who had experienced the remarkable results referred to in the *Annual Report*. To begin with, there was Fay Francis, a middle-aged manic-depressive woman (with some additional schizoid features), who had seen at least eight of the leading psychiatrists and physicians in Boston in the years before her admission to McLean in 1941. Harry Solomon had been brought in for a personal consultation. "The main point," Solomon wrote in the clinical note following the visit, "is that spontaneous improvement is not to be expected," and that "the chances of this are so small that it needs really no consideration." His conclusion: "Lobotomy is advised." Operated on in October 1945, Mrs. Francis was discharged to the care of her husband in 1948. A year later, the husband wrote to the staff that the patient was once again leading a normal life. Except for one seizure, he stated, "the operation has been a complete success."[33]

Two other women with manic-depressive conditions, both elderly, also seemed to do well following their operations in 1947 and 1948, respectively. Before lobotomy, Mrs. Abigail Banks was overwhelmed by having to make even the smallest decisions and would pace the hallways, mumbling, "O God, O God, why don't they let me go home?" Following a lobotomy, Mrs. Banks was in fact sent home. Her husband, a prominent judge, reported to the staff: "She is, and has been, in excellent condition. She engages in all the activities she formerly did – church, shopping, lectures, seeing friends, etc. The results of the operation performed by Dr. Mixter seemed a miracle to me. It still does."[34] Then there was Mrs. Ruth Ignatius, a middle-aged housewife with a neurotic depression, who was haunted by morbid thoughts and her own desire to die. After long courses of psychotherapy, insulin shock, and electroshock had failed, psychosurgery was tried. A year or so after her discharge from the hospital, her husband wrote that his wife was fine, and that they had just returned from a summer vacation which they both enjoyed. "We want to thank the hospital for making her well," he closed.

The staff also encountered some good results with several types of severe psychoses. Lenora Hutchins, a young woman admitted to McLean in 1947, was described as a schizophrenic with a "ten-year story of bizarre behavior and delusions." A year after the lobotomy, her father told the staff that she was active in her church, sang in the choir, and was employed in a factory forty-eight hours a week. In short, he was happy to report that his daughter "leads a normal life." Two women diagnosed as catatonic, Gladys Randall and Adelaide Hitchcock, also were judged to have had good results. Mrs. Randall was described as greatly relieved of tenseness, depressive feelings, and feelings of apprehension. Her husband reported that she was doing all the housework and shopping, and was maintaining a cheerful mood; it was his opinion that she was now better than she had been for years. In Miss Hitchcock's case, the operation was judged to have made a "tremendous improvement," as she was active, social, and coherent in her thoughts. As she had been a piano instructor, it was particularly significant that her musical abilities were spared by the operation; the hospital's own music instructor formally evaluated her playing ability as exceptional and unchanged since the lobotomy. A year after discharge, the condition of Miss Hitchcock was reported to the staff by her personal physician, who was pleased to note that she was, on the whole, greatly improved and free of any evidence of psychosis; Miss Hitchcock was once again gainfully teaching piano.

There were also several examples of paranoid schizophrenia responding to psychosurgery. The husband of Elizabeth Hanley was enthusiastic about the results of her operation, stating that in all respects his wife was entirely the person of previous years, before her illness had begun. Mrs. Anna Winthrop was a housewife and mother described as having been mentally ill for ten years. The staff, as well as her husband, noted that the operation had caused a profound change in her personality. Although her behavior was far from perfect, and she had some difficulty following through on her duties, the husband emphasized that should he be given a choice of his wife in her current condition or the way she had been even before her illness developed, he would select her as she was today.[35]

Mrs. Mary Sullivan was in her late thirties, an Irish Catholic housewife who had led an active social and intellectual life, writing the occasional paper on poetry and philosophy. Her troubles began when her husband was shipped overseas during the war, and she was forced to move home to her parents. At first restless and irritable, she became increasingly suspicious and began to talk about telepathic experiments. When her parents no longer could cope with her, she was sent to a state hospital where she remained for half a year. Released, she eventually rejoined her husband, now stateside, but the mystical experiences returned. Growing terrified of her hallucinations, she eventually committed herself to McLean Hospital. Then, discharging herself against the physicians' advice, Mrs. Sullivan returned home, but only briefly. She would pace the floor for days on end, forgoing sleep, would refuse to bathe or let others touch her clothes, and gradually lost all interest in her surroundings. After she was shipped back to McLean Hospital, various treatments such as ambulatory insulin were found to leave unchanged her "paranoid, stubborn . . . and essentially hostile personality," and she remained tense and experienced constant hallucinations. Mrs. Sullivan bitterly resisted the decision that she should have a lobotomy, and on the day of the operation fought and struck the nurses as they tried to prep her.

Only two weeks after psychosurgery, the staff physicians were amazed at what they saw. To their astonishment, Mrs. Sullivan was active and outgoing, playing cards, going on field trips with her husband, and with much zeal planning to redecorate her apartment. "The change in the patient's psychiatric condition following the operation was dramatic and remarkably extensive," her physician at McLean somewhat breathlessly reported. After a few days of postlobotomy lethargy, Mrs. Sullivan began to take a great deal of interest in all hospital activities. She gave no further evidence of hallucinations and became much more friendly. Her husband felt that she had essentially regained her pre-psychotic personality. In interviews with the doctor she discussed her period of psychosis with amazing insight. . . . She even admitted that the operation had helped her a great deal as she now could keep these ideas out of her mind. Her only complaint about the effect of the operation was that she seemed to be able to enter into the reading of books a little less completely. She expressed this by saying that the emotions when reading had previously been in colors and were now more black and white. She appeared genuinely to feel that this loss was more than compensated by the gain in comfort, ability to concentrate, and efficiency.

"From the standpoint of the doctor observing the patient," Dr. James Harmon concluded, "the change away from paranoia, poorly controlled hostility, and unreasonable stubbornness, was remarkable."[36]

The same doctor also was quite taken by the results of psychosurgery in the case of Mrs. Catherine Birmingham, a divorcee in her late thirties with several small children to support. Upon her admittance in 1946, Mrs. Birmingham was given month after month of insulin shock treatments. For a time thereafter, her behavior was usually pleasant and friendly, though changeable. She spent the summer months at library teas, movies, and sunning herself on the grounds. The most disagreeable moments surrounded the visit of her mother. Gradually, though, she retreated from hospital life and shunned psychotherapeutic interviews with the physicians. The clinical notes indicate that, in general, "she presents a complete picture of cynicism, bitterness and withdrawal." By October 1947, her vulgar outbursts and verbal abuse caused her to be transferred from Codman to Wyman, where she would spend the day "just sitting and passing out caustic comments to the world as it flows past her." A lobotomy was performed upon her in the following month, and by April, Harmon reported that "She has undergone a major and truly remarkable change for the better." In the course of her psychotherapeutic interview, the patient

exhibited none of the highly defensive, sarcastic, cynical conversation which had been so consistently present at all other times during her present hospitalization. She spoke of the various events of her life during the past few years in what seemed to be an eminently reasonable fashion. For the first time during the year and a half that the observer has known her, she spoke of herself in a serious fashion, and did not in any way indicate contempt with her surroundings or with the general set of rules and regulations by which the world operates. In discussing her operation, she stated that she felt it had done her a great deal of good, in that her swings of mood were not as great as they had been before. . . . in practically all respects, the patient's attitude and behavior during this interview were almost diametrically opposed to everything which she has shown during her year and one half in this hospital. Her excellent behavior during the past month would suggest that the improvement noted during this interview was not just a fleeting change, but represents a sustained change in the patient's personality. It is difficult to find words to describe this change, but one can not help saying that it is one of the most dramatic changes which could be imagined in an entire personality as a result of a pre-frontal lobotomy. The patient is literally a different person than she was during all of her hospital stay prior to the operation. . . . She might adjust very well outside the hospital, although one would certainly have hesitated to predict or even imagine this three months ago.

The following month, Harmon added that "Perhaps the best indicator of the patient's improvement is the fact that her mother seems to have lost, during a period of three or four weeks, almost all of the considerable apprehensiveness which she previously had with regard to the patient's behavior." The mother later confirmed this rosy assessment. She reported to the hospital, a year after the patient's discharge:

I am very glad to give you a good report of my daughter. In 1948, she remarried her former husband, the ceremony performed in a Roman Catholic church, in the presence of the necessary witness and their little children. [My daughter] has no outside assistance in the house-work, takes great interest in cooking, . . . and keeps the house in excellent order. She appears equable, cheerful, and responsible, defers to her husband, who seems to be very wise with her, drawing her into outside activities, music, lectures, etc. The relationship between the two appears to be very harmonious. . . . Another marked improve-ment since her remarriage is the gentle tone of her talk, now kindly. . . . We are all amazed at the improvement which her treat-ment at the hospital achieved, and which should be an immense hope for other sufferers.

Not just families but patients themselves might communicate with some passion the positive changes in their life following a lobotomy. Mrs. Sarah Worthington, a housewife and mother in her forties, was admitted in the fall of 1947 with what was described as a neurotic depression. In the previous half-decade or so, Mrs. Worthington had shown a gradual emo-tional decline that culminated in a suicide attempt in 1946. At the staff conference in September that was held to determine her course of treat-ment, she was described as aggressive and paranoid; the general consensus was that neither insulin nor electroshock would do much for her. Neither would psychotherapy, for as Dr. Herbert Averbuck commented, "about five years of analysis might or might not help," for "there is nothing to go back to in her case." That winter, she was discovered on the ward in a barbiturate-induced coma, a suicide attempt from which she eventually recovered. Over the next few months, the treatment plan consisted of electroshocks followed by psychotherapeutic interviews. The physician who conducted the interviews with Mrs. Worthington described them as extremely depressing events, in which the patient would replay every distressing moment of her life, drenching herself with tears. The fact that Mrs. Worthington remained so depressed following electroshock was evidence that "the problem remains an extremely difficult and dangerous one, for which no ready solution is apparent at the present time."

A lobotomy was performed in the late spring. The patient's progress was considered so exceptional that a staff conference was arranged in which the patient might be exhibited to the whole staff. (Such *post-treatment* conferences were rare events.) After she left the room, one physician present declared that Mrs. Worthington was obviously quite friendly and responsive, with a "good deal of pleasure and spark." In the clinical note following the conference, her assigned physician ventured an explanation for Mrs. Worthington's excellent condition. "The patient seems to have derived a good deal of protection from the overwhelming accumulation of her depressive feelings," he elaborated. Moreover, he added, "It seems justifiable to say that the lobotomy has given her a chance to solve these problems in a way which no previous therapy had succeeded in doing." The clinical records also indicate that her postsurgery IQ was measured at 134 – higher than it had been before lobotomy.

In the year after her discharge from the hospital, Mrs. Worthington continued to meet with Dr. Harmon for weekly psychotherapeutic interviews held in an office at Massachusetts General. She was employed by a retail store to demonstrate merchandise before women's clubs; she had done so well there that she was due for a promotion. Several years later, her improvement seemed to be continuing; she had even been advanced to a supervisory position in her job. The patient wrote to Dr. Harmon:

> I have been wishing to write to you a note of appreciation, not a sentimental gushing expression of gratitude but an honest expression of how I feel in regard to your work with me over these many months. In my usual inarticulate manner I can not find the right words for the right places and will be forced to fall back upon concrete pictures and expressions. When I first came to the hospital I was in a room with no doors, no outlets. My only companions were Fear and Hopelessness. It was grim. Gradually throughout all of this time you have made me

see for myself that particular room (which actually seems to have been of my own choosing) has doors. I am the one who must open them. I, myself.

The picture emerging for the staff at McLean Hospital, of the therapeutic possibilities of psychosurgery, was its extraordinarily broad range of utility, results seen with their own eyes across a wide variety of conditions and ages. What was so interesting to the staff about Sarah Worthington was the operation's helpfulness in the case of a patient whose mental capacities were generally well preserved before the operation but whose inner torments had crippled her daily living. If it was psychotherapy that enabled her to cope once again with the stresses of everyday life, it was the emotional change in her nature brought about by psychosurgery that was assumed to have made the psychotherapy possible.

The case of Rose Whitehall Thorner demonstrated to the staff what psychosurgery could do to reclaim (even if partially) a patient who existed at the far end of the spectrum – that is, one who had deteriorated so far in her mental state as to be hardly recognizable to her former self, if such a hypothetical meeting might ever be arranged. Truly, for Mrs. Thorner, as in her descent, there were not many rungs left before she would reach hell itself.

### Rose's Story

Rose Thorner was one of the more troublesome patients on the ward. A middle-aged woman diagnosed with involutional melancholia, by 1947 she was already a ten-year veteran at McLean, with no end in sight. At her original admission, her eldest son detailed her life history in a three-hour interview. The highlights are as follows. Born to a financially secure family, Rose Whitehall was shepherded through the usual parade of boarding schools, the natural endpoint of which was an active life as a young socialite in New York City, where plans for gala parties were interspersed with trips abroad. She was known both as a charming hostess, often becoming the life of a party, and as a very religious High Episcopalian. Married in her twenties to Harry Thorner, a successful professional, Rose was soon occupied as the mother of several children, one of whom was described as mentally deficient. Her emotional troubles began during the Great Depression and were intensified when her husband killed himself after a period of despondency. In the months following the suicide, family and friends expected it was but a matter of time before she too would "crack." In fact, shortly thereafter Rose "went to pieces" during a game of bridge and was shuttled through a series of sanitaria. Found by them to be too hard to handle, she was shipped off to McLean Hospital in the summer of 1938.

After Rose's admission, the staff at McLean Hospital received a report from the superintendent of the prior institution she had been in, which filled in a few more details of the anamnesis. Apparently, the marriage had been strained from the outset, in that Mr. Thorner married Rose only because he was "on the rebound" at the time and because she came from a wealthy family. Harry later would accuse his wife of being frigid and unduly jealous, even though it was evident he was in fact having affairs. The referring superintendent was doubtful about the existence of a true mental illness, in that Rose "dramatized her incapacity and exaggerated her problems." Rather, "it was a picture of undisciplined character, selfish and vain, rather than a very ill state." He also noted that Rose had violently resisted entering his sanitarium, afraid that she might end up in a mental hospital.

The son who had assumed the role of informant reinforced this unflattering picture. Returning by mail a signed contract in which he agreed to pay for his mother's care at McLean, the son took the occasion to expound upon a similar theme. "I am quite sure," he announced to the staff, "that many of mother's outward manifestations or symptoms are artificial and acquired rather than natural and uncontrollable by her." As proof, he continued (in a rather cold tone), "For example, sir, several things she does such as wringing her hands, and pacing up and down, . . . she saw my father do in the month just prior to his death." Moreover, as his mother had been reading popular books on mental illness (such as Overstreet's *About Ourselves*), the son's personal theory was that she would incorporate whatever symptoms she fixed upon and that these would last only as long as she could remember them. He recalled that, after she read a chapter titled "Regression to the Infantile," his mother exclaimed: "You see that's what's the matter with me. I've regressed to the infantile."

The staff at McLean were not so optimistic. In the original case formulation generated after her admission, Rose's most recent breakdown was blamed primarily on the news that her eldest son was engaged, which threatened her "pathological" dependence upon him. Even with this knowledge, her prognosis was considered poor, however, as she did not have much family to return to and she had already alienated most of her friends. It was predicted that "she will have to be ill for a long time and gradually work out of it more or less on her own with the care and regulations which a hospital of this sort can provide." One of the persisting problems was the patient's level of self-accusation, and her constant fear of being moved to a "worse building."

At first, Mrs. Thorner fit comfortably in the hospital routine. Placed in the relatively unrestricted Belknap I, she was described as making a good if not model adjustment. She was comfortable and sociable, taking up bridge, golf, and needlepoint, and attending teas. At the end of her first month of residence, Dr. Elliot Austin began a biweekly correspondence with her son that would continue for some time. Mrs. Thorner, Austin stated in the first of these communications, had been pleasant and cooperative at all times, and she was beginning to join in the hospital activities. After a few more months had gone by, Austin was no longer so optimistic. The son was informed that of late his mother had been doing poorly and was preoccupied with the notion that all of her children were dead. As letters from them did not suffice to quell her fears – she claimed they were all forgeries – Austin suggested firmly that a personal visit would help greatly. In response, the son did make a visit in March, which appeared to ease matters – but only temporarily. During this period, Rose also initiated something of a letter-writing campaign, in which she described to friends and relatives in gruesome terms all sorts of tortures and indignities to which she was exposed at McLean, in the hope that they would investigate and liberate her. After a flurry of monogrammed stationery landed on Austin's desk, he resorted to the standard institutional response of a mail embargo; henceforth, all her letters would be sent to her son, who was to read them and return them to McLean if necessary. Rose's file grew thick with intercepted correspondence.

As she grew increasingly agitated, Rose's apprehension and misery began to upset the other patients in Women's Belknap. The decision was made to transfer her to East House II. Placed almost daily in the continuous baths, Rose at times would become calm and dress up in sporty clothes; at others, she would fret about ending up in a state hospital. In October, her agitation returned unabated. Mrs. Thorner was observed pacing up and down the hallways, pulling her hair. When a strong odor of feces emerged from her room, she was immediately sent down to a lower hall. Rose's response was to become resistant and combatant; at night she would cry out in her sleep. In March of 1939, Rose began to reveal her delusions and fears about being interred under Wyman Hall, "hermetically sealed." She sent out a new round of letters pleading for rescue. Of one friend she asked: "Please answer me this one question – must I be virtually buried alive? . . . To be just thrown away and eaten up by rats and bugs, never even have a decent burial. . . . You have no idea of the cruelty of it all. . . . I want so to be able to sit out in the sunshine and see the birds and summer again." She also admitted to a physician that she felt she was being punished for having had premarital sex with a man other than her husband. Overwhelmed by guilt, Rose sent a letter to her staff physician that stated simply: "I choose to give up. Please have arrange-ments made to put me away today. It is unfair to many others for me to stay in Codman any longer. Thank you." At this point, the physicians ordered a series of sodium amytal and then benzedrine trials.

In October, at the patient's request, a series of psychotherapeutic inter-views were begun with a woman physician on staff. Talking about her past in depth for the first time, Rose confessed that her marriage was born out of human weakness, not love. At the time, Harry had recently been jilted, and, as far as she was concerned, she married him for the security he represented. The marriage had not been happy, and she had been hurt by his extramarital affairs. Rose expressed particular concern for the welfare of her children, who had to live with the dual burden of a father who had killed himself and a mother currently in a mental institution. It was Rose's expectation that she would never fully get well; her goal was to improve enough so that she might leave McLean, which was expensive, for the less costly arrangement of a boardinghouse and nurse. At least then some money might be saved for the kids. At about this time, Rose sent a letter to Director Austin. "I wish to make a very frank confession," it began. "My husband contracted a venereal disease from me, went insane, and commit-ted suicide, making me a murderer. I am a thief, a liar, a traitor, a drunk-ard. I have deserted [my family], one a mentally deficient cripple. I have hurt patients and nurses at McLean. I am the most wicked, cruel, de-praved woman in the world, without one element of human emotion. I have denied God . . . the wages of sin is death. . . ." To her assigned physician, she wrote, "For the sake of humanity, in order that there be no more deaths and suffering on my account, that innocent people may go to their houses for Christmas, that my children may be spared any more suffering, may I *please* give up my life this afternoon. Facts must be faced. I have *no* rights in this world any longer. If death is not possible may I *please* be put in restraint in complete isolation this afternoon."

In January 1940, Rose was again transferred to the lower hall of Cod-man, due to her assaultive behavior toward the other patients. There, she begged for the "ultimate punishment" and to be told how to "give up." Deteriorating further, she began to bite the nurses, expose herself, and tear her clothes. Her latest demands were to be sent to Wyman "for further punishment of her sins," where she might be the recipient of a mercy killing.

The physicians' response was to start a series of metrazol shocks. Ap-parently, Mrs. Thorner was "somewhat startled by the severe treatment," which had the ultimate effect of calming her down so that she even began to socialize with the other patients and to converse with the doctors. Obviously dreading the treatments, Rose expressed a desire to learn what was expected of her so that she might ultimately be discharged. In further interviews, she revealed that shortly after menstruation had begun she had been seduced by an older neighbor of the family. She wondered how her mother could have allowed this to happen. The psychiatrist also learned further circumstances surrounding her unfortunate marriage. During the cruise home from her last international trip, under the influence of alcohol she had had intercourse with a stranger and was terrified that she might become pregnant. It was this fear that prompted her to marry Harry. Moreover, not long after their marriage, both parties began to have affairs. She had developed the notion that she had contracted syphilis and had infected her children with it; subsequently, each of her doctors, she believed, had conspired to hide this fact from her. In the months ahead, Mrs. Thorner again became fixed on the theme that her children were all dead. No amount of reassurance could convince her otherwise. The interviewer noted that it was rather discouraging to talk to her because her psychotic ideas remained intractable and added that "one feels that there is very little frontal lobe to work with." Metrazol was continued until June, when a shoulder was dislocated – a fairly frequent complication of metrazol, which causes violent muscular contractions.

In the fall of 1940, Mrs. Thorner's condition worsened and she was returned to the lower ward in East House. The nurses stated that she was "now back to her infantile, immature stage showing more deterioration all of the time." She would wander the halls crying out, "They are all dead, aren't they?" or "It wasn't my fault, was it? I was born queer, wasn't I? Why doesn't someone tell me? . . . I'm a sacrifice to science." Rose had also become "very untidy about her room and person," the nurses' polite shorthand for the fact that she would lie in bed all day, picking feces out of her rectum or masturbating. The staff tried to counter these "obnoxious habits" by locking her out of her room all day and by applying daily enemas. Sometime during 1941, the bank that managed her trust was legally appointed conservator of her estate and person.

Rose had bottomed out, transformed into a grotesque caricature of her former self. Over the next half-decade, she never strayed far from this level. Almost as a rule, the nurses' notes began with the stock phrase, "has remained the same," which in her case indicated a rather horrifying condition. All during this time she maintained the "disgusting habit of consistently smearing feces on the bedsheets, floors, hallways, woodwork . . . and filling the registers with it, no matter how often she is reprimanded." She filled her days pacing the halls, muttering constantly the same phrases, such as "Nobody knows what it's all about, do they?" and generally pestering the patients and staff, who objected to her rank odor and tendency to cling to them physically. At night she would masturbate whenever awake. The clinical notes indicate that Mrs. Thorner remained concerned about her children being dead, a fear the physicians felt was not thoroughly unjustified, as the children never visited or wrote. Indeed, as if Rose's life was not filled with enough tragedy, by the end of the war she was informed that two of her sons had been killed in action – a partial lie that disguised the brutal fact that the eldest son had shot himself while on leave.

The year 1946 passed like those before. Rose would alternate between being pleasant and being vicious, going so far as to strike another patient in the eye with a rock. The nurses' notes in May, for example, began with the almost obligatory "has shown little or no change in the past month." We learn that Rose "continues to pace endlessly up and down the corridors all day long," "goes into the other patients' rooms and takes or destroys anything she sees lying around," and "continues to pick at her rectum and smear feces and has a very offensive odor to her body and her room." At the end of the year, the clinical notes described her as growing even *more* offensive and agitated. During the day, Rose continually harassed the other patients, bumping into them as she paced; still parked her feces; and developed a new habit of stuffing hairpins, grass, or pieces of paper into her ears, which had to be medically removed. There was no respite, even at night. "Most of her waking hours," wrote the night nurse, "are spent masturbating, which creates an offensive stench that permeates not only her room, but the entire lower corridor." At the time this last note was written, the patient's worst fear had in fact been realized, as she had finally been transferred to Wyman, the "lowest" ward at McLean. All of her family was either dead or deformed, and now here she was, "regressed to the infantile." Buried alive, in the end.

In November 1946, a decision had been reached to give Mrs. Thorner a prefrontal lobotomy. Dr. Austin wrote to the judge overseeing her conservatorship:

> Mrs. Thorner has been in the hospital for a good many years and has not responded to any of the previous treatments administered to her. We are now applying to many patients such as Rose, an operation called a bilateral pre-frontal lobotomy which in many cases enables the patients to return essentially to normal living, and in about eighty percent of the cases this makes them much more comfortable. Rose is still quite clear intellectually, has no memory defect or other organic changes which would argue against such an operation. We feel that she is a very good candidate for it and therefore, I am enclosing a permit with the request that you sign it. . . .

The judge was also informed that the expense would be between six and seven hundred dollars, and that if he had any further questions, to ask.[37]

To the conservators, Austin wrote: "The operation itself does not involve any great discomfort and there is considerable hope that it might make her more comfortable and able to live in a better environment inside or outside of the hospital depending on the degree of success."

The operation was performed by Mixter on 22 January 1947, in a converted room at McLean Hospital. The first clinical note indicated some hopeful signs. Within a week after the operation, Rose occasionally was sociable enough to attend occupational therapy, and to even play cards with some of the other patients. The nurses' notes reported that "she displayed none of her former habits." With her condition improving, Rose was sent to live on Codman I. In June, additional progress was noted. She was friendly and cooperative almost all the time, and only on one occasion did she hide some feces. In August, the nurses described her as "gracious upon approach – mixes in very well with the other patients." The following month, Rose was considered so improved as to warrant a transfer to Codman III, an open ward, an event that greatly satisfied her. The nurses' notes indicated that she took advantage of her grounds privileges, going to movies in Waverly and visiting a beauty salon for a "badly needed" manicure and permanent. Her staff physician reported that "She is always pleasant, cooperative, and agreeable on approach. She spends her days in the occupational therapy and greatly enjoys playing bridge in the evening."

Over the course of the following year or so, Rose presented a picture of slow, gradual improvement. Described as happy, pleasant, and sociable most of the time, her major deficits seemed to be carelessness, irresponsibility, and inattention to personal grooming. By April, Rose had regained sufficient presence of mind to hold classes in which she would instruct other patients on how to play contract bridge. "Mrs. Thorner is doing very nicely," Austin wrote to a family friend in August, "she has been going out to shop, to the theater, and to baseball games." He concluded, "It is really remarkable how she has improved in the last few months." By January 1950, Rose Thorner was living at a level of existence that several years earlier would have been inconceivable to the staff and friends who knew her in her deteriorated condition. She would attend movies in Waverly alone, go on buying sprees in Boston, and meet her friends for the occasional lunch or dinner in town. Idle time was spent reading books, some of which were described as "serious" in quality. One night she was invited by the staff chauffeur and his wife to ride with them to a church social. Entering the bridge tournament held that evening, she triumphantly won first prize.

In the following months, Rose was described in the nurses' notes as becoming more adventurous about leaving the hospital for day visits.

From Austin's perspective, such outings proved a little too adventurous, especially when on one trip Rose consulted a lawyer about the possibility of obtaining release from McLean. The lawyer took the case, feeling that "from my own observation, she seems to appear 100 per cent normal." Austin strongly disagreed, believing that Rose's inadequacies of judgment were simply hidden from casual observation, her normal appearance notwithstanding. Although Austin managed to fend off the lawyer, Rose's action had in fact forced his hand. In short order, Rose was placed "on visit" (the equivalent of parole) and sent to live at a boardinghouse near the coast that was run by a retired psychiatric nurse.

The caretaker reported to Austin that Rose seemed comfortable and contented in her new environment. She enjoyed long walks and going to church, movies, concerts, and square dances. "Whatever the occasion," the caretaker added, "she seems to take it in stride and be prepared to find pleasure in it." At one point, Rose's surviving son (the mentally deficient one) had a chance to visit her, with mixed results. Rose herself sent a postcard to Austin, which read: "The [resort] is very pleasant. Feeling well, have quite a tan, enjoy the swimming. My friends have been so nice to me." Such niceties belied Rose's determination, however, to obtain release from the hospital's oversight. In another letter, she inquired of Austin: "If my stay down here is a probationary period I would like to know how long it is to last. I would appreciate it if I could have control of my money as I find it troublesome to have it go through so many channels. Hope you and Mrs. Austin had a pleasant vacation."[38]

In February 1951, the caretaker wrote a very long letter in which she described life at "the manor." Rose appeared to be in excellent health and spirits. "She keeps up and on the go whenever there is anything of interest to her," she reported. Such activities included church, sewing groups, and volunteer work as a Gray Lady at the local hospital – for which she proudly earned a red cross. It was also noted that Rose went on vacation to stay with her son for a week, a visit that was emotionally trying for her but enjoyable nonetheless. It was the caretaker's judgment that, positive as was Rose's overall condition, she lacked good sense and was still unable to handle by herself the many little challenges that crop up in the course of a day. Fully independent living was not yet possible. In May, two cousins of Rose visited her, after which they reported to Austin that they were delighted to find her in such excellent shape. "We had expected trying scenes," they feared, yet, "on the contrary, she seemed perfectly satisfied to stay where she is, at least for the present." During the visit, Rose (with the consent of the caretaker) "went to a friend of ours for cocktails, and drank one . . . , enjoying herself." After this, "she engaged rooms for us at the Inn, and introduced us there with all her old poise." The letter ended with the note, "We both feel that her recovery is a great tribute to your care."

The next few years continued in this manner, with Rose mostly content in her life with the caretaker (whom she genuinely liked and for whom she felt great affection) but never abandoning her quest to gain freedom from Austin and the long reach of McLean Hospital. The last note from Rose to Austin, written in January of 1955, asked for permission to take some silver out of the bank to give to her son and new daughter-in-law. It was written on personalized stationery bordered in tasteful blue ink and headed, in elegant lettering, "Mrs. Harry Thorner."[39] Rose had returned, at least partially, to her former station in life.

### Poor Results

Such dramatic results as those described above were more the exception than the rule, however, as even the staff would be quick to admit. The physicians at McLean witnessed their share of operative failures in which no lasting change for the better could be found. Some postoperative patients were judged to be in even worse shape. (Indeed, of the first eight women operated upon, seven were still in the institution five years after surgery.) Mrs. Frances Lee, the very first woman selected for lobotomy, was considered more manageable and less depressed immediately following the operation. But it was not long before she sank back into her prelobotomy condition. In fact, a year later a second lobotomy was performed upon her, to ill effect. Eight years later, she was described as amiable at times but sullen and sarcastic at others, and, in general, depressed and clearly retarded. The nurses' notes describe her as being "cared for as a small child would be, except that she is uncooperative, often resistant," and that "the only thing she does well is eat." She was discharged to a state hospital in 1948.

For Mr. Robert Parkhurst, a young man diagnosed with schizophrenia, the operation proved disastrous. Considering Mr. Parkhurst's postlobotomy condition, Austin advised the family that visits to the hospital were no longer necessary. "I have taken the matter up with the staff," he wrote, "and while we shall cooperate with you whenever you visit we must say that it does not make any difference to Robert whether or not you visit," for "he does not seem to be interested in his surroundings, his personal appearance, or anything else." Mrs. Grace Farmer, a widow in her late thirties, was diagnosed as catatonic. After her lobotomy in 1947, she was described as poorly oriented, noisy, apathetic, prone to combativeness, and likely to misidentify people. "She is often content in a rather silly way," Harmon noted, "but at other times becomes disturbed by her hallucinations and is difficult to manage." "All in all," he concluded, "the results of the operation are not impressive."[40] Following their operations, Kay Levitt and Helaine Strauss did so poorly that they soon ended up in local state hospitals. Like Mrs. Lee, the hospital's response to Mrs. Strauss's condition was to attempt a second, more "radical" lobotomy. Here, too, the attempt only made a bad situation worse. The discharge summary for Mrs. Strauss indicated that "the prognosis for improvement is nil." In addition to the poor result in her mental condition, the operation had caused a total loss of sphincter control. Between 1949 and 1951, another four patients fared so badly that a second round of surgery was given.[41]

Perhaps the most despairing cry was that of Annabel Simms, who following the operation was so depressed as to attempt suicide after her discharge home. Her brother-in-law reported that after the operation she was "decidedly off the beam, more so than prior to the operation, if that is possible," in that her "general attitude toward life and conduct has been practically in complete reverse of that formerly." Her own words provided poignant testimony to the hopelessness of her situation. In a strongly worded complaint sent to her physician at McLean Hospital, Mrs. Simms declared, "I cannot do anything that will make me happy," and "NOTHING interests me." These cases were not the only poor results.

More common than the clear failures or successes, however, were the instances in which the operation was judged to have had some good effects and some bad, yielding mixed and uncertain evaluations. Clara Northrup, an elderly woman with involutional melancholia, was operated on in 1949 and returned to the care of her relatives the following year. At first, the odd habits of Mrs. Northrup were rather trying for her cousin and niece who looked after her, as she might urinate in a vase or refuse to wash or change her clothing. Her condition improved somewhat, and in a follow-up note her staff physician observed that Mrs. Northrup was "leading a very active and pleasant existence," even if "some of her social graces had probably deteriorated." After this consultation, the niece sought advice from the physician as to her aunt's status, which puzzled her. "I am more confused than ever before in regard to her mental condition," she began. "In many ways, particularly in conversation, she seems alert, seems to know about current events, and talks coherently and well," yet, she continued, "one senses something is not quite right." Most troubling to the niece, it appeared that Mrs. Northrup had "turned away . . . from her old friends and wants nothing to do with them." The hospital staff did not have much advice, other than to state that "she is, after all, an old lady," and that "there are bound to be certain changes in personality after a lobotomy."

Hilary Wise was a young schizophrenic woman who was already on her third admission to McLean Hospital. After a long series of electroshocks and insulin shocks, the staff recommended a lobotomy. Her father assented, hoping that this new treatment will "make the thing 'stick' so that she will be able to lead a normal or semi-normal life without these setbacks." Although Miss Wise was judged sufficiently improved to return home, the results were not unambiguous. In the father's opinion, his daughter had been "lowered" by the operation. Admitting that his daughter was in fact freer of the disease than she had been for many years, on the other hand, he pointed out, since the operation she had not been able to regain in her best moments her former personality. "She cannot rise as high nor does she go as low as formerly," he explained. Although she had been ambitious to return to a normal social life again, she no longer had the capacity to get along with people. In short, "She just can't make the grade."

## The Overall Assessment

The cumulative weight of these case histories – good, bad, and mixed – was sufficient to persuade the psychiatrists at McLean Hospital that psychosurgery was a useful therapeutic option, a judgment which was shared by most institutional physicians who had publicly commented upon the procedure.[42] The cases of remarkable recovery, however diffuse, were hard to deny for those who had witnessed them. Howard knew that the numerical tables and summary judgments he presented in his conference talk, necessary as they were, somehow missed the essence of what the psychosurgery program was all about. "You can't exactly measure human misery in statistics," Howard cautioned his audience. Instead, he described a patient who had suffered ten years of depression, seven years of which were spent in great distress and perplexity, "walking about, wringing her hands, asking to be annihilated and in complete social withdrawal except for annoying other patients." Three years after her operation, "she has gradually shown a degree of social improvement consistent with her previous rather shallow social life and emotionally dependent attitude." As to her intense agitation, it almost immediately ceased following the operation. He then brought into the room Mrs. Thorner, for the staff to question and observe in person.[43] For Howard (and by extension for the other doctors at McLean), as far as the potential positive effects of lobotomy were concerned, seeing was believing, even if they appeared only in selected cases.

That such good results were only rarely achieved was not considered sufficient reason to brake the program. Although the Waverly group labored in a superior professional environment and drew from a higher profile of training, nonetheless they saw the clinical world in fundamentally the same way as did hospital psychiatrists elsewhere, and worked through the therapeutic calculus in much the same manner. The patients at McLean clearly were not subject to the kinds of abusive conditions that existed in some of the larger state hospitals, yet for many the inner torment was surely no less. Thus, we find Howard in his staff conference speech characterizing lobotomy as a treatment "of last resort," to be used only after psychotherapy, social manipulation, extensive hospitalization, and insulin or electric shock had all failed. "Last" did not imply trivial, however, for as Howard emphasized, "it really is very important to have some treatment in mind for those cases where all other treatments have failed." Without such a recourse, patients were de facto consigned to a life of endless suffering. For them, psychosurgery represented, in Howard's analysis, not only the physician's last resort, but these patients' last true hope.[44] As Howard pointed out, the real value of the operation derived from the fact that virtually none of this group were expected ever to leave the hospital. Statistics indicated, Howard informed his audience, that of patients hospitalized for more than two and a half years only 3 percent would ever recover. Yet of the McLean psychosurgery patients, for which his figures showed an average of seven years' hospitalization, almost one-third of the schizophrenics and three-fourths of the manic-depressives were improved enough to be discharged.

Here we see that Howard employed the same clinical equation, that of *human salvage*, which was described in the previous chapter. "One statement we frequently make to relatives about the suitability of the patient for the operation," Howard stated, is that "she has very poor chances of getting better without it," but with it, she has "a definite chance of – if not being entirely well – at least in having a marked amount of suffering relieved." Such suffering might be in the form of "very painful anxiety, depression, tension, feelings of guilt, hallucinations, delusions, and lastly confinement in the hospital with the disease picture separating her from her family." On the negative side, there was a real chance that it might "take away something from the personality." Nonetheless, "it may relieve distressing symptoms and put the patient partly on the road to social contact." And so it went, back and forth. As elsewhere, however, the deficits and risks of the operation were fed into the same equation as were the positive outcomes; and, as elsewhere, the overall equation reported a marginal benefit in favor of the intervention. "Any loss in sensitivity," Howard concluded, "will be made up by an increasing ability for the patient to enjoy what she has." Or, as Tompkins concluded in his paper on the effects of lobotomy on thirty-six patients, "None can be said to have no trace of the former illness but many can be said to have made an adjustment which pleases both the patients and their families."[45]

It is clear that others on the staff worked through the same reckoning process and had arrived at a similar conclusion in the case of many patients: there was no hope without lobotomy, and a partial salvage was better than none. In the discussion of Anna Winthrop, Addison declared that hers was the kind of case "you are justified in doing it on because you have nothing to lose." "I second the motion," Green added, for she could live outside the hospital, and "if it is not done, she will have to be hospitalized the rest of her life." Burdett concluded, "I don't think we are going to make her any paragon by lobotomizing her, but it is a difference between a person who is activated by delusions and one who is much less that way."[46] Similarly, Stanley Cobb informed Rourke that the hospital and family had only two choices left in regard to treatment for Mrs. Emily Marr, which were "1. to go as we are indefinitely," and "2. to have a lobotomy." In light of the patient's poor response and emotional hardships caused by electric shock, Cobb went so far as to argue that "I am inclined to believe that the last is perhaps the most humane thing to do because it might relieve her tension."[47]

An especially clear rendering of the partial salvage offered by lobotomy is found in a letter by a staff physician seeking operative permission from the husband of Eleanor Lowell:

> We have found that this operation, which severs nerve tracts from the front, that is higher elements of the brain, affects the emotions so that as a result these people do not worry and are much more happy and contented, and consequently do not have such temper tantrums, do not quarrel so much with those about them, and are much more tractable and life for them is much easier and more livable. The operation also clears up to an astounding degree mental depressions. Such an operation would not remove the delusions, she would still think that she was being poisoned or that her thoughts were being read and she would hear voices railing against her as she does now, but she would not worry about it, she would throw it off with a shake of their head and perhaps smile at her persecutors. In other words, this operation has the effect of removing the anxiety and painful emotional feelings that torment such people endlessly from their persecutory and other false ideas. Therefore, I would not expect that this operation would cure her insanity or affect her insane ideas in any way, as far as content is concerned, but it would deprive those ideas of the distressed feelings and she would be comparatively content and happy where she is now continually anxious and miserable.

When all is said and done, the operation "would make life much more tolerable in her confinement." In the realities of life on the wards in 1948, even at the very best facilities in the country, such a small chance of even a moderate gain, or an exchange of altered personality for relief of misery, was considered sufficient rationale to perform a lobotomy.

## "What the Lobotomy Would Help"

The physicians at McLean Hospital entered into the use of psychosurgery in the same way as they did any other new therapy. Relying upon what they had learned from careful and extensive reading of the medical literature, and from any personal communications they might have had with its leading exponents, they worked up a series of guidelines to shape their selection of patients. As Howard explained in his lecture on the subject, the first order of business was to answer two questions: (1) What did the operation do for the individual patient? and (2) What kinds of patients were suitable for it? It was these kinds of practical, bread-and-butter therapeutic issues that were the mainstay of clinical discussions at McLean: the need to better understand what their therapeutic tools might accomplish as well as the logic behind their application.

Such "clinical frames," then and now, constitute the stock-in-trade of medical practice, the major resource utilized by physicians when deciding which therapy to try next. When considering the available treatments – in this instance, perhaps, vitamins, hydrotherapy, hormones, electroshock, insulin, or lobotomy – clinicians must associate each with a series of predefined criteria. The patient is viewed against each of these, seriatim: this treatment is ruled in (e.g., the patient exhibits the right cluster of symptoms and has been hospitalized more than a year), that treatment is ruled out (the patient exhibits the wrong cluster of symptoms or is too old), until one or two options remain.

The first year or so of the extensive use of lobotomy at McLean was thus an anxious affair of setting up both a rank-order list of the kinds of problems for which it worked better than any other mode of treatment available; a list of inclusion rules; and an opposing list of exclusion rules, the clinical boundaries of when the treatment was not to be used. Then there was the matter of fitting the new therapy into the overall logic of the existing treatment strategies, taken as a whole. The staff never did become content that a satisfactory account of psychosurgery's utility or safety had been reached or that their frameworks were anything but provisional. Nonetheless, they came to believe that their personal experience had yielded an understanding of the procedure that was sufficiently clear-cut and reliable to proceed forward with new cases.

The staff conferences represented just such a space in which the practitioners could demonstrate their understanding of the various clinical frames then in use: it was not just the patients who were on display, but the physicians and medical students as well. In the give-and-take of these discussions, the staff wrestled over what they thought was the matter with any individual patient and what might be the best treatment plan. At the same time, however, such meetings served as forums in which the staff reshaped the clinical frames by which they all practiced. Thanks again to McLean Hospital's obsession with record keeping, which extended as far as the transcription of all such professional meetings, it is possible to listen in on these discussions.

When the physicians at McLean Hospital first experimented with psychosurgery, discussions tended to be highly theoretical in nature. For example, at the staff conference held for Mrs. Pauline Stanton in May of 1941, one physician in favor of using the operation argued that "Frontal lobotomy . . . might succeed in separating the site of hyperactivity from the effector system and thus eliminate the clinical manifestations of overactive behavior." At the outset of the second wave that began in 1945, it was clear that the staff was still venturing into territory with which they were personally unfamiliar and were groping around for clues to direct them. When discussing the advisability of lobotomy for Mr. William Brandford, speculations dominated the discussion:

Murphy: Do you think he should have a lobotomy, Arthur?

Burdett: I think it would be interesting to speculate what we would expect it to accomplish. . . . There is no thinking it is going to make him any worse except it might make him incontinent of urine.

Murphy: It might make him dead or have convulsions.

Burdett: I don't think that is very much worse than his present situation. I favor lobotomy, not with great enthusiasm, but still I favor it.

Murphy: Dr. Green, what do you say?

Green: I do not feel qualified to express an opinion.

Swadley: I don't know what lobotomy would accomplish. . . .

Maddox: From what I have read about lobotomies, those done on patients with real inner drive are more successful so this man might benefit.

Averbuck: Seems to me the fundamental disorder is not changed and I am opposed unless there is some very urgent need for it. . . .

Murphy: One argument against the lobotomy is that he does not have a decent personality to go back to. . . . [On the other hand,] if we do not do a lobotomy the chances are he will just go along on Bowditch in this same state for many years.

Kellogg: All the data in this record is on the hopeless side, but I do not have any definite opinion. I am rather against it as the risks are too great and the results too small. I wonder if he could be kept from deteriorating so rapidly by total push means.

The discussion ended with Dr. Murphy putting it up to a vote; the decision was against lobotomy.

At the January 1946 meeting of the Boston Society of Psychiatry and Neurology, Tillotson and Wyatt took advantage of the occasion to share notes with Walter Freeman, the procedure's most vocal advocate. In describing the hospital's renewed interest in the treatment, and its focus on chronic schizophrenics, Tillotson prodded Freeman on what were the range of conditions suitable for the procedure. Wyatt, also in discussion, raised the issue of the lack of information concerning what were the operation's effects on the patient's personality. In his opinion, the work done to date by Freeman and his colleague, psychologist Thelma Hunt, which had been based on various kinds of neuroses and agitated depressions, was of limited generalizability to the chronic invalids at McLean; the failure to measure dramatic changes in personality was due to a sample that was skewed by its inclusion of mostly well-preserved individuals. In response, Freeman admitted that Wyatt's criticisms were apt, reflecting an unavoidable limitation of existing intelligence tests. As to what kinds of patients were suitable for the operation, Freeman indicated that the emotional component of the mental illness was the target; agitated depressions, schizophrenia, obsessive tension states, and hysteria all responded.[48]

Over the course of the next few years, the McLean psychiatrists in fact worked largely within the flexible guidelines articulated by Freeman. The particular clinical target the psychosurgery was aimed at was precisely this emotional component of the mental illness. When recommending the procedure in the staff conferences, the physicians repeatedly referred to its ability to lower "tenseness" or "anxiety." In discussing Mr. Everett Daniels, for example, one physician noted, "He is tense and a lobotomy prognosis might be good"; on the day the operation was performed, the clinical note explained, "It was felt that a prefrontal lobotomy would circumvent the cumulative tension." The procedure was found to be of some use across a wide variety of diagnostic divisions. In schizophrenia, it might diminish the problems triggered by delusions and hallucinations or bring the patient closer into interpersonal contact. When Partridge noted that "the schizophrenic picture often changes after a lobotomy," this was saying a lot, for no other treatment then available seemed to have much impact on the course of a chronic psychosis, whether for good or ill. And in agitated depressions of various kinds (involutional melancholia, psychoneurotic reactive, or manic-depression), it might stem the misery that otherwise was unrelenting.

In time, the staff accumulated sufficient experience with the operation – seventy-three were performed before the end of 1951 – to feel reasonably confident in their ability to assess the operation's suitability and effects. The McLean physicians began to state outright what sort of symptoms the "ideal lobotomy patient" presented, or they might identify a given individual as "perfect for a lobotomy, clinically." This was not based on abstract standards but on their direct experience. When arguing for a lobotomy on Mr. Howard Peckler, Harmon directed the staff's attention to the number of their patients "who were a great deal worse off than he" who had made striking improvements. Moreover, the staff now worked within lines sharp enough to state when patients did *not* fit the profile. Even its strongest advocates, such as Burdett, were not averse to arguing against an operation if they felt the patient did not possess the right characteristics for a good result.[49]

On the one hand, the staff now had close enough contact with psychosurgery patients to discern a pattern of unfortunate side effects, which had become a syndrome of its own. In the case of Mrs. Gladys Randall, for example, the clinical notes indicated that she demonstrated a typical "acute lobotomy syndrome," which was characterized by "lethargy alternating with undue vivaciousness and a tendency to be abrupt and flippant in a pleasant way." Such deficits, however striking, were thought to subside to manageable levels over time. On the other hand, the staff had also become that much more certain about its benefits. "The only thing I think would make any mental change for the better," Burdett now was heard to say, "would be a lobotomy." Harmon wrote in the clinical notes for Miss Claire Mulvahill, a paranoid schizophrenic, that "There is no reason which the writer can see how any form of treatment short of prefrontal lobotomy will influence the patient's psychiatric condition." Experience has shown, he argued, "that lobotomy is the treatment of choice in this type of case." Already sure in their knowledge of what a lobotomy might do, the physicians might open a staff conference with the question "What we want to know is whether we should do a lobotomy," as Richardson did in the case of Howard Peckler, or interject, as Simpson did in the discussion about Mrs. Adelaide Kerr, "We should try to benefit her with a lobotomy." In the case of Mrs. Helaine Strauss, Murphy summed up discussion by asking, "Is anybody against lobotomy?" As a last example, during the staff conference on Mrs. Mary Montero, held in March 1948, Harmon's terse assessment, "Get on with a lobotomy," spoke volumes about the change in the staff's position.

The staff had also found a ready place for lobotomy within the institution's existing logic of therapeutic deployment. As elsewhere, psychosurgery became a technique of "last resort," to be employed when the other available treatments were perceived to have been exhausted. When Everett Daniels returned home following a series of insulin treatments, Partridge warned his parents about the strong possibility of relapse; they were advised that "in the event of another hospitalization, lobotomy should be generously considered." In the case of Mrs. Heloise Ann Rathburn, when the family was apprised that electroshock treatments were not working, they were at the same time informed that "a definite recommendation of lobotomy might be made in the future." The benefit of having a treatment to fall back on was a psychological resource not to be underestimated. Psychosurgery thus took on a role as a faithful standby, never far from the clinician's thoughts in the case of patients who had taken a turn for the worse. Indeed, for recently admitted patients who had mental illnesses of long standing, this "last resort" was in fact first in mind. "After a preliminary period of observation, electric shock and or insulin shock should be tried," Burdett wrote in the clinical notes on Mrs. Elizabeth Moorehouse. "However," he cautioned, "the prognosis in either therapy with this patient is not good and she may well become a candidate for lobotomy." Psychosurgery had filled in the last gap in the therapeutic armamentarium. Should a patient fail to improve permanently in response to shock treatment, psychotherapy, or socialization programs, there was indeed a final recourse – psychosurgery.

Here, too, the structure of the therapeutic armamentarium in this period led patients to slide almost inevitably into the pool of candidates considered suitable for the operation. In the case of Mrs. Anita Payne, the staff recommended a series of shock treatments, but "keeping the possibility of lobotomy in mind for later on." For Simpson, the temporary improvement of the patient in response to electric shocks automatically triggered the next decision. "A lobotomy is considered to be a very desirable procedure," he wrote in the clinical note, "to be employed as the next step." For patients whose combination of age, sex, diagnosis, and mental history placed them in the pool of possible candidates, the meter was ticking as to the eventuality of receiving a lobotomy – a race between improving enough to be discharged from the hospital and being brought before a staff conference at which they would be recommended for surgery. For example, the clinical note for Miss Annette Draper simply stated that, as "this patient has now had ample treatment of electrical and hormonal nature and been depressed sufficiently long," "prefrontal lobotomy should be performed." Also in line with the national experience, the expectation of curability brought about by the introduction of the somatic treatments had the paradoxical effect of lowering patience for those who did not respond. By way of contrast, when Rose Thorner first entered McLean in the 1930s, the presumption was that she would spend the coming years, or even decades, on the wards, playing out whatever was to be her psychiatric fate. By 1946, however, Burdett argued that, should Mrs. Annabel Simms not respond to a moderate amount of shock treatments, then "I think you are entitled to be bold."

The end result of the McLean initiative in psychosurgery – in which the staff paid close attention to the wide variety of patients undergoing the procedure and took advantage of the opportunity for close follow-up evaluation – was a certain confidence in clinical decision making. Psychosurgery was no longer mysterious and hypothetical, but a familiar (though still elusive) entity. When Mrs. Adelaide Hitchcock was brought before the psychiatric staff for a treatment evaluation, Dr. Simpson simply responded with the judgment that "she has what the lobotomy would help." A clinical frame for the use of psychosurgery had emerged.

### The Essential Tension: Medicine as Art or Science

Just what was this clinical frame that the McLean physicians applied so confidently when deciding whether a particular patient should undergo psychosurgery? And what does it reveal about the kind of medicine they practiced?

Curiously, the route followed by the McLean physicians in their quest for medical certainty led them to a position filled with contradictions. As narrated above, the McLean staff had entered the psychosurgical arena unsure of their current understanding of the procedure yet fully expecting that a reliable medical framework would develop soon enough. Indeed, the zeal exhibited in the discussions of the staff conferences (which drew upon the staff's wide reading of the scientific literature, their own research, and individual clinical experiences) clearly demonstrated their intent to identify a set of medically defensible standards for the use of the procedure in the near future.

Yet, at the very moment when these physicians felt reasonably secure in their judgment of whether an operation was in fact necessary or desirable, the *basis* for this decision was not so easily articulated in the kinds of clearcut scientific protocols that were often referred to in their professional discussions. A large portion of these conversations consisted of far more mundane concerns such as whether a patient had recently become violent, had gone on a successful shopping trip, or was more upset than usual. Indeed, if the example of Dr. Simpson is any indication, the rise in therapeutic confidence of the physicians at this hospital had *not* been tethered to any obvious concomitant increase in their scientific understanding. When Simpson delivered his judgment on the suitability of psychosurgery for Mrs. Hitchcock, he did so without reference to any standardized list of symptoms, etiologies, or laboratory findings – the sorts of criteria associated with medical science. The sketchiness of his rationale did not, however, imply that he was any less sure of his clinical judgment. On the contrary, that some patients presented a clinical target best hit by psychosurgery, of this he *was* sure – even if he could not put its precise parameters into words or formulas.

Ironically, even as these physicians settled into a working framework with which they felt comfortable enough to order psychosurgery on an almost routine basis, some tended to deny its existence or to portray it in forthrightly nonscientific terms. For example, in the only published report of the lobotomy program at McLean Hospital, J. Butler Tompkins stated that no formal criteria existed for the identification of lobotomy patients. "Selection for operation," he wrote, "was an individual matter." And, as quoted earlier, other physicians at McLean simply waved the banner of "any and all" and left it at that.[50]

At first appearance, this example of the obvious gap between the psychiatrist's idealized image of him- or herself as a kind of applied scientist and the cruder reality of everyday practice further undermines the profession's already shaky reputation. The psychiatrists' swagger, one might editorialize, was not backed up by performance. It is easy enough to attribute the origin of this disparity – a kind of cognitive dissonance at the professional level – to the historical circumstances besetting the field of psychiatry in the 1940s. As described in Chapter 1, in general medicine, new scientific methods and laboratory products were rapidly transforming the medical ideal. In contrast, the psychiatric world of the asylum was perhaps the slowest-moving area in medicine. Psychiatrists interested in advancing their field, in making the discipline as medical as any other, found themselves caught in the crosscurrents. For them, ideal and reality threatened to grow further apart, not closer, and the lure of medical science was too compelling to ignore – even if it did not yet apply to their own specialty. In this scenario, whatever clinical frame was being used by the psychiatrists as they selected candidates for lobotomy was certainly inferior to their own medical goals – and thus, in retrospect, necessarily suspect.

Another scenario can be invoked, however, that considers this disparity between the ideals of medical science and the reality of psychiatric practice in a different light, and that treats the psychiatrists more favorably. To Tompkins and many of his colleagues, the abstract, generalized guidelines found in medical textbooks seemed only distantly linked to the murky, protean problems that confronted them on the wards. Each of the eighty lobotomy patients constituted an experiment of one, a unique mix of personality traits, faculties, emotional attributes, and formative experiences. Categorical statements about which kinds of patients were or were not suitable for lobotomy (or any other treatment) were to be rejected outright. Psychiatry was not about curing a patient in the abstract, but the distressed patient facing them. It was not a biological entity called schizophrenia that they were directly confronting, but a deeply troubled Mrs. Blithedale and her concerned family.

As in the prior account, the model of the physician as a scientific worker who deduced what next to do from published formulas simply did not correspond to the reality of medical practice as psychiatrists knew it. But here it was the poseur scientists who were suspect, not the workaday clinicians. Medicine, in important ways, was still an art and not yet fully a science, dependent more upon knowledge of the individual than the general case. The McLean physicians thus could plausibly maintain the belief that they understood when and how to use lobotomy, even if not in scientific terms. Navigation by sighting stars and feeling the wind can get the job done, depending on the skills and personal experience of the mariner. And so too in medicine.

From today's perspective, the fact that the McLean psychiatrists were using a clinical frame based more on art than on science is a sort of qualified reprieve. These practitioners may have had genuine faith in their ability to detect good lobotomy candidates, but this is no reason for us to place much stock in their medical skills. The underlying narrative of medical progress remains unchanged, the only question about the relation between the art and science of medicine being when the latter would displace the former. The story of psychosurgery, then, is most useful for dating just how archaic psychiatry was at the time.

Another strategy exists, however, that takes an alternative look at what the participants actually were doing as physicians and sees the supposed conflict between the art and science of medicine as a false dichotomy. The account of psychosurgery at McLean Hospital thus becomes useful for its broader lessons, an occasion to reexamine our assumptions about what it means to be an effective physician and what constitutes valid medical knowledge.

As will be shown in the following sections, the clinical frames used by the McLean psychiatrists differed from the formulas of science in three significant ways. First, although the frames did conform to certain clinical parameters, they were not equivalent to the formulas of science. Because they were constructed in a dialectic that drew from both domains – the universalized models of science and the localized reality of medical practice – the resultant clinical frames were *mediated* forms. Second, the kinds of variables that entered into a decision were far broader than the kinds reported in medical textbooks. Good medicine meant more than just understanding how the body functioned, but how the world worked as well. Third, to be a practicing psychiatrist implied the responsibility to wear not one hat but many, each entailing a different set of perspectives and obligations. Medical decisions necessarily involved the balancing of conflicting human interests, a thorny problem that had no easy resolution – and certainly no formulaic one. An attempt to reconstruct the shape of these clinical frames, and the logic of their application, will illuminate the human dimensions of medical decision making and the consequent limitations within which physicians must labor. A physician's practice is forged in the *intersection* of medical art and science.

### The Clinical Frame: The Macroview

Was Tompkins right? Was the selection of patients for psychosurgery entirely an individualized matter, a decision that had to be made without reference to any predetermined frame? As a matter of historical prudence, global statements of this kind must be taken with a grain of salt. Even in the putatively rational world of medicine, self-perceptions and behavior do not always correspond.[51] How, then, do we make visible the set of inclusion and exclusion rules that might have guided these psychiatrists? How do we begin to reconstruct the clinical frame by which patients were selected for psychosurgery at McLean Hospital? In this task, the power of hindsight provides a perspective not available to any one person who was on the scene and may bring out any discrepancies between a person's thoughts and actions. A macroscopic view has its advantages. In this manner, we may hope to recover the unseen "rules" that, much like traffic lines, guided but not did determine individual behaviors.

The first step toward a reconstruction of this clinical frame is to characterize the pool of patients operated upon. Between 1938 and 1954, the year of the final operation, a total of eighty patients at McLean had received a lobotomy.[52] As Figure 6.4 indicates, if you were recommended for a brain operation at McLean, you were most likely to have received it sometime between 1945 and 1951, the period when over four-fifths of the total were performed. The odds were similarly stacked that you would be female. Just fourteen – about one-sixth – were male. The median age of the lobotomy patients was fifty years at time of operation, with only a small

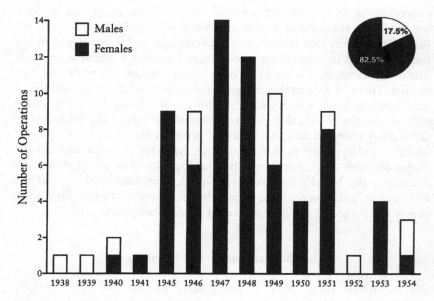

Figure 6.4. Psychosurgery at McLean Hospital, 1938–1954. Years in which operation was performed, by sex (n=80: 66 females, 14 males). (Source: McLean
Hospital, Belmont, Massachusetts)

difference between sexes. Ages ranged, however, between a low of nineteen years and a high of eighty-three, and the distribution by age category
approximated a normal bell curve.[53]

The average length of stay for all eighty patients was about five years of
total prior hospitalization, a figure less than that reported by Howard and
Tompkins, who were basing their statistics on earlier portions of the
series. Even so, their numbers are misleading, as the *median* lengths of stay
show quite a different story: half of the patients had less than 2.1 years of
total hospitalization.[54] There also appears to have been a gender disparity
in the length of stay. For males, the median length of all prior hospitalizations was as high as six and a half years; for females, less than two years.
And whereas one-fourth of the women had one year or less of hospitalization, this could be said of only one of the fourteen men. Conversely, one-
tenth of the women as compared to one-third of the men were hospitalized
for more than ten years.[55] However, the wide variance washes out any
clear pattern, as males were operated upon with as few as thirty-three
weeks of hospitalization, and females were selected with a total length of

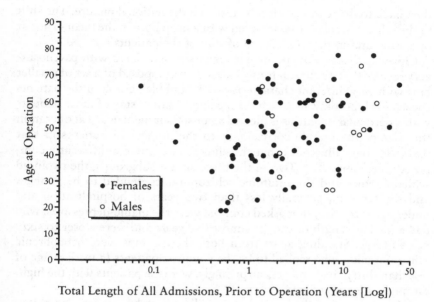

Figure 6.5. Psychosurgery at McLean Hospital, 1938–1954. Hospitalization (this admission) versus age at operation, scatterplot (n = 80). (Source: McLean Hospital, Belmont, Massachusetts)

stay of as much as thirty-seven years. Indeed, a scatterplot of age at operation versus length of stay (plotted on a log scale of years, as such stays varied from 26 to 13,681 days) reveals that, for both men and women, among the short-term patients as well as the long-term, the young as well as the old were operated upon (see Figure 6.5). A first glance thus supports Harmon's aside that "any and all" were considered appropriate for the operation.

Some patterns do emerge, however, when the patients are analyzed in terms of diagnosis. To begin with, it appears that the clinical frame went through several distinct phases. As mentioned previously, in the first wave that ended in 1941 all five patients were diagnosed with forms of agitated depression. The expansion during the second wave was clearly due to the introduction of the operation's use for the various kinds of schizophrenia; the decline in the lobotomy program in the final years between 1952 and 1954 was a consequence of a falloff in the numbers of schizophrenics. This "diagnostic crossover" – from depression to schizophrenics, and then back to depression – closely mirrored the national picture. The shift to the schizophrenias corresponded with a drop both in the median age at operation and in the total length of stay of the patients selected.[56]

Closer analysis of the particular diagnoses associated with psychosurgery reveals that its clinical frame was in fact composed of a set of smaller bins with very different characteristics. A "bubble" graph of the patients chosen for lobotomy, in which the median length of stay of those patients with a particular diagnosis is plotted against their median age at operation (the size of the bubble corresponds to the number of patients in that particular bin), illustrates that the clinical targets were differently composed (see Figure 6.6). Two of the three largest subgroups, the paranoid schizophrenics and the catatonic schizophrenics, tended to be younger and shorter-term, generally less than two years of hospitalization and under age forty-five. In marked contrast were the manic-depressives, who had a median length of stay of almost five years and were closer to sixty years of age. Standing apart from both these camps were hebephrenic schizophrenics, who tended to be the youngest patients (a median age of less than thirty-five) and yet, surprisingly, were the patients with the highest median length of stay.

A breakdown of the psychosurgery diagnoses by gender also shows some striking differences (see Figure 6.7). Whereas more than half of the female lobotomy patients were either paranoid schizophrenics or catatonic schizophrenics, these categories amounted to only a small portion of the males (2 out of 14). And although the categories of involutional depressions and psychoneuroses together accounted for a significant number of female patients, none of the males had these conditions. For their part, the males were almost exclusively either manic-depressives (6 patients) or hebephrenic schizophrenics (5 patients). The latter category is particularly interesting, in that only 1 out of the 66 women were hebephrenic schizophrenics. It appears that, not only was the decision to consider lobotomy heavily gender-biased, but so too was the particular pattern of its application.

An analysis that focuses exclusively on the pool of patients who received psychosurgery can only go so far, however. What it cannot do is offer any insight into the prior process by which patients were first selected as candidates for the procedure. Perhaps the reason more females were lobotomized than males was that at McLean Hospital there were more of them to begin with; similarly, the differences in the median age and length of stay between the various diagnostic groups of psychosurgery patients may indicate no more than that these were the characteristics of those

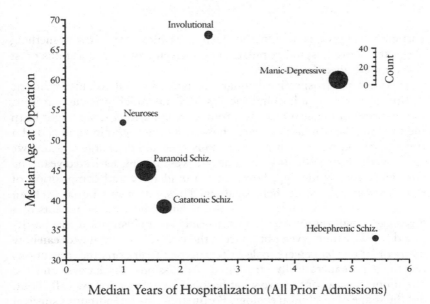

Figure 6.6. Psychosurgery at McLean Hospital, 1938–1954. Hospitalization (all prior admissions) and age, by diagnosis, bubbleplot (n=75). (Source: McLean Hospital, Belmont, Massachusetts)

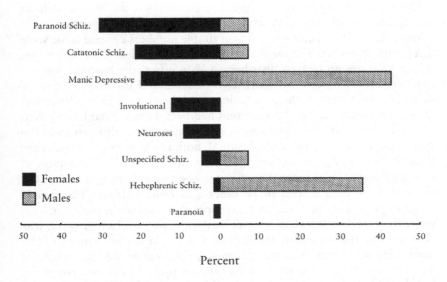

Figure 6.7. Psychosurgery at McLean Hospital, 1938–1954. Diagnosis by sex, bar-chart (n=80). (Source: McLean Hospital, Belmont, Massachusetts)

particular subgroups within the hospital. Unless we know something about the entire hospital population on a given day, such questions must remain mere speculation.

This kind of retrospective demography is not a trivial task in psychiatric institutions, even in a hospital such as McLean which was vigilant in its preservation of medical records. From an *Annual Report* we might learn the total number of patients in the hospital at the beginning and end of a fiscal year; and from the preserved admissions and discharge registers we can identify those patients who came and went during a selected year. The vital piece that is missing, however, is the identity and composition of those patients who were there all along. Thus, nowhere – not at McLean nor at any other mental hospital – was it tallied how many patients of a given age, diagnosis, or length of stay resided in an institution on a particular day. (We cannot even obtain from the *Annual Report* at McLean how many of its residents were male or female.) At their core, the institutions remained bureaucratically structured. Admissions, discharges, and the remaining census count were what hospital administration was all about, not the shape of its clinical ecology. Fortunately, the serendipitous survival of several months' worth of canteen bills in 1948 enables us to recapture these long-term patients at McLean, and, with the addition of the registers, an accurate re-creation can be made of the entire hospital population.[57]

On 1 January 1948, there were 195 patients on the wards with an average age of almost sixty and a length of stay (not counting prior admissions) of over eight years. These simple numbers conceal some wide disparities, however. The median length of stay was less than four years, which indicates an uneven distribution.[58] In effect, the hospital population was split between the short-term patients and the very long-term. Whereas one-fourth of the population at McLean were in residence less than six months, an equal proportion had been hospitalized longer than ten years. Of particular significance, however, were the differences in the way the sexes were utilizing the hospital, both in the number of beds they occupied and in the patterns of their stay. In fact, women outnumbered men on the wards by more than a two-to-one ratio (133 versus 62). On the whole, women tended to be older and more chronic. The female median age of sixty-one was six years more than that of the male patients, while their median length of hospitalization, at four and a half years, was almost twice that of the males. Indeed, a much larger percentage of the male population was short-term; almost 40 percent of the male residents had been at McLean less than six months, compared to 20 percent of the females.[59] McLean's reputation as a holding facility for elderly, long-term female patients was in large measure true.[60]

The baseline population on 1 January 1948 also provides a stable point from which to test the received opinions regarding the poor prognoses of the chronic patients, by following their fates prospectively. A linear regression between the patients' prior length of stay (all prior admissions) and their future time until discharge does reveal a strong, direct correlation.[61] The longer you had been in a hospital, the longer you were going to stay. Furthermore, if the 195 residents are partitioned into cohorts with different prior lengths of hospitalization, their respective "half-lives" can be charted by calculating the median times until discharge. Such an analysis determines that a sharp change for the worse did in fact take place for those patients so unfortunate as to be hospitalized for longer than two years. A patient's chance of ever leaving the hospital alive also declined precipitously. Patients hospitalized less than three months had a survival rate of 95 percent, but for those already in the hospital between five and ten years, this dropped to a grim 37 percent. In fact, of the 195 residents in the hospital on our census day, as many as 41 percent would eventually die still hospitalized.[62]

A basis now exists from which to discern some of the pressures bearing upon the selection of patients for psychosurgery. The fact that the hospital housed twice as many women as men is a first step toward explaining the wide gender disparity in the lobotomy program. This statistic alone can account for half of the skewed 3.8 to 1 ratio between the female and male lobotomy patients. A breakdown of the diagnostic categories by sex also reveals some interesting differences that were reflected in the psychosurgery program. Figure 6.8 illustrates that the major clinical subgroups for women were (in descending order): paranoid schizophrenics, manic-depressives, seniles, catatonic schizophrenics, and then involutionals. Other than the seniles – who were considered to suffer from an "organic" brain condition and thus to be unsuitable for psychosurgery – this progression corresponds to the relative frequency of lobotomies (compare to Figure 6.7).

The male residents had a dissimilar diagnostic profile. For example, proportionally, many more men than women entered McLean for a drug or alcohol problem, or for counseling to overcome a psychoneurosis. Of note here, the differences in the diagnostic patterns presented by the male and female patients can shed light on the variance in the rate at which the genders were lobotomized. The number one diagnostic category among male residents, for example, was manic-depression, which also happens to have been the most frequent diagnosis among the male patients operated upon. The population of male residents also had significantly lower proportions of paranoid schizophrenics, catatonic schizophrenics, and involutionals – all categories represented by lower proportions among the

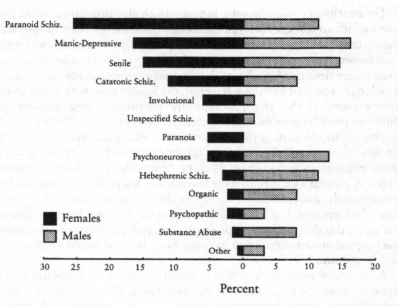

Figure 6.8. Patients in residence at McLean Hospital on 1 January 1948. Diagnosis by sex, bar-chart (female n = 133, male n = 62). (Source: McLean Hospital, Belmont, Massachusetts)

males chosen for lobotomy than were the females. It is also significant that the other major category of males selected for operation, the hebephrenic schizophrenics, was in fact ranked fourth in the categories of male residents, immediately trailing the psychoneurotics and the seniles – of which neither category was considered a good bet for psychosurgery. In contrast, very few women hebephrenics were operated upon; this corresponds well to the fact that only 3 percent of the women residents were in this category.[63]

The number of patients in residence on a given day gives us only a partial picture of the long-term hospital burden imposed by a patient with a particular diagnosis, however. Rather, of more immediate concern to the institutional staff was the relative rate at which the beds were emptying. For example, by the end of the year, all seven substance-abuse patients had already been discharged; this could be said of only about two of the eleven hebephrenics. One strategy is to count the number of days each patient occupied a bed in the course of the following year, and then to calculate for each diagnosis the percentage of the total "bed-days"; next, this figure is matched against the percentage of all patients who had that diagnosis. The resulting ratio provides a rough index of how much of a drain upon institutional resources the hospital staff could expect from a patient with a given diagnosis. Such an analysis reveals that, in the case of the males, the hebephrenic category accounted for more bed-days than did any other diagnosis and, at the same time, that it did so with the relatively fewest number – in other words, it also averaged the highest number of bed-days per patient. In the case of the women, the results correspond to the rankings already observed: paranoid schizophrenics both constituted the highest absolute number of bed-days and also held a very high average number of bed-days per patient.[64]

Although this kind of analysis helps to pin down why particular categories of patients were selected for psychosurgery, it does not account for why certain groups were passed over. In particular, one puzzle that emerges is the lack of paranoid schizophrenics among the males chosen for lobotomy. There were as many of them as there were hebephrenics, and they certainly accounted for a significant number of bed-days – with a high bed-day average per patient, in addition. An answer may be found in a closer examination of who these patients were at McLean. Compared to the female paranoid schizophrenics, who had a median length of stay (all prior admissions) of over eight years, the males in this diagnostic category had a median stay of almost thirty years, an extraordinarily high number (indeed, it was the highest among all of the male diagnostic categories) – a figure that put it far afield of the usual lobotomy profile.[65] Such a situation also pertains to the female hebephrenics, who also were extremely long-term, with a median hospitalization of more than twenty-five years.

After establishing some sense of what were the multiple frames with which patients were identified as candidates for lobotomy, the next matter is to ascertain the overall selective pressure – that is, to ask what were a person's odds of being recommended for a lobotomy? On the whole, of the 195 patients in residence on 1 January 1948, only seven (less than 4 percent) would receive psychosurgery during the next year, which does not look particularly significant. An additional eleven would receive it in the following years, however, raising the total to over 9 percent. If the other eighteen patients who *already* had had a lobotomy are added, one finds that thirty-six – 18 percent – were at some point in the past, present, or future captured within the psychosurgery program. And if a patient fell into the right "bin," his or her odds grew even higher. For example, of the thirty-four female paranoid schizophrenics, eight (23.5 percent) received a lobotomy by the end of 1948. (Patient records reveal that an additional three were recommended for the operation, but for various reasons did not have it.) This endpoint was also true for three out of the eight involutionals (37.5 percent), and for seven out of fifteen catatonics – a remarkable rate of almost 50 percent. If the "bin" is narrowed to particular ranges of age and length of stay, even tighter fits emerge. For example, of the seven female catatonics who were neither very short-term nor extremely long-term (those who were in residence for a period between six months and fifteen years), only two did *not* have a lobotomy. In the case of the males, out of the seven hebephrenic schizophrenics who were in residence on 1 January, three would receive a lobotomy in 1949; if the frame is further narrowed down to those who were hospitalized for less than twenty-five years, this yields four residents – three of whom would soon receive a lobotomy, while the fourth was considered for it.[66]

The picture presented by this analysis of the 1 January population is literally only half the story, however. In one of his essays in the *Annual Report*, Dr. Paul Howard described the "two worlds" in which the hospital clinician worked, in that "the static picture of a given moment is different from the impression of the clinical work to be done on the total annual load of cases." Although the view of the wards on any given day looked rather bleak, as the hospital was filled mostly with chronic cases, in fact there was a rather rapid turnover in the beds that were not permanently occupied. In a year's work, Howard noted, the psychiatrist actually treated twice as many acute patients as he did chronic.[67]

A profile of the 303 patients admitted during the year does reveal characteristics quite different from that of the resident population. Compared to the resident population, the new admissions were on average ten years younger, with a distribution skewed heavily in the opposite direction.[68] There was also less disparity among the new admissions in how the sexes were using the inpatient services. Of these, 169 were female and 134 male, a far more even ratio; moreover, the median age of forty-four was the same for females and males.[69] A breakdown by diagnosis does show some differences, although not as dramatic as those among the residents. Apparently, the most popular use of McLean by males was as a place to dry out from alcohol or drug problems. At the same time, men entering McLean were far less likely to be diagnosed with senility or involutional melancholia than were women.[70]

When a comparison is made between the ratio of new admissions to residents for each diagnostic category, some suggestive patterns emerge.[71] Such a ratio gives a rough approximation of the rate at which the beds were turning over or, contrariwise, were stuck. (In interpreting these figures, it should be noted that, as McLean was a private hospital, the staff had the luxury of deciding which patients to admit.) Among the males, only in the senile and hebephrenic categories did the residents outnumber the admissions; it was the hospital's experience that, should one of these patients stay, it would be for a very long time. In the case of women, once again the paranoid schizophrenics stand apart, with far fewer new admissions than residents, which is suggestive of a very high retention rate. The same might be said for the catatonic schizophrenics, though not as extremely. In contrast, the new admissions of manic-depressives and involutionals far exceeded the number of residents; apparently, the beds turned over far more rapidly for these conditions. As shall be evident, these differences had visible effects on the way in which the psychosurgery patients were selected.

By merging the two worlds of the resident population and that of the new admissions, a complete portrait can be drawn of the patient universe from which the psychosurgery patients were chosen. By comparing the lobotomy patients with an entire year's worth of patient profiles, further insight can be gained into the process of selection. Patients fell into the right "bin," not just because they were already on the wards at the moment when the psychiatrists first went out looking for likely candidates, but also because they were admitted afterward with the appropriate clinical history or had stayed long enough to "mature" into the right profile even if they had been passed over earlier.[72] To accomplish this statistical task, some assumptions and artifices were employed. In the case of the "hospital-year" population of 498 cases – 195 residents plus 303 admissions – length of stay was calculated as the number of days hospitalized as of 31 December 1948. The pool of psychosurgery patients was enlarged to include all patients operated on between 1946 and 1950, for the reason that the number of operations in any given year was small and by itself not particularly representative.[73]

An age versus length of stay scatterplot of the two populations is not immediately revealing (see Figure 6.9). Some patterns do emerge, however, if the raw data are first broken up by sex and then by diagnostic categories, and the resulting scatterplots are transformed with a density estimation function to yield a contour map.[74] The males are especially open to such analysis, as during the peak of the psychosurgery program all seven lobotomy patients were diagnosed with various forms of schizophrenia. If these male psychosurgery patients are superimposed upon a contour plot of all schizophrenic patients in the hospital-year population, two patterns are suggested (see Figure 6.10). First, apparently the procedure was used on those patients who had arrived at the "edge" of the short-to-moderate-term population and who were still relatively young. Second, it was also used on younger members of the very long-term population. This indicates that two separate strategies were in play: the "noth-

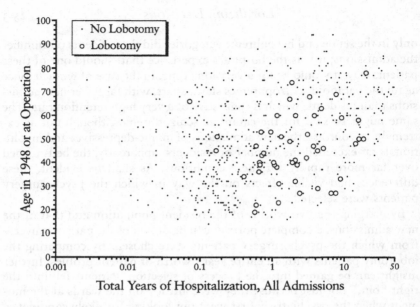

Figure 6.9. Patients in residence at McLean Hospital during the 1948 calendar year. Comparison of nonpsychosurgery population with patients operated on between 1946 and 1950, scatterplot (residents n=458, psychosurgery n=49). (Source: McLean Hospital, Belmont, Massachusetts)

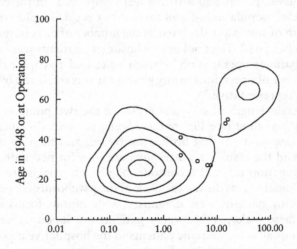

Figure 6.10. Male schizophrenic patients at McLean Hospital during the 1948 calendar year. Comparison of nonpsychosurgery population with similar patients operated on between 1946 and 1950, contour plot (nonpsychosurgery n=50, psychosurgery n=7). (Source: McLean Hospital, Belmont, Massachusetts)

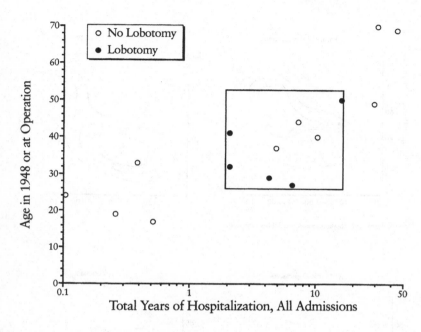

Figure 6.11. Male patients with hebephrenia at McLean Hospital during the 1948 calendar year. Comparison of nonpsychosurgery population with similar patients operated on between 1946 and 1950, scatterplot (nonpsychosurgery n = 10, psychosurgery n = 5). (Source: McLean Hospital, Belmont, Massachusetts)

ing left to lose but still something to gain" scenario for the long-term males, and the goal of preventing moderate-term patients from crossing over the "point of no return." The tightness of the clinical frame for men is revealed by an inspection of just the hebephrenic schizophrenics, who accounted for five of the seven patients operated on: there were only ten nonlobotomized hebephrenic men in our sample year. Figure 6.11 indicates the small region of the clinical map into which the lobotomy patients fell. Only three patients in this region did *not* have a lobotomy.[75]

The pattern of use of lobotomies on female patients reveals, not one story, or even two, but multiple ones. A contour map of the paranoid schizophrenic patients, for example, shows a pattern of operating upon the younger and short-term members of a population that was concentrated toward the longer term (see Figure 6.12a). A picture of the catatonic schizophrenics resembles the example of the males, in which the procedure was used on young but longer-term members of a population

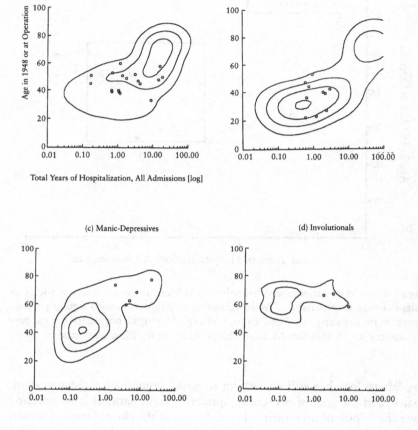

Figure 6.12 a–d. Female patients in residence at McLean Hospital during the 1948 calendar year. Comparison of nonpsychosurgery population with similar patients operated on between 1946 and 1950, contour maps: (a) paranoid schizophrenia; (b) catatonic schizophrenia; (c) manic-depression; (d) involutional. (Source: McLean Hospital, Belmont, Massachusetts)

that was mostly short term (see Figure 6.12b). The next two populations, the manic-depressives and the involutionals, yield a very different picture, however (see Figures 6.12c, d). The manic-depressive population was generally short-term, but the patients selected for lobotomy were the very old and very long-term; the involutional psychosurgery patients were like-

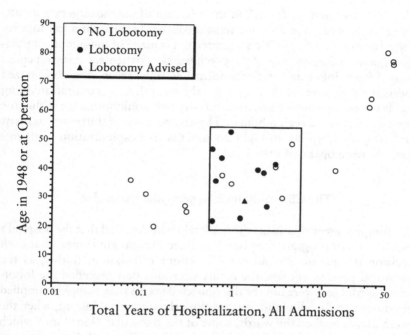

Figure 6.13. Female patients with catatonic schizophrenia in residence at McLean Hospital during the 1948 calendar year. Comparison of nonpsychosurgery population with similar patients operated on between 1946 and 1950, scatterplot (non-psychosurgery n = 16, psychosurgery n = 10). (Source: McLean Hospital, Belmont, Massachusetts)

wise very old and very long-term, having been chosen from a population that was relatively short-term in stay but very old nevertheless. Significantly, virtually none of the psychosurgery patients landed "on the peak" of any of the diagnostic categories. The procedure apparently was in fact a procedure of last resort, not to be used as the mode of routine therapy for the average patient.

As to the selective pressure within each particular frame, the numbers are suggestive. The ten female lobotomy patients who were diagnosed with catatonic schizophrenia all fit within a boundary of six months to five years of total hospitalization; only six catatonics within this boundary did not receive such an operation, and one of these was in fact recommended for the procedure (see Figure 6.13). And of the involutional population of twenty-one patients, there were only four who matched the three chosen for psychosurgery in long-term stay yet who were not extremely old. The most active "frame" in the selection of psychosurgery patients, however, was the one used for female paranoid schizophrenics. In a reverse contour graph, in which a scatterplot is made of the sample population against a density map of the psychosurgery patients, the region encircling fifteen lobotomy patients identifies only seven nonlobotomized individuals. A count of the subjects in the second, more concentrated ring yields ten psychosurgery patients and only two nonlobotomies; within the peak – a very small region bounded by an age range of thirty-five to forty, and roughly from six to eighteen months of hospitalization – *all five* patients were operated upon.

### The Clinical Frame: General and Particular

Dr. Tompkins was clearly off the mark when he declared that the hospital's psychosurgery program contained no fixed clinical guidelines, that each decision to operate was an entirely unique calculation. Rather, as the statistical portrait reveals, the eighty decisions that preceded the lobotomies at McLean were not the disconnected events that Tompkins implied but did generally fall within certain clinical parameters. Indeed, when the psychiatrists walked the wards, some of the particular "bins" into which patients were segregated by age, sex, length of stay, and diagnosis were certainly destined for consideration for lobotomy. For a number of patients, the decision to operate did follow set guidelines and was predictable.

This said, the frames that the McLean psychiatrists used were not equivalent to the kinds of formulas that appeared in scientific textbooks, in which the ingredients are assumed to be standardized and the results the same regardless of the location of the laboratory. To begin with, psychiatrists knew all too well that no two hospitals were exactly alike in their combination of patients and conditions. The respective clinical maps were shaped in contrasting ways by very real regional variances. Patients in northeastern hospitals presented an altogether different mixture of nationalities, economic resources, and mental conditions than those in the southern institutions, for example. At the same time, there was the disturbing reality that in psychiatry the practice of diagnostics itself varied widely from place to place. Moreover, a hebephrenic schizophrenic at a private institution was not the same kind of problem that it was at a state hospital, which had different resources and limitations. The institutions' diverse problems generated varied solutions.

This plurality of contexts pertained to more than just the differences among hospitals, however. It also played out within each institution. In the present example, it was discovered that the clinical frame for psycho-surgery was not defined in reference to a single idealized clinical type but was varied in accordance with the region of the hospital's clinical ecology in which the patient happened to be located. Tellingly, within each of these different sectors the procedure was used *for different functions*. Experience had taught the McLean staff that, for the kinds of female patients they referred to as involutionals and manic-depressives, their mental disturbance was likely to clear up on its own and was unlikely to lead to very long-term institutionalization. As there was no immediate pressure, the use of the operation was thus limited to those patients for whom even longer periods of hospitalization were unlikely to yield further hope of discharge. In the case of male schizophrenics and female catatonic schizophrenics, however, an opposite tactic appears. Such patients were operated on after only a moderate waiting period had elapsed, in the hope of preventing them from slipping into the pool of chronic schizophrenics which, in the hospital staff's experience, was considered certain doom. The most extensive selection was of female paranoid schizophrenics, who presented the worst clinical scenario, with the large majority of the total hospital-year population being elderly and long-term; the strategy here was to operate early and often. (The males, it should be noted, had a significantly longer waiting period.) Remarkably, then, even within the same facility the frames were multiple, not single, and were applied for widely varying and even contrary strategies. In short, the treatments in a doctor's black bag are often akin to the tools in a carpenter's chest: the value and particular use of any instrument depends on the nature of the problems that arise and the inventiveness of the user, regardless of what the manuals instruct.

This multiplicity of frames takes on greater significance due to the lack of any clear congruence between the profession's diagnostic map and the inherent logic of how the patients were scattered through the wards. Each ward at McLean was uniquely defined by the kind of behavior tolerated, the level of nursing provided, the treatments available, and so on. For whatever reason, patients on Belknap I presented a very different kind of problem than those on Appleton III, and invited different solutions. As the clinicians introduced new treatments into the hospital, then, they tried to ascertain the therapy's utility within each of these local regions. What looked like a "good" lobotomy patient – or for that matter, a likely candidate for insulin shock, Total Push, or psychotherapy – thus varied from building to building, and from floor to floor. Whether being applied among wards within a single institution or between hospitals, the psychiatrists' tools, perspectives, and store of knowledge all had to be recalibrated.

The clinical challenge for practicing psychiatrists, then, was precisely the process of abstracting – the medical literature, national meetings, or even staff conferences within the home institution – the kinds of information that did seem relevant to their clientele, and weighing this against their personal experience while working within their own clinical backyard. Confronted by a range of pressing problems (that might or might not exist elsewhere) and yet having on hand only a limited set of therapeutic tools with which they felt comfortable, the doctors' response had been both flexible and adaptive. A clinician's work is defined exactly in this intersection of the general and the local: both are needed to find the path to therapeutic action. Eventually, the frames themselves become tailored to fit the local geography. Clinical handbooks that spelled out when to use what type of treatment were like compasses without a map, or cookbooks without the ingredients listed. It was the doctor's own experience on the wards that filled in the guiding landmarks.

In sum, the fact that the patients who received lobotomies at McLean did, in large measure, fit within a particular set of clinical boundaries is not proof that the physicians had applied a kind of scientific formulary. A repertoire of specific clinical frames was in place, but its utility was localized, a product of the interaction between a particular group of McLean physicians and the clients they served.

## Expanding the Frame

The image of the clinician as a form of applied scientist led to another kind of distortion in our understanding of what doctors must consider. The frames which physicians used to sort out likely candidates for a particular treatment were by no means limited to such strictly "clinical" factors as diagnosis, duration of illness, and age, but incorporated a far broader range of dimensions. The goal of returning a patient home to a life of work, love, and play, was altogether a different kind of challenge from that of patching up a broken organism; individuals had to survive within complex social realities that were spun by families, friends, employers, and the wider community. Indeed, it was this task of tending to this social matrix that presented some of the most critical difficulties for the psychiatrists in our current example. Thus, as much as the McLean physicians might concern themselves about the appropriate medical response to a clear case of "biological schizophrenia," yet another responsibility entered into their occupation: the need to understand and manipulate the social environment from which the patient came, and to which he or she would have to return if discharged from the institution. The modern psychiatrist was necessarily also a kind of social worker.[76]

The initial success of the lobotomy program, for example, brought out the sad truth that unless family members were willing to welcome a patient back home, an operation could be a success but the patient still might never leave the institution. Experience taught that McLean occasionally served as a dumping ground for unwanted relatives. The staff bitterly noted, for example, that, as the husband of Mrs. Helen Stoddard wanted to "get on in life" socially and professionally, he had brought his wife to McLean with the idea that "there is not much to do and that this is the nicest way of getting rid of her in a decent fashion." In this situation, the potential for cure only raised additional problems. When it came time to recommend for or against lobotomy, these realities were factored in. In the case of Anna Winthrop, for example, one argument presented against lobotomy was the fact that the patient had "worn down" her husband's enthusiasm so much that he did not want her returned home; even with the operation, it was felt, "we would still have quite a problem on our hands as to what to do with her."

The prospect of preparing for discharge patients with long periods of hospitalization, many of whom had no family left or who required some degree of supervision, prompted the hospital to explore alternative social solutions. In the 1940s, however, no "halfway" or "transitional housing" programs for former mental hospital inmates existed. The problem was further exacerbated by the use of the new active treatments, which were sending home patients who previously would simply have remained institutionalized.[77] McLean's creative response was to place such patients in boarding homes run by its own former or retired nurses. Many of the lobotomy patients thus were farmed out to an informal network of establishments scattered about the New England seashore. (During his summer vacations, Director Wood himself would drop by these facilities to check up on things.)

Another unintended consequence of the lobotomy program was an appreciation of how changes in the basic personality of the patient could result in a realignment of the overall family dynamics – changes for good or ill, depending on the local circumstances. In the previously quoted letter from the mother of Catharine Birmingham, for example, it is evident that an important factor in the judged success of the operation was the patient's newfound deference to her husband. The staff also learned that the improvement in a patient's personality might in fact lead to strained relations where none had existed before. When Sarah Worthington returned home, motivated and able to seek employment, her husband rebelled at the change in his wife's ambitions.

Every family had its own rats' nest of problems with which the individual patient had proven unable to cope. The postoperative personality, it was hoped, would provide a second chance. For example, Mrs. Eliza Wigglesworth had felt inadequate compared to her daughter, who was described as a bright, capable person. Before the operation, she could not face the thought of returning home to live with her daughter. As a result of lobotomy, however, "her pre-operative inability to accept the idea" changed into "a complete acceptance of the situation." What previously had been "a source of great concern, no longer disturbed her."

It was this feel for the circumstances of an individual patient's life upon which psychiatrists at McLean prided themselves, and which they often relied on in the search for clues as to what treatment route was most appropriate. When the staff wrestled over what to do with Adelaide Hitchcock, the deciding factor was actually the status of her *father's* physical health. Now at the end of a very long life, the father had expressed to the staff his desire "to get her straightened out if possible before he dies." The Waverly physicians saw only a bleak future ahead for this particular patient. The father was in fact irreplaceable, as he had devoted a considerable portion of his life to taking care of his unbalanced daughter. The daughter, having led a necessarily restricted, overprotected life, was sure "to go all to pieces when he's not there to watch her." As the father was aware that "he won't be able to help her forever," the solution was to inform him of the potential of a lobotomy if performed while there was still time.

In short, the kinds of factors that were used to identify good lobotomy prospects were not restricted to clinical indicators, narrowly defined. When the psychiatrists scrutinized their patients for indications as to what course of treatment might prove successful, they looked to any and all characteristics by which to predict good results. In so doing, the physiological or psychiatric signs, such as age, length of stay, or frequency of hallucinations, became shuffled in with the social factors, such as the willingness of the family to receive the patient home and the amount of money available for an extended stay. For a treatment to be adopted with some regularity, it would have to satisfy all of these other considerations as well. At a pragmatic level, then, boundaries collapsed between the clinical and what are usually regarded as extraclinical factors. A treatment either made sense for a particular kind of patient or it didn't. In consequence, the clinical frames employed by physicians were multidimensional, expansive constructs that interwove diagnostic and cultural maps.

## Women Troubles

The heterogeneous nature of these clinical frames had important ramifications for what kinds of persons would be perceived as in need of a particular treatment. Indeed, what looked like a good candidate reflected the special qualities of the world in which the patients and physicians lived. An enduring mystery of the psychosurgery story, for instance, is why women were lobotomized nationally at a rate twice that of males, a fact made public in 1949 by the USPHS psychosurgery survey. There was certainly nothing in the theoretical or physiological justifications undergirding the procedure that pointed to a higher therapeutic value for women than for men. Indeed, as a rule the authors who wrote articles on the use of lobotomy never posited the idea that female brains or constitutions were somehow more suited for this treatment.

The USPHS survey was a conspicuous exception to the silence maintained on gender issues, devoting an entire paragraph to the phenomenon. "Persons familiar with the administration of hospitals," it reported, had suggested to the statisticians that the higher proportion of females operated upon was related to "the greater administrative difficulty in providing adequate nursing care for agitated females."[78] If this were true, one might expect the beleaguered state hospitals to lobotomize women in greater proportion than the private hospitals, which had ample nursing resources. The report itself published the exactly opposite finding, however.

More recently, the gender bias in the use of lobotomy has been cited as proof of how sexism pervades medicine. Such accounts contend that doctors preferentially routed women into the psychosurgery programs because they malevolently adhered to social prejudices that tolerated less autonomy in women than men. Lobotomies were the latest equivalent of the Victorian-era fad for clitorectomies.[79] However, the example of McLean Hospital, a place where the gender bias was skewed substantially more than the national average, reveals that such direct linkages are oversimplistic. The men clearly were also targeted for psychosurgery, though in different areas of the clinical grid. Indeed, within some of these regions they were lobotomized at a rate equal to or even higher than the women.

This is not to say that the medicine of the day was gender-neutral. Rather, issues of gender, as well as other social or cultural lines of demarcation, were so inextricably woven into the basic structures of medicine as to yield gendered results even when the medical apparatus was applied neutrally. The question of why men and women received psychiatric treatments at varying rates depended upon the prior issue of why, for example, schizophrenic women happened to be perceived as presenting a different kind of problem than schizophrenic men. There are two major sources of these disparities.

First, as was evident at McLean Hospital, the sexes were utilizing the hospital in divergent ways. For whatever reasons, social or biological, they came in with different rates of mental pathology and were dissimilar in their lengths of stay – even within the same diagnostic categories. (As much as half of the gender skewing in this facility's use of lobotomy, we have seen, could be accounted for on the basis of such differences in clinical ecology.)

Second, given the social realities of the day, the route to mental health was understood to be different for women than for men. Thus, although the psychiatric criteria for psychosurgery on the surface might be considered gender-neutral, nevertheless the medical algorithm would yield one-sided results. Of especial importance was the perception of how the two genders might make their way in the world after the operation. "We have based our work more on the social than on the psychiatric findings," Freeman wrote, for "we have performed operations when the patient faced prolonged or permanent disability and when the type of occupation did not require much constructive imagination."[80] In short, the fact that women's work was not considered to require much intelligence relative to men's no doubt accounts for much of the gender bias. It is suggestive that at a private hospital like McLean – where the men typically came from the ranks of professional and skilled workers, careers not easily regained, and in contrast the women were so well provided for that a return to even housework was not always expected – the disparity in the gender bias was much higher than at the state hospitals.[81]

In either case, it made little practical difference to the psychiatrist on the wards whether the gender differences in clinical ecology or prognosis were due to errors of biology or social convention. The highest priority was simply to return the patients home. They saw that lobotomy did just that, though more for certain kinds of women than for other kinds of patients, and adjusted their clinical frames accordingly. Whether or not the psychiatrists agreed with the notion that women should have more fulfilling job opportunities, or even blamed a number of nervous breakdowns on the lack of good career paths for women, the matter of who looked to them like a good lobotomy candidate came out the same, given the circumstances of the world as they knew it.

## Multiple Hats

It was not just the methods and skills of the clinicians as they went about their daily practice which distinguished their work from that of an applied scientist, but their goals. The decision to follow this or that course of treatment necessarily involved trade-offs – for the patient and his or her family, for the institution that housed them, and for the professionals involved. Physicians – then as well as now – must balance all the competing interests that arise, trading in the messy stuff of human values. These kinds of equations are not easily routinized, further complicating the process by which physicians must reach their decisions.

As important as were the clinical frames, they were of course only one of the many possible routes that brought patients into the pool of psychosurgery candidates – or that ruled them out. The physicians at McLean Hospital wore several hats in addition to that of clinician. First, as members of a psychiatric elite, they took on an additional responsibility of adding to the store of existing medical knowledge: they also considered themselves *researchers*. Thus, some patients might be selected for a brain operation for the precise reason that they stood *outside* the usual or known guidelines, becoming test cases for future revisions to the existing clinical frames.[82] In 1946, for example, the staff viewed Mrs. Annabel Simms as "an opportunity to study further . . . what the bilateral prefrontal lobotomy might do for a higher function" patient, as had been suggested by the work of Freeman and Watts.[83] And when a good result was obtained in a well-preserved psychoneurotic, Cowes saw this as an occasion to congratulate Harmon, who "has made an important contribution" to the subject. In effect, some patients became experiments waiting to happen. In the case of Adelaide Hitchcock, for example, Murphy noted that "She might be a good candidate for one of the lower quadrant lobotomies which we were thinking about doing." As a last example, when the staff dithered back and forth about the advisability of a lobotomy for Howard Peckler, Norcross noted that the evidence weighed equally for and against it; the hopelessness of the case spoke for taking a chance just to see what would happen. The lobotomy was justified, he stated, "from an experimental point of view."

The medical staff at McLean were proud of their clinical and scientific hats, wearing them as signs of professional commitment. However, several other hats went along with the job of being a hospital physician, some of which did not fit so comfortably. More than they cared to admit, even to themselves, physicians had to compete within a larger fee-for-service economy that answered to those who paid the bills. The truth of this had already registered with Tillotson when he defended the hospital's adoption of the shock therapies on the ground that family pressures could no longer be resisted. And once psychosurgery became known to the public, it was only a matter of time before it too would be demanded by anxious families. In the case of Mrs. Harriet Palmer, for example, the operation was originally the husband's idea. In time, patients entered McLean for the sole purpose of having a lobotomy.[84] Apparently, the lobotomy program was its own advertisement. For example, the parents of Lenora Hutchins had occasion to meet one of the discharged lobotomy patients and were so impressed with the results that they asked the hospital to do one on their daughter. The postoperative condition of Miss Hutchins in turn convinced the sisters of Grace Farmer to arrange for Mixter to operate on her at McLean.

In the above examples, the family viewpoints happened to match those of the staff, favoring "active treatment." This was not always the case, however. The flip side of the reality that medicine was a market commodity was the fact that the final decision about treatment belonged to the purchaser. No matter what the physicians recommended, the families retained veto power. (Although physicians held more sway in the state hospitals, they still needed signed permissions for any major medical interventions.) "The family may object right now," Harmon noted after recommending a lobotomy for Mr. Everett Daniels, "but maybe in a year or two we could get it done."[85] In several instances the family refused, and that was that.[86]

The staff was equally aware that, should a family insist upon a particular procedure, their refusal to comply would result in the patient's transfer to a facility whose physicians saw things differently. When Mrs. Jane Bremerton was being discussed at a staff conference, it was noted that the family doctor had asked for a lobotomy to be performed on her. The hospital declined. A staff physician (a lobotomy supporter) noted how this incident demonstrated that the hospital was being "forced by families into doing more for them." In acquiescing to such pressure, the hospital staff might tell themselves that if the patient was to undergo the specified treatment, at least at McLean it would be done right.[87]

Paradoxically, the more technical psychiatry had become, the less control psychiatrists had over individual treatment decisions. In the days when hospital resocialization programs were the major therapy, decisions about who was admitted to which ward remained firmly in the grip of the institutional physicians; families did not have much say in such judgments. Individual technologies are commoditizable, however, and in the medical marketplace can be ordered on demand by the buyer – especially when the buyers are the resourceful and motivated families that frequented McLean. Tempering this awkward circumstance, however, was the fact that the lay public usually was exceptionally deferential to the wishes of The Doctor. For example, when permission was sought for shock treatment on Annabel Simms, her son wrote to the staff physician, "I do not know what the treatment consists of and nor do I know what the consequences might be." The son assented nevertheless, as his mother had considerable confidence in her doctor's judgment, and "everything should be done to maintain that confidence." "I can only ask," he closed his letter to the doctor, "that you should use your best judgment."

Patients thus came to be lobotomized at McLean through a variety of routes: they fit the right clinical frame, or looked like an interesting research subject, or perhaps their family had committed them with the operation already in mind. Another major pathway existed, however, which touched upon an unpleasant aspect of psychiatric reality: the need to maintain order on the wards. As was illustrated in the previous chapter, the selection of a particular psychiatric treatment often was not dependent upon a patient's diagnostic label but upon his or her behavioral features. Manic-depressives, catatonic schizophrenics, psychoneurotics, any of these might be either agitated or calm, noisy or quiet, resistant or compliant. It depended on the individual case. At McLean, as at the largest of state hospitals, "troublemakers" had to be dealt with. Here, too, psychosurgery was sometimes recommended not just for what it did for the patient but what it did for the institution. Indeed, a familiar refrain seen in the folders of the patients chosen for lobotomy was that they had become "difficult to manage." Or, as one physician stated in the staff conference held to determine the fate of Mrs. Judith Loewy, "We usually do a lobotomy to quiet people down."[88]

To the physicians who practiced at McLean, the challenge of medicine lay in wearing all of their various hats at once, balancing one perspective against the others. In the case of Judith Loewy, for example, they saw a choice between what was indicated from the standpoint of the hospital, which was a lobotomy, and that of the patient, for whom continued custodial care was enough; they opted for the operation. At times, however, the clinical frame eclipsed the administrative one. Anita Payne, a middle-aged schizophrenic, was judged by the staff to be one of the most aggressive individuals in the entire hospital. In spite of her prolonged hospitalization, unrelenting belligerence, and a hopeless prognosis, the staff ruled her out of bounds for psychosurgery: she simply did not possess the right kind of "emotional tone."[89] As another illustration, some of the patients diagnosed with nonpsychotic paranoia or with psychopathic states surely fit the right psychosurgery profile, if judged on behavioral terms alone. Yet, they were ruled virtually off-limits on the clinical grounds that the underlying personality was inappropriate for the procedure.[90] In the case of Mary Montero, the choice was perceived as being between the clinical needs as presented by the patient and the social harmony of the family. Dr. Burdett argued that, although the patient would in fact be "more comfortable," "she would not fit into the family well after a lobotomy . . . creating a bad social situation." In this instance, concern for the family prevailed.

Unlike doctors in some of the other medical specialties, psychiatrists did not have the luxury of retreating into the professional confidence that their work focused exclusively upon fixing up this or that part of a broken body. Rather, the factors that piled onto the scales of the therapeutic decision necessarily included personal concerns as well, which in spite of their relative intangibility were no less important in determining where the balance eventually came to rest. Perhaps a patient had a parent like that of Everett Daniels. "His mother says she wants him to go home," Murphy reported in the staff conference; "I agree with insulin and lobotomy." Or maybe the patient was in the same predicament as Annabel Simms, whose money was running out. The ideal situation, the staff concluded, would be to discharge her home in the care of a practical nurse, but this option was financially impossible; and in light of her deteriorating condition, even so, she might end up in a state hospital. The hospital was in a quandary. "She can not afford to stay at a hospital like this and she can not go home and would not be more comfortable in a state hospital," Dr. Rourke agonized, "so what else have you left but a lobotomy."

During staff conferences, the physicians abruptly shifted among the various hats. One moment they spoke with great compassion of the need to alleviate a patient's inner distress, and the next they were excited about having identified in her a likely prospect for a pet research project; arcane medical discussions of differential diagnosis between manic as opposed to reactive depression soon drifted off into more banal queries as to whether or not the patient had recently bitten a nurse. (Further compounding the confusion were the multiple clinical philosophies then circulating within the field of psychiatry, from psychoanalysis to endocrinology.) The various perspectives swirled back and forth; there was no absolute hierarchy by which to predict which one might ultimately prevail. The staff conferences resembled, in this respect, an elaborate game of scissors-paper-hammer, in which who would win was a matter of which particular combination happened to show up at the moment.

The meaning of this apparent fragmentation must not be overstated, however. When consulting with a patient, the psychiatrists were faced with a single decision: the choice of the next therapeutic step to take for the individual in front of them. Regardless of how many different kinds of perspectives they brought to the task, or how numerous the dimensions of the patient's psychopathology, the fact remained that this patient represented one situation to be dealt with. To try to divide this problem into separate spheres simply made no sense to them. *That* was the underlying message of Adolf Meyer's psychobiology, and the reason for its widespread professional appeal. To the physicians at McLean, the holistic vision of modern psychiatry was not just a matter of academic philosophizing about the underlying unity of mind and brain in the patient. Rather, it was an articulation of what it meant to be a practicing psychiatrist, to have to shuttle across a wide range of perspectives and responsibilities and yet never lose sight of the original problem that sat there in its messy, organic wholeness.

What psychiatrists responded to was not an illness defined in unambiguous and rigid somatic terms, but *problems* – problems of the patient, the family, the hospital, and society, as well as the underlying biological organism, all melded together into one disaggregatable plexus of which no two human beings had the same exact combination. The simple truth was that the therapeutic calculus unavoidably added up a very unlikely assortment of clinical and nonclinical factors. From the perspective of the practicing psychiatrists, to pretend otherwise was to abdicate their responsibility as physicians.

## Conclusion: Psychosurgery and the Art of Medicine

In brief, the sensibility of the working physician is very different from that of an applied scientist whose consciousness is trained to think in terms of a few well-defined variables at a time. Rather, the clinical challenge is located in the "booming, buzzing" confusion and noise of everyday life (to borrow William James's phrase), in which the variables are infinite and uncontrolled. Through the construction of what has been designated here as clinical frames, doctors attempt to impose some form of order on the chaos. What is required is a talent for shifting back and forth between a dizzying number of often contradictory conceptual grids, and an eye for the multilayered contours of human life that are formed in the intersection of the physical and cultural domains. What results is a form of knowledge quite unlike the formulas of the laboratory, even though it depends in important ways upon medical science.

The challenge facing the McLean psychiatrists as they met with their patients and decided what to do next was essentially the same as that in any other area of medicine. They came into the situation armed with an extensive knowledge of a wide array of therapies and the general guidelines for their use; the clinical task involved figuring out which of these treatments was most appropriate for the particular sufferer in front of them. Should the presenting problem happen to be a disease or condition that was easily recognized, and for which a reliable course of treatment was known, the decision could be a simple one, reached almost by rote. "In case of disease X," a physician could look up in a medical textbook, "give 50 milligrams of compound Y until the blood pH is normal." At times, then, the practice of medicine did resemble an applied science. Often, though, textbook formulas that looked neat in theory proved inadequate to the tasks of everyday medical practice. Just what was wrong with a patient was not always obvious or unambiguous. (This was especially true for psychiatry, which labored under a nebulous diagnostic system.) Moreover, as each person's physiology was as unique as a fingerprint, the effect of any drug or procedure was rarely identical to the textbook description and could range widely and unpredictably. Out of necessity, then, physicians resorted to a complex process of reasoning-by-analogy to match treatments to patients.

Would Mrs. Smith be recommended for a lobotomy at McLean Hospital? The answer hinged upon a series of determinations by her staff physician. The first task was to locate Mrs. Smith within the overall clinical ecology, identifying which group of patients she most closely resembled. The next step was to ascertain the need for further medical intervention. If the kind of problem posed by this population was known to respond well to mild interventions, or even to resolve on its own over time, the question of lobotomy might never come up. A poor prognosis, however, advanced the case to the next round of considerations. If her physician understood that, on balance, members of this group were known to benefit from psychosurgery, then Mrs. Smith might very well become viewed as a candidate for the procedure.

In the case of some patients, the perceptual grid that determined whether or not psychosurgery was appropriate derived entirely from the published medical literature. Indeed, for some regions of the clinical ecology, the textbooks were explicit. Certain conditions ruled the operation out-of-bounds, such as senile dementia or brain tumors, and others in-bounds, such as agitated depression. At McLean Hospital, as elsewhere, a recommendation of lobotomy would have to make sense within the accepted boundaries of medical knowledge that applied throughout the profession. As a practical matter, however, the grids that appeared in the medical literature were of only limited utility. On the one hand, they were both too broad and inclusive to identify, for example, which of the many manic-depressives in a hospital might benefit from a given treatment. On the other hand, they were too dependent upon the conditions that existed at a particular institution – the place where the study had been conducted – to allow for reliable generalizations to other facilities. Thus, the specific regions of the clinical ecology upon which the articles focused might or might not have corresponded to what the physicians at McLean were concerned about. Given McLean Hospital's particular combination of resources, patient mix, and physician training, *its* manic-depressives might have presented a different kind of challenge from that seen elsewhere – and thus required different treatment strategies.

To address the problem of applicability, the doctors at McLean worked up their own set of clinical frames tailored to local circumstances. Irrespective of what was reported from other institutions, if involutional melancholics remained a pressing problem at McLean, then psychosurgery would receive additional consideration there and the staff's frames would adjust accordingly. As to the matter of specificity, the grids were fine-tuned for more precise sorting, tightened through the overlay of additional variables. Indeed, it was shown earlier that certain subregions of the clinical ecology at McLean – defined in the intersection of such variables as age, diagnosis, sex, and length of stay – became identified as particularly hot areas for the operation. These combinations were only of local significance, however, having been established in relation to a *specific area within this hospital's clinical ecology*. At McLean, although a short length of stay might have been considered a sufficient reason to exclude a manic-depressive from the psychosurgery program, the same factor might have had the opposite effect elsewhere on the wards, targeting as a likely prospect, for example, a paranoid schizophrenic.

To the practicing psychiatrist, the formulaic grids that appeared in the medical literature were inadequate in other significant ways, and thus needed to be supplemented by additional kinds of filters. First, the variables that were used to define the clinical region often were not easily expressed or quantified in strictly scientific terms, especially in the field of psychiatry. Indeed, due to the lack of congruence between the diagnostic system and the actual behavioral and emotional problems that surfaced on the wards – for example, schizophrenics might be euphoric or depressed, withdrawn or extroverted, combative or compliant – an additional set of frames evolved to guide the psychiatrists' decisions. Such considerations as the patients' capacity for violence, depth of despair, incoherence, and so forth, extended the list of including and excluding factors – all useful indicators, but hardly the stuff of scientific exactitude. Advocates of psychosurgery, for example, routinely pointed to a patient's "emotional tone" as the single most important indicator for a successful operation. This particular quality, though, was something each physician would have to assess for him- or herself. Second, the psychiatrists were acutely aware that the outcome of a given course of treatment often depended upon features of the social environment in which a patient normally lived and worked. When pondering the prognosis for a female patient, for example, the staff might have paid attention to such factors as the husband's interest in other women, her fondness for housekeeping, and the existence of a trust fund. Such considerations were equally as important as the putatively more medical ones in predicting final results.

The question of identifying which patients might benefit from psychosurgery thus was resolved through a set of filters applied in combination, each of which had been derived from a separate base of experience. From their basic medical training, the doctors at McLean learned how to sort the patients on the basis of current physiology and general classifications of disease. Their more specialized background in psychiatry yielded additional filters concerning the treatment of mental disorders. And the years on the wards at McLean provided an opportunity to observe patients who had undergone the latest innovations in treatment; at the same time, it led to an intimate acquaintance with the everyday affairs of persons who inhabited a very narrow section of the social strata. The decision to operate was formed in the intersection of these various filters, which, added together, demarcated similarities among those patients who did well with the procedure and those who did not. If Mrs. Smith could be sited within the appropriate clinical frame, then her physician proceeded with confidence. It did not matter whether the patient's "emotional tone" was due to a hormonal imbalance, the delusion that aliens were trying to abduct her, the real fear that her husband might sue for divorce, or a distaste for institutional life – or all of the above. Her case seemed similar enough to others who had gone before; Mrs. Smith had what a lobotomy was expected to cure.

A doctor's knowledge, then, was only partly expressible within the framework of laboratory science. To be sure, a vital portion could be communicated in medical journal articles and laboratory protocols. The rest, however, was often ineffable: physicians might not have been able to describe a clinical grid fully in words, but they believed that they intuitively knew it when they saw it and could point it out to others. Furthermore, any given clinical frame was inextricably linked to the original site of its generation and thus was not immediately portable. It was without contradiction, therefore, that a particular clinical frame might work at one facility, and not at another – certainly not the case with, say, the formula for gunpowder, which should work in any reputable lab. Moreover, psychiatrists knew all too well that the business of figuring out *what* a treatment does was inexorably linked to the particularities of *who* the patient was. As no two individuals were identical in their personal history or life circumstances, it was also without contradiction, therefore, that two patients who otherwise matched in diagnosis and medical history might have received altogether different treatment recommendations – even within the same institution and with the same psychiatrists making the decisions. Similarly, two different physicians – each with their own unique professional history and perspectives – could reasonably arrive at varying conclusions as to whether a specified treatment might work for a given individual. (And even in retrospect, as it was not possible to use a person as their own experimental control once the individual had been irrevocably altered, there was no sure way to determine whose recommendation had in fact been right.) Certainty was never attainable.

Working with clinical frames thus required that the physician possess a range of intellectual and emotional skills very different from that needed for applied science. To begin with, the knowledge necessary to match patients to treatments was not something that could be passively assimilated, as a chemist might rely upon a set of formularies that had been handed down. Clinical frames, localized in time and place, imposed special burdens on the medical practitioner. Unlike the bench technician, who might simply apply the guidelines set by nameless others, every physician had the unshirkable responsibility of fabricating his own personal set of clinical frames for daily use, and of devising a unique logic for their application. No two physicians followed precisely the same mental route when examining patients and arriving at treatment decisions. Moreover, as the world of medicine was in constant flux – for example, changes were always occurring in patterns of hospital administration, patient demographics, knowledge about particular treatments, and the local ecology of disease – the usable shelf life of any clinical frame was unpredictable. Physicians had to remain ever vigilant.

The construction and subsequent readjustment of clinical frames was no simple task. As mentioned above, the practice of effective medicine necessitated that the physician be competent in several disparate domains. Sometimes it was necessary to think like a physiologist, bringing to bear a general knowledge of how compounds and fluids react under well-defined conditions. At other times, though, it was not the skills and instincts of a laboratory scientist that were needed, but those of a field biologist, trained to make sense out of what occurs under the normal conditions of life. Then again, as human disease and suffering also reflect disturbances in the social matrix, sometimes what was required was a feeling for the inner workings of human culture. The physician on the wards at McLean had to be comfortable in all three domains.

Moreover, because clinical frames were continually evolving, formed in the intersection of the abstract general case and the particular one facing the physician, a special facileness of mind was required to resolve this peculiar dialectic. Indeed, it was *after* the treatment was performed on a given patient and the results assessed that the true complexity of the clinician's work was revealed. The thirtieth candidate for lobotomy at McLean was chosen on the basis of clinical frames that had been fabricated on the findings of what transpired with patients one through twenty-nine. The thirty-first, however, would be based on a newer set of frames, altered in accordance with what had happened to patient number thirty. This process of abstracting useful information from the individual case required the proactive deliberation of the physician. Perhaps the operation on Mrs. Smith did not yield the expected results. Was this further evidence that schizophrenics were poor risks, that this particular clinical frame should be phased out? Another possibility was that most schizophrenics did fine with the operation, just not those of her advanced age. If this were proved true, the correct action would simply be to tighten the grid for schizophrenia. Alternatively, the physician might judge that the clinical frames were fine but wrongly applied. The error might have been in the original diagnosis; Mrs. Smith was more like a manic-depressive than a true schizophrenic. Then again, it was conceivable that the clinical frame and the diagnosis were in fact both correct, and it was the operation that had been botched. Finally, even a well-chosen and well-executed operation was no guarantee of success. Perhaps the patient's family was unwilling to accept her postoperative condition and subjected her to undue stress, thus neutralizing any chance for positive gains. In reasoning through Mrs. Smith's case, the clinician might also mentally revisit any of the preceding cases that seemed similar to hers. The experience with each new intervention, therefore, might occasion a reshuffling or redesign of the various grids that made up the overall clinical frames.

The ability to navigate back and forth among these perspectives, finding useful patterns within the kaleidoscope of possibilities, was not something that could be taught didactically in medical school. Rather, the line that separated good physicians from bad ones was based on the individual physician's powers of observation and intuitive sense. Moreover, the tactic of waiting until rigorous controlled experiments might be able to identify the relevant variables was not an option. It was then – and remains today – the doctor's responsibility to make fateful decisions on the basis of knowledge that somehow is always incomplete and in a constant state of revision. Not everyone has the temperament or talent for such a task.

Lastly, it was not just the cognitive challenges that differentiated the laboratory scientist and the clinician, but their goals. When considering the choice of therapy, such important issues as the amount of risk worth chancing, which side effects are unacceptable, and even the purpose of the intervention itself were all matters of personal choice. The scientific method could generate new kinds of treatment and more reliable predictions as to outcome, but it had little to offer in the way of personal advice. *Physicians,* however, were looked to by patients and their families precisely for their role as counselors who were wise in the affairs of men and women, and who might guide them in making such difficult choices. If bodies are the temples of the soul, we look to physicians to construct a more perfect edifice. Such work necessarily involves a strange alchemy that merges an understanding of how the body works with a sensitivity to the demands of human convention.

Today, when one hears it said that medicine is an art, it is most likely on those occasions when there is a need to explain away a conspicuous mistake. Artful medicine thus becomes that portion of a physician's work which is sloppy, ill-founded, and specious. One is thus left with the implication that it is an art because it is not fully a science – yet. This is an unfair characterization of what it means to be a practicing physician. As argued above, medicine is an art not because it is watered-down or incomplete science; rather, the challenge facing physicians is very different from that which faces laboratory scientists, and constantly draws upon a unique combination of perceptual talents. And, like architecture, medicine is formed in the junction of technical expertise and human values, a domain in which decisions must meet physical as well as human standards. Even in current times, then, physicians necessarily engage in the medical arts – as understood in their positive connotations, that is.

## Epilogue

In the early 1950s, McLean Hospital's psychosurgery program began to decline. To some extent, the hospital had had its fill of lobotomy patients. In the years between 1946 and 1950, as many as 85 percent of the lobotomy patients operated on in a given year were discharged within eighteen months of the date of operation. The remainder stayed on the wards, however, and began to accumulate. In December 1948, for instance, nineteen female postoperative patients were in residence at the same time – almost 15 percent of the entire women's population. Within the particular "bins" earmarked for lobotomy consideration, the number of patients not operated on was rapidly dwindling. The salvageable deadwood had been logged out. Moreover, as the beds of long-term inhabitants were freed up, they were being replaced by patients with a very different profile from that of those who had entered a generation before. The new admissions tended toward milder and shorter-term mental disturbances that fit with a general shift toward psychotherapeutic intervention; the rest were patients with organic brain syndromes. At the same time, the long-term resident population was aging beyond what even psychosurgery was thought to be able to reclaim. In 1952, Sutton noted, there were a hundred patients with an average age of seventy-seven, a third of whom were diagnosed as senile.[91]

Indeed, the seventeen patients operated upon in the final phase (the years between 1951 and 1954) had a median age of sixty.

Even as the hospital garnered additional experience with lobotomy, the decision to operate remained difficult. Although the psychiatrists could point to an increased number of operative successes, the failures also continued to mount. The procedure's reputation was further tarnished by the stream of patients who, discharged as improved, nonetheless suffered a relapse, some returning to McLean, some going to another institution.[92] In the case of Annabel Simms, the gap between what the hospital had hoped to accomplish with lobotomy and what actually resulted was best expressed by the patient herself. In a letter to her doctors at McLean, Mrs. Simms went right to the heart of the matter when she shouted at them in a sentence underlined three times: "My mind is not adjustable!"

In the individual case, whether or not psychosurgery would prove useful was still too unpredictable for comfort. The closer the staff looked into it, the more confused the subject became. Speculation reigned, for, as Dr. Howard noted in his staff conference talk, "there are a variety of types of operations done on diverse kinds of patients observed by different techniques, by people with different points of view, in a field in which matters of measurement are rather inexact." Indeed, the fact that psychologists could measure no intellectual deficit in postlobotomy patients was proof to Howard, not that the operation was benign, but that existing psychological tools of measurement were inadequate. It was up to future tests to reveal the "defects in initiative, motivation, planning for the future and creative thinking."

One can sense that, by the time of Howard's talk in 1950, the advocates of psychosurgery were already on the defensive within the profession. Too many patients apparently had lost "some of the important characteristics of personality integration." Howard was quick to reassure his audience that at McLean such patients showed only a "minimum of the bad results," all thanks to the hospital's policy of doing the least extensive kind of cutting. Less was more. "I think our cases are more spry after operation than the usual lobotomy," Howard stated. It was obvious to him that the only real solution was "to discover the operation which produces the most relief of symptoms and tension and the least bad results." His audience was treated to a brief survey by Howard of the efforts currently under way in the nation's research institutes to find this better lobotomy. He also informed them about Walter Freeman's latest innovation, the "ice-pick" procedure, which enabled psychosurgery to be performed rapidly and even on an outpatient basis. A "probably fictitious story" was making the rounds, he related, that patients were seen going into Freeman's office for shock treatment only to descend in the elevator a few minutes later with black eyes, the sign of such a lobotomy having been performed.⁹³

The staff at McLean would have to await further developments, however. Whether a new kind of operation would emerge from the results of neurophysiological research or from Freeman's rough-hewn approach, the future of lobotomy lay elsewhere.

# 7

## The Politics of Precision
### The Quest for a Better Lobotomy

As in the night all cats are gray, so in the darkness of metaphysical criticism all causes are obscure.

William James, *Principles of Psychology* (1890)

Beginning in 1943, the *American Journal of Psychiatry* dedicated a section of its annual literature reviews to the fast-growing field of psychosurgery. After the war, the number of publications on the subject increased dramatically (see Figure 7.1). Nolan D. C. Lewis, an influential professional leader, reported in the 1948 review that psychosurgery was universally under way, "for better or for worse."[1] With this phrase, Lewis nicely captured the ambivalence that dogged the use of lobotomy even during the height of its postwar heyday. The controversy surrounding the operation – which dated from the moment Freeman and Watts first reported on their surgical forays – had not been dispelled by the procedure's remarkable ascent within clinical practice so much as it had simply been bypassed, muted in the hurry to provide the nation's mental hospitals with the latest in therapeutic advances. Moreover, the many psychiatrists and administrators who established psychosurgical programs in the postwar years were no doubt emboldened to ignore the critics as their own trial experiences with the procedure revealed that the threatened worst-case scenarios were off the mark. Nonetheless, the collective wisdom was indeed slowly recognizing that the actual results of lobotomy were often equivocal. Although programs of psychosurgery did not reduce every patient to the state of a "vegetable" or drooling "zombie," over time they did produce a stream of disastrous results that demanded attention.[2] The "price paid" by even the better-off lobotomy patients for their behavioral or emotional changes was no longer a hypothetical conjecture, limited to discussions in the professional literature, but had a definite meaning to all those who had occasion to walk the wards of a mental institution.[3]

In the case of psychosurgery, a pervasive unease had settled on the profession that something had to be improved, and soon, as the programs were visibly accelerating in growth. Complaints surfaced that the original

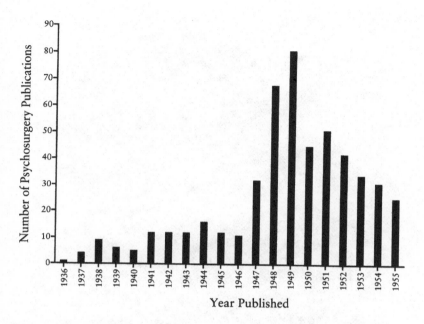

Figure 7.1. Psychosurgery publications in U.S. medical literature, 1936–1955

Freeman and Watts procedure, now referred to as the "standard" prefrontal lobotomy, was unnecessarily drastic: some critics likened it to the neurosurgical equivalent of a blunderbuss. Even an observer friendly to the operation, in a prominently placed editorial in the 1949 *Psychiatric Quarterly,* depicted the use of psychosurgery up to that date as having been little more than a stab in the dark.[4] The rush was on to devise operations with a minimal extent of cortical damage: the salvation of the psychosurgery industry – and by implication, the nation's severely mentally ill – would be found in the search for greater operative *precision.*

The neuropsychiatric literature soon brimmed with psychosurgical variations that were advanced by their innovators as the latest in "selective," "limited," or "fractional" lobotomies. Psychiatric and neurosurgical centers in Minnesota, Massachusetts, Pennsylvania, Connecticut, Kentucky, New York, and Toronto thus introduced such procedures as lobectomy, bimedial lobotomy, stereoencephalotomy, orbital undercutting, topectomy, and gyrectomy – to name only a few. Each technique was championed as representing a therapeutic advance based on greater precision or control. For example, some neurosurgeons visually exposed the

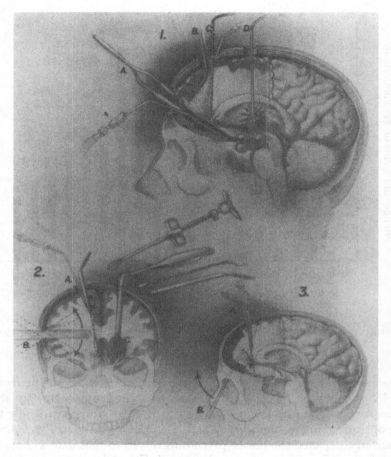

Figure 7.2. Variant forms of psychosurgery. (Source: *Proceedings of the Second International Conference on Psychosurgery,* 1972. Courtesy of Charles C. Thomas, Publisher, Springfield, Illinois.)

brain surface and employed weight scales, so that specific anatomical areas could verifiably be removed in equivalent amounts bilaterally (top-ectomy); others devised a stereotaxic surgical apparatus to control point of entry (stereoencephalotomy). So eagerly pursued were these kinds of innovations, that symposia on lobotomy afterward became populated by neurosurgeons hawking their individual wares.[5] One participant sardonically described how neurosurgeons "persist in inventing instruments for particular purposes each one of which we fondly imagine is better suited to achieve its end than anything that has gone before." There was no finer example of this tendency, he noted, than the "astonishing creations" yielded by those performing psychosurgery.[6]

## Cut to Measure

Did the use of psychosurgery grow in an appropriate manner? At first glance, the overall picture roughly conforms to the growth cycle one intuitively assumes governs any new medical technology. The first, small clinical trials were superseded by a period of rapid expansion, if not overenthusiasm. In turn, the treatment became a target for criticism as its shortcomings were revealed, leading to a final stage in which investigators scrambled to devise an enhanced therapy. Described in another way, progress in medical therapeutics derives from the give-and-take between laboratory researchers, whose theories and discoveries result in unanticipated medical applications, and clinicians, whose explorations define the uses of the new treatments. In due course, a treatment's "field" results become fodder for new laboratory investigations that ultimately yield further applications.[7]

In actuality, however, medical progress is rarely so straightforward. Production of medical innovations is in itself no assurance of clinical gains; divisive conflicts may also erupt concerning the best route to an improved treatment, or over what constitutes a therapeutic advance.[8] The disjuncture between the idealized image of how science works and its not-so-pretty reality was brought home to Harvard neuropsychiatrist Stanley Cobb when he wrote to his close friend John Fulton: "Where are we coming to in all this brain cutting? Some of it is a little wild. . . . So knowledge grows!" The root of the current mess, Cobb believed, was traceable to the peculiar circumstances of the treatment's development, which in his view had been prematurely applied to patients.[9] Cobb thus raised the troubling point that perhaps psychosurgery's ascendancy into clinical practice was so rapid as to break the bonds that normally bound laboratory-based researchers and clinicians in a common venture. Psychosurgery, it was feared, had entered a kind of free-fall, its eventual destination unknown. With at least five thousand such procedures being performed each year in the late 1940s, such potential rifts between the world of the laboratory and that of the clinic could not be ignored.

Perhaps the best example of an attempt to restore credibility to the psychosurgical enterprise, through a search for operative precision, was provided when the eminent scientist John F. Fulton redirected his research enterprise to such a task in the years immediately following the war.

Fulton had little doubt that a full-throttle research program in neu-rophysiology would result in the discovery of more exact, limited pro-cedures that would be better matched to specific kinds of mental dis-orders. Lobotomies would no longer be random affairs of hit-or-miss, but, in Fulton's words, "tailor-made."[10] Moreover, Fulton believed that from the moment responsible scientists spoke out clearly on the issue in professional as well as public forums, the current excesses of the lobotomists would quickly disappear – clinicians would naturally heed the guidance of scientific medicine. In time, he believed, psychosurgery would command respect as a fully established component of scientific medicine.

The target of Fulton's campaign was clearly Walter Freeman, now enshrined as dean of lobotomy. Freeman's own response to the need for improved lobotomies presented, if anything, the inverse image of Fulton's call for laboratory-guided investigations. He discovered his own answer not in an elite, state-of-the-art laboratory, where the latest in sophisticated neurophysiological equipment might be found, but in a hospital morgue where he went to work with an ordinary ice pick – coming up with the now infamous procedure known as the transorbital lobotomy.[11] Paying little heed to any notion of slowing down his own operative pace, Freeman instead found in the new form of "ice-pick" surgery the very means of vastly increasing the number of lobotomies that might be performed.

Fulton the elite laboratory scientist and Freeman the in-the-trenches clinical innovator were thus headed toward an inevitable showdown. In retrospect, what is to be learned from this confrontation? It is tempting to apply the simple standards of good or bad science and thus cast Fulton in the role of the noble "pure" scientist and his adversary as a reckless opportunist. Yet the two were in some ways hauntingly similar. Freeman, for example, was equally committed to the betterment of psychosurgery through increased specificity in surgical technique. He too was interested in lobotomies being "cut to measure," and grounded his own innovations in recent neurophysiological theory.[12] It is equally tempting to cast *both* of them as antiheroes, to condemn all efforts in this era to find a better lobotomy as dangerously misguided. Perhaps Fulton, Freeman, and everyone else involved should have heeded the danger signs the moment they had become visible and have simply abandoned the enterprise before getting in even deeper. The concept of hubris, after all, was first pinned on a technological innovator whose combination of arrogance and naiveté proved fatal (at least to himself). This kind of categorization, however, presupposes that our judgment is somehow more perfect than that demonstrated by the participants. Perhaps it is our own arrogance that is on display here.

A better historical strategy, I contend, is to abandon the familiar frameworks of good and bad science and instead use the story of Fulton and Freeman as an opportunity to reexamine how medical science actually works. Freeman and Fulton were also far more different from one another than might at first be assumed. Embedded within their common quest for more precise operations were thoroughly distinct visions of what should be the proper relations between the domain of the laboratory and that of the clinic. An account of their separate and conflicting solutions to the problem posed by psychosurgery's inadequacies will bring out the strong tensions that arise whenever laboratory-derived knowledge and the needs of real-world medicine interact. Neither party, experimentalist and clinician alike, was happy to advertise this unpleasant reality. The situation pertains today.

## Fulton's Prefrontal Blues

In 1952, a former research associate sent John Fulton the following squib from *The New Yorker,* identifying it as evidence that Fulton was now appreciated in the highest court of American humor:

> Mrs. Snyder will review *The Biography of Harvey Cushing, A Brain Surgeon,* by John Fulton, introducing and concluding it with appropriate selections on the piano – *Daily Californian*
>
> [Editors:] The "Prefrontal Blues?"[13]

The editors had touched upon what had been a source of great concern to the Yale physiologist. Over the years, Fulton watched with increasing frustration as his original proposal for small, scientifically administered clinical trials of lobotomy was ignored with the advent of the large postwar programs. On the one hand, his initial faith in lobotomy's clinical utility had only grown stronger. He stated before a variety of professional audiences that psychosurgery was probably one of the foremost discoveries of modern scientific medicine, on a par with insulin, penicillin, and cortisone. Such groups learned from Fulton that, thanks to lobotomy, "innumerable" patients, most of whom had been considered hopelessly ill and were confined for life in institutions, had been sent home, some even to useful occupations. The procedure's inherent possibilities, in his view, promised "a new phase of scientific medicine." Fulton's enthusiasm derived in part from personal observation. As previously mentioned, although medically trained, he was not a practicing physician and was never directly involved with lobotomy in human beings. His close professional relations with a broad network of research-oriented physicians, however, provided him ample opportunity to witness firsthand many such therapeutic interventions. William German, for example, a professor of neurosurgery at Yale, presented a psychosurgical patient to Fulton's Neu-

rological Study Unit in November 1948. Fulton described the event in his
diary:

> An artistic woman, widely read and musical, became over-agitated
> some years ago and following a superior quadrant lobotomy three
> weeks ago she has become completely calmed down, and today be-
> fore the students she gave a most eloquent account of her illness and
> what had happened to her since the operation. She said immediately
> Dr. German had made the section in her second hemisphere she felt
> completely relieved from all the pressure that she had been under
> during the previous years.

Fulton concluded, "It was a most dramatic demonstration."[14]

On the other hand, Fulton was alarmed by the widespread use of psychosurgery, the fact that "countless thousands" of mental patients had
been subjected to overextensive operations. He reasoned that lobotomy in
its present form, which involved as much as one-fifth of the total brain
mass and the excision of a range of anatomically and functionally discrete
regions of the brain, most likely caused indiscriminate and unnecessary
damage. Neurosurgeons, Fulton observed, had indeed been busy developing a bewildering array of surgical procedures which they proposed as
more limited operations. By and large, however, such modifications were
devised "empirically" (that is, unscientifically) through trial and error.
Especially distressing to Fulton was the neurosurgeons' indifference to
their own ignorance of brain physiology, letting "zeal . . . outrun their
knowledge of function." Real progress in the form of a less destructive
procedure would not ensue until such time as advances in neurophysiology might illuminate the way. Fulton aired his fears at the 1947 meeting of
the AMA, stating his belief that, before the procedure could be intelligently applied in man, far more information was needed from the scientific study of animal brains. "And so we leave the physiologist at this
point," Fulton mused, "impatiently attempting to keep pace with the
daring of our contemporary neurosurgeons."[15]

Fulton felt compelled to intervene, to assume the responsibility for
correcting the growing imbalance between scientific knowledge and clinical practice in the case of psychosurgery. To begin with, a sense of culp-
ability gnawed at him as he remembered his own strong role in advancing
the procedure on the basis of the putative connection between Moniz's
initial reports and the chimpanzee experiments that were conducted
within his Yale Primate Laboratory. Moreover, any substantial exploration of lobotomy's neurophysiological basis necessitated an unlikely combination of neurosurgeons, physiologists, and lower primates. A short list
of available locations in the United States would reveal only one such
location – Fulton's.[16] Further, the task of incorporating the many opera-

tions into a coherent neurophysiological scheme required a breadth of disciplinary vision few others were in a position to exercise. Fulton thus turned his full attention to the lobotomy issue and personally took up the role of scientific leader who – if anyone could – would bring scientific prudence and rational guidance to the psychosurgical enterprise.

Beginning in 1946, Fulton put into motion a multipronged strategy that dominated his professional life until his retirement from the world of academic science in 1951. One tactic was to campaign hard, through addresses, lectureships, monographs, and professional meetings, to educate the lay as well as medical public about the importance of these issues. Complementing these efforts, Fulton took advantage of his unique position as a respected authority spanning the many fields associated with psychosurgery – in touch as he was with an unequaled network of correspondents and professional associates – both to remain at the forefront of lobotomy-related investigations and to focus attention on those research avenues he himself considered most promising. Finally, he committed his own laboratory resources to the problem of establishing a sound neurophysiological foundation for psychosurgery. He expected an arduous road ahead and went to work.[17]

## The Campaign

Fulton had wished to extend his original frontal-lobe research ever since first learning of Moniz's operation in late 1936. Such plans were stymied by Yale's inability to match an academic offer that lured away Jacobsen in 1938, and soon thereafter by Fulton's involvement in war-related projects. In addition, between 1942 and 1946, Fulton was engaged in several time-consuming literary projects.[18] When his desk cleared in late 1946, he returned to experiments on the frontal lobes of primates, "spade work" for his planned lobotomy research.[19]

Encouraged by his preliminary findings, Fulton spoke in January 1947 to the House Officers Association of Boston City Hospital on the "Physiological Basis of Frontal Lobotomy." This talk served as a blueprint for more than a score of later addresses and published papers. Between 1947 and 1951, Fulton toured the country, from the American Philosophical Society in Philadelphia to the Los Angeles County Medical Society in California. International stops were also added to the tour.[20] Newspaper and radio journalists publicized his talks, identifying him to the public as the "trail-blazer" whose expertise on brain surgery had led to the operation, or as "the foremost authority" on psychosurgery. Wherever he spoke, Fulton marveled at the interest and size of the crowds. "The world," Fulton noted in his diary, "seems to have become interested in the frontal lobes."[21]

Like any politician on tour, Fulton delivered a standard speech, elaborated upon to incorporate recent developments or local flavor but otherwise substantially the same in thrust and content. The body of the talks emphasized four main points. First, his addresses invariably began with a well-honed account of how chimpanzee experiments at Yale had encouraged Moniz's "bold" step. In addition to establishing scientific priority, this approach also neatly provided Fulton with credentials on the subject in spite of his lack of clinical experience. For example, the published version of one of his lectures contained a blurb (written by Fulton himself) stating that "Dr. Fulton is well qualified to deal with the subject since the operation of frontal lobotomy originated in his laboratory."[22]

Next, Fulton publicized the treatment's inherent social as well as scientific value. In the early speeches, he pointed out that, whether the operation returned 5 or 50 percent of patients to their homes, it clearly had "wide economic significance." In the later forums, he confidently predicted a net savings to American taxpayers of a million dollars a day resulting from a nationwide program of lobotomy.[23] But to Fulton the importance of the brain operations extended far beyond mere economic considerations. Within the field of neurophysiology, lobotomy's development had dramatically increased both the quality as well as quantity of research material.[24] Fulton argued that if this new clinical material were correlated with animal studies (which allowed more extensive lesions and the routine use of postmortem examination to verify excision sites) a new era would occur in neurophysiology. Scientists would come that much closer toward the Sherringtonian imperative to understand the brain as "the matrix of the mind" – the dictum that had guided his entire scientific career.

Third, the pressing cause for his campaign lay not in psychosurgery's anticipated benefits, however, but its current deficits. Woven into his talks were "earnest pleas for caution" on the part of neurosurgeons, lest irremediable harm occur. Fulton hoped to shame "the lobotomists" into holding back until a physiological rationale had been established. He cynically observed that neurosurgeons had built up large programs of lobotomy, all based on a single chimpanzee experiment, whose results were not published in detail until at least a decade had passed.[25] Neurosurgeons, Fulton admonished, "being what they are were unwilling to wait." At the minimum, he argued, the "blind" operative approach of Freeman and Watts's operation must be abandoned.[26] Even Fulton's terminology for the operation was a deliberate rebuke to lobotomists for their anatomical imprecision. In his opinion, the term *prefrontal* literally referred to the area between frontal lobes and sinuses – a misnomer. Unfailingly, Fulton referred to the operation as *frontal* lobotomy.

Lastly, Fulton mapped out specific cortical regions and surgical approaches that current research suggested were the most promising for neurosurgeons to pursue. He anticipated that smaller operative lesions, precisely matched to the patients' individual symptoms, would yield all the benefits of the standard operation but avoid unfortunate damage as to intellect and personality.[27] In the early speeches, his advice consisted mostly of a warning to avoid infringement of the posterior orbital surface (Brodmann's Area 13), which he believed was often cut by the standard lobotomy. Fulton's advice was based on a study devised by Henry Shenkin, a practicing neurosurgeon in Philadelphia who had been a Yale Visiting Fellow in 1941–2, and on corroborative findings that this region had been spared in the chimpanzees Becky and Lucy.[28] In his later speeches, Fulton communicated more positive suggestions for improved lobotomies based on recent neurophysiological findings.

Fulton's addresses detailed the heady challenge presented by the development of psychosurgery and placed the Yale physiologist at the forefront of future discussions, public as well as professional. His campaign was decidedly upbeat, spreading the message that the operation had not only "scientific, ethical and practical justification," but "broad philosophical implications" as well. Fulton, retaining deep reservations about current as well as past psychosurgical practice, nonetheless invested heavily in its future.

## Showdown in New York

Fulton's lecture tour provided visibility for his platform, but preaching alone would not succeed in significantly altering the direction and rate of lobotomy. Rationalization of psychosurgery was more than a matter of accumulating additional medical knowledge or of promoting new attitudes. Somehow, its leading proponents would have to be convinced to abide by higher standards. One professional forum in particular provided Fulton an exceptional opportunity to advance his plan, the December 1947 meeting of the Association for Research in Nervous and Mental Disease (ARNMD). The association events, held annually, were attended by distinguished scientists from many disciplines who discussed a single theme related to neurology or psychiatry; each conference was published as a definitive volume that commanded wide attention and respect.

The subject in 1947 was the frontal lobes, and Fulton was awarded the honor of serving as both association president and chair of the Program Committee. Under his guidance, the meeting was by all accounts a great success, with a record attendance by three hundred members and five hundred guests. Fulton recorded in his diary that he had never seen a larger or more enthusiastic meeting. The resulting published volume, *The Frontal Lobes,* edited by Fulton with the aid of Charles Airing and S. Bernard Wortis, included thirty-seven papers by seventy-two contributors, filling nine hundred published pages.[29] Fulton "agitated" over this particular event for more than a year, self-consciously orchestrating its structure and content to address the psychosurgical issue. In early 1947, he wrote to John Eccles that he had been having a "high old time with the lobotomists," who he felt lacked any knowledge of what they were doing to the frontal lobes; he especially looked forward to the ARNMD meetings, where he hoped to rein in their unthinking enthusiasm. Here was an ideal forum at which to call into question the treatment's neurophysiological rationale. With Walter Freeman's participation assured, "fireworks" were expected.[30] Indeed, as moderator of each session, Fulton steered discussions and set the tone of the often lively debates, going so far as to single out and instruct Freeman in the audience to respond to statements that raised significant doubts about standard lobotomies.

Viewed in its entirety, the conference mirrored the concerns of Fulton's speeches. It, too, began with an account of the Becky and Lucy experiments, though this time in full – and as yet unreported – detail. It also contained convincing reports on the treatment's potential to empty the state mental hospitals and concluded with the inspirational message that the proceedings marked an important step toward a realization of Sherrington's challenge to elucidate how "the brain is the organ of the mind."[31] Most importantly, addresses by Gosta Rylander, a leading Swedish psychiatrist, and neurophysiologist Arthur Ward (a recent alumnus of Fulton's Laboratory) focused attention on the critical thrust of Fulton's campaign tour.

For an exposition of the psychological dangers posed by lobotomy, Fulton could have found no better performance than that delivered by Gosta Rylander, an honored foreign guest. Rylander's analysis of his patients' personalities before and after frontal lobotomy led to the meeting's most heated discussions. He commenced by stating his unequivocal belief in lobotomy's power to lessen the symptoms of mental disease. "But is anything of the original personality destroyed," Rylander wondered aloud, "do any nondesirable mental changes occur after the operation?" During the course of his investigation, negative effects did surface. Disappointed families of lobotomized patients in Sweden, Rylander discovered, might remark: "She is my daughter but yet a different person," "She is with me in body but her soul is in some way lost," or "His soul appears to be destroyed." Rylander formed his own negative opinion of the operation's hazards after he had hired a lobotomized woman as a cook in his own household, in order to allow close observations of her reactions to daily tasks. He discovered that although she could satisfactorily prepare old recipes, any deviation from established routine would be hopelessly distracting. As a consequence of this experiment, Rylander chose thereafter to restrict the use of the operation to severely psychotic patients.[32]

In the discussion period that followed, and after Richard Brickner's emphatic thanks for Rylander's "note of caution," Fulton rose to prod Rylander further:

> President Fulton: I had rather hoped that Dr. Rylander might tell of still another case of a Salvation Army worker who had certain troubles of a religious nature. The case seems to me of very great significance.
>
> Dr. Rylander: I think you can do it better than I.
>
> President Fulton: I think you must tell it.[33]

Rylander's arguments were obviously no surprise to Fulton. Several days before, he had been a guest at Fulton's home and had been feted at Mory's, an eating club at Yale, where he had previewed his talk for Fulton and twenty of his colleagues.[34] He continued:

> Dr. Rylander: For years she lay in the hospital constantly saying that she had committed sins against the Holy Ghost. . . . When the operation was finished, she was quite silent. . . . I asked her, "How are you now? What about the Holy Ghost?" Smiling, she answered, "Oh, the Holy Ghost; there is no Holy Ghost."[35]

Freeman, aware of the severity of the criticism implicit in Rylander's anecdote, immediately challenged the Swedish psychiatrist once the laughter had subsided:

> Dr. Walter Freeman: If I understood correctly one of Dr. Rylander's conclusions, it was that something is taken away from the mind of the patient which is more important than the relief afforded. Is that a correct quotation from Dr. Rylander?
>
> Dr. Rylander: That is right.
>
> Dr. Freeman: . . . It is a serious matter. . . . It seems to me that Dr. Rylander's conclusion that lobotomy takes something from an individual should be judged in the light of what lobotomy gives back to the individual in relation to his prepsychotic adjustability in his social surroundings.[36]

At this point Fulton intervened on Rylander's behalf, stating that the speaker's point was merely to raise, not answer, the question as to whether in some cases the operation's costs outweigh its benefits. Freeman, psychosurgery's foremost advocate, had been placed on the defensive in front of an august body of scientific peers. In his diary, Fulton singled out Rylander's contribution, saying that he could not imagine a better performance. To Rylander, he later wrote: "you sounded a welcome, cautious note which I think has been heeded, and we are most grateful to you for it." Indeed, Rylander's critique expressed in vivid form deep reservations which many physicians – including supporters – had felt but had not discussed publicly. Rylander's story of the lobotomy patient "losing his soul" rapidly circulated within the profession and was repeatedly cited, though later its origins were forgotten.[37]

Fulton's hope that neurophysiology might soon provide suggestions for improved operations was fulfilled by Arthur Ward's presentation. Ward described how lesions restricted to the anterior cingulate gyrus (Area 24) affected personality in monkeys, specifically reducing "social fear and anxiety." An initial trial of such a limited lesion, performed on an institutionalized woman, proved encouraging. Ward ended his paper with a plea for less destructive operations, such as those suggested by new research findings.[38] Fulton began the discussion:

> One of the purposes of this meeting has been to find out more concerning functional localization in the frontal lobe and more particularly with regard to the operation of frontal lobotomy. It is clearly suggestive. Dr. Ward just pointed out that this profound change in behavior occurs when a lesion is limited to the cingulate gyrus, and I am hoping that Dr. Freeman and others will comment on the possibility which Dr. Ward has just mentioned, that perhaps the major results seen following the larger operation are due to encroaching upon this part of the rhinenchephalon.

Fulton admitted that this region was particularly difficult to get at surgically, but he had "intimate confidence" that his neurosurgical colleagues could meet this challenge.[39]

The ARNMD meeting placed Fulton at the epicenter of the psychosurgery debates. Given prominent display at the symposium were the historical and continuing contributions of Fulton's frontal-lobe research to the development of lobotomy. It was this occasion that prompted the observation that "'the shot fired' at the Yale Lab. into the frontal lobes of Becky and Lucy was ultimately 'heard round the world.'" In addition, the influence of Fulton's current research program was demonstrated by the array of conference papers that originated in his own laboratory. In fact, complaints were voiced that too many contributors to the meeting were or had been directly associated with Fulton's laboratory.[40] Lastly, the ARNMD provided Fulton with a forum to express his unique multidisciplinary authority. When Fulton talked, neuroanatomists, neurophysiologists, neurosurgeons, neurologists, and psychiatrists all listened. Affectionately called "the father of all frontal lobes" and "the world's greatest physiologist," Fulton thus established himself as the foremost adjudicator of the psychosurgery disputes.[41] In short, for Fulton the ARNMD was a resounding success. The campaign was in full swing.

### Gathering the Forces

Fulton was at the zenith of his professional influence and was well aware of the impact he might have on the direction of future research on psychosurgery. Fulton's strengths derived from several sources. His unit at Yale had matured into a research program of international standing, whose participants represented the cream of neurophysiology, neurology, and physiology, and were drawn from all corners of the map. It was an honor to spend a year in Fulton's shop, and those who had done so had performed handsomely. By 1950, the total number of research papers that originated in his laboratory had neared the one-thousand mark. Moreover, as author of the classic textbook *Physiology of the Nervous System* (which achieved three editions and was translated into five languages) and editor of *Howell's Physiology* (which would soon become *Fulton's Physiology*), Fulton held a commanding view of research accomplishments past and current. Through his service to numerous scientific societies, editorial boards of research journals, and various governmental committees, Fulton put together a wide range of contacts that he maintained through a personal correspondence of truly Olympian proportions. He was in close contact with those pioneering major scientific advances in a wide range of fields. As just one example, Fulton's role in brokering the development of the penicillin trials in wartime America (which has been likened to medicine's equivalent of the Manhattan project) has only recently come to light.[42]

Fulton's original contributions to science are less impressive, it is true. He was personally responsible for no single major discovery or research breakthrough. Rather, he deeply affected his students, his colleagues, and those who looked to his own exemplary career as an inspiration for scientific research, for a model of how to investigate human biology. Those who knew Fulton credit him, more than anyone else, with bridging the gap between clinical and experimental medicine and with setting the dimensions of modern neurophysiology. Illustrative of this role was Fulton's extraordinary impact on a generation of neurosurgeons who learned from him the value of experimental physiology. He maintained this influence through a continuing involvement with the Harvey Cushing

Society and the presence at Yale of the *Journal of Neurosurgery*, a publication founded by him in 1943.[43]

As far as the medical study of brain and behavior was concerned, it was clear that no other scientist had forged the kinds of extensive professional connections John Fulton had. Indeed, his dense web of networks had always kept him apprised of developments concerning lobotomy. During the war, several of his correspondents had been actively involved in lobotomy programs and research, and had kept Fulton in touch with their work.[44] Beginning in 1946, Fulton tentatively aired to this group his new theories concerning the dangers of damage to the orbital surface and the possibilities of safer, more limited operations. Once he had committed himself to reentering the fray, his information-gathering network turned into a mechanism for action. He was soon informally discussing the latest developments in operative technique and the implications of recent neurophysiological findings for improved lobotomies, dispensing advice in some cases and receiving it in others. He was in direct communication with nearly all those who promoted major psychosurgical variants, including Solomon in Boston; Spiegel and Wycis in Philadelphia; Pool and Scarff in New York; Scoville in Hartford, Connecticut; Livingston in Portland, Oregon; Grantham in Louisville, Kentucky; Penfield in Toronto; Sjoqvist in Sweden; and Cairns in England.[45] A substantial portion of Fulton's queries and discussions about psychosurgery took place in correspondence with his extended family of former students and research associates, many of whom were directly involved in lobotomy studies. Fulton carefully nurtured this group, maintaining friendly relations and commanding strong loyalties in return. Included in these discussions were Harold Buchstein, Paul Bucy, James "Pete" Campbell, Robert Livingston, Frank Nulsen, Karl Pribram, A. Earl Walker, Henry Widgerson, Yale Koskoff, C. G. Mahoney, A. A. Ward and, of course, James Watts, as well as foreign visitors Derek Denny-Brown and Carl Sjoqvist.[46]

Nationwide publicity surrounding Fulton's speeches indirectly reinforced his network's preoccupation with lobotomy. After each public appearance, he usually received numerous entreaties from distressed families for advice about the appropriateness of the operation for their sick relatives and about where such a treatment could be obtained. Fulton invariably declined to provide direct medical advice, but he would refer the families to a local neurosurgeon whose operative skill and judgment he could personally endorse. Between 1947 and 1951, what Fulton termed his "fan mail" had led to dozens of such referrals nationwide and at least one overseas. Watts himself half-facetiously suggested to Fulton that, as his efforts were generating so many patients, it might be the time to open a clinical practice.[47]

## New Research Gains

The final component of Fulton's strategy was the redirection of his own laboratory toward research in neurophysiology that might lead directly to an improved lobotomy. In 1948, he successfully argued to the NRC's Committee on Veterans Medical Affairs that his was the best laboratory for such primate research; a large three-year grant was awarded.[48] As a result of this contract, Fulton was able to add to his staff a group of talented young researchers who were to conduct a wide range of primate studies. Their investigations included reconfirmation of the effects of the Freeman-Watts lobotomy, as well as trials of new surgical approaches and broad physiological studies of the effects of various kinds of cortical ablations.[49] At least twenty-two articles and three monographs resulted from the VA grant. Fulton later commented that the work of the Lobotomy Project in the years between 1948 and 1951 had constituted the most productive period of his laboratory.[50]

In the final stage of Fulton's career as a physiologist, the several components of his campaign to rationalize psychosurgery would neatly dovetail. The result was a series of prominent lectureships, most notably the William Withering Lectures delivered at the University of Birmingham in England, in June of 1948, and the Thomas W. Salmon Lectures, given in New York, in January 1950, which afterward were published as the important monographs *Functional Localization in Relation to Frontal Lobotomy* (1949) and *Frontal Lobotomy and Affective Behavior* (1951).[51] In such addresses and subsequent publications, Fulton reviewed the history and recent progress of frontal-lobe research, incorporating lobotomy studies into his analysis. To Fulton, such research gains had broad scientific implications that stretched far beyond psychosurgery's domain.

With the delivery of his Salmon Lectures, Fulton was satisfied that he had achieved some measure of success in bringing order and responsibility to the psychosurgical programs. First, his quest for specificity in lobotomy operations had indeed resulted in specific, neurophysiologically sanctioned recommendations. True to his physiological convictions, Fulton conceived of psychiatric disorders as an imbalance in the operational level of a dynamic system, either behavioral or emotional. Medical cures came from stimulating the system, if abnormally inactive, or slowing it down, if overactive. Thus, the key to a satisfactory lobotomy would be to understand which areas of the brain, when cut, increased emotional or behavioral levels, and which lesions had an opposite effect. In Fulton's view, lobotomists had assumed, wrongly, that improved operations were simply a matter of better surgical technique or anatomical precision, thereby overlooking more fundamental considerations of precise neurophysiological *function*. He attributed the operation's unreliability to this igno-rance. Psychosurgeons blindly sliced through areas that yielded effects contrary to those desired, with the result that a given procedure might inadvertently cut areas that both stimulated and depressed emotional behavior. Compounding the error was the fact that patients were selected arbitrarily for different lobotomy procedures, rather than carefully matched by whether they needed to be "reactivated" or slowed down, making interpretation of clinical results exceedingly problematic.[52]

Relevant neurophysiological studies, Fulton argued, would have to come from animal rather than human investigations, for unless an au-topsy was performed, there was little certainty as to exactly which part of the brain had in fact been cut. He had discovered his initial clue in the previously mentioned animal experiments of Smith and of Ward, which first gained wide notice at the 1947 ARNMD meeting. Damage to the cingulate gyrus, their research indicated, led to "tameness" and affected the animals' "social consciousness." Work from Fulton's own laboratory, as reported in the Salmon Lectures, confirmed that lesions in this area led to profound emotional changes in chimpanzees yet had little effect on intellect. Standard prefrontal lobotomies cut through both this area as well as the cortical surface, a region which other studies clearly indicated did affect intellectual performance. Here, then, was the foundation for an optimistic conclusion. Fulton surmised: "if these animal studies are appli-cable to man, and I think they are, it seems clear that the undesirable side effects of the radical lobotomy are due to unnecessary encroachment upon the neopallium [cortical surface] and its projections."[53]

On the basis of these prior animal studies, Fulton had proposed a new form of lobotomy to the Society of British Neurological Surgeons in late 1947, and again when delivering his William Withering Lectures in the summer of 1948. By the time of the Salmon Lectures, his suggestion had already led to a number of small clinical trials. In the published version of these lectures, Fulton reported a personal communication from his friend Sir Hugh Cairns, England's most prominent neurosurgeon. Cairns had performed forty-one cingulectomies, Fulton noted, which led to con-spicuous improvement in cases of anxiety neuroses and obsessional states. Fulton was especially encouraged by the results described in another per-sonal communication, this time from Kenneth Livingston (the brother of Fulton's research associate, Robert Livingston). Fifteen of twenty-eight cingulectomized patients were shifted to privileged wards or discharged; improvements were found in none of the control patients, who had under-gone sham operations. Evaluators were not told which patients were in the control group. Livingston added that results in violent and aggressive psychotic cases were strikingly similar to Ward's description of postopera-

tive monkeys. Most gratifying of all were the results in his private patients, who had come from a "higher milieu." Livingston found them to be
happier, more emotionally stable, but without intellectual impairment.
Such results were all the more impressive because of Livingston's extensive experience with the Lyerly-Poppen operation while at the Lahey
Clinic.[54]

For patients whose emotional lives needed to be "reactivated," as in
depressed schizophrenics, Fulton looked to the posterior orbital surfaces,
areas known to yield hyperactivity in animals. A British psychiatrist, F.
Reitman, applied such findings in his operations on twenty-two schizophrenics and observed no instance of mental impairment. In a different
report, anatomical examinations of 122 prefrontal lobotomy patients
who had come to autopsy revealed that interruption of the central segment of the radiations between the thalamus and posterior orbital cortex
had led to the best results. Fulton then described what he felt was the most
promising operation to date, Grantham's technique of electrocoagulation
that targeted precisely these ventromedial projections. Fulton read from a
letter sent to him by Grantham that described 73 percent effectiveness
with no evidence of intellectual impairment. Rylander and Sjoqvist's own
studies of ventromedial lobotomy – also directly communicated to
Fulton – confirmed Grantham's findings. Fulton was heavily influenced
by the fact that Rylander himself could detect no significant intellectual
deficits following the new form of psychosurgery.[55]

"It would thus appear," Fulton concluded in the Salmon Lectures, "that
whereas cingulate ablation is indicated for the aggressive, hyperactive
psychotic, orbital gyrectomy or mid-ventral quadrant coagulation is indicated for schizophrenics and depressed patients with subnormal psycho-
motor activity. Neither operation is followed by undesirable side effects in
the intellectual sphere."

Thus, Fulton had reached – at least to his own satisfaction – his primary
goal by 1951. He had discovered possibilities for new, more limited operations that avoided the cortical surfaces and that could be specifically
designed to suit the characteristics of a patient's mental illness.[56] The
following year, he declared to the American Philosophical Society that "it
now seems highly probable that a small lesion . . . is all that is needed to
break the vicious cycle which underlies certain psychoses."[57] His confidence in the ingenuity of neurosurgeons, as expressed in his discussions at
the ARNMD meeting, had already paid full dividends. True, the development of new techniques was but one-half of his campaign. Fulton, however, also felt confident that his "castigation" of the lobotomists' "casual
methods" had had some salutary effect. Watts himself partly confirmed
this.[58]

Fulton's faith in the revised procedures was more than just academic. Indeed, he went so far as to suggest lobotomy as a viable alternative for a crisis that arose in his own extended family. In 1951, a relative sought advice from Fulton about an alcoholic wife whose perverse life-style, it was feared, might ultimately lead to tragic consequences. Fulton was aware of the situation, as he had followed her progress in and out of several mental hospitals, and was pessimistic. His only advice was to suggest that a "limited lobotomy of the medioventral quadrant of the frontal lobe would probably do more for her than anything." His reasons for saying this, he stated, would be found in his Salmon Lectures.[59]

Fulton's Salmon Lectures had struck a sympathetic chord in the professional as well as the public arena. A psychiatric team in Cincinnati, for example, was so impressed by his argument that they at once set out to perform the Grantham operations, soon accumulating a series of several hundred patients. Their surgeon, Frank Mayfield, had had previous experience with over two hundred standard operations and could personally attest to the lack of complications when using the new procedure. The team described Fulton's recommendation as "prophetic."[60] Fulton's address also stimulated more than the usual "fan mail." For example, a Bronx man with a schizophrenic daughter read an account of Fulton's lectures. When her doctors requested permission to perform a lobotomy, he first read some material by Freeman and Watts and then personally inspected several psychosurgery patients at the mental institution housing his daughter. This experience was enough to dissuade him. However, Fulton's description of a procedure that reduced fears and anxieties without harming personality and intellect "opened a ray of new and positive hope for me." He wrote to Fulton that his discovery "sounds like a reward for my hope and confidence in science." Fulton must have felt the same.[61]

## Freeman's Bold Stroke

Proudly displayed on the dust jacket of Walter Freeman and James Watts's first edition of *Psychosurgery*, published in 1942, was a powerful message: "This work reveals how personality can be cut to measure, sounding a note of hope for those who are afflicted with insanity" – good advertising copy, perhaps, but at the time hardly an accurate assessment. As psychosurgery entered its heyday after the war, Walter Freeman himself, psychosurgery's most prominent supporter, became dissatisfied with the standard lobotomy's lack of precision. He was anxious to find a less destructive operation for several reasons. First, his confidence had been shaken by several dramatic instances of severe personality damage. Second, he was eager to operate on a "better grade" of patient than chronic schizophrenics; he wanted to treat patients within the first year of mental illness, before severe deterioration had set in. Freeman knew that if the profession were to tolerate lobotomies on recently or nonhospitalized patients, a safer, less destructive operation would have to be devised. Lastly, he grew impatient with what he considered to be an inadequate rate of lobotomy, which he blamed on the fact that neurosurgery was a monopoly. Neurosurgeons were too few in number and too expensive for most state hospitals. Indeed, Freeman's own professional relationship with Watts had become strained, as Watts, the more conservative of the pair, often exercised his "veto" power and rejected patients who did not appear to be disabled by their illness. As many operations as the two accomplished together, they were not enough for Freeman.[62]

Freeman's encyclopedic knowledge of the psychosurgical literature led him to an obscure report of an Italian psychiatrist, Amarro Fiamberti, who injected alcohol or formalin directly into the frontal lobes of the brain by inserting a thin cannula through the bony orbit above the eye.[63] With his restless drive to innovate, Freeman at once set out to improve the procedure, choosing to destroy the brain tissue not through chemical means but through the direct surgical action of moving the cannula itself. In Freeman's words:

> I worked out details in the autopsy room at Gallinger Municipal Hospital. There was no surgical instrument available that was tough enough to perforate the orbital roof in some cadavers, though in others a spinal puncture was sufficient. I selected an icepick as being the only instrument possessing the necessary qualities of sharpness and toughness to do the job. It was with some trepidation that I operated on my first patient. . . .

Freeman named his technique "transorbital lobotomy" and eventually replaced the ice pick with a specially forged instrument – a stronger, blunter, and calibrated version – which he termed a "transorbital leucotome."[64] The technique never fully shed its origins, however, and remained widely known as "ice-pick" surgery (see Figures 7.3, 7.4).

Freeman, operating without Watts's knowledge, performed transorbital lobotomies as an office procedure on a small series of patients between January and March of 1946. When Freeman at last demonstrated it to his colleague, Watts was so upset that he threatened to dissolve their partnership unless Freeman abandoned the project. Freeman relented – for a while. He did not perform any transorbitals in Washington, D. C., for a year, but he did begin trial runs in remote West coast state hospitals during the next few summers. When the second edition of *Psychosurgery* was published in 1950, Freeman had already accumulated experience with

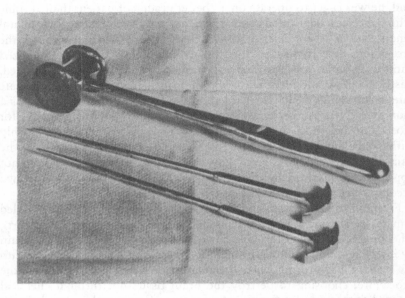

Figure 7.3. Transorbital lobotomy tools. (Source: Walter Freeman and James Watts, *Psychosurgery*, 2d ed., 1950. Courtesy of Charles C. Thomas, Publisher, Springfield, Illinois)

four hundred transorbitals and had committed himself totally to this new procedure. He went so far as to declare publicly that he could no longer recommend the standard prefrontal lobotomy except as a fallback.[65]

Transorbital lobotomy fit Freeman's requirements for a limited brain operation. First, total brain tissue destroyed was far less than in prefrontal lobotomy. Indeed, he blamed the failures of transorbital lobotomy on inadequately extensive lesions, and he soon devised a "deep frontal cut" for intractable cases.[66] Lesions were well placed to interrupt connections between frontal poles and thalamus, which Freeman had become convinced was the ideal operative site. Second, he argued that the new operation yielded no significant intellectual or personality deficits, and thus could be justified for use on even "well-preserved" patients. Transorbital lobotomy, he declared, was in fact a *minor* operation. Astonishingly, patients were ambulatory within an hour and might even be ready for the next meal.

Freeman's surgical chutzpah did not end there. In his opinion, the true roadblocks to more extensive use of psychosurgery in the nation's mental hospitals were not technical hurdles but professional ones: there simply

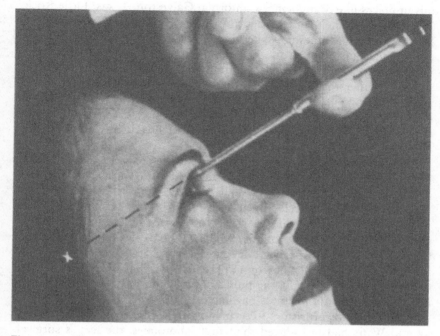

Figure 7.4. Woman receiving a transorbital lobotomy. (Source: *Proceedings of the Royal Society of Medicine*, 1949. Courtesy of the Journal of the Royal Society of Medicine)

were not enough certified neurosurgeons to go around. According to him, transorbital lobotomy was so "safe, simple, and quick" that this problem could now be circumvented: simply dispense with the neurosurgeons altogether. Freeman, with a renewed evangelistic vigor, took up the mission of training hospital psychiatrists and even psychiatric residents to perform the procedure on their own, and without special operating facilities or anesthesia. Freeman's new operation could be performed directly following electroshock while patients were still unconscious.[67] Prefrontal lobotomy, which might take as many as two to four hours of surgical time, was thus replaced by a procedure that was limited only by the speed with which patients could be wheeled in for regular shock treatment, perhaps as little as twenty minutes per case.

Starting in 1948, Freeman barnstormed through the nation's state hospitals, equipped with a pocket set of transorbital leucotomes and motivated by an unflagging drive to operate on as many patients as time and patient supply permitted. He crisscrossed the country, stopping at hospitals in places like Mendocino, California; Galveston, Texas; Little Rock, Arkansas; Lincoln, Nebraska; Sedro Woolley, Washington; Independence, Iowa; Hastings, Minnesota; Sykesville, Maryland; Milledgeville, Georgia; and Ogdensburg, New York. Liberated from his restrictive association with Watts, Freeman succeeded in dramatically increasing his lobotomy series. Together, the two had recorded 625 operations between 1936 and 1948; Freeman, on his own, had lobotomized an additional 2,400 patients by 1957. At his peak, he operated on as many as 225 patients in just twelve days. *Time* magazine, taking stock of Freeman's activities, heralded the dawn of "mass lobotomies."[68]

Freeman had found his métier. His nationwide program of transorbital lobotomy demonstrations had placed him center-stage in a medical drama of his own design, where he would perform modern medicine's latest miracle cure while encircled by attentive trainees and hospital staff. The casual observer was not likely ever to forget such operations. Brain surgery itself stirs uneasy emotions, while the image of ice picks jammed through the orbits of the eyes added a visceral charge to such memories. Freeman thrived on the "horror and fascination" that accompanied such demonstrations, especially the publicity and notoriety they engendered. His concern was not neatness but impact.[69]

Once again, unsurprisingly, Freeman battled intense opposition. When he and Watts had introduced their first lobotomies, the team's surgical credentials were impeccable, thanks to Watts's unsurpassed neurosurgical training and reputation. Now, however, Freeman himself was lobotomizing away at full speed, without benefit of any formal neurosurgical training – or *any* kind of formal surgical training, for that matter. Not all neurosurgeons went so far as to deny Freeman the right to operate solo, as his vast neuroanatomical knowledge and extensive experience performing lobotomies in association with Watts provided strong qualifications. What was impossible for them to abide, however, was the image of untrained mental hospital psychiatrists and medical residents performing such procedures. For example, they would lack the most rudimentary knowledge of how to stop a hemorrhage should one occur.[70]

Freeman, true to form, had little interest in placating the fears of neurosurgeons. To the contrary, he seemed intent on antagonizing them, displaying an insensitivity toward the conventions of their profession. Watts himself had been aghast that Freeman did not even bother to drape patients in sterile linen before beginning his operations. Others soon decried Freeman's introduction of yet another "blind" approach when the trend was clearly toward more "open" operations. In that neurosurgery was the medical specialty which came in closest contact with the complex stuff of self, its execution required meticulous, almost reverent, surgical technique. Freeman's rough treatment of the patient as akin to a "piece of ice" was viewed as an affront to the specialty's carefully built reputation.[71] Freeman brushed such criticisms aside, dismissing them as the self-serving "hokum" of a professional group trying to maintain monopolistic control. He presented his technique as a means of breaking that hold. He went so far as to argue that transorbital lobotomy did not require an elaborate aseptic surgical field because fluid surrounding the eye is already sterile, and that the method had a far lower mortality rate than more sophisticated operations. Such a procedure, he claimed, yielded precise lesions and was indeed so simple that medical residents untrained in surgery could operate after a single afternoon's instruction. *Every physician his own lobotomist.*

Lost in all the handwringing about transorbital lobotomy's neurosurgical propriety, Freeman contended, was the more important consideration of whether it got the job done. Sophisticated techniques such as topectomy and undercutting were, he admitted, impressive operations. Nonetheless, he claimed, their results were not superior to those found in the simpler transorbital lobotomy. Freeman felt that, though his own method might appear crude, its statistical results provided ample justification. His vindication would come in the form of grateful thanks expressed by the distraught families of mental patients and by beleaguered state hospital superintendents. More importantly, he maintained, this technique alone stood the best chance of adoption in areas where it was needed most, remote state hospitals. Otherwise,

> at the present rate – an operation a week in a hospital of 10,000 patients – they would never get around to the fellow who is being admitted now. Something has got to be done. . . . Patients in isolated hospitals should not be denied the benefits of a lobotomy because a ukase is handed down that lobotomy should be done only by a certified group.

Freeman, confident of the treatment's future, boldly declared that the neurosurgeon "had better get busy" with it "before he folds up completely." To him, transorbital lobotomy was unequivocally the "method of choice in institutional practice."[72]

Freeman's energetic promotion did succeed in stimulating many trials of the new treatment. Now even remote state hospitals, such as the Western State Hospital in Fort Steilacoom, Washington, might share in the dual benefits of "active treatments" as described earlier.[73] Reports from participating state hospitals counted their lobotomy series by the hundreds. The largest use of transorbital lobotomy occurred in Texas and in Freeman's West Virginia Lobotomy Project.[74] Already by 1951 this particular procedure had escalated into the fastest-growing of the variant lobotomies, amounting to approximately one-third of all operations performed in the previous few years, and an even higher percentage of those attempted in the state hospitals.[75]

## Collision Course

Freeman was experimenting with his transorbital method at the precise moment when Fulton went public with his deep concern about reckless lobotomizing. Their collision was certain. Fulton fired the first shot in October 1947, well before Freeman had even published his new technique. Incited to a rare display of bitter sarcasm, Fulton wrote to Freeman: "What are these terrible things I hear about you doing lobotomies in your office with an ice pick? I have just been to California and Minnesota and heard about it in both places. Why not use a shot gun? It would be quicker!" Freeman replied that the operation was "much less traumatizing than a shotgun and almost as quick." His straight-faced response reflected his defensiveness, however. Freeman untruthfully added that he did not recommend the technique as an office procedure and that Watts was cooperating.[76] Once his nationwide lobotomy crusade was under way, he dispensed with any such pretenses, and the rift between him and Fulton grew wider.

Battle lines were first drawn on the occasion of the 1947 frontal lobes meeting of the ARNMD, beginning even with Fulton's distribution of paper topics. Although Freeman and Watts jointly delivered two papers, neither communication focused on lobotomy's effectiveness for relief of mental illness: one was on its use in cases of intractable pain (a less controversial topic) and the other was a neuroanatomical essay. Freeman felt shackled by these assignments. Intent on presenting results of his as yet unpublished method, he wrote to Fulton: "How about transorbital lobotomy or some exciting new theoretical work about the frontal lobes in relation to the time mechanism? This is really *research*."[77] Unfortunately for Freeman's request, Fulton's precise goal as orchestrator of the conference was to prove that it was *not*.

Freeman had no chance to advance or defend his cause other than in the meeting's discussion periods. Never shirking from opportunities for public debate, however, Freeman held his ground at the meeting and established himself as the most vocal discussant. The sparring match began immediately following the first paper, Jacobsen's long-awaited description of Becky and Lucy, which suggested that lobotomy did yield considerable intellectual deficits. Freeman contentiously declared Jacobsen's findings irrelevant, explaining the supposed deficits as nothing more than insignificant artifacts produced by the testing situation. The face-off continued throughout the symposium. When Freeman delivered his own paper on the connections between thalamus and frontal lobe, Fulton himself challenged an implicit suggestion that it was necessary to damage the orbital surface (which happened to be the effect of transorbital lobotomy) for psychosurgery to work; this had been disproved earlier in the morning, he stated, by the report on Becky and Lucy.[78]

It has already been shown how Fulton directly attacked Freeman's position, using the papers by Ward and Rylander as a springboard. They suggested that more limited operations were effective and that prefrontal lobotomy did cause personality damage.[79] In defense, Freeman argued that Ward's conclusions, which were based only on animal experiments, were inconsistent with results in several of his own clinical cases. Fulton, in rebuttal, dismissed Freeman's particular examples as irrelevant and poor arguments against the thesis. In response to Rylander's claim of extensive personality damage, Freeman noted that Rylander had not factored in the benefits of the operation, the improvement in social adaptability usually shown by patients. Freeman found a golden opportunity to reinforce this latter point. Spafford Ackerly delivered a follow-up study to his classic case of a man who since childhood had had severe bilateral damage to his frontal lobes. "I think," Freeman noted, that "Dr. Ackerly's presentation shows one thing that hasn't been mentioned, and that it is the extraordinary ability of this man with a profound organic defect to make his way in society and not become too much entangled with the law and the mental institutions." Freeman concluded, to widespread laughter, that "apparently it doesn't take much frontal lobe to hold a job."[80]

The debate continued with Fulton's later lectures. In response to criticisms in the Withering address, Freeman requested that Fulton use his influence to arrange trials of transorbital lobotomy in Connecticut's state hospitals. Fulton replied that his neurosurgical training had made him suspicious of such blind approaches. Instead, he argued, his own group was trying to determine the exact tracts involved and correlate them to specific mental disorders. This necessitated an open approach and a precise knowledge of what was being cut. Freeman's response was to forward a reprint describing four hundred successful cases. After a final exchange of letters occasioned by Fulton's Salmon Lectures, the two ceased direct communications on the issue, agreeing to disagree.[81]

## Science Pure and Medicine Applied

Fulton and Freeman's conflict stemmed not from personal antagonisms – relations between the two had been otherwise congenial – but from their contrasting professional identities. Fulton was the academic scientist par excellence, confident at the helm of a diverse, internationally recognized university laboratory supported by prestigious grants and fellowships. His assemblage of professional activities provided a vantage point from which he surveyed a panorama of research developments. At heart, he was a systematizer and a theorist. His secondary professional career as a bibliophile and historian of medicine led to a measured, steady manner of placing new developments in broad, historical perspective. And if Fulton had been able to grade his own life as a scientist, he would have calculated it by the reverence his laboratory alumni bestowed upon him at his retirement party.[82] Himself childless, he treated those passing through his laboratory as de facto members of an extended family. The flip side of Fulton's devotion to the insular world of academic science was a resultant isolation from the workaday realities of clinical practice. The ivory tower suited Fulton just fine.

Freeman, too, lived and breathed academic medicine, expending truly fearsome amounts of energy keeping abreast of the latest technological and experimental findings reported in the literature; appearing before innumerable local, national, and international medical and scientific societies; publishing scientific articles by the score; and maintaining a heavy university course load. The primary concern of all his restless, even manic, workaholism was quite different from that of Fulton's, however. Freeman's driving motivation – if not compulsion – was to be the instrument that radically altered the desperation and suffering he personally observed in his patients and their families.[83] The clinic, not the lab, anchored Freeman's life, though the two were indubitably linked, even from the outset of his career in medicine. As mentioned earlier, for example, he was a member of the Army Medical Corps at Fort Dix in 1918, where he was responsible for the care and then postmortem examination of the scores of soldiers who succumbed to the flu epidemic. This experience awoke him to the power and mystery of disease, a story that was played out in the destruction of the body's tissues, and which was visible to Freeman in all its gruesome detail on the microscope's slide. Unlike most in his medical school class, Freeman had a strong stomach for spending countless tedious hours in the pathological examination of specimen slides, in time modifying a stain here or a photographic technique there, all in the absolute conviction that an advance of practical consequence – however minor – was within reach.

Although consumed by the researcher's passion for advancing knowledge, which brought him into close contact with the world's scientific leaders in medicine, Freeman's true professional identity never strayed far from that of a private-practice clinician ever anxious to maintain a viable livelihood, either in his own office or through a steady presence on the wards of the various local hospitals. Freeman's experience was quite dissimilar from that of an elite university scientist. He had no cadre of well-qualified graduate students, postdoctoral fellows, or research associates, no elaborate research facilities to attract extramural researchers. His own laboratory existed more in name than in reality, and what neuroanatomical or neuropathological facilities he did obtain were either wrested from medical school administrators or personally subvented. He blamed his isolated clinical career for the fact that virtually every foundation or philanthropy he approached rejected his applications. Thus immersed in the incessant demands of everyday medical practice, Freeman exuded what he termed a "no-nonsense" approach, always remaining on the lookout for the latest techniques that could meet these immediate needs. His sympathies lay not with those within the ivied walls but with those who fought on the battlefronts of disease – for example, state hospital superintendents who labored under impossible conditions and who, unlike laboratory researchers, lacked the luxury of working to their own schedules. Freeman himself was always a man in a hurry, wanting to accomplish things now, not later. Patients came to his office in pain and torment, demanding if not begging for quick relief.

The distance between the world of the laboratory scientist and that of the practicing clinician thus split Fulton and Freeman on many points central to the lobotomy issue. To Fulton, the most far-reaching and reliable medical knowledge stemmed from a combination of basic animal research and a few clinical trials exhaustively studied. Criteria for patient selection and evaluation had to reflect the standardized, objective qualities of good science rather than the untrustworthy, subjective reports filed by practicing clinicians. Freeman, as one might surmise, had an altogether different set of standards. To begin with, animal experiments were to him interesting but potentially misleading exercises because of the unbridgeable gaps between anthropoids and man. Small clinical trials, for their part, were indeed important but were not to be considered a treatment's acid test. Investigations of clinical efficacy were routinely confounded by such factors as variability in the environment, patient condition, and therapeutic technique, influences that might be overcome only through large-scale trials and elaborate long-term follow-ups.

Most important of all to Freeman was the question "Did it work?" He was skeptical of the ability of putatively objective, laboratory-based evaluations to settle the issue in the case of lobotomy. What mattered were not the arbitrary criteria of intelligence tests, but the successful reintegration of patients back into the stream of everyday life. In Freeman's view, a treatment's value was best judged by blending the opinions of the patient and his or her family with the sensitive observations of the clinician. At professional meetings he would bring along testimonial letters from former patients and simple charts of the number of them employed or keeping house, forceful – if "unscientific" – testimony of lobotomy's real-life benefits.

The gulf between the two points of view is also evident in the disdain each side displayed in regard to the other's attitude toward patients. Fulton was truly appalled by the lobotomists' failure to appreciate that each psychosurgical operation was "in the truest sense a physiological experiment." Historically, neurophysiology had been constrained by a lack of appropriate human material. Yet, Fulton charged, literally here were tens of thousands of patients having their brains haphazardly sectioned, without a single case being studied adequately. Waste of such precious scientific material, gained at so grave a cost, was from a neurophysiological standpoint nothing less than unconscionable. Freeman, in contrast, bemoaned to Fulton the vast human "wastage" caused by insufficient deployment of lobotomy.[84] Although the technique had already proved itself clinically valuable, Freeman argued, overconservatism on the part of the scientific community was impeding its adoption, causing untold harm as numerous patients were allowed to deteriorate further. There was little chance that either Fulton or Freeman would be convinced by the other's position, no matter how intensive or prolonged their discussions.

Who held the high ground in this debate? Psychosurgery, it has been shown, was employed in a spectrum of conditions ranging from remote state hospitals to elite research institutes. One might wonder at which end of the scale patients were better off: at the low end, in Freeman's bailiwick of ice picks and severe hospital conditions, or at the other extreme, in the nation's most prestigious research institutes, such as the New York Psychiatric Institute and its state-of-the-art topectomy? Not surprisingly, many psychiatric leaders at the time singled out the topectomy group as the most likely to shed new light on the lobotomy issue. They were reassured by its rational design, along with its exhaustive research protocols, which included a "highly impressive battery of examinations," and were clearly taken by its greater surgical precision. Here was something that was "scientific, logical and understandable by neurologists, psychiatrists and neurosurgeons."[85] Such sentiments speak to the foremost issue that separated Fulton and Freeman, and their respective followers: how to find the most trustworthy path to medical progress.

In Fulton's perspective, a true, lasting therapeutic advance would above all else have to make sense scientifically, conforming to experimental protocols. Operations such as topectomy, or his own recommendation of cingulotomy, at least stood a chance of fulfilling this desideratum. Within this framework, the advance of knowledge was a virtuoso performance of intellectual method, fundamentally a *process*. Implicit in the worldview of the elite academic was the corollary assumption that the connection between laboratory-derived knowledge and its application in the external world was unproblematic. Investigators, boldly following a blend of inner intuition and well-formed guesses, would chart out new territories of knowledge, stake out claims, and then refine them until something of value was obtained. Only afterward, when the science and its derivative technology had stabilized, should clinicians have widespread access to laboratory products (a sort of trickle-down model of therapeutic advance). Possibilities for danger arose only if the process was hurried, either by investigators abandoning their high standards or by clinicians acting prematurely, not waiting for the scientists' go-ahead signal. In his William Withering Lectures, Fulton thus hoped to ridicule Freeman by publicly airing the psychosurgeon's declaration that through "ice-pick" surgery an "enterprising neurologist" could lobotomize ten to fifteen patients in a morning.[86]

Yet what Fulton viewed as a professional embarrassment, Freeman pointed to with pride. Freeman argued that such enterprising neurologists were exactly what current conditions demanded. He was not at all worried about leaving therapeutic innovation in the hands of clinicians. The simple truth was that virtually all recent therapeutic advances in the fields of neurology and psychiatry had been discovered by practicing clinicians, not bench scientists.[87] In any case, to Freeman, the true test of medical progress was not the process of how new knowledge was derived but whether a practicable advance was in fact produced. The proof was in the pudding, not the publication. He noted with some satisfaction that though the procedures of topectomy, undercutting, and stereoencephalotomy at first glance looked far more sophisticated than were his own procedures of transorbital and standard prefrontal lobotomy, their much vaunted precision was so much rhetoric. The proponents of these procedures, he argued, foolishly believed that complicated techniques or equipment automatically translated into greater operative control or result. (Freeman derided Scoville's electrocoagulation technique, for example, as having all the fine control of applying a vacuum hose to a tub of spaghetti.)

A more important issue for Freeman was the fact that the technical encumbrances often made such procedures irrelevant to standard psychiatric practice. Available at only a handful of well-equipped facilities, they would perforce have little impact on the vast numbers of hospitalized mental patients in America. Should these sophisticated procedures alone turn out to be the only current options, then in actuality no real therapeutic advance had occurred for the mentally ill in America. What was the good of a treatment that was not deployable? In contrast, transorbital lobotomy, in his opinion, had brought surgical relief of mental illness to whole new categories of patients and had proven its value for institutional practice.[88] It wasn't pretty, and it had a suspect pedigree, but it got the job done.

It should be noted that some of Freeman's criticisms were indeed on the mark. Pool's operation, for example, in spite of its sophisticated appearance and progressive psychiatric research design, clearly subjected patients to far greater operative hazards than did simpler procedures; its postoperative rate of epileptic complications was found to be startlingly high. In fact, its beneficial results did not appear that much different from those following other procedures. Why, then, was this particular technique chosen? Pool admitted that his was not the ideal operation from the *clinical* standpoint, but was selected because the operative procedure provided an opportunity for certain electrical stimulation experiments.[89] The moral is evident. Although patients in remote state hospitals may have been at the mercy of institutional expediency, their brethren in prestigious research institutes may have fared no better, their fate being determined instead by research protocols – a different kind of procrustean bed, but no more forgiving.


The clash between Fulton and Freeman was not new in the annals of medicine. Beginning in the late nineteenth century (as the story usually goes), laboratory-based medicine embarked upon its triumphant march, knocking out one disease after another and placing medical practice at last upon a stable empirical foundation. There were losers, of course. According to the new standards, what the best clinicians had previously had to offer – in the combination of a trained eye and hand, sound professional judgment, and an irreplaceable store of personal experience – was no longer sufficient. Rather, further progress would involve scientific analysis of data, instrument-assisted diagnosis, physiological studies of function, and laboratory-produced therapeutics. The transition to the new scientific medicine thus was not a smooth, natural upgrading of method and belief. On the contrary, every step of the way was bitterly resisted by trusted medical authorities who voiced grave doubts as to whether the new scientific medicine was more flash than substance, a promise of things yet to come rather than as yet realized, and often blatantly wrong, posing real dangers to the welfare of patients. From the clinicians' perspective, those working in the isolated laboratories failed to comprehend the actual conditions of life: there was something about in vivo that was unreproducible in vitro. Such sentiments were not unfounded. As recent scholarship in the history of medicine has indicated, the new scientific medicine was indeed often oversold, still something of a pig in a poke.[90]

The battle between Fulton and Freeman had all the important hallmarks of this now traditional confrontation between scientist and clinician. Indeed, it will become evident that neither one of the two was entirely correct – or dismissable. Each simply had been true to his own respective professional context. It is too easy to adopt Fulton's demarcation of responsible and irresponsible medicine, to divide the good lobotomists from the bad with no intervening shades of gray. Such an overly clean rendering obscures the ongoing debates within the psychosurgical literature about what constituted a therapeutic advance, debates based not just on matters of scientific fact or physiological interpretation but on professional perspective. Ironically, one advocate of lobotomy aptly captured the incommensurability of the two positions by quoting from Fulton's own mentor, Sir Charles Sherrington, in support of the clinician's irreducible perspective: "Science, nobly, declines as proof anything but complete proof; but common sense, pressed for time, accepts and acts on acceptance."[91] Neither the clinician nor the researcher has any prior claim to virtue. Indeed, the fate of the two domains of the laboratory and the clinic are linked in ways not usually publicized.

## Reciprocal Legitimation

In the course of half a century, however, something significant *had* changed in the way the tension between the clinic and the lab was worked out. By the end of World War II, the issue of the laboratory's practical utility to society had been resolved, in science's favor. Through such displays of power as the awesome atom bomb and the miraculous penicillin pill, the laboratory had proven itself as a resource of seeming limitless potential to transform the material circumstances of life. The nation was convinced to invest heavily in experimental research, and the era of large-scale government funding of science commenced. By the time of Fulton and Freeman's dispute, the medical profession (by and large) had been persuaded that laboratory science was indeed the bedrock of medicine – at least in its idealized form.

This victory did not ease the tension between the world of the clinician and that of the scientist, however. Oddly enough, although the two domains were in many instances as incommensurable as ever, in the new state of affairs the fates of the scientist and the clinician nevertheless had become thoroughly interdependent. Intraprofessional disputes were just as bitter, though more tightly controlled in site of conflict. What had changed was the necessity to present to the public, as well as to the rest of the medical profession, a system of medical science that was not separate but unified, with clinic and lab as joint partners in a single, socially valued mission.

On the one hand, Walter Freeman's lobotomy trials were not arbitrarily constructed, mere flights of clinical fancy, but were deliberately fashioned by him to conform to prevailing scientific theories and laboratory findings. In this new era of scientific medicine, Freeman indeed would have had little chance of inspiring other clinical trials of lobotomy unless the procedure had, at some level, the imprimatur of the scientific community. He and the other lobotomists were not obligated to provide this scientific justification themselves. It was sufficient that trusted scientific authorities could be identified and cited who would either condone its use or vouch for its potential. In the early years, the justification was Fulton's assertion that Moniz's patients had responded in a manner similar to his chimpanzee's loss of experimental neurosis. Later, a glut of neurophysiological and neuroanatomical research related to the topic – not to mention, once again, Moniz's Nobel Prize – was sufficient proof of backing by the scientific community.

On the other hand, John Fulton and those committed to research programs that studied lobotomy were able to sustain concerted laboratory efforts only because of the perception that the targeted problem was of extensive clinical importance. Without this kind of proven clinical potential, scientists were unable to justify the purpose and expense of such research to their patrons. Wedded to a program of expensive primate research, at a university medical school that for two decades had been unwilling to allocate sufficient funds for educational let alone research purposes, Fulton was acutely sensitive to the need to cultivate patronage.[92] During the 1930s, he had relied upon a series of private philanthropies to equip and maintain his laboratory. The war, however, had been a watershed in the realignment of funding sources for medical as well as for all scientific research, when the federal government stepped in as the dominant provider of research monies. The future had been intelligible to Fulton: university departments were increasingly obliged to depend on governmental support if they were to compete as active centers of research. Fulton was quicker than most to realize a subtle but significant consequence of this transfer of economic responsibility from the private to the public sector. Medical scientists, individually as well as collectively, were now directly dependent upon the public's perception of their work as being or not being of immediate social relevance.[93]

Fulton solved his own funding dilemma by applying to the NRC's Committee on Veterans Medical Affairs (CVMA) to underwrite the costs of his lobotomy research. The "VA Lobotomy Project" became the largest undertaking of the Yale Laboratory between the war and Fulton's retirement, spending $200,000 between 1948 and 1951. Fulton not only maintained his laboratory but expanded it. His proposal was shrewdly calculated. He played upon governmental contacts established during the war and upon the VA's interest in developing an aggressive medical research and treatment program, especially in psychiatry. (The total resident population of VA psychiatric facilities at the time was second only to the state hospitals.) Most significantly, a top VA priority had been the provision of all forms of modern psychiatric treatment, which resulted in psychosurgery being utilized by all of the thirty-seven VA psychiatric hospitals. Fulton successfully argued to the Committee on Veterans Medical Affairs that, as the VA lobotomy program had already been "conspicuously successful" in reducing the amount of hospital care needed, discovery of an "optimum" operation would lead to even greater benefits. Fulton declared to the CVMA's chairman that the problem was "one of considerable urgency and its economic significance cannot be overstressed."[94]

Whereas Freeman at times was forced to bend a knee to scientific authority in justifying his clinical forays, Fulton himself was hard-pressed to promote his own ties to Freeman's domain. Out of a need to justify his research projects, Fulton went so far as to point to the results of precisely those large-scale clinical trials that in the professional forums he had previously denigrated as unscientific. The experience of Fulton and Freeman is not unique, but generalizable, indicative of a widespread and continuing phenomenon. In short, the separate and often opposed domains of the clinician and the laboratory scientist nonetheless became jointly linked for purposes of survival. Indeed, the pursuit of medical progress was dependent on successfully projecting a dual image of scientific validity and social utility, if the profession were to be mobilized and the public were to underwrite the costs. Still strange bedfellows, the scientist and the clinician found political strength through a sort of moral division of labor, what might be termed a system of *reciprocal legitimation*. One party provided the scientific rationale and the other the social significance. Fulton and Freeman (and their later parallels) were thus far more dependent upon one another's work than either might have cared to admit.

The argument can be advanced, however, that Freeman does not well represent the typical clinician in everyday practice, a point underscored by his university post, long record of publications, and drive to innovate. Perhaps he should be categorized instead as a lesser academic, a shadow of Fulton. Freeman indeed was different from most rank-and-file clinicians in the intensity of his quest for the advancement of knowledge and technique, but this should not be interpreted as proof that he was more a scientist than a clinician. As previously touched upon, until the late nineteenth century what was considered scientific within the field of medicine still had multiple meanings. In this regard, Freeman was simply following in the footsteps of an elite in clinical medicine who assumed the responsibility for advancing knowledge, and who slowly were incorporating laboratory-defined standards – though not necessarily in the same manner as their counterparts at the bench. In the first few decades after 1900, a category of physician was emerging who hoped to apply the new experimental method directly to the problems of clinical practice; thus emerged the field of *clinical investigation* as a specialty of its own. Advocates of this approach, for example, founded the American Association of Clinical Research. "The crux of the matter," they inveighed, "appears to be that experimental laboratory proof is not sufficient clinical proof."[95]

Freeman might conceivably be more accurately located somewhere within this trend, though his service role still fundamentally remained that of a private-practice clinician, not an academic researcher.[96] The incorporation of experimental method into clinical practice was also much slower to reach fulfillment than is generally recognized, and certainly had not gained much headway until after Freeman's time. The attempt to marry experimental method to the real-world conditions of the clinic remains incomplete; the new field of *clinical* science did not resolve the tensions between the two domains so much as transform them into a less noticeable form.

## Heart of Darkness

What does this model of reciprocal legitimation imply about the overall story of medical progress? Optimal science is traditionally presumed to be disinterested investigation, research that is free from the supposedly distorting influences of politics, financial obligations, or professional rivalries, and instead is wholly attuned to "internal," purely disciplinary interests, guided only by intellectual curiosity and intuition. Often contrasted to this noble pursuit of pure knowledge is the grubby business of clinical practice. It is not surprising when individual clinicians are found to advocate particular therapies the scientific basis of which proves lacking. After all, this is what is expected of professionals who must labor in an environment beholden to "external" influences. Temptation will sooner or later claim a willing victim. Freeman's own excesses – something of the carnival huckster clings to him – seem less shocking due to their familiarity. His is not a new story, it would seem. The case of Fulton, however, may seem more disturbing, as it suggests that considerations of research funding might have led him to promote research in a field that perhaps would have been ignored had its merits been disinterestedly weighed.

In pursuing a line of research that responded to a great need, Fulton was not necessarily acting as a bad scientist, however, just a normal one. Indeed, it was a combination of forces arising out of a context that was simultaneously social as well as scientific which motivated the neuroscientific community to direct its resources to lobotomy research. First, several research trends within neurophysiology and neuroanatomy were converging toward a new model of cerebral function, one into which the lobotomy studies fit naturally. Second, the societal import of lobotomy did not distort these trends away from a more rewarding path. In fact, the opposite is true: it galvanized the field by underscoring the important ramifications of a new model of brain and behavior. Without this added significance, researchers might not have been so motivated to pursue this particular line of investigation.

This interplay of factors is evident in the development of Fulton's own research enterprise, in the way in which a set of scientific ideas came to fruition in a specific social and professional context. A major contribution of modern medicine, Fulton believed at the outset of his career, was the growing evidence that human behavior is a product of anatomical structure and physiological function. A past generation of researchers, including his teacher Sherrington, had formulated the principles of neuronal integration, in the process mapping out intricate motor, sensory, autonomic, and reflex systems. As previously mentioned, these systems were subdivided according to an evolutionary hierarchy, whereby the anatomically oldest structures (known as the archipallium or diencephalon) governed the most "primitive" bodily functions, such as respiration, blood pressure, and so on, while the newest structures (neopallium or neocortex) were assumed to govern "higher" functions such as thought and voluntary movements. Progress had been achieved mostly in the lower systems, as scientists filled out the details of the autonomic nervous system and those areas with visceral (bodily) effects. The relation between the brain and bodily functions was growing ever clearer. This was not the case with the frontal lobes – evolutionarily the highest brain structure – knowledge of which had remained scant. They were still referred to as "silent" in function. The biology of human thought remained cloaked in mystery.[97]

Elucidation of frontal-lobe function, and its ties to the rest of the brain, remained the central research problem of Fulton's laboratory throughout his tenure. Looking backward in 1950, Fulton would claim that the previous fifteen years had seen a remarkable advance in neurophysiology: investigators had begun to discern significant connections between the old and new brain systems. Fulton stated that one of the most significant developments in modern medicine – if not all science – had been the recent achievements in relating human behavior to anatomical structure and physiological function, the first step toward reaching the elusive goal of establishing the brain as the organ of the mind. Indeed, a similar sentiment of Fulton's on a slightly earlier occasion had prompted an editorial in a prominent medical journal, which stated that "nowhere is the pursuit of knowledge more exciting than in the correlation of structure and function in those areas of the cerebral cortex traditionally termed 'silent.'"[98]

Two lines of brain research yielded the richest discoveries. First, scattered experiments revealed that the supposedly silent frontal lobe did have direct effects on the autonomic nervous system, both stimulative and suppressant. On the basis of the suggested connections between neocortex and diencephalon, and the patterns of resultant behavioral effects, Fulton had generated his first recommendations concerning improved lobotomies. A unified theoretical model was still lacking, however.[99] Second, a breakthrough in neurophysiology had occurred when attention shifted away from a direct emphasis on the frontal lobes to studies on midbrain structures, which were discovered to make intermediary connections between neocortex and diencephalon. The significance of these structures was publicized in 1949 in a paper of Paul MacLean, a young investigator in Stanley Cobb's Boston psychosomatic medicine group. MacLean, exploring relations between emotions and epilepsy, had chanced upon a 1937 paper by a Cornell neuroanatomist, James W. Papez, that had fallen into obscurity. In this admittedly speculative article, Papez had boldly hypothesized that the midbrain structures of hypothalamus, anterior thalamic nuclei, gyrus cinguli, and hippocampus were interconnected into a harmonious mechanism that was nothing less than the means by which *emotions* were expressed and felt. He termed this network the "limbic lobe," following Broca's nineteenth-century designation.[100] MacLean fastened this model onto Paul Yakovlev's conception of a tripartite brain that envisioned a middle (mesopallium) level mediating between old and new cortex. MacLean's resultant new concept of a "visceral brain," based on the limbic lobe, in essence represented the neurophysiological equivalent of a "missing link." Here was the meeting ground of thought and bodily action, the bridge between our primitive and civilized selves, a central problem that had dominated much of neurology and psychiatric thought from John Hughlings Jackson to Sigmund Freud. Emotional life had at last found a structural basis – an exciting if not revolutionary proposition at the time.[101]

MacLean's rediscovery of Papez, it should be noted, was not a random event but occurred within a specific historical context. Cobb's research program at Massachusetts General Hospital was the showpiece neuro-psychiatric institute funded by the Rockefeller Foundation in this period. His research program, in consonance with foundation aims, was deliberately targeted toward exploring the relations between emotions and disease, and, by extension, how scientific medicine might lead to greater social stability through an understanding of human behavior. True to the interdisciplinary flavor of the psychosomatic school, MacLean concluded his essay by framing the tripartite division within the Freudian model of superego, id, and ego. Moreover, if MacLean's interest in psychosomatic medicine had placed Papez on the scientific map, it was Fulton's concern for discovering a unifying model for lobotomy that brought MacLean's own work into wide circulation.[102] For Fulton, MacLean's article crystallized in a single model the many lines of research he had been following on the connections between neocortex and midbrain structures. The visceral brain, Fulton wrote, was no less than a "distinct functional entity concerned primarily with the regulation of visceral organs and elaboration of affective [emotional] behavior."[103] Of special significance to his own research program, Fulton found in MacLean's model a neurophysiological mechanism for lobotomy's effects and a basis for the procedure's improvement. For example, the model predicted that the cortical surfaces could indeed be bypassed in successful operations, thus sparing the patients' intellectual abilities.

The challenge of discovering the structure and function of this hypothetical third brain system provided a new focus for Fulton's research program. He redirected the thrust of the VA lobotomy project toward the problem of working out the parameters of the visceral brain. It was also no accident that MacLean was added to Fulton's team just as his paper was reaching print. Ultimately, Fulton's VA contract provided a platform for a large number of important investigations concerning the limbic lobe. In fact, the modern term *limbic system* was first coined in a paper by MacLean as part of the VA project. Young investigators who were involved in this project, or who had had strong connections to Fulton's laboratory, would play prominent roles even into the 1980s in shaping the conception of the limbic system. In today's neuroscience, this brain structure is considered to be the bridge that links "brain, mind and behavior in a functional continuum."[104]

Historians of psychosurgery have explained that newer operations of the early 1950s were weighed against emerging theories of the limbic system and even yielded information that was to influence these conceptions. My point here is to go one step further, to emphasize that the innovative cerebral theories were driven forward by lobotomy programs, which had created what one investigator of the day termed a "mighty stimulus" for such research. Gerhardt von Bonin, a leading neuroanatomist, wrote at the time that the anatomy of emotion was the least understood chapter of neuroanatomy, yet "its importance, in these days of psychosurgery, is hard to overrate." It was precisely *because of the lobotomy studies* that many of the day's neuroscientists felt they were entering a new era in research of cortical function. Fulton unequivocally promoted the role of lobotomy as an important catalyst in neurophysiology. "Prior to the introduction of the operation of frontal lobotomy," he stated in his introduction to his substantially rewritten third edition of *Physiology of the Nervous System,* "the literature of the frontal areas was confused and conflicting."[105] As Fulton approached the end of his career as a neurophysiologist, the development of the new field of limbic system research came as a welcome added bonus.

Choosing which research venture to pursue is always a human choice, with external consequences; it is only natural that scientists incorporate social and cultural considerations into their motivations. Scientists, in framing the intellectual boundaries of their next research project, face an infinite number of possible choices to pursue. The decision of which research path to develop – a matter not so much of finding the right answer to a particular problem but of defining an interesting question – is made that much easier when something has become visibly *at stake* in the venture. (The lore of science is laden with the metaphors of discovery and conquest; scientists like to portray themselves as a special form of explorer. This stipulated, let us note that Columbus and the rest were hardly on "disinterested" voyages.) In our own story here, it was only when the social – as well as intraprofessional – need for an improved lobotomy had become clear that a particular line of neurophysiological research also snapped into focus. Something of great value had become at stake in exploring the brain's own heart of darkness, and the investigators responded to the call, claiming their discoveries en route.[106]

### The Perils of Progress

The passage of time eroded claims to monumental achievements in therapeutics by either Fulton or Freeman. Ice-pick operations, along with topectomies and orbital undercutting, have since all faded from the scene. That some operations were at one time "physiologically justified" thus provided no lasting foundation. Opinions as to which procedure were the most scientifically valid, based on current fashions in scientific theory, proved to be as ephemeral as judgments made only on clinical or empirical data. Fulton's strategy may indeed have been more sophisticated and scientifically informed than Freeman's rough-and-ready approach, but this in itself was no guarantee that it would be the more certain. The simple truth is that a decade later no psychosurgical operation remained as a therapy with widespread clinical application.[107] Hypothesis is often the secular name for Holy Grail.

The possibility that psychosurgery might fail to achieve full validation at some point in the future was hardly an unforeseen circumstance. Although neurophysiology was quickening its pace of advance and practical experience with the technique was quite broad, it was still clear to all that a complete scientific justification for the operation did not yet exist. The wholesale use of the procedure in the late 1940s had raised the spectre that a treatment some might call experimental was in fact being deployed on a routine basis.

Why didn't the proponents of lobotomy research abandon the enterprise at the earliest moment when they became cognizant of the grave hazards associated with the procedure? Even Fulton and Freeman, we have seen, were dismayed by the personality deficits that appeared in numerous cases. This line of inquiry misconstrues how science operates, however. Fulton's and Freeman's response to this challenge was uniform insofar as both believed that the solution lay not in abandoning the procedure but in refining it. In reaching this decision, they were simply following through on their faith in science. It would have been out of character for them as innovators to have acted otherwise. That the brain operations had achieved almost miraculous cures in even a handful of cases was sufficient proof to them that *something* significant was occurring, a fact that could not be walked away from in good conscience. In 1939, psychiatrist Abraham Myerson commented on a comparable situation in regard to the shock therapies. "We need not be discouraged by the fact that these drugs have not lived up to their early promise," Myerson advised. Admittedly, "the airplane has flown ten yards" and then "it has crashed." Nonetheless, "the fact remains, it has flown ten yards."[108]

As the brain was becoming understood as a collection of discrete though interconnected functional units, it seemed only logical that increased precision in surgical intervention was a likely route to further progress.[109] It was only natural to assume that with each additional investigation science would hone in on which part of the brain, if damaged, produced hazardous side effects, and which areas would lead to symptomatic relief. In time, the wheat would be separated from the chaff and an effective as well as safe operation would remain. This is what science does best – learn from its mistakes.[110] Freeman and Fulton differed only in their interpretations as to where to begin the search for a more precise operation and in their evaluations as to what constituted a workable medical advance.

The bevy of investigators who joined with Fulton and Freeman in the quest for a better lobotomy walked a fine line in delicately balancing the need to cut "as little as possible" and "as much as was necessary."[111] Alas, with the benefit of hindsight one might question whether this search for an "optimum" procedure was not itself tragically misguided. In Carlyle Jacobsen's final, private report to Fulton on the effects that the original brain operations had on the chimpanzees Becky and Lucy, a pessimistic hypothesis can be found concerning lobotomy's future which was based on an important argument others had overlooked. Jacobsen observed that, after surgery, anxiety had disappeared in the animals along with some loss in their intellectual faculties. Over the span of a few years, however, the chimpanzees did begin to recover some problem-solving abilities that had been lost. At the same time, Jacobsen discovered, some of the frustrational behavior also returned. "It is my opinion," Jacobsen concluded, "that the same mechanism – namely impairment of higher functions characterized by impairment of abstraction, tendency to respond concretely, inability to organize several elements of a problem, and distractibility – is responsible for alleviation of the anxiety state in human beings. As recovery approaches normal state, I should expect the capacity for anxiety to rise also."[112] If this were true, any attempts to whittle away the unfortunate consequences of lobotomy and yet retain its clinical benefits would be doomed to failure. Tragically, they were two sides of the same coin.

It is all too easy to judge this headlong rush to redouble psychosurgery's efficacy at the first signs of doubts about its worthiness as a classic example of hubris. Fulton, Freeman, and their followers, it is presumed, should have known better than to stake their careers on the search for an optimal lobotomy. Such a judgment must be tempered, however, by the consideration that most of science is in fact a giant gamble, a point that has been discussed here and elsewhere. Sometimes the experiment works, and sometimes not. With benefit of hindsight, the future winners and losers stand out in high contrast. Participants at the time, however, have no such basis to guide them in distinguishing potentially useful avenues of research from worthless ones. This line of argument already arose in an earlier chapter, in the account of why Fulton and Freeman originally decided to invest their professional energies and reputation in Moniz's bold suggestion. The two had been at this fork in the road before. The same lessons still applied. One might expect that their initial investment in the procedure should have made them leery of a second round. In practice, the exact opposite tends to hold true, as the participants have convinced themselves that hard experience has granted them special insights into the situation.

Sadly for Fulton's and Freeman's eventual reputation (and for all those patients on whom an operation was tried and failed, as well as for all those potential patients for whom a truly improved operation might have yielded relief), the scientific groundwork for the widespread use of lobotomy never did emerge. This is not to say that positive or long-lasting influences upon scientific knowledge could not emerge from the search for operative precision. As demonstrated earlier, for example, our modern theory of limbic function owes more to its legacy from psychosurgical research than is generally explained in current medical textbooks. Clearly, the belief that something of immense social value was at stake within the inner convolutions of the brain proved a significant stimulus for productive neurophysiological research.

There is another kind of hubris, though, which I would like to explore, that refers not to the intellectual underpinnings of Fulton's and Freeman's missions but to the professional issues embedded in their separate campaigns, especially in regard to the issue of how new knowledge in science affects medical practice. Fulton's campaign proceeded, not only on the assumptions of Sherringtonian neurophysiology, but also on the basis of a particular model of how medical science itself functions. As mentioned earlier, Fulton believed in a trickle-down model of scientific medicine, in which the field clinician patiently awaits for laboratory-based technologies to be certified by academic scientists; and should the academic scientist publicize an update as to a therapy's true medical value, the clinician at once follows suit as instructed. Freeman, for his part, lived within the parameters of the laissez-faire model of private-practice medicine in America, in which every physician was his own king, beholden to no one in the choice of therapeutics – not even to the AMA. Science offered additional choices, but it was clinical wisdom that remained in control. Both men, however, ignored the changing parameters of contemporary reality and in time saw their visions collapse.

That the enterprise of psychosurgery had grown into such a huge industry was in itself proof that clinicians in the field were untethered to the proscriptions of scientists cloistered in academe. Fulton in the early years clearly had been naive in assuming that he could vigorously promote psychosurgery and yet pay little attention to the matter of whether the clinical trials would adhere to rigorous guidelines. Its subsequent migration into mental hospitals should not have come as a surprise, either. He set the stage, and turned away. Equally simplistic was his later assumption that the torrent might be reversed simply with the ex cathedra announcement of the academic scientists that the procedure was not yet validated and should be decelerated. This did little to address the true factors propelling the operation's diffusion into hospital practice. Moreover, relying upon each clinician to follow his or her own conscience as a means of insuring compliance within the profession was quaintly honorable, but ineffective.

In several respects the laboratory was indeed colonizing the world. As many an imperial leader has discovered, however, simply legislating orders and goals is a world removed from having them put into effect once one is away from the center of power. Regardless of how substandard the practices of the clinicians were, their services were irreplaceable. And, as a practical matter, the rapid increase in the number of possible new treatments to examine stretched beyond what the limited resources of the academic laboratories could supervise, even if researchers were so motivated. The evaluation of any new therapy, therefore, even one explicitly labeled "experimental," was necessarily going to end up in the hands of a small band of physicians distributed around the nation, filing individual case reports.[113]

Many of Freeman's later difficulties, too, would stem from a naive misreading of how science affects medical practice, though his oversight was of a different kind. The challenge posed by lobotomy was, for Fulton the research scientist, truly "academic," an occasion to push back the limits of known neurophysiology as it applied to human psychopathology. His identity as a research scientist, and his commitment to certain fundamental intellectual paradigms, were essentially unchanged by the later plunge in psychosurgery's popularity – though perhaps his stellar rating as a visionary scientist has since been downgraded. In this regard, Freeman and Fulton were fellow travelers, as the two shared the belief that physiology was the master science of all human experience. Freeman's workaday world was additionally that of a clinician, however, and his own fatal blunder was to assume that the structure of the private-practice neuropsychiatrist would hold constant in the face of science's relentless advance. New therapies would replace old ones, he thought, but the rules of the game would stay fundamentally the same. The challenge posed by psychosurgery within the clinical domain was far more dramatic than that in the research arena, however, where its effect was limited to focusing attention on problems that were ripe for future investigation. In contrast, the need to evaluate the exact *clinical* utility of lobotomy brought to the

# The Politics of Precision

361

surface long-simmering disagreements within the psychiatric profession
as to what were the proper criteria for judging any and all therapeutic
efforts. This already contentious issue arose at the very moment when the
profession was also forced to address the issue of whether psychiatric
practice ought to be regulated.

The new era of scientific medicine plunged the profession further into
crisis and the resultant state of affairs was no longer as supportive of
Freeman and other physician-kings. Neither Freeman nor Fulton had
foreseen that the standard of what constitutes valid medical knowledge
was itself undergoing a dramatic evolution. Nor did they anticipate that
the particular scientific model of human behavior within which both labored would be seriously challenged by competing models that also laid
claim to the problem of mental disorder. It should be remembered that the
professional locations of Fulton and Freeman, respectively that of physiologist and neurologist, lay outside the central realm of psychiatry, and
that their arrival on the mental health scene had been by invitation – an
invitation that was historically contingent and hence revocable. The ultimate fate of psychosurgery thus became intimately bound up in the erupting warfare among psychiatrists, a story that returns to psychiatry itself.

# 8

## Medicine Controlled
### Psychiatry's Evolution as a Science and a Profession

"The decision for or against prefrontal lobotomy," declared Lothar Kalinowsky and John Scarff in 1948, "is a difficult one and more serious than any other decision psychiatrists are called upon to make."[1] To predict whether or not the procedure would lead to a beneficial result in a particular candidate was a vexing problem, one that severely strained the art of clinical decision making. A physician's stance on the efficacy of the brain operations reflected a great deal more than was suggested by the circumstances of an individual case, however; it also touched upon the inner core of a psychiatrist's belief as to what were the most effective means of altering the mental or behavioral structure of patients, a question of treatment philosophy or orientation. Indeed, the decision to support or denounce the use of psychosurgery became an exercise in self-identification, an occasion for physicians to define what *kind* of psychiatrists they were.

Psychiatry, as previously described, had never been a truly unified system of practice. It remained, rather, a loose confederation of very different kinds of clinical orientations and occupational locations. And, in the post–World War II years, this most heterogeneous of medical specialties became even more fractious and unruly. Whatever bonds that did exist to hold this group together were severely strained. Thus, arising at a historical moment of intense politicization, the psychosurgery question was parlayed by both advocates and critics into a referendum on what should be the future shape and substance of American psychiatry.

Indeed, as the disjuncture grew between psychosurgery's dual image as a bona fide therapeutic breakthrough and a triumph of laboratory science, and the disquieting reality of the technique's often unpleasant results and its persistent opacity to physiological scrutiny, the current state of affairs became increasingly untenable for its foes as well as its friends. Vocal supporters of lobotomy increasingly were held accountable for the procedure's conspicuous failures, yet they lacked a stable base of scientific knowledge that might adequately address the situation. *Let the results testify for themselves* was the usual response, a mixture of bravado and defensiveness. Any individual case of operative failure was attributed to conservatism on the part of the responsible physicians; "too little too late" has been the favorite such explanation for centuries. Detractors, for their part, were chagrined by their own inability to explain away the equally conspicuous examples of the procedure's success. In either case, the source of the unease lay deeper, indicating a more structural issue facing contemporary psychiatry and medicine.

## Psychiatry at the Crossroads

Following World War II, psychiatry as a profession entered uncharted territory. In 1946, then APA president Sam Hamilton poignantly titled his farewell address "Our Association in a Time of Unsettlement." Other psychiatric leaders shared the perception that the profession was at a "crossroads." In the previous decade, APA membership had doubled in size and dramatically changed in composition. Even as late as 1940, as many as two-thirds or more of the association were employed in institutions. A 1948 survey, however, revealed a dramatic shift: state hospital psychiatrists comprised a surprisingly low 17 percent. The change was due not to a precipitous decline in the numbers employed by the state hospitals, a level which held relatively constant, but to the expansion in opportunities for office-based practice and for various governmental or industrial posts.[2]

The erosion of the APA's traditional base in the institutions, resulting from this influx of new and different kinds of mental health care workers, in turn set in motion a powerful dynamic for change that would eventually transform every aspect of psychiatry. In the old order, a slow-moving if not stolid world of civil service rules and hospital bureaucracies, a minimal level of harmony was enforced within the profession, even among those holding to different treatment philosophies. Enemies from without – enterprising neurologists, muck-raking journalists, predatory politicians – posed more immediate dangers than what were viewed as intrafamilial, private spats. In any event, the tight congruence between the realities of state hospital practice and the boundaries of American psychiatry led inevitably to a certain homogeneity in the definition of what constituted mental illness and its proper treatment. In the new order, however, all the old arrangements and implicit understandings were no longer operative. Coming under pressure for renegotiation were such fundamental issues as the placement of the line that separated normal from pathological, the agreement about what were plausible causes of insanity, the range of acceptable modes of treatment, and even the conception of what the psychiatrist's proper role in society as a knowledgeable and responsible expert was – these elements represented the very bedrock of the profession. An unstable, turbulent period of transition ensued in which a diverse mix of constituencies battled for the right to set psychiatry's agenda.

The structure and function of the association itself became a prime target of concern, as it represented the logical starting point for any serious attempts at professional reform. Whoever controlled the APA was likely to set the course for decades to come, once the infighting abated. No matter who prevailed, however, the immediate business at hand for the association was to put its professional house in order. If psychiatry were to command the respect and legitimacy one might expect of a major medical specialty, it was clear to all that its corporate body, at the minimum, would have to assume responsibility for vigorously defending its borders from nearby specialties and for establishing some means of disciplining wayward members. The impetus to assume such tasks was not limited to internal forces but would also arise from the external realities imposed by the sudden entrance of the federal government into the mental health care domain.

The need to define and enforce standards of practice – the primary responsibility of any mature profession – in turn brought into play another destabilizing dynamic. APA leaders set out to fulfill these tasks by importing contemporary standards of medical validation, which recently had undergone their own transformation, with scientific verification now being favored over clinical judgment. In so doing, psychiatrists discovered the harsh fact that their own methodology needed a drastic overhaul. Indeed, the closer the psychiatric leadership examined any particular matter before them, the worse the situation appeared. Attempts to banish even the most flagrant charlatans dangerously backfired; demands fell alike upon heterodox and unorthodox practitioners – and doubly so upon each of the various warring factions – to validate their therapies in "controlled" experiments that might separate real effects from spurious ones. Although the application of scientific standards to psychiatric investigation proved no easy task, psychiatrists were left few options. Should the profession fail to reach a consensus on how to evaluate psychiatric treatments scientifically or how to conduct a bona fide psychiatric experiment, no single faction could claim superior validity – and thus all would become equally suspect. Psychiatry's development as a profession became dependent upon its further coevolution as a creditable science.

It was only natural that psychosurgery – the most fiercely debated and closely scrutinized psychiatric treatment of the time – would become a focal point for developments along both fronts, political as well as methodological. On one front, lobotomy's conspicuous image as the boldest form of somatic intervention meant that its fate was inevitably linked to the coming showdown between the psychoanalysts and their physiologically oriented rivals. (Walter Freeman, for example, was a walking lightning rod for such disputes.) The debates over the appropriate use of psychosurgery also became a convenient proxy for fights along other political axes that polarized the profession. Such battles were not limited to disputes about particular therapies, but were also about competing visions of what constituted modern psychiatry. On the other front, the fact that psychosurgery was considered by psychiatrists to be the first tool in their therapeutic armamentarium capable of causing grave, irreversible damage entailed that its use would be subject to an unprecedented level of scrutiny. (The opening comment of Kalinowsky and Scarff was in large measure motivated by precisely this concern.) Something was finally at stake for the average psychiatrist in knowing whether or not a particular psychiatric therapy *really* worked, with evidence that could be defended to the general medical community as well as to the public. "Well, there's no harm in trying this out, and then that" simply would not do anymore.

The matter of evaluating psychosurgery's effects thus became a paramount concern for the profession to an extent that surpassed any other mode of treatment in this period. Forced to reevaluate such matters as how they measured personality changes, judged therapeutic success, and designed experiments, psychiatrists discovered along the way that conclusive answers to the difficult issues posed by lobotomy would require advances in every aspect of psychiatric investigation. The problem of psychosurgery developed into an exploration of the future meaning of psychiatry as a *scientifically* based medical specialty, and thus motivated the evolution of the profession's research methodology in unanticipated ways.

As the history of psychosurgery illustrates, a medical specialty's professional history often intertwines with its scientific development. In the current example, the need to present an image of political cohesiveness merged with an equally compelling need to construct a coherent methodology. Issues of professional control and experimental control converged.

### A House Divided

By the 1940s, the accord among psychiatrists that had existed, if only on the surface, began to break down into factional strife. The vision of Adolf Meyer, Thomas Salmon, and Alan Gregg of an all-encompassing profession that would unite such diverse worlds and worldviews as those of the state hospitals and urban clinics, physician and social worker, bacteriologists and psychotherapists, was unraveling from within. Some gains had been achieved, especially in convincing individual states to upgrade their mental health care systems through packages of civil service reform; in selling the public, through comprehensive education campaigns, on the need for closer attention to the problem of mental health; and in bringing the isolated world of mental health into the fold of general medicine, through new bridges to university medical schools and general hospitals. The problem of mental illness was no longer strictly separated into nervous ailments, meliorated by family physician or neurologist, and insanity, managed by asylum superintendents. A basis had been forged, in both the public's expectations and the medical student's training, for a single type of medical professional to deal with all of life's problems, from the minor to the severe. *Psychiatry* was launched. What type of psychiatrist would prevail, however, became the next bone of contention.

The arrival of the émigré psychiatrists fleeing from Nazi oppression in the 1930s injected new vitality into the American psychoanalytic community. Previously, basic precepts of the Freudian canon had already been incorporated into the reigning psychiatric paradigm, but in a neutered and simplistic form: the Americans had been rather selective in their interpretation of Freud's work, borrowing only that which fit within the native framework of eclectic psychobiology. The European analysts, on the other hand, were not content with subordinating psychoanalysis, but set their sights on establishing Freudian analysis as the master discipline in the United States.[3] Even among those psychiatrists who espoused the psychodynamic model of psychiatry, such as Edward Strecker, the advent of a new class of high priests on the scene did not sit well, and open opposition flared. The reaction to these developments was even more severe within the large camp of psychiatrists who placed little trust in anything but a straight physiological understanding of mental illness.

The fault lines stratifying the profession were growing increasingly strained, and the subject of psychosurgery became one of the more visible areas in which tensions between the camps periodically erupted. Even at the very outset of work in the late 1930s, for example, Walter Freeman received his harshest criticism at the hands of psychoanalysts such as A. A. Brill and S. E. Jelliffe. To the analysts, lobotomy was yet one more throwback to the predynamic era, a time when spurious models of nerve function had led psychiatrists to apply worthless somatic treatments and to ignore the importance of faulty interpersonal relations in mental illness. What made psychosurgery especially damned, from their perspective, was the inability of the lobotomized patient to introspect constructively; the road to therapeutic insight was thus irrevocably destroyed. For example, H. S. Sullivan in 1940 was enraged by the lobotomists' assumption that it was better to be a "contented imbecile" than a schizophrenic. As another example, David Rioch, an analyst on staff at Chestnut Lodge (an elite Freudian enclave), publicly derided lobotomy in 1947 as nothing more than a form of "partial euthanasia." Those on the receiving end of such attacks gave them little notice, dismissing their critics as too far removed from the concerns of the mental hospitals. Indeed, the bitter tone of the psychoanalysts' complaints suggests their impotence to affect this issue.[4]

It is important to note that such polarization between the two camps was by no means a necessary event; there was nothing inherent in either the somaticists' position or the analysts' that precluded collaboration. One of the central tenets of Meyer's platform of psychobiology, in fact, was precisely the integration of such disparate theoretical orientations. As mentioned earlier, centers of Meyerian psychiatry such as the Institute of the Pennsylvania Hospital and McLean Hospital proudly advertised that analytic work went hand in hand with the somatic therapies. Moreover, the psychodynamic model of human behavior ruled psychiatry almost by default, as the somaticists had yet to field a conceptual schema of equal richness. Ironically, even the most physiological accounts of human behavior would at some point fall back upon Freudian terms and concepts to get their point across. Thus, when Walter Freeman explained the mode of action of lobotomy, he praised its success in "whittling down the superego" – no doubt one of the more egregious mixed metaphors in medical history.[5]

Meyer's platform for the profession's future was built upon certain assumptions concerning how workers in the disparate sites were to be integrated into a confederated whole. However, with the dramatic shift away from the profession's traditional base in the asylums – a trend that Meyer and his followers stimulated and which gained momentum following World War II – larger forces were set into motion that eventually undermined the confederation.

## Ten Minutes That Shook the Psychiatric World

In May 1948, the APA embarked upon its second century of annual meetings on an inauspicious note, as a political confrontation erupted during its usually low-key presidential elections. C. C. Burlingame, flamboyant director of the Institute of Living, an elite private mental institution in Hartford, Connecticut, was the lone candidate slated by the Committee on Nominations and was expected to win the presidency without incident. Burlingame's candidacy did not go unchallenged, however. Dexter Bullard, a prominent figure in the psychoanalytic community, rose from the floor to nominate George Stevenson, director of the NCMH. Bullard provocatively contrasted the choices offered to the membership. There was his candidate, "who has long been associated with the preventative aspects of our work," and then there was the original nominee, "whose current views frequently lean toward psychosurgery." Karl Bowman, a recent president of the APA, stood up to defend Burlingame, outraged by the "highly improper" nature of Bullard's remarks. Unfortunately for Burlingame, the deck had already been stacked against him when at the last minute the meeting's location had been changed to Washington, D.C., Bullard's home city. With only 792 members voting – less than 20 percent of the total membership – Stevenson narrowly defeated Burlingame. Burlingame's unprecedented defeat brought to a head political undercurrents that had been mounting for several years. Later, Bullard would describe this event as "ten minutes that shook the psychiatric world."[6]

The attack by Bullard was a combination of happenstance and hidden agendas. He had received, not long before, Burlingame's latest *Annual Report* from the Institute of Living, which described the institute's erection of the world's first operating suite dedicated to psychosurgery. Bullard, no friend of Freeman's, had regarded lobotomy as akin to a criminal act ever since Freeman described to him the results of an operation on a fourteen-year-old. Convinced that Burlingame's election would spell disaster for the profession, Bullard grew sufficiently outraged to perform the one overt political act of his career. He was not speaking for himself alone, however. He had been cajoled and flattered into performing an act that others desired but dared not carry out personally. Members of a psychiatric "action group" had in fact pressured Bullard into making the nomination, hoping to elect a president sympathetic to their cause while at the same time avoiding the unpleasant political consequences that might ensue if the deed were somehow directly linked to them. Bullard was a willing pawn.[7]

The conspiracy to derail Burlingame's election was orchestrated from Topeka, Kansas, home of the famous psychiatric brothers William and Karl Menninger. The pair had inherited a sleepy, family-run sanitarium and had transformed it into America's largest psychiatric training institute in the postwar era, an institution whose influence on the future course of the mental health care system is hard to overestimate. Serving as Brigadier General of Army Psychiatry during the war, "Dr. Will" had positioned himself as the country's most powerful psychiatrist, with an unmatched network of professional connections and governmental influence. "Dr.

Karl," through his writings for the lay audience and media appearances, achieved prominence as the nation's best-known and trusted mental health authority. The two would prove adept at capitalizing upon the lessons and opportunities provided by the war, not least of which was the future importance of governmental funding for the reorganization of traditional patterns of medical care and education, and the ability of centralized authority to transform organizational blueprints into action. At a local level, through adroit political maneuverings and well-managed community liaisons, they succeeded in commingling the resources of the nearby Topeka State Hospital and the Winter VA Hospital with their own facility. Looking to the APA, they saw in it the possibility of extending their hegemony nationwide.

The attraction of the Menninger school was its uniquely American blend of eclectic, often contrasting, values. The family's evangelistic, strict puritanical upbringing had instilled in its sons a lifelong zeal to do the Lord's missionary work; at the same time, however, the boys had acquired a parallel thirst to achieve social prominence through commercial savvy. Dependent upon immediate family ties and culture as the central organizing principle in their life and work, the Menningers nonetheless made the transition from managing a family business to overseeing a large corporate enterprise and directing complex bureaucratic systems. Projecting an image of folksy, rural American wisdom, the Menninger tradition at the same time also placed great stock in cosmopolitan, European-based education. In its psychiatric orientation, the Menninger school relied upon the American legacy of pragmatic eclecticism. Looking to the psychoanalysts to provide new tools of psychiatric intervention and theory, the Menningers felt no need to hold to strict analytic dogma, rejecting whatever they felt uncomfortable with, such as the emphasis on sexuality. And if a somatic tool like electric shock or lobotomy seemed especially applicable to a particular patient, they used it. The Menninger model was thus well suited for a nation that was entering into the postwar era, as it was both forward-looking in its deference to technocratic expertise yet comfortably grounded in an idealized pastoral past of town meetings and neighborly interactions. The brothers Menninger peered into the nation's future and saw themselves.[8]

The first direct efforts of the Menningers to reshape the profession began in 1945 when Karl, as chairman of the APA Committee on Reorganization, drafted a revised constitution. The need for some kind of comprehensive change was evident. Even though association membership amounted to more than four thousand, there still existed no permanent facility, and no salaried officers. Up to this time the APA was little more than a facade, a federation of halfhearted committees that revolved around a yearly set of meetings and the sponsorship of a single journal – a level of activity insufficient for the needs of a large medical specialty. Will's own involvement in reform activities also began at war's end, when he deplored the lack of training opportunities for the increasing numbers of young physicians who had hoped to pursue a career in psychiatry; he attributed the problem to APA inaction. Others, concerned about psychoanalysis's postwar status, wrote to Will Menninger suggesting the need for a "young Turks" movement that might galvanize the association. Influential figures, such as Frank Fremont-Smith of the Josiah Macy, Jr., Foundation (a major medical philanthropy), encouraged him to convert this recently gained political strength into concrete action. Dr. Will was a natural choice to lead any such reform efforts, as his stature was already sufficient to ensure his rapid ascension to the presidencies of the American Psychoanalytic Association as well as the APA – the first individual to hold both offices simultaneously.[9]

At the 1946 APA meeting in Chicago, William Menninger informally broached the idea of a reform-oriented group to a handpicked few, who soon formed The Group for the Advancement of Psychiatry, or GAP. Envisioned as a collection of "action" committees, GAP grew over the next few years to seventeen committees drawn from one hundred and fifty members. Many of GAP's committees, such as its Committee on Therapy and the Committee on Research, had direct counterparts in the APA. GAP also formed such innovations as the Committee on Social Issues and the Committee on International Relations. In Will's own words, GAP was to be a "mobile striking force for American psychiatry," flexible where the association was rigid, outspoken where the association remained silent. Journalist Albert Deutsch, who frequently addressed mental health developments, closely followed GAP's ascendancy. His favorable reports in the press described how a group of young, dedicated psychiatrists, who shared a common military background and an enthusiasm for the new "dynamic" psychiatry of Freudian psychotherapy, had come together to do what the APA would not: that is, work for the field's immediate progress. The old guard, in contrast, were presented as a conservative if not reactionary elite who had risen through the bureaucratic ranks of the state hospital system, who were generally preoccupied with somatic therapies to the exclusion of psychotherapy, and who were suspicious of public exposure.[10]

With considerable deftness, Chairman Menninger quickly established GAP as a dominant political force in American psychiatry. Within two years, its representatives held most of the top APA executive positions, starting with Menninger himself as president, Howard Potter as treasurer, and Leo Bartemeier as secretary. Menninger and his allies comprised the entire Executive Committee, and beyond that they filled the new post of medical director, two-thirds of thirty-one committee chairmanships, and the majority of the seats on the organization's council. GAP's influence was not limited to the APA. In 1948, Menninger reported to the Commonwealth Fund (which had underwritten the majority of GAP's costs) on his success in placing many chief psychiatric advisors throughout important government and military agencies.[11]

Some APA members ruefully observed that activist groups often spawn opposition groups. As it happened, resistance to the Menningers' goals for the APA arose as soon as details of Karl's proposed constitution leaked out. Some of the old guard, including Clarence Cheney (APA president 1935–6), James May (APA president 1932–3), and C. C. Burlingame, who were staunch supporters of institutional psychiatry, reacted strongly against key provisions of the plan. In their minds, the lack of a mail ballot was undemocratic, as it limited voting to those who could afford to attend meetings; the proposed creation of a delegate system was a blatant effort to gerrymander political power for a proposed "Topeka District"; and, worst of all, the appointment of a medical director would allow enforcement of a minority clinical viewpoint – most likely psychoanalysis – through executive fiat. "Just as sure as God made little fishes," Burlingame wrote to Winfred Overholser in the spring of 1945, "a schism and fights are being started in the APA, which is an awful high price to be paid for doubtful progress." Burlingame was skeptical of assurances by Bowman, then association president, that the analysts were not attempting a takeover through the reorganization plan.[12]

GAP's subsequent debut and initial efforts confirmed opposition fears. The success of GAP candidates in the 1947 APA elections at first elicited a lighthearted but sarcastic response, as old guard representatives such as C. B. Farrar (editor of the APA's *American Journal of Psychiatry*), Samuel Hamilton (previous APA president), and Winfred Overholser (outgoing president) proclaimed themselves the "Group of Unknowns in Psychiatry," or GUPpies. Burlingame bemusedly played along with the rest of the "little fishes." Visible resistance broke out, however, upon GAP's release of its first official publication, a report prepared by its Committee on Therapy that sought to discredit and limit the use of shock therapy. The report began with an indictment of "promiscuous and indiscriminate use of electro-shock therapy." Casting doubts upon the treatment's actual therapeutic value, the statement went on to proscribe its use in private practice. Comments such as "overemphasis and unjustified use of electro-shock therapy short-circuits the training and experience which is essential in modern dynamic psychiatry" left no doubt as to the committee's own therapeutic orientation. Defenders of electroshock therapy responded in public and private tirades against what they considered ill-advised "pontification" by analysts who had little if any experience with the realities of institutional psychiatry. The initial publication of GAP's Committee on Research, a report on psychosurgery, similarly portrayed somatically oriented psychiatrists as irresponsible at worst, outdated at best. Circulated in February 1948, it stated that lobotomy "represents a mechanistic attitude toward psychiatry which is a throwback to our pre-psychodynamic days."[13]

Although Will Menninger carefully specified that GAP pronouncements were not to be interpreted as official APA policy statements, and that his official APA work was not an expression of GAP sentiments, such neat distinctions were ignored by GAP's opponents, who resented what seemed to be a takeover of the profession by a self-appointed elite under Menninger's direction. The opposition's worries were justified. Many prominent GAP members, such as those on its Committees on Therapy and Research, were also members of the APA counterpart. Over time, the APA committee meetings degenerated into rehashes of work that had transpired at GAP, and distinctions between the rosters of the two organizations grew increasingly faint. It is understandable that the old guard was concerned the public might mistake GAP statements as representing the entire profession.

The choice of Menninger's successor to the APA presidency, to be decided at the May 1948 meeting, became a test of wills between the two camps. The old guard closed ranks behind Burlingame, sure of his dedication to "uphold the traditions of the Association," and to be a "forceful president" able to rebuff "a minority group . . . that is trying to tell everyone else what to do and how to live." Although Burlingame was officially chosen by the APA Committee on Nominations, his selection originated during a meeting of the Vidonian Club. Described by its members as "an illustrious gang of good fellows," this elite drinking and dining society of psychiatrists and neurologists, limited to twenty members, met a half-dozen times a year in Manhattan's fine restaurants. A. A. Brill, in his introductory remarks on the occasion of Samuel Hamilton's outgoing Presidential Address, described how he and Hamilton had been founding members of this club back in 1914. In the past generation, Brill boasted, Vidonians had filled seven APA presidencies, including those of Overholser, Bowman, Cheney, and Chapman. At their October 1947 gathering, after some discussion of GAP's failings, a resolution was passed that Burlingame – one of Vidonia's most lively participants – should be nominated. By January 1948, the APA Committee on Nominations had been sufficiently electioneered by the Vidonians to submit Burlingame's name without opposition to the APA membership.[14]

Menninger, kept apprised by his informants of all significant political developments within the profession, interpreted the campaign to nominate Burlingame as the handiwork of those who had been incensed by the GAP shock therapy report, a message that the "group of young upstarts known as GAP" should not be allowed to take over the association. In response, Menninger mobilized the GAP committee chairmen as soon as the nominations were officially released to elicit suggestions for ways of stopping the considerable momentum behind Burlingame's election.[15] Any counternomination would have to come from outside GAP; Bullard was identified as a sympathetic figure of sufficient prominence to carry out the deed.

### Backlash

Bullard's ambush of Burlingame inspired his defenders to open rebellion. After the dust settled at the convention, the anti-GAP faction met in Overholser's hotel room to plan a counterattack. That the political pendulum would at some point swing in favor of the analysts was admitted by those present as an inevitable development of history. Even so, they felt, the APA must not become "a tool for the promulgation of psychoanalytic principles alone." Proposals were fielded for an opposition group, perhaps called the "Friends of Psychiatric Democracy," that might herald a return to a "middle of the road position" where advocates of any treatment program, "pure psychoanalysis at one end of the scale, psychosurgery at the other, and all the various modifications in between," would receive the proper dignity and recognition worthy of any scientific endeavor.[16]

After this initial strategy meeting, reaction to Burlingame's defeat continued to ferment, leading to an emergency session of the Vidonian Club. Several members expressed feelings that GAP had proven a "dangerous, undemocratic" movement. Those present, recorded Secretary Robert McGraw, deplored how Vidonian Burley was underhandedly defeated in a small ballot, thus spiting the efforts of the Committee on Nominations that had "gone to great pains to find out the sense of the Association membership" before acting. All indications, the Vidonians worried, pointed toward the APA fracturing along the lines of psychoanalysis as opposed to shock treatment or lobotomy. Burlingame recorded his own fears that a secessionist movement was at hand.[17]

Calls for organized opposition eventually resulted in the formation of the Committee for the Preservation of Medical Standards in Psychiatry

(CPMSP), or "Preserves," led by McGraw. The battle commenced in January 1949, when the Preserves circulated the first of a series of inflammatory newsletters that delineated in hyperbolic and somewhat distorted form the questionable aspects of Menninger's reform campaign. A typical page illustrated the APA administrative chart for the past few years, with smiling GAP faces soon reducing frowning non-GAP faces to "extinction." Preserves appealed to the "rank and file" of the APA membership who, in their estimation, faced certain demotion to the status of a disenfranchised underclass unless the Menninger-backed elite was blocked. The Preserves were especially suspicious of what was hidden from view, such as GAP's influence on appointments to psychiatric posts in university medical schools and its guidance of the new federal grants in mental health. CPMSP's basic demands were for the repudiation of the current reorganization plan and the resignation of all GAP members currently holding APA posts. The opposition group was to self-terminate when GAP dissolved.[18]

The root of the Preserves' fears was a belief that the APA, as controlled by GAP, would turn away from efforts to establish psychiatry as a discipline able to command respect as a scientific medical specialty. Recent hard-fought gains in this regard would thus be abandoned. For example, opposition members observed that the "Scientific Forum," the constellation of proposed APA committees in the Menninger reorganization plan, conspicuously failed to include provision for sponsorship of biologically based psychiatric research. GAP's initial reports on therapy and research, attacking electroshock and lobotomy, undermined what Preserves considered to be their armamentarium's most visibly medical tools.

Also, the campaign against Burlingame was interpreted as more than just a provocative character assassination; it was an indication of a widening gulf between psychiatric philosophies. In the first CPMSP newsletter, the psychiatrist who nominated Burlingame's rival was derided as someone who "publicly announced that the election of his candidate would frustrate people who are interested in medical research, particularly the further studies of lobotomy operations and shock therapies." The editor wondered, "is this further evidence of a trend away from medicine?" By the fourth newsletter, Preserves had grown even more bitter over Burlingame's defeat and what it signified. "Should the APA endorse the viewpoint that we are opposed to medical or surgical treatments for psychiatric purposes?" It continued, "Should we penalize our members because they are also physicians?"[19]

If Will Menninger was the ideal leader for the young, assertive, dynamically oriented psychiatrists, then Burlingame was an equally appropriate representative for those who espoused a traditional conception of psychiatric progress, seeing psychiatry's future instead in stronger ties to general medicine. Appointed as director of the moribund Hartford Retreat in 1931, which a century earlier had been one of the most prestigious asylums in the young nation, Burlingame soon launched a "Neuropsychiatric Institute and Hospital," styling the one-time retreat into the new "Institute of Living." Within a decade, the institute regained its status as one of America's foremost private mental facilities.[20]

Burlingame's plan was to fulfill simultaneously the needs of fine living and medical science. First, the institute was to be more an exclusive country club than a hospital, a self-described "campus" of charming cottages that sprawled across a wooded estate, where "guests" – not patients – applied themselves to sculpture, drama, individual music lessons, and perhaps a daily swim in the outdoor terraced pool. At day's end residents gathered for elegantly appointed meals. At the same time, Burlingame's intention had been to construct state-of-the-art facilities for medical research and treatment, convinced that "the complete intellectual unification of psychiatry with all the other branches of medicine must be our goal if we are to be in the vanguard of progress." Psychiatry, he felt, could no longer exist independently of the other medical specialties. Burlingame's early introduction of psychosurgery at the institute in 1939 and the construction of specialized psychosurgical facilities in the late 1940s were thus logical extensions of his goal to offer the latest medical treatments and research opportunities. The 1948 *Annual Report,* which so incensed Bullard with its description of the institute's lobotomy program, also proclaimed that psychiatry's destiny, "beyond any shadow of a doubt, must be cast with medicine."[21]

From Burlingame's perspective, the two goals were complementary. The institute's therapeutic philosophy was thus one part "sound physical medicine" added to one part "re-education therapy," a place which taught the "art of successful living."[22] Living right and good medicine, in this worldview, were melded into a single seductive vision. To Burlingame, here was a habitat that offered residents safe harbor from the world and yet at the same time was infused with the latest scientific knowledge. In short, Burlingame had the rare opportunity to bring into reality the treasured ideal of every state hospital superintendent.

Although based within an elite asylum setting and tending to a separate bluestocking private practice in Manhattan, Burlingame maintained close contact with his fellow administrators in state hospitals, becoming an important advocate of institutional reform in Connecticut. Indeed, his speeches on the need to revitalize the public's interest in mental health, in order to increase legislative appropriations, were syndicated in newspapers nationwide. At the time of his nomination, Burlingame was regarded as a national spokesman for institutional psychiatry. That a director of an elite private hospital was selected as a leader of state hospital psychiatry was not a contradiction, but followed a pattern first set by Thomas Kirkbride, whose exclusive Pennsylvania Hospital for the Insane provided a model for the construction and operation of state mental hospitals in mid-nineteenth-century America.[23] Burlingame was only the latest example of a long tradition of symbiotic support between the leaders of private and public asylums.

Burlingame had also established himself as a prominent advocate of psychiatry's continued medicalization. As chairman of the APA Committee on Public Education, he was prevailed upon to defend psychiatry's status as a medical specialty not only to the lay public but to the general medical community as well. For example, a 1947 speech published in the *Journal of the American Medical Association,* "Psychiatric Sense and Nonsense," drew praise from physicians across the country. Burlingame lamented the recent overselling of psychiatric cures and in particular castigated the endless discussions of psychotherapy that, in his opinion, served only to conflate psychiatry with the occult or metaphysics. The emphasis of psychoanalysis on deep-rooted sexual drives and unconscious primal fantasies, he declared, was so much "bunk," neither medical at root nor particularly effective in training patients to reenter society. Echoing the American penchant for self-help and reeducation, he reinterpreted valid psychotherapy as constituting no more than "personal tutoring" – a tradition that had dominated psychiatry in the United States since the time of Austen Fox Riggs. Although he admitted that somatic methods, such as psychosurgery and shock therapy, must be used in moderation, their value nevertheless was something only a "stupid person would decry." Elsewhere, Burlingame advocated that every opportunity must be utilized "to consolidate our professional interests with the other branches of medicine."[24] In Burlingame, opponents of GAP had found a strong champion for their traditional conceptions of medical psychiatry.

For several years, conflicts among the various camps erupted in psychiatric journals, society meetings public and secret, and heated private correspondence. GAPs traded blows with Preserves, analysts fought shock therapists and lobotomists, and the old guard battled the upstarts. Deutsch reported the Preserves' formation in a newspaper article titled "Revolt May Split Ranks in Psychiatry." The Preserves had gained some ground. Several important psychiatric leaders, including some sympathetic to the Menningers' reform plans, believed that GAP's continuation was not worth the price paid in APA disharmony. Daniel Blain, who had already resigned a high post in the VA in anticipation of his appointment as the first APA medical director, seriously considered withdrawing his name rather than face continued opposition. The reorganization plan became bogged down in the controversy, placing the Menningers in the awkward position of having it shelved rather than face certain defeat at the 1949 APA meeting. Similarly, Will Menninger instructed the GAP Committee on Therapy to revise its original electroshock report in accordance with its critics' wishes.[25]

Menninger was genuinely surprised by the negative response to his plans, "never dreaming" that such a high level of antagonism would be generated. His lapse of political insight was typical of the mixture of naiveté and arrogance demonstrated by GAP members who ignored the implications of their committee proclamations. Victory in APA elections had lulled reformers into believing that their opinions were in fact representative of the whole profession. Convinced of the justness of their cause, they could not have anticipated the sharp distinctions between the interests of the APA and their personal viewpoints. GAP members assumed that their opponents held regressive beliefs, not variant ones; all that was needed was further education and enlightenment. In this view, the APA had to be modernized, not reconstituted. Menninger himself maintained that GAP was an "action group," but not a political one.[26] There seemed to be little chance, however, that GAP and its opponents might easily settle their differences.

## A Crossroads

The debate was not simply personal, nor should it be reduced solely to disagreements among therapeutic camps, or a struggle between analysts and somatotherapists. As previously mentioned, for example, Will Menninger himself was not wholly opposed to somatic therapies. Indeed, at the very time when GAP was circulating its electroshock therapy report, Menninger was attempting to obtain facilities for outpatient shock treatments at his own facility; and the Menninger Clinic's own staff neurosurgeons performed lobotomies. To Menninger, the primary issue was not which therapy was employed but the practitioner's competence. Imprecision on this point, he felt, was the unfortunate error of the original electroshock report. Likewise the Preserves, who were skeptical of psychoanalysis, nonetheless were reconciled to the enduring presence of Freudians in their midst and, when pressed, would admit that psychotherapy had its uses. Rather, the "crossroads" facing the profession were the apposite choices concerning the profession's future. Coded within the debates between GAP and the old guard were real differences of opinion as to what constituted valid psychiatric practice. At stake was nothing less than the delimitation of the psychiatrist's role in society, the nature of his or her social responsibilities and powers. GAP initiatives met with such belligerent responses precisely because they threatened the foundations of traditional psychiatry.

To Preserves, the most repellent aspect of GAP's reports was not issues of language or content, which were objectionable enough, but what was implied by the manner of their preparation and release. GAP publications, they asserted, could claim neither authoritativeness nor objectivity, as prominent experts on the treatments under consideration had not been consulted. Furthermore, the status of such reports was shamefully ambiguous. Were they medical advisories? As such, their audience was unclearly defined. Were they simply the distilled opinion of a select group? If so, no such qualifications were stated. Nor were they official statements of APA policy, or even consensus judgments of the profession. No such authority had been established. Preserves feared that, in spite of the diffuse intent of the reports, certain concrete results were sure to follow. The lay public, as well as the general medical community, were ignorant of the fine distinctions among psychiatrists and would view the findings as comprehensive guidelines. Consequently, patients or their families might hesitate to give permission for certain treatments, leading to untold numbers of unnecessary hospitalizations and suicides. Confirmation of the opponents' worst fears was provided when the Los Angeles County Medical Society, on the sole basis of GAP's report, ruled that any physician who used shock treatment as an office procedure would be subject to immediate expulsion. This incident alone was sufficient to sway Karl Bowman – who all along had been a vocal critic of Preserves tactics – to demand GAP's immediate dissolution.[27]

Opponents of GAP were scandalized by its assault on the principle of clinical autonomy, what had been a doctor's most basic freedom and responsibility. Preserves thus bitterly objected to this attempt by a self-appointed group to dictate if and when a particular therapy could be used. Not to fight back would be equivalent to abandoning their jobs as physicians. In any event, Preserves argued, if the time was appropriate for professional discussion concerning a given therapy's safety or efficacy, under no circumstances was the public press an appropriate forum. Surely, they wondered aloud, GAP members were aware that their public pronouncements would elicit statements opposite in conclusion? The ensuing spectacle of open debates would lead only to an overall decline in public confidence, thus undermining every psychiatrist's effectiveness. Psychiatry's recently gained prestige as a medical specialty was nowhere near firm enough to hazard such risks.[28]

GAP members, however, were setting off on a rather different path, one based on the assumptions of dynamic psychiatry concerning the social and intrafamilial etiology of mental illness. GAP literature called for "development of criteria of social action, relevant to the promotion of individual and communal mental health." Through application of psychiatric principles to "child and adult education, social and economic factors which influence the community status of individuals and families, intergroup tensions, civil rights and personal liberty," psychiatry would be carried "out of the hospitals and clinics and into the community." One strategy for accomplishing this expansion was to create a pyramid of professions, with the few psychiatrists on top. Underneath them were the nonmedical workers such as clinical psychologists and social workers, through whom psychiatrists might extend their reach. GAP also was not unduly troubled by establishing close ties to the media, as their new conception of mental health was predicated on the psychiatrist's intervention in community and world affairs, a social role that in fact could be built only through extensive public-relations efforts. With public attention to problems of mental health at an all-time high due to psychiatry's role in the war effort, the conditions were ripe for professional action.[29]

GAP members, reminiscent of Progressive Era social activists, saw no contradiction between a psychiatrist's political role and a medical one. In their vision, society's aggregate mental health depended upon particular social policies and viewpoints. If anything, they argued that the old guard's "reactionary" or "conservative" conception of psychiatry was overly narrow and willfully aloof from such larger concerns. If progressive psychiatry could not fit into the traditional view of medicine, then the answer was not to constrain psychiatry's reach but to widen the general conception of what medicine was about and to reorganize its internal structure, if necessary. To GAP's opponents, however, such broadened concerns as world affairs, politics, and the melioration of social ills were no business of the psychiatrist. And to the extent that public perception linked them together, they feared, psychiatry as a profession would become "dislocated" from its status as a medical specialty.[30] GAP's proposed inclusion of nonmedical members in the APA, even at a lesser status, was viewed as proof that a desire for political power would ultimately undermine psychiatry's medical authority. From their perspective, democracy was a good thing within the ranks of established psychiatry, but beyond that, dangerous; GAP advocates held to the opposite position.

The profession's choice was not an easy one; there was something to be said for the arguments of both camps. GAP members contended that their actions were necessary because the APA, left to itself, would retreat into a "do-nothing policy."[31] Dynamic psychiatry, when combined with the creation of the psychiatrist as social interventionist, was their preferred route to professional revitalization. The conservative or even reactionary opposition, for their part, also sought "action," but via a different program. The old guard were convinced that the best means of professional advance lay in improving state hospitals by narrowing the chasm that still separated psychiatry and general medicine: that is, funding intramural medical research, establishing ties to medical schools, and upgrading facilities to the standards of the general hospitals.

Many within the institutional camp, in fact, adhered to the Meyerian platform of psychiatric reform that also campaigned for the extension of psychiatry into society and the active participation of the psychiatrist at the front lines of social maladjustments. The GAP position had gone one step further, however, in disengaging the future of psychiatry from its historical home in the mental hospitals. Moreover, the two frameworks had different conceptions of psychiatry's function as subset of public health. Meyerians saw the social consequences of individual maladjustments and advertised the psychiatrist's ability to readapt malfunctioning citizens. In contrast, GAP members concerned themselves with the larger issue of a maladapted social system and recommended policy changes for a more perfect society.

A workable truce between the two groups was not likely to be easily reached. GAP's efforts, for example, appeared to undermine the opposition's own platform of reform. When Lothar Kalinowsky (a prominent electroshock expert) was brought in as a consultant for the revised GAP report, he declined to sign an initial draft for fear of sabotaging state hospital psychiatrists who were then fighting "for active treatment against great odds." "It would also offer a good excuse to some state hospital superintendents," Kalinowsky further noted, "to give up the only active treatment which many of them have introduced half-heartedly, and to return to their old custodial care attitude."[32] Worse yet, there existed a more fundamental breach in the mode of professional discourse: the two camps were unable to agree even on how to disagree. The old guard relied upon a laissez-faire model of therapeutics based on tolerance of each psychiatrist's clinical choice; insulated from public exposure, professional disagreements would not undermine psychiatrists' collective authority. In contrast, GAP reform efforts, a blending of medical and social policy objectives, relied upon the consensus of committees, a strategy intolerant of dissent; once the vote was over, minority opinions were marginalized.

No neutral forum existed in which to settle the differences between their two approaches.

Once the battle started, it was unclear where or when it might end. Neither GAPs nor Preserves could marshal sufficient strength throughout the profession to force a quick resolution. Indications, however, were pointing to an eventual victory by the GAPs and their followers. Clearly, Menninger's vanguard was in close step with the larger social forces that were greatly expanding psychiatry's role in American culture and social affairs. Also of importance was the rapid penetration of Menninger alumni into the newly created academic posts at prestigious universities and medical schools, gains that set the stage for a relegitimation of psychiatry that was based on neither the laboratory nor the asylum but on the social sciences, which at that moment were reaching their political zenith. In contrast, the sun was setting on Vidonia, as meetings degenerated into a mutual admiration society preoccupied with eulogizing members who were departing at an increasing rate. The sudden death of Burlingame himself in mid-1950 dealt the final blow. "The old spirit" had left, surviving members confided to one another in 1950. "Psychiatry," they noted, "has changed a great deal in the last dozen years. It has become broader, more involved, and has had a tremendous mushroom growth. The founders were unique. They set the pace for the whole psychiatric world, were king makers and master politicians." They concluded, "We live in a different world now."[33]

On the other hand, the fading away of organized opposition did not mean that GAP would win the war. It would prevail, perhaps, but would it triumph? Menninger's troops soon discovered that achieving political success within the APA was not the same thing as actually advancing the profession. In 1951 the chairman of GAP's Committee on Therapy confidentially suggested to Menninger that its continued existence must be reviewed, insofar as every member was an analyst; so one-sided a panel held little actual authority within a profession whose methods of treatment remained diverse.[34] Also left unspecified was what the new party in power would actually accomplish for what remained the major psychiatric burden in America – namely, how to raise standards of care in the mental institutions. And although the Preserves were waning as a political force, the matter with which they were so concerned, establishing psychiatry as a respected medical specialty, did not disappear so easily. If anything, pressures were mounting for psychiatrists to demonstrate that their black bag of treatments was medically valid, proven scientifically to be safe as well as effective. As Menninger and the rest of the psychiatric leadership would soon learn, a storm was rising that would threaten all ships regardless of what flag they were flying.

### The Necessity for Validation

In 1948, Robert S. Morison prepared for his fellow directors at the Rockefeller Foundation a confidential analysis of psychiatry's status as a medical specialty. Ever since the foundation's reorganization in 1929, mental health projects had received the majority of funds expended by its Division of Medical Sciences, the largest medical grants program in America. In Morison's view, psychiatry's medical prestige had fallen to a "disappearing point" in the 1920s and 1930s but had since regained lost ground, a success built largely upon foundation funds that had been spent across a wide variety of promising areas. One of these, psychoanalysis, was credited by Morison with having convinced open-minded physicians that psychiatry, with its potential to explore the depths of human behavior, "deserves a hearing." Morison warned, however, that the general medical community's acceptance of psychiatry was merely tentative, based on an unfulfilled promise. To date, psychiatry's increased respect stemmed from the psychotherapists' virtuoso rhetorical efforts, not from advances in genuine medical knowledge. It was disconcerting to Morison, therefore, that many psychiatrists underrated the importance of scientific verification to the profession's ultimate standing. He feared that psychiatry would remain vulnerable until it presented some conclusive, scientific proof for its claims. Initially, the foundation had focused on construction of psychiatry departments in university medical schools. Perhaps now was the time, Morison suggested, to switch priorities from training to real research.[35]

Implicit in Morison's critique was a fear that foundation grants had somehow artificially distorted this field's pattern of development from what it otherwise would have been. What began as a series of well-intentioned efforts, perhaps justified by the acute shortage of psychiatrists, might have had the unintended effect of extending the profession beyond what its store of experimentally derived knowledge could rationally support. Although it was not specifically mentioned in his memorandum, Morison was no doubt also alluding to the foundation's imaginative funding of psychosomatic medicine, a school of thought that blended psychoanalysis and physiology in the name of philosophical unity. Through the foundation's conspicuous philanthropic awards, for example, psychosomatic studies did become sufficiently respectable to legitimate psychotherapy's presence in medical schools. Indeed, the first psychoanalytic program formally associated with a medical school in America was approved only because its title included the phrase "psychosomatic studies."[36]

In Morison's scenario, psychotherapists had deluded themselves into mistaking such professional inroads for true gains in medical science. GAP's committees, he scoffed, apparently believed that psychiatric authority ultimately rested upon majority votes rather than experimental findings. Morison's memorandum concluded that, at this point in psychiatry's evolution, "it is critically important to do all that we can to encourage scientific validation of modern psychiatric procedure." Morison's concerns shortly proved prophetic. For psychiatrists, professional success became a two-edged sword. Along with the increased benefits came the obligation of having to abide by the same standards as other medical specialties. Psychiatry's long heritage of hands-off eclecticism was no longer viable. The public as well as the general medical community looked to the APA to differentiate quacks from medical regulars, and to communicate which of the many available therapies met scientific criteria increasingly in vogue in other medical fields. Indeed, circumstances soon brought exactly these kinds of issues directly before the APA, and its leaders discovered just how ill prepared psychiatry was for the new scientific era.

## Boxed In

When Wilhelm Reich scandalized the profession in the late 1940s with his bizarre "orgone therapy," APA officers were embarrassed by their subsequent inability to enforce even minimal guidelines. At the 1948 meeting of the APA Executive Council, Berkeley Gordon, medical director at a New Jersey state hospital, testified that several of his staff had become converts to the new Reichian "cult." (In Reich's orgone therapy, patients were placed, nude or seminude, in a large cabinet that was ringed with aluminum and other materials alleged to focus cosmic energy.) After some deliberation, and a consensus that the association must "put a stop to all this," the council referred the matter to the Committee on Research. However, as members of this committee were unpaid volunteers, none of them was willing to expend the personal time or money necessary for a field investigation. The case was remanded to council.[37]

It fell upon William Menninger, current APA president, to find some means of adjudication. Menninger tried, unsuccessfully, to spare the APA any further trouble by transferring jurisdiction over the matter to the investigative arms of the AMA and the local medical society. It wasn't their problem, he was told. Exasperated, he contacted the original informant for suggestions about what might be done, other than stripping Reich of his APA membership. Menninger quickly backtracked on even this largely symbolic gesture, suggesting that such an action might be beyond his official powers. Even though personally convinced that Reich was a "fakir," Menninger noted that "if we are going to be scientific we ought to investigate it and I probably shouldn't be even expressing such an opinion." Menninger's predicament was real. The council would not act until the matter had been investigated, yet the association possessed no investigative apparatus. The APA was paralyzed.[38]

Gordon had inadvertently stumbled upon a central problem in American psychiatry, the lack of professional machinery appropriate to a mature medical specialty. Writing to Menninger, Gordon stated that the "ambiguous" status of Reichian therapy must be resolved. "If it has merit," he judiciously reasoned, "it should be endorsed and used more extensively for the welfare of our patients." Otherwise, "it should be definitely condemned, the matter should be brought out into the open and settled once and for all." Gordon's plea could have been just as easily stated for any of the disparate therapies then employed by psychiatrists, orthodox as well as heterodox. Previously, the association had not been expected to oversee clinical practice, or to evaluate psychiatric therapies. It came as a rude awakening to the APA that it had neither bureaucratic means of controlling professionals nor agreed-upon methods by which to measure the clinical effectiveness of a given therapy.[39]

Reich's case acutely embarrassed the APA, but the underlying problem remained chronic: replacing a system of clinical evaluation based on personal judgment with one of uniform scientific criteria. Furthermore, the need for such change was made more urgent by the dramatic entrance of the federal government as the dominant provider of research monies in the postwar years, and by its unprecedented funding of the elaborate system of VA hospitals that rapidly were built up into the nation's most advanced system of psychiatric facilities. The arrival of the federal government as a major player in mental health care had the unanticipated consequence of thrusting the APA into the unsought role of referee.

When the VA hospital authorities wanted to establish general treatment guidelines, for example, they did not leave this for each staff physician to decide personally, but looked instead to the association – and thus also to its surrogate, GAP – to set policy in questionable treatment areas. Indeed, GAP's first report, the statement on shock therapy, was produced in response to a direct request from a VA administrator. The world of the VA hospital was neither that of private practice nor that of the state institution; physicians had become answerable to a centralized *external* authority.[40]

Of special significance was the influx of federal funds for psychiatric research that had supplanted the contributions of the private philanthropies. This trend began with the 1946 National Mental Health Act that enabled the construction of the National Institute of Mental Health (NIMH), which began as the National Advisory Mental Health Council (NAMHC). Between 1947 and 1951, government expenditures for psychiatric research rose from $87,000 to $1,380,000, overshadowing the role of private foundations.[41] Competition for funds in the government arena, however, was a far different enterprise from that transacted in the closed-door deliberations of private philanthropies. Whereas the Rockefeller Foundation was free (within limits) to champion whatever projects its directors saw fit, publicly supported government agencies had to have some means of accounting for their decisions. The NAMHC turned to APA and GAP committees to provide guidelines.

Psychosurgery became a special concern of the NAMHC, which had been stymied by the task of ranking submitted applications. The large number and diversity of lobotomy proposals had been particularly distressing. In response, the NAMHC commissioned a member of GAP's Committee on Research to prepare a comprehensive survey of existing lobotomy investigations, with attention to details of experimental design. It requested the same GAP committee to provide guidelines for future lobotomy studies, which resulted in GAP *Report No. 6,* "Research on Prefrontal Lobotomy." It also converted a proposed Sub-Committee on the Evaluation of Therapy into a Sub-Committee on Lobotomy to deal with the special problems raised by psychosurgery. Unsatisfied by APA or GAP efforts, the Sub-Committee on Lobotomy suggested an unusual government-sponsored series of conferences, from which practical guidelines might emerge.[42]

The resulting federal Research Conferences on Psychosurgery met annually in New York, between 1949 and 1951, with approximately twenty-five distinguished participants at each session. (Fred Mettler, the coordinator of the New York State Brain Research Projects, presided over the meetings.) One immediate consequence of the conferences was a new appreciation of psychosurgery's importance as both a therapy and a research subject. Surveys commissioned for the conferences enumerated an unexpectedly high lobotomy count, as well as an extraordinarily diverse field of psychosurgery studies conducted throughout the empire of academic medicine. Treatment surveys conducted in this extensive detail were in themselves an innovation in American psychiatry.[43]

Of all the psychiatric treatments of the day, psychosurgery would be scrutinized to a degree far beyond that visited upon any of its alternatives.

The research conferences had become the focal point for the convergence of several powerful currents. The gravity of the procedure, as compared to the other therapies in use, demanded that a definitive answer be determined as to both its efficacy and safety; prevailing empirical standards of evaluation were revealed as insufficient to the task. In addition, as previously shown, the erupting warfare between the various psychiatric factions had catapulted the question of the brain operations into a highly charged atmosphere of intraprofessional politics. Lastly, the shift to the era of federal funding had placed the profession's corporate body in the awkward spotlight of having to set publicly accessible standards of psychiatric practice, an unwelcome responsibility it could not eschew.

Yet when psychiatrists, hospital administrators, neurosurgeons, and others scoured the medical literature for clues on how either to improve upon the use of the procedure or to resolve the heated debates, they quickly lost their scientific bearings. The startling heterogeneity of the literature was confounding. Lobotomy reports differed widely, not only as to surgical approach or site of cortical incisions, but in such important factors as the category of mental disorder treated, the patients' socioeconomic and demographic status, the criteria and length of follow-up period used in therapeutic evaluation, the quality of the mental institution, and even the degree of postoperative care. Faced with the task of discovering coherent neurophysiological or psychiatric themes in such material, a diligent investigator, if not intimidated by the literature's sheer bulk, could only be bewildered by its diversity and distressed by its variability. Counterintuitively, then, the publication of every new positive clinical report would simultaneously augment the prestige of lobotomy as a significant psychiatric therapy, and yet further cloud ongoing discussions about how the procedure worked or what type of patient was clinically appropriate. As the publications piled up, the procedure grew that much larger in importance – and yet less, not more, about it was certain.

The published proceedings of the research conferences reveal that American psychiatrists, though divided into disparate therapeutic camps, were earnestly attempting to find a common ground upon which to construct a rational policy for the use of psychosurgery. Honest intent by conferees, however, proved ineffectual in the face of methodological problems that eventually undercut any attempt to formulate a conclusive position. Every target of discussion, such as diagnosis, therapeutic evaluation, adequate controls, or prognostic indicators, faded into a confusing haze of semantics or conflicting opinions. Each session concluded with desultory comments on the vital need for further investigations before any conclusions might be proffered.

Quite unexpectedly, the conferences had stumbled upon something of consequence for the entire profession. It slowly dawned on the participants that the difficulties plaguing the lobotomy studies were equally applicable to *all* psychiatric investigations. In the final conference, Mettler proffered the sobering thought that attempts to resolve the psychosurgery problem had failed because "psychiatry has not yet advanced far enough to provide the objective data necessary." Psychiatry remained, he noted, "in an atmosphere of opinion."[44] Realization of this fact was in itself a defining moment for the profession. Through these meetings, psychiatrists became aware of the critical need to reassess their basic methodologies, to become more sophisticated in reporting research results. Mettler remarked: "It seems to me that if we have gotten nowhere else in this conference we have gotten to a place where publications, from here on in, which make any pretense for evaluating therapy, should at least be urged to present this kind of data for the sample presented."[45] Another participant noted that the precedent set by the conference was "one of the healthiest things" in psychiatry; he regretted that other areas of research did not have comparable forums.[46] Afterward, the conferences were praised for achieving "progress in establishing criteria for evaluating any form of therapy for psychotic patients." A first tentative step had been taken toward the further evolution of psychiatric methodology.

## Mental Measurement

The discussions in the USPHS conferences indicated that psychiatrists' conceptions of what constituted good experimental design had run ahead of existing tools. In particular, psychosurgery studies had shown the complete inadequacy of available psychometric tests (the tools for the measurement of intelligence or personality), revealing a "basic contradiction." Patients clearly lost some aspect of practical intelligence, yet their scores on personality and intelligence tests failed to clarify what – if anything – had been changed. The psychological tests may indeed have yielded "objective" measurements, but in practice such numbers proved to be of limited value. Some state hospitals, skeptical of such cursory examinations by extramural personnel, chose instead to rate patients in staff conferences where clinical changes were determined in a show of hands by hospital workers who best knew the patient.[47]

The considerable gap between what investigators knew subjectively through simple observation and what they could capture with available scientific instruments produced a reservoir of frustration. Gosta Rylander's memorable presentation in 1947 to the Association for Research in Nervous and Mental Disease, in which he described impressions of lobotomized patients in fearlessly subjective terms, created so much stir precisely because it tapped into this broad animus. One discussant noted that Rylander's personal observations, based on living and working with the patients, deserved emphatic approval. Because his studies were not limited to psychological tests, there was "a flavor and a knowledge that cannot be derived from tests alone, a point that should be particularly stressed in days when formal tests are getting to dominate the scene more and more." Another investigator acclaimed Rylander's characterization that a patient "had lost his soul" as the finest assessment of psychosurgery, as it encapsulated what laboratory tests and ward examinations missed.[48] Simply by stating in subjective, *unscientific* form what could not be expressed in current laboratory language, Rylander was greeted by thunderous applause from a community bound to scientific conventions. In effect, the use of psychological tests had created a type of cognitive dissonance at the professional level. Psychiatrists expressed a desire to introduce the standards of objective, quantifiable measurements into their profession; at the same time, however, practical decisions about the use and effectiveness of psychosurgery could be decided only through traditional clinical judgments – now denigrated as nonscientific. It had taken a foreigner to break the taboo.

To some extent, the psychometric tests were flawed simply because they were designed before investigators had worked with lobotomized patients. Whatever such instruments did measure was not relevant to the case at hand. Or, in the words of one researcher, the phenomena produced by psychosurgery simply were not "caught as yet in a net of reliable tests."[49] Indeed, a subtle dialectic is at work in the development of all medical technologies. New therapies yield unpredictable effects for the reason that, as a result of physiological manipulation, the organism has been not so much altered in familiar ways as it has been *transformed* into something qualitatively different, requiring new modes of conceptualization. The lobotomy experience brought home to psychiatrists the point that experimental treatments necessitate a coevolution in the tools researchers use to evaluate and make sense of such interventions.

The cognitive difficulties in applying the descriptive power of science to the phenomena of mental illness were compounded by the profession's structural isolation from other disciplines. Reminiscent of the problems encountered when attempts were first made to bring psychiatry up to the standards of general medicine, the initial contacts between the disciplines of psychology and psychiatry, too, reflected the historical consequences of their separate development. Until World War II, when clinical psychologists began to appear in state hospitals and then, in large numbers, in VA hospitals, the two professions did not significantly overlap. However, as a new breed of clinical psychologist came into increasing contact with seriously ill mental patients, a cross-fertilization of methods occurred. American psychiatrists, who had had little formal training in scientific methods or experimental design, developed from their collaborations with clinical psychologists an awareness of statistical analysis, matched control populations, baseline measurements, and the like – exactly the kinds of scientific tools so admired by Morison.[50]

Conversely, psychologists were forced to change their own methods in accordance with mental hospital realities. Psychological tests, for the most part, had been screening devices applied in schools and offices, useful in identifying deviant characteristics such as psychoneurosis, low intellect, or overemotionality. Self-applied tests, however, were impractical in state hospitals filled with chronic agitated or withdrawn schizophrenics. Moreover, as psychological tests had been normalized against distributions of characteristics found in the general population, they proved insensitive to changes in the condition of psychotics. Sooner rather than later, psychologists improvised tests specially designed for mental hospital environments, with rating scales based on overt behavioral and emotional conditions, normalized against chronic institutionalized populations. Several of these new tests were designed in conjunction with lobotomy studies.[51]

The exchange of views between psychologists and psychiatrists in the psychosurgery discussions thus led to a heightened appreciation of the kinds of evidence necessary if "scientifically valid" studies were to be produced. At the same time, it revealed the difficult, unfamiliar nature of the task. In 1950, the APA held a roundtable discussion on "Evaluation of Effectiveness of Treatment." Joseph Zubin, a clinical psychologist on the Columbia-Greystone psychosurgery project, outlined the vital need for standardization of diagnosis as well as evaluation in a field that had grown comfortably haphazard. "Without such standard reference points," Zubin warned, "both the therapists and the scientists are lost on a dark sea without a compass or a chart."[52] The precise means by which such order was to be imposed on American psychiatry was not, however, spelled out.

## Model Science

After the last USPHS Research Conference on Psychosurgery in 1951, the APA itself stepped in and assumed the responsibility for bringing the needed scientific coherence to modern psychiatry. Policy and method thus converged in an unprecedented manner. Its plan was to sponsor a model research project performed under the association's imprimatur. Such a

demonstration was intended to establish minimum standards and guidelines for the scientific evaluation of psychiatric treatments, thereby tran-
scending all political and clinical schisms within the profession. In February 1952, a formal proposal was submitted by the APA to both the
Department of the Navy and the NIMH for "An Investigation of the
Effectiveness of Psychiatric Therapies through the Establishment of a
Commission for the Development of Criteria, Methodology, and Standards." The application argued that there existed "a critical need for a
scientific evaluation of the effectiveness of psychiatric therapies for the
mentally ill, military and civilian." Lack of such standards had made it
difficult for the profession to choose future courses of action "with a
confident sense of direction." "Not only has there been no comprehensive
scientific evaluation of therapies," the application continued, "there have
not even been established sound criteria, methodology, or standards under
which such validation might take place" – an extraordinarily frank admission for a profession that staked its legitimacy on the availability of such
knowledge. The APA proposed an ambitious five-year project that would
evaluate a wide selection of therapies. The goal was not to yield any
ground-breaking experimental results but to establish the framework itself for conducting such investigations. It was intended, in effect, to be the
discipline's first valid experiment, the master template from which a new
scientific psychiatry might be cast.[53]

Although the applications were rejected as overly ambitious, the NIMH
did fund an intermediate step, a conference that might formulate the
protocols for such a model experiment. The conference, the revised application optimistically forecasted, would "determine in a definitive way the
extent to which psychiatry as a basic medical science is now sufficiently
advanced that it is in a position to review and evaluate its scientific practices and their relative efficacy. This in itself would constitute a significant
contribution to the further development of psychiatry."[54]

A three-day "Conference on the Development of a Research Program
for the Evaluation of Psychiatric Therapies" was held in Princeton, N.J.,
in March 1953, with twenty-five participants comprised of a broad mix of
constituencies, including the APA, GAP, the VA, the NIMH, major philanthropies, and an array of psychoanalysts and somatically or eclectically
oriented psychiatrists. Daniel Blain, APA medical director, was the official
grantee for the project; Paul Hoch, chairman of the APA Committee on
Therapy and principal investigator of the prestigious New York State
Psychiatric Institute, presided over the conference.

The conference minutes indicate that its origins lay in the exasperation
psychiatric administrators felt when called upon to decide whether a particular investigation or treatment deserved support, a judgment greatly

complicated by the lack of clear, standardized criteria. William Malamud, a member of the APA Committee on Therapy, complained that the organization was "placed behind the eight ball" whenever it had to determine a particular treatment's efficacy. Hoch, committee chairman, added that "again and again and again this comes up." Unless a "practical" method of evaluation was soon found, they noted, the association would face the unfortunate prospect of abandoning any such responsibilities. The NIMH was said to be in a similar predicament. Hoch also remarked that state legislatures, besieged by requests from departments of mental hygiene to fund assorted therapeutic programs, were eventually going to demand some proof of psychiatrists' claims. As Hoch dispiritedly noted, however, "there is no proof, gentlemen, for any of these things."[55]

Frank Tallman, director of California's Department of Mental Hygiene, echoed Hoch's fears. Tallman remarked that in past years psychiatric programs had been supported by the public solely on the basis of the personal advice of experts. A newly educated public, though, was prone to ask embarrassing questions. Recently, the California legislature had offered Tallman an opportunity to "write his own check" for a complete state hospital treatment program. "This is really heaven," Tallman initially thought, "all the money needed to hire nurses, to hire all the doctors I need, all the psychiatrists, all the gadgets and everything." Tallman eventually declined the support, as further deliberation exposed dangerous implications. Without any means of conclusively demonstrating that the increased expenditures had led to measurable clinical improvement, the offer in fact represented "a gallows for the doctors in California to hang themselves on."[56]

The need to formulate such demonstrable psychiatric standards was the primary purpose of the conference. For example, Hoch noted that, as every hospital followed an individual course, attempts to compare existing psychiatric studies would inevitably prove futile. The aim of the proposed project would not be to determine whether a particular therapy was either good or bad. Rather, it was to "get some basic methodology," to ask "what models can be constructed in this field?" Robert Morison, representing the Rockefeller Foundation, captured the spirit of the event:

> Mr. Chairman, as a sort of sympathetic outsider I should like to emphasize that this has very vast importance, this idea of just setting up a standard which everybody can look at. I do not think it is giving away any secret to say that psychiatry among the medical professions is not perhaps the most admired in this respect, and if this could be done in a better way, say, than in gall-bladder statistics, it would certainly increase the prestige as a whole of the American Psychiatric Association. . . .

Morison's remarks were met with a resounding "Hear! Hear!" In response, conferees who had participated in the Columbia-Greystone psychosurgery experiment noted that, only five years earlier, extreme difficulty was encountered in their attempts to introduce controls into the project's design. Psychiatry was already to be congratulated, they stated, for the progress in attitude since achieved. Daniel Blain summarized the main thrust of the APA's proposed pilot investigation: "We are learning to carry out a controlled experiment which we have not done so far."[57] The possibility was thus entertained that the much maligned field of psychiatry, by the end of their demonstration project, would in fact be at the vanguard of scientific methodology in medicine. Forced to start from scratch, psychiatry might end up leading the way among its medical brethren.

The project's design was deceptively straightforward. Hospitalized chronic schizophrenics, America's most significant psychiatric problem, were targeted as experimental subjects. From the standpoint of researchers, patients in this category of mental illness had the administrative advantage of being a captive population easy to locate and then follow up, and also such disturbed patients might exhibit the most noticeable indications of clinical improvement. The venture itself was divided into three institutionally separate but methodologically consistent experiments. Establishment of a baseline rate of improvement in a patient population was given first priority. At the same time, a standardized hospital population was to be constructed, a guide by which other hospitals could then select candidates for trials of particular therapies. Without a baseline rate of spontaneous remission, measured in uniform populations, therapeutic evaluation would remain little more than conjecture. Zubin presciently noted that this initial project would prove of considerable utility should the profession stumble upon innovations such as new drugs (one year later, the discovery of chlorpromazine, the first major tranquilizer, would indeed revolutionize the field). The core of the APA project was its second phase, a demonstration of the scientific evaluation of psychiatric treatments. Shrewdly, the APA proposed simultaneous investigations of psychosurgery and psychoanalysis, "the two extreme poles of the therapeutic approach," thereby effectively encompassing the full range of political as well as clinical disparities within the profession. If successful, the association would have established jurisdiction over all its diverse elements, putting in place a kind of science court for the forced arbitration of all future disputes.[58]

Discussants readily immersed themselves in the task of designing an ambitious psychosurgery experiment. Many conference members had served as consultants to lobotomy projects or had discussed the subject in previous conferences, and their collective experience showed. Elaborate experimental designs were suggested and dissected, complete with provisions for mock operations and careful matching of controls. In comparison, enthusiasm for the psychotherapy project quickly waned, as its prohibitive cost (analysts were expensive) and extreme methodological difficulties came to light. Not at all evident, for example, was what constituted an adequate control in psychotherapy. (One participant suggested in all seriousness that perhaps the analysts might provide some patients with wrong interpretations.) Issues of definition, uniformity, evaluation, and follow-up somehow seemed far more complicated here than in the parallel trial of lobotomy.

That psychoanalysis and psychosurgery were being seriously considered within the same forum – and with even a determined attempt at uniformity – was indeed a remarkable event. Hostilities between GAPs and Preserves had by this time already receded, and the profession was bending to pressures to present a unified front. A kind of scientific parley, the conference had transformed the nature of the debate between Freudians and somatotherapists. Opponents of psychosurgery appeared to welcome the lobotomy project, convinced that close scrutiny would undermine the claims of fervent lobotomists; once pinned down, the procedure's true benefits would appear less glamorous. And unlike at the USPHS research conferences, here there was no Walter Freeman present to sidetrack detractors with baited criticisms and exaggerated claims. The matter would be weighed soberly.

At the same time, analysts too were placed noticeably on the defensive in the discussions of the psychotherapy project. One conferee hesitated to compare psychotherapy of chronic schizophrenia (then a relatively new idea) to "a more concrete procedure like lobotomy." After several attempts to clarify the psychotherapy project had ended in frustration, another participant challenged: "At the risk of sounding nasty to the planning committee, why do we want this? Why do we want to study psychotherapy at this time?" Hoch responded that indeed it would be a "happy thing" if the whole issue of psychotherapy could be ignored and the commission were free to concentrate on something more "tangible." Nevertheless, he noted, psychotherapeutic treatment was in fact rapidly expanding nationwide, as evidenced by the construction of large training programs. The profession had no choice but to face the question "Is the whole thing worthwhile or not?"[59] Analysts at the conference put themselves in the awkward position of exempting themselves from the new methods of experimental investigation and yet defending their record of clinical effectiveness. Joseph Wortis, a steadfast biological psychiatrist, pressured analyst Ben Watterson: "You seem to suggest, sir, that it is rather futile to define a psychotherapist in the terms that would permit an experiment. Do I understand you correctly?" Freudians as well as psychosurgeons faced an uncertain future in the new scientific framework.

The conference closed on a discordant note. Although participants sensed that psychotherapy had overtaken psychosurgery as the dominant mode of innovative psychiatric practice, it was clear that lobotomy investigations more closely conformed to their present attempts to validate psychiatry as a scientific discipline. Indeed, Morison went so far to as to suggest that, tactically, the psychotherapy project should be run as a separate endeavor lest it detract from the "prestige" of the psychosurgery investigation. The summary of the conference presented to the association concluded that, in contrast to the "harmonious, straightforward" discussions on how to evaluate psychosurgery, attempts to approach psychotherapy "disclosed more uncertainty and differences of opinion."[60] With benefit of hindsight, it is apparent that the conferees' frustration was generated by the deep structural changes then working their way through the profession. Whereas psychosurgery evoked the past legacy of an institutionally based psychiatry with which they were all intimately familiar, psychotherapy reached forward into an uncertain future in which office-based practitioners would set priorities.

## The Benefits of Bureaucracy

Although the APA experiment was never directly realized, an approximate version of the psychosurgery project had already begun under the aegis of the Veterans Administration. Model science thus found its home, not within a national professional organization, but within a branch of the federal government that had greater direct control over both practitioners and patients.

By 1950, each of the thirty-seven VA neuropsychiatric hospitals had used lobotomy, with an aggregate total of more than fifteen hundred such operations. Richard Jenkins, chief of research for the VA Division of Neurology and Psychiatry, along with psychologist James Holsopple, decided to pioneer a large controlled experiment that might improve this program and, in addition, serve as a pacesetter for all future comparative experimental studies in psychiatry. Between 1950 and 1953, surgeons at six participating hospitals in the VA Lobotomy Study performed operations on a total of 373 patients, utilizing an array of surgical techniques. Patients were matched to controls by diagnosis, age, sex, and length of hospitalization. Follow-up evaluations were performed between 1953 and 1958; in 1955 the team coordinating the VA Lobotomy Study formed the basis for the new VA Central Neuropsychiatric Laboratory in Perry Point, Maryland.[61]

The VA's ambitious psychosurgery program was a natural extension of its commitment to psychiatric progress. Under the leadership of General Omar Bradley, the federal government reinvigorated the system of veterans hospitals as part of its commitment to services for returning servicemen. In something of a repeat performance of what transpired following World War I (the label of *neuropsychiatric* hospital evidenced these roots), the United States committed itself to funding an elaborate program of outpatient as well as inpatient services for veterans. Unlike the state hospitals, the new VA facilities were rebuilt from the ground up, adorned with the latest in medical equipment, and staffed with an enthusiastic and highly trained medical corps. In their prime first years, the network of VA hospitals, for example, set the pace in the utilization of such innovations as clinical psychologists and psychiatric social services.[62]

The VA Lobotomy Study's unique contribution was its interhospital design, an attempt to standardize patient selection and evaluation for cross-hospital comparisons. Previously celebrated lobotomy studies, such as the Columbia-Greystone experiment and the Connecticut Cooperative Lobotomy Project, had already boasted "cooperative" research design. Their innovations, however, were limited to the administrative oversight of multidisciplinary research scattered across several institutions and did not extend to the kinds of careful interhospital standardization described in the conferences. At each of the various psychosurgery symposia, for example, researchers had pointed to the need for a central lobotomy registry to maintain uniform records. In spite of repeated pleas, such suggestions were never followed. No single agency – not the APA, NIMH, or any individual department of mental health – had the resources or the authority to bring even this minimal level of standardization into the decentralized world of American psychiatry. In contrast, Congress had constructed in the VA an "almost perfect framework for cooperative research." For example, clinical records were not the property of any given facility but were open to all investigators; and patients could at any future time be located through the regular veteran tracking service.[63] Jenkins and Holsopple looked to the special circumstances of government-sponsored and -located research as the key to successful experimental design in medicine.

Historian Harry Marks has argued that the impediments to the introduction of controlled experiments in general medicine were as much institutional and organizational as they were intellectual. Although the concept of what might be termed the modern clinical trial was largely understood by the 1930s, its execution in practice was not easily achieved. As Marks recounts, it was only when such bureaucratic organizations as the Medical Research Council (UK), the VA, and then the USPHS stepped forward in the 1940s to conduct experiments on their own behalf that research protocols were taken out of the hands of individual clinicians and could conform to the needs of good experimental design. Indeed, Jenkins and Holsopple had used the VA's recent study of tuberculosis treatment as a basis for their own experiment.[64]

In short, the introduction of modern experimental design into American medicine was not just a matter of controlling the experimental conditions within a laboratory setting or hospital ward, but of controlling the researchers themselves – a situation that only came about with the entrance of centralized bureaucracies. The rush of government support of science that followed the war thus had far-reaching consequences, not just on the size and variety of research projects funded, but on the inner culture of medical research as well. Researchers no longer needed to match their projects solely to the interests of the private philanthropies, but now scrambled to fit them into the priorities of a democratic nation; at the same time, within the profession the previous laissez-faire organization of medical practice, which was guided by a social as well medical elite, no longer held sway in the new era of peer review. The only useful data was nationalized data.

A final report on the VA lobotomy project, published in 1959, indicated that patients given a lobotomy did exhibit statistically significant improvements when compared to control populations. Discharged psychosurgery patients were rated as having made a better social adjustment in the community. Among the patients who remained hospitalized, the psychosurgery patients also fared better than the controls, showing a lower "psychotic morbidity" rating. This said, it should be noted that a 1955 preliminary paper detailed the many unexpected problems that had confounded the researchers. Although patients had been carefully matched to controls for many factors, none of these selected variables yielded any prognostic value. The realities of hospital life soon negated investigators' "double-blind" design, as information regarding who had undergone an actual lobotomy was quickly communicated via the "grapevine." Poorly trained, harried staff members inaccurately filled out "objective" rating sheets. And patients had not been randomly scattered between control and treatment groups – a consideration inadequately understood at the time of the experiment's inception – leading to serious skewing of results; the most disturbed patients, in general the lobotomy candidates, would naturally tend to exhibit the greatest improvement. To Holsopple, the VA Lobotomy Project had been a sobering lesson: "Thus we admit, however we may dislike doing so, that our experimental methods in psychiatric therapy have much more in common with the sciences of astronomy, archaeology, and history than they have with physics or chemistry." Lobotomy had taught psychiatrists invaluable lessons – some heartening and others disappointing – concerning the application of scientific methods to the study of mental illness and its treatment.[65]

## Conclusion: Psychiatry in Transition

Commentators on the history of psychosurgery in America generally blame the procedure's rapid growth on the failure of American psychiatrists to exercise available professional controls or to apply proper scientific rectitude. Such characterizations oversimplify the true nature of psychiatry's professional and scientific status in this earlier period. The critics assume, first, that the contemporary research tools were of sufficient power to reveal the treatment's inherent faults and, second, that once such information was uncovered, the professional infrastructure in place already held the authority to brake further use of the procedure. Neither consideration was true.

Before World War II, the APA was a figurehead organization with only minor responsibilities. In practice, psychiatry was a matter of individual physicians acting wholly autonomously, beholden to no one. Indeed, any attempt to dictate which therapies a particular psychiatrist might employ would have been decried as a violation of the fundamental rights of clinical choice. In the American laissez-faire medical tradition, physicians collectively claimed total corporate control of the right to practice medicine, and only slowly would they tolerate regulatory interference within the profession. Every man was not his own physician, but every physician was surely his own man. In general medicine, firm boundaries delimiting what physicians could or could not do in their own practice had arisen mostly out of the need to draw a distinct line separating heterodox from orthodox practitioners. It would hardly do, for example, for a respected member of a medical community to perform some chiropractic on the side.

Psychiatry had been even slower than other medical specialties in developing its own standards and procedures for professional self-regulation. In the grueling, mostly homogeneous world of state hospital practice, the need for even this kind of disciplinary apparatus was redundant. There were not many noninstitutionally based psychiatrists interloping into the asylums, and those physicians employed by the hospitals did not have many therapeutic options upon which to deliberate. In sum, it is unlikely that the wide use of psychosurgery could have been halted by executive decree even if its putative "unscientific" basis had been revealed, for the simple reason that at the time no such brakes existed. The threat most feared by today's investigators, a cutoff of research funds, was obviously not yet an option.

The matter of psychosurgery's scientific merit has also been misinterpreted. When recent observers harshly denounce the original psychosurgery studies as having contained "virtually zero" scientific value, or of being "pitifully poor" in experimental design, they are anachronistically judging past efforts by current standards of scientific medicine.[66] Our current standard of scientific validity, the double-blind experiment with adequately matched controls, is of surprisingly recent vintage. Certainly before World War II the final arbiter in psychiatry was not controlled experiments but clinical reports, filtered and aggregated by often arbitrary standards. Even more unexpected is the fact that *no* medical specialty had yet begun to assess its therapeutic armamentarium through a systematic regime of controlled experiments. Virtually all of medicine, on the eve of the war, was crudely unscientific according to today's standards.[67]

This is not to say that the rise of psychosurgery was wholly disconnected from what is recognized today as modern psychiatry. To the contrary, the story of lobotomy is so telling precisely because its heyday in the decade following World War II coincided with a remarkable transition period in which psychiatry rapidly evolved as both a profession and a science. The evolution was occasioned by forces both internal and external to the field. A rapid influx of new kinds of mental health care workers destabilized traditional conceptions of psychiatry, leading to open factional warfare that in time developed into a battle for political control of the profession's organizations. Yet, the field's dramatic growth in membership and a parallel gain in acceptance as a bona fide medical specialty meant that its professional organization, the APA, would have to begin acting like other comparable medical organizations. The intraprofessional strife had to be resolved or all parties would suffer. At the same time, the impact of the federal government and its massive resources on the mental health scene, through such avenues as the construction of the NIMH and the system of VA neuropsychiatric hospitals, placed additional pressures on psychiatric leaders to discipline their ranks and to proceed to the next step of certifying which of the many competing modes of treatment then available were both safe and efficacious, proven so by the latest methods of medical science. The prewar, traditional way of doing things was no longer an option. In both its mode of professional organization and its scientific methodology, psychiatry was forced to seek new structures and resolutions. The issues of professional control and experimental control were inextricably linked.

More so than any other treatment of the day, psychosurgery was intimately bound up in the events that impelled psychiatry to evolve along both fronts, political and scientific. As the procedure was the most dramatic physiological intervention then in use, at a time of high tension between somatically and nonsomatically inclined practitioners, and as it was the first treatment considered to result in occasional instances of grave, irreversible damage, the subject automatically invited an unprecedented level of scrutiny. Debates over the use of the brain operations were thus seized upon as pivotal occasions for the various factions to fight over the current and future direction of psychiatry as a profession. Moreover, attempts to ascertain the true clinical value of the operations became defining moments for psychiatrists to learn just how ill-prepared they were to apply the new methods of experimental science to the problem of mental health. One might conclude, echoing Roger Cooter's account of phrenology in the nineteenth century, that psychosurgery was truly a "provocation to progress."[68] Ironically, the model of modern psychiatry that was to emerge would soon downplay the important contributions made by psychosurgery as a catalyst for change. For within a short period of time, the story of lobotomy would no longer be usable as an exemplar of the future triumphs of psychiatry, becoming instead an unwelcome reminder of the new psychiatry's own uncomfortably recent past.

# Epilogue
## The New Synthesis

> This is what I know. The ward is a factory for the Combine. It's for fixing up mistakes made in the neighborhoods and in the schools and in the churches, the hospital is. When a completed product goes back out into society, all fixed up as good as new, *better* than new sometimes, it brings joy to the Big Nurse's heart; something that came in all twisted different is now a functioning, adjusted component, a credit to the whole outfit and a marvel to behold. – Chief Bromden.
>
> Ken Kesey, *One Flew Over the Cuckoo's Nest* (1962)[1]

The era of psychosurgery as a widespread hospital therapy ended with the introduction of the drug chlorpromazine in 1954. Synthesized by a French pharmaceutical firm in the search for a new form of anesthesia, Thorazine (its brand name) was discovered to have remarkable "tranquilizing" powers for a wide range of psychotic conditions. Psychiatrists nationwide described the miraculous conversion of locked wards into open halls and the replacement of bars and gates by drapes and screen doors. Everywhere peace and quiet was breaking out. (One facility went so far as to publish oscilloscope recordings of the noise level on the wards before and after chlorpromazine.) Within a year of Thorazine's introduction, hospital reports indicated the first-ever decline in resident populations. Just as impressive was the rapid falloff in the use of the older somatic treatments. The sharp decline was true for lobotomy as well. By the 1960s, the brain operations all but disappeared in the state hospitals.[2] Lobotomy had become redundant.[3]

Although the actual use of lobotomy was comparatively moribund in the years that followed, the *story* of what had happened during the heyday of psychosurgery took on a life of its own. History was not kind to the lobotomists. As quoted in the Introduction, C. C. Burlingame expressed a heartfelt fear that one day he and his psychiatric peers would be ridiculed for their strong advocacy of the physical treatments, in spite of the fact that such therapies looked so effective to them at the time. His apprehensions were well founded. Within a generation after his sudden death in

1950, the evaluation of lobotomy underwent a startling reversal, sullying
the reputations of all those who had been involved with it, Burlingame
included.

The turnabout resulted from the convergence of several factors. To
begin with, hospital psychiatrists were genuinely astounded by the effectiveness of the new drugs. In convincing others – and themselves – that the
psychopharmaceuticals were revolutionizing psychiatry, the profession
draped the new developments in a rhetoric of progress that heightened the
differences between past and present practices. New psychiatry was portrayed as scientific, liberating, and humane; conversely, previous efforts
were represented as irrational, enslaving, and cruel. As was shown earlier,
a similar logic had ushered in the physical treatments in the late 1930s.
Insulin, electric shock, and lobotomy were originally each put forth as
state-of-the-art medicine, the introduction of which was supposed to replace the barbarism associated with past eras of institutional practice.
Ironically, when the wheel of technological progress rotated once again,
these previous emblems of success were transformed into icons of failure
and shame. No longer high watermarks of what psychiatry might achieve,
the physical treatments now indicated the distance from which psychiatry
had even more recently advanced.

In due course, Moniz and his Nobel prize-winning leucotome were
quietly dropped from the introductory pages of psychiatric textbooks and
consigned to the museum that housed the whips, chains, dunking chairs,
and magic amulets of yore. Moreover, the falloff in brain operations
produced a secondary effect that amplified the profession's distaste for the
procedure. The only experience of lobotomy for those psychiatrists who
entered the profession in the late 1950s and after consisted of attending to
those patients who had received the surgery long before yet were still on
the wards – namely, the failures. As the years passed, and fewer psychiatrists remained who could instruct their younger colleagues about the
occasional miracle cure that he or she had personally witnessed, the procedure became enshrouded in purely negative connotations. No one of
prominence was left to defend the notion that lobotomy had ever had its
uses.

The public's regard for psychosurgery similarly plummeted. With increasing frequency, this and other psychiatric treatments were met with
skepticism and even outright fear. A chorus of dissenting voices was emerging in popular books, plays, and movies that derided the image of the
psychiatrist as benevolent healer. Indeed, in such celebrated works as
Tennessee Williams's *Suddenly Last Summer* (1958), Ken Kesey's *One
Flew Over the Cuckoo's Nest* (1962), and Elliott Baker's *A Fine Madness*
(1964), lobotomy was singled out as a particularly frightening form of

medical abuse. Kesey's character Chief Bromden, for example, explained the hazards of lobotomy. When done wrong, the patient ended up "like Ruckly sitting there fumbling and drooling over his picture." If done right, the patient was transformed into "a sleepwalker wandering round in a simple, happy dream." "A success, they say," Bromden added, "but I say he's just another robot for the Combine and might be better off as a failure."[4] Lurid science-fiction tales, such as the chilling *Planet of the Apes* (1964), further poisoned the idea that any good might be associated with lobotomy – not now, not in the past, or even in the distant future.

Soon thereafter, the fate of psychosurgery's reputation was sealed when popular and professional currents collided in a controversial exchange about the desirability of a new round of psychosurgery. In the aftermath of the Detroit riots of 1967, a group of heretofore respectable physicians published a letter in the *Journal of the American Medical Association* proposing a novel solution to the endemic problem of urban violence. It seemed plausible to these physicians that the social disturbances originated in the handiwork of a few rabble-rousers whose violent ways stemmed from identifiable brain pathologies, most likely focal epilepsies that might be removed through sophisticated and precise brain operations. If these assumptions were to prove true, then medicine could offer an answer to the political problem: cull the leaders of these uprisings and wheel them into the nearest neurosurgical suite. Although the proposal was more speculation than a practical blueprint for action, the proponents for what was called the "second wave" of psychosurgery did manage to elicit support for a corollary proposal, namely, to operate on habitual criminals. A small number of prison inmates were in fact operated upon. In the tumult of 1960s politics, such activities sparked a firestorm of harsh criticism within the medical as well as lay community. The spectre of politically motivated doctors hacking away at the brains of unpopular citizens branded psychosurgery as a form of bad, if not evil, medicine. The controversy eventually led to an investigation by the President's Commission for the Protection of Human Subjects of Biomedical and Behavioral Research. Although the commission's findings were rather muted – it reported that psychosurgery actually might have some benefit – the damage had been done to the procedure's image.[5]

The reputation of psychosurgery has never recovered since for any of the psychosurgeons, whether they were proponents of the second wave or participants in the first. Although the two phases had little in common (the procedures were technically very different, and the earlier patients were mostly long-suffering mental patients, not criminals or sociopaths), their stories merged into a single narrative. From this point onward, Burlingame and his brethren would be likened to Nazi doctors, too.

John Fulton and Walter Freeman lived long enough to see their respective disciplines evolve away from what they had known during the high point of their careers. The rapidly changing world of medical science was no kinder to Fulton than it was to Freeman, and both were forced to the periphery as events passed them by. Their reactions could not have been more different, however, as each played out his life true to character. Fulton, throughout his career, was always as comfortable in the rare-book room as he was in the operating theater. When it came time to retire, he gave up his active scientific endeavors, finding solace in historical contemplation. Freeman, in contrast, was never one to look backward in his work. Even during his twilight years, to Freeman history was not something to embrace but an enemy to fight to the bitter end.

After two decades of chairing Yale's physiology department, a job that involved constant wrangling with a succession of medical school deans, Fulton had had enough. In 1951, the annual skirmish over budget appropriations turned especially nasty. When the dust had settled, Fulton graciously relinquished control of the department in exchange for an appointment as Yale's first Sterling Professor of the History of Medicine. It was time to move on. Although no longer a productive member of the research community, Fulton kept abreast of developments, maintaining his important behind-the-scenes role as confidant, mentor, and broker of information to the legions of scientists and physicians whose lives he had touched. Nevertheless, the exchange of titles was more than symbolic. Fulton settled into his new primary seat of residence, the library chair. His remaining years were noted mostly for his publications on the history of science and medicine, his editorship of the *Journal of the History of Medicine,* and his travels to collect prestigious honorary degrees and governmental medals.

If a list is prepared of the most important medical scientists from the past, there is little chance that Fulton's name will be mentioned. Indeed, considering the high luster of his promise and opportunities, one might fairly assess his direct contributions to scientific knowledge as disappointing. Certainly, his involvement in seeding the development of psychosurgery did not bring the kind of lasting fame Fulton had desired. The plunge in the procedure's fortunes was already evident by the end of his career, and in his last addresses, he felt it necessary to distance himself from its origins. At one talk given in 1959, for example, Fulton noted that Freeman had "proclaimed me the father of lobotomy," but if that was so – and Fulton intimated it was not – "it was really an instance of unplanned parenthood!"[6]

Fulton's true influence within the discipline, however, was more subtle than that of a brilliant scientific thinker or innovator. A generation of leaders in medicine and science had relied upon Fulton's wise counsel. Some came into contact with him through the symposia over which he presided, the medical journals he edited, and the textbooks he wrote; others came under his personal care at Yale, within the premier postgraduate program in the nation. (One of these was Freeman's son, Walter Freeman III, who eventually went on to a distinguished research career in neuroanatomy.) At the outset of his career, Fulton believed that his most lasting contributions would be indirect, taking the form of identifying and nurturing the careers of junior scientists who would someday make their mark. He was right.

Although Fulton himself made no major discoveries, his role as an enabler of others' work should not be discounted. His special talents were his capacity for seeing both the content and the future structure of medical research and a synthesizing ability to link past traditions to emerging realities. For all of his bookish ways and studious worship of heroes past, Fulton was one of the few medical leaders of the day who had a practical feel for what lay ahead. Under his astute directorship, the Yale program evolved into an exemplar of how prewar programs of medical research, which at the time were mostly small affairs dependent entirely upon the whims of private philanthropies, might successfully make the transition to postwar reality, in which the winners were large programs supported by public funds. Fulton's intimates in science passionately believed that his career was indeed something to celebrate, even if it did not fit the mold of the heroic investigator. In him, they found a comrade and leader who best exemplified the perspectives and ideals of medical research, one who could be trusted to guard these interests within the uncharted world of the government committee room. One might say that Fulton was one of the first of the new breed of scientist-administrators, a less romantic role, to be sure, but one just as equally vital to the future of university research in America.

Fulton died in 1960, at age sixty.

Walter Freeman, for his part, watched in disbelief and consternation as the psychiatric order changed around him. The immediate future belonged to his arch rivals, the psychotherapists. Of the four junior colleagues whom he had hired into his own neurological practice in Washington, D.C., three went over to the other side. They too had become analysts, courtesy of the G.I. Bill. ("I lost them," Freeman confided in his autobiography.) Sensing the end of an era, Freeman retired from his post at George Washington University in 1954 and headed west to Los Altos, California, hoping for greener – and less obstructed – pastures. In the years ahead, he often took

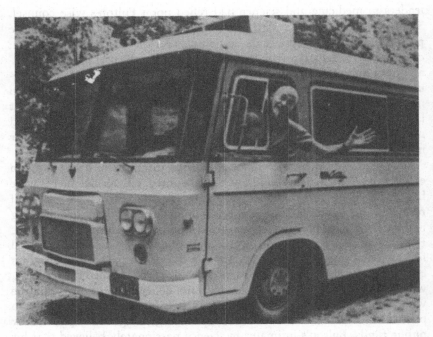

Figure E.1. Walter Freeman's postcard. On reverse: "Greetings from my home to yours! Following my retirement a year ago I drove around the country greeting friends and relatives." (Source: Archives of the American Psychiatric Association)

to the road to visit his former lobotomy patients and to perform some transorbitals in the remote state hospitals whenever local authorities permitted – a circumstance that was becoming increasingly rare. Over time, Freeman's refusal to adjust to the new medical climate led to a tragic reversal in professional fortune. Once a national figure in medicine, by the early 1960s he had become a pariah. Even his home-base institutions, such as Los Altos Hospital, eventually felt compelled to strip him of his medical privileges.[7]

Freeman never did give up the battle to convince the world about lobotomy. For him, the subject remained, in the words of his former partner Jim Watts, a "magnificent obsession." He gamely carried on, publishing elaborate follow-up studies based on information obtained during his road trips. One article that appeared in the 1957 *American Journal of Psychiatry,* for example, reported on the current status of three thousand patients that he or Watts had operated on between 1936 and

1956. A decade earlier, the weight of such numbers might have caused some in the discipline to take notice. But no longer. Still an attendee at professional meetings, Freeman never tired of badgering his medical colleagues to perform more brain operations, or of delivering rancorous papers that communicated his contempt for the prevailing trends. (One of these, for example, was entitled "With Camera and Ice-Pick in Search of the Super Ego.")[8] On these occasions, Freeman would bring with him some shoe boxes crammed full of Christmas cards sent him by grateful lobotomy patients and their families; and, when the opportunity arose, he would dump these on the tables in front of skeptical physicians. His exhortations had little effect, however. Nobody was listening any more.

Freeman died in 1972, at age seventy-six.

## Past and Present

What lessons can be learned from the story of lobotomy's dramatic rise and fall? To date, most commentators have focused on the sheer enormity of the tragedy and its luminous aura of horror. *Tragedy,* from the perspective of today's neuropsychiatry, because so many of our citizens were permanently reduced in their capacity to think and feel by being subjected to a procedure of dubious therapeutic merit – all on the basis of a great need that was soon met with the discovery of tranquilizers. If only their doctors had waited for the right treatment and shown more faith in science to point the way! *Horror,* because the procedure originated without any semblance of scientific method and then was quickly adopted into practice, mostly in response to the petty expediencies of ward management. If only they had acted more responsibly as physicians!

The usual accounts of psychosurgery in America thus draw their inspiration from the subject's standing as a medical mishap of epic proportions. The plots generally conform to one of two basic patterns. For some observers, the primary value of the lobotomy story (as well as that offered by comparable misadventures) lies primarily in its high emotional shock value, its potential to shatter our complacent regard for the safety and benevolence of modern medicine. These tales are deliberately sensationalistic, written with the aim of awakening the citizenry to just how bad things can – and will! – get if scientists and physicians are trusted to police themselves. In contrast, authors of the second kind of story seek a more dispassionate form of analysis, asking us to look past the lurid details to the important lessons buried within. Their emphasis is not on the immorality or irresponsibility of the individual protagonists but on identifying where the process of medical science itself malfunctioned.

Somewhere, it is assumed, there must have been a lapse in the normally efficient checks and balances that are part of the scientific method. The hope here, then, is to put in place a more reliable set of procedural firewalls that might prevent the misdeeds or errors of scientists and clinicians before they can proliferate.

Although the two approaches disagree about the specific lesson to be learned, they nonetheless are in broad agreement upon the larger issues. Tellingly, even though the subject matter is of great potential embarrassment to the medical establishment, few of these reports have been inspired by a strong desire to undermine our collective faith in the medical science ideal. That good things happen when science is done right and when physicians act appropriately is a basic tenet that most of these authors affirm. Indeed, the gravest problems, as they see it, derive not from any flaws in the ideal itself but from those occasions when its standards are abandoned in practice. Moreover, as the scientific method is believed to be inherently self-correcting, the expectation is that any such deviations inevitably will be exposed and eliminated by members of the discipline themselves, even without public or external oversight. But this is not to say that the process cannot or should not be accelerated. The major impetus for these historical efforts thus derives from the assumption that, with the right kinds of interventions, a wayward treatment can be terminated before many casualties have accumulated – and perhaps even before the first human trials have begun.

If there is a single message offered it is this: unless we start paying more attention to what goes on at the shadowy *periphery* of the medical establishment, needless deaths and injuries will occur. History will repeat itself, with tragic consequences. The real danger ahead, such stories further imply, is the public's unrealistic conception of the extent to which the practice of medicine and medical science in this country actually measures up to the ideal. Clearly, our culture has already been saturated with stories that extol the wonders of medical science. Each of these is a laudable endeavor, perhaps, but in the aggregate they have imparted a false sense of security. We remain far too ignorant – or willfully forgetful – about what happens when the wrong types of people are allowed on the wards or in the labs, or when the right types act incorrectly. As a counterbalance, it seems that what is needed is a well-promoted rogues' gallery, the exhibits of which prominently display the psychosurgeons and their ilk, and which also chronicle the devastating effects of their handiwork. Maybe then responsible members of the lay as well as professional communities will be prodded into action, insuring that any looming deviation from the medical science ideal is immediately hunted down and brought back in line with the highest standards, as fast as is humanly possible.

It seems pointless indeed to challenge the notion that with the introduction of lobotomy something went terribly askew in American medicine. The evidence of gross malpractice is intuitively obvious and compelling, provided by the psychosurgeons themselves in their descriptions of what they did. Lobotomy, as performed in the 1940s, was a crude and reckless procedure devoid of any scientific justification that has stood the test of time. This fact is as clear-cut as any. Who today has seen the photos of a transorbital lobotomy and not cringed? Who can read the accounts of lobotomized housewives, operated upon for the mere reason that they were depressed by their lack of options in life, and not give in to outrage and pity for the victims? It is hard to imagine a medical activity of the recent medical past that stands out in starker contrast to what we consider good medical practice. Moreover, it seems equally unclear why anyone might even *want* to cast doubt on the usual story. Any rewriting of the familiar narrative smells of whitewash and invites the accusation that it is an apology for the establishment.

Nevertheless, to challenge the presumed history of psychosurgery in America has been the exact purpose of this book. This said, let me state first that the conventional goals expressed by the previous commentators are ones that I heartily endorse. As a historian, I too am committed to the general notion that forward progress sometimes is aided by a retrospective vision, as well as to the specific idea that a case study of psychosurgery might help to thwart future calamities. The similarities end there, however, especially in regard to what are considered the facts of this particular case and what are thought to be its noteworthy conclusions.

To be sure, the accepted storyline of what happened during the lobotomy years has become so well known to us today that it appears patently correct and beyond dispute. Nonetheless, it is mistaken. As I have tried to demonstrate in the preceding chapters, our understanding of what occurred during psychosurgery's heyday is based on a series of representations that suffer from significant distortions, anachronisms, and omissions. The story just doesn't hold up. "The great tragedy of science," T. H. Huxley once wrote, "is the slaying of a beautiful hypothesis by an ugly fact." Sometimes this adage pertains to the stories of science itself.

My severest criticisms, though, pertain not to how these portrayals go awry in their representation of past events but to their shortcomings when used to prepare for what lies ahead. Noble intentions notwithstanding, such accounts share a set of assumptions which I believe to be inherently misguided. And their advice, I fear, consequently will leave us *more* vulnerable to future tragedies, not less.

The central weakness of these histories, moreover, is not an isolated incident. The same might be said about any of the stories typically used to account for occasions of failure – or success – in science. Thus, a reexamination of the case of psychosurgery, one that seeks to understand why the familiar stories tend to steer us in the wrong direction, is also an opportunity to consider new ways of telling this as well as other such stories of science. In so doing, perhaps a more satisfying or useful history will be achieved.


The central historical riddle posed by the psychosurgery story is this: how could a therapy so highly valued at one point in time later be considered wholly useless? Clearly, a significant discordance exists between past and present perceptions. The manner in which an examiner goes about healing this breach, I propose, is perhaps the single factor that most structures the resulting narrative.

The usual accounts respond to the riddle by drawing upon a powerful historical argument implicit in the current widespread belief that medicine is a form of applied science. The reasoning runs something like this: the true value of any therapy – like other laboratory-based standards – is something that transcends time and place. For we know that if a chemical formula works here, it should work there; and if it is demonstrated to succeed today, then it must have worked yesterday – and will do so tomorrow, as well. The first step, then, is to examine the claims made by psychiatrists in the 1940s in light of what is believed now. Thus, from the mere fact that today's medical scientists reject lobotomy as a worthless procedure, one can deduce that the procedure *never did* have any real medical function. The earlier positive testimonials to the procedure's efficacy are revealed to be illusory and can be dismissed as being of no historical consequence. The case of psychosurgery is but one example of how the medicine-as-applied-science model neatly eliminates the paradoxical tensions that ensue when practitioners in the past and those in the present disagree. It is the nature of scientific progress that prior conceptions of truth are necessarily subordinated to later ones.

In the narratives that follow this approach, the original puzzle is thereby transformed into a more manageable and less potentially disturbing issue: explaining how a *worthless* therapy was widely adopted in practice – albeit temporarily. An immediate consequence of this shift is the placing of a severe limitation on the range of scenarios that might account for the rise and fall of psychosurgery. Indeed, by force of logic, the only possibilities remaining are the two alluded to above. For a time, either a number of bad doctors must have plied their trade without proper professional oversight, or a group of otherwise good doctors fell asleep on the job. In either instance, the story concludes at the inevitable moment when knowledge about the procedure's true effects broke free, thus rousing the profession as a whole to come to its proper senses. Rendered in this manner, the parable of lobotomy no longer threatens to separate the past and the present, but offers yet another opportunity to join them: human weakness is something shared by people everywhere and in any epoch. This is a story we can easily assimilate.

An observer who inspects the past history of psychosurgery in such a way will have no trouble finding tangible evidence that this scenario is indeed what happened, at every stage. Bad science, it seems, was followed by worse medicine. From today's perspective, the original alcohol injection experiments of Egas Moniz on human beings appears to have been patently ridiculous, and the subsequent attempts of Fulton to construct a scientific rationale for psychosurgery on the basis of the available chimpanzee data were equally implausible. Certainly, nothing was proven that justified the extensive clinical use of this dangerous procedure; the zealous promotion of lobotomy by Freeman, and others, is reminiscent of the hawking of patent medicines in the previous century. An argument can be advanced that in these early years, when the fate of the procedure was in the hands of an ego-driven few, common sense and prudence gave way to venality and a lust for professional notoriety.

The second half of the story appears equally shameful, the period when lobotomy was launched into widespread use. Adopted within the nation's vast system of state mental hospitals, which were professional as well as geographic backwaters, the procedure indeed flourished at the periphery of reputable medical practice. Its usage can easily be linked to the non-medical interests of administrative expediency; incidents of casual and even punitive use of psychosurgery in the back wards are there to be found. And so too are cases of patients being reduced to "drooling zombies." Finally, the perception that the psychosurgery enterprise was sustainable only as long as the responsible center of the profession ignored what was happening is in fact substantiated by how the story ended. In the mid-1950s, as soon as an effective alternative treatment such as Thorazine surfaced and a handful of experimental studies reported negative findings about the operation, the use of lobotomy collapsed. The profession had come to its senses at last. It all fits.

But does it? In following this line of inquiry, such accounts restrict their attention only to those instances in which the treatment appears unjustifiable, worthless, and marginal in use. Another possible side to the story exists, but it has been deliberately unexplored. Indeed, as indicated in the course of this book, a revisit to the scene of the events discovers much that does *not* fit this tidy scenario.

To begin with, the original justifications for the operations were clearly

persuasive to the community of scientists working at the time. The awarding of the Nobel Prize to Moniz cannot be written off as a temporary
delusion, but must be accepted for what it was: a measure of scientific
validation. Second, as revealed earlier in this monograph by a review of
patient records, the idea that all or even most lobotomy patients were
vegetablized is clearly fictitious. Indeed, there is ample reason to believe
the psychiatrists when they claimed that some of their patients greatly
benefited from a lobotomy. To think otherwise, one must reject not only
the testimony of hundreds of physicians but *all* of the statements made by
the patients' families – and, in some cases, even by the patients themselves.
Lastly, the image of lobotomy as having been at the periphery of medical
practice is simply wrong. We have seen that it was a favored mode of
treatment not just in the remote state hospitals but in the most expensive private asylums that offered state-of-the-art care. Physicians who
promoted the procedure as both effective and humane were scattered
throughout the mainstream of the profession and were not just on the
margins. Some even came from the ranks of psychiatry's most respected
leaders.

What, then, are we to make of this unexpected image of lobotomy as a
viable therapy? Although such news may be surprising, it is not necessarily
unwelcome here, for it leads to a different means of resolving the historical
tension surrounding the subject. There remains the outside possibility
that, even by today's standards, it was not the judgments about lobotomy
made by practitioners of the past that were in error, but ours. (This would
not be the first time, after all, that our medical forebears have been falsely
maligned as incompetent or unknowing.) Perhaps lobotomy as practiced
by Freeman – and apparently, the main body of the psychiatric profession – was indeed an advantageous treatment, one that should immediately be made available to suffering patients today when the need arises.
Should these facts prove true, the disjuncture between past and present
perceptions simply dissolves, thanks to the power of revisionist history to
set the record right.

Yet the facts as we know them today do not support even this alternative plot. To accept it would mean overturning substantial portions of our
present-day understanding of neurophysiology, brain functioning, and
therapeutics. Nothing in this story, though, even remotely hints at the
necessity for such a massive correction of scientific knowledge. The current rejection of the standard Freeman-Watts lobotomy, upon reinspec-
tion, remains grounded in good scientific sense. Any physician today
attempting such a procedure would face malpractice losses, if not criminal
charges. (And rightfully so, in the opinion of this observer.)

Epilogue

13

It appears, then, that these efforts at a corrective history have not yet solved the historical paradox with which we began. If anything, the rift between current and past medical perceptions is only that much greater. Indeed, it would be comparatively easy to understand how a treatment could have been considered effective in 1949 and not now if we assumed that its supporters were incompetent or unscrupulous. The standard historical accounts may have suffered from the defect of being inaccurate, but at least they made sense. The emerging narrative, in which so many trustworthy physicians in the 1940s believed in the safety and efficacy of lobotomy, still does not.

A solution to the riddle does exist, but it requires that we turn on its head the way we approach the matter of failed therapies. If, as in the case of psychosurgery, the particulars stubbornly refuse to fit into the existing model, then perhaps the source of the problem lies not with the facts but with the framework. In casting the story of lobotomy as a case study of marginal medicine, the usual accounts presume that all the later salient events diverged from a common historical source: the fateful point at which the protagonists failed to abide by the scientific ideal. Right here at the outset, I contend, such depictions go decidedly wrong.

The characterization of psychosurgeons as practitioners who did not live up to the best standards of medical science, as we currently define them, is certainly valid. Used as a historical point of reference, however, this fact is both irrelevant and gravely misleading. As I have tried to demonstrate in the course of this book, medicine most assuredly *was not equivalent to laboratory method,* and even the supposedly timeless standard of medical science *did not remain fixed, but evolved.* The idealized model thus falsely represents what it was that physicians were able to do at the time. In requiring these practitioners to have possessed abilities and knowledge that they did not and could not have, the model has led to ahistorical readings of their actions. And, by misconstruing the past in this manner, it reinforces an untrue image of the nature of medical practice today.

The only way out of the historical paradoxes, I suggest, is to substitute for the approach of using our current idealized models of medical practice to interrogate the past, the reverse strategy: to see in an examination of prior events an opportunity to revamp present understanding of how medical therapies appear and disappear. We should not impose on the past our idyllic versions of what biomedicine can achieve, but confront its very real temporal and human constraints. To date, the value of the psychosurgery story has been limited to what, as a conspicuous example of medicine gone extraordinarily wrong, it can tell us about what goes on at the periphery. The strategy I suggest here, instead, is to consider such events as a unique chance to dissect the workings of normal medical science and practice that usually remain hidden. This alternative approach will lead to a different, fairer reading of how we judge researchers and physicians in the past, and to a more accurate measure of what can reasonably be expected from their successors upon whom we currently depend.

For some time now, the story of psychosurgery has served as a persuasive vehicle for those agitating for the reform of the medical establishment. To go against these tales, then, might seem to be a bald defense of the status quo. Ironically, the reverse case applies. For it is the polemical accounts which, in internalizing the scientific community's clean divisions between worthless therapies and sound ones, end up reinforcing the traditional ways of seeing things. Rather, to retell the story of psychosurgery from an opposite perspective – in a way that breaks down the boundaries between it and other therapies, and that relocates the narrative from the periphery to the mainstream – puts to a close test the actual powers of medical science to deliver us from human tragedy. To do so, I propose, will ultimately lead to the conclusion that our faith in the benevolence and safety of modern biomedicine is constructed upon even less stable ground than the one these critics portray.

## What Works?

The breach between the past and present perceptions of psychosurgery originates in our assumptions about how physicians determine that a treatment works. The body of this book, therefore, has been structured to engage three kinds of historical distortions that have been interjected into this issue by the familiar notion that medicine conforms to the laboratory ideal.

The first kind of error arises from the hard-to-suppress sentiment "They should have known better!" What does or does not make sense to medical science today, it is felt, should have been equally perceivable to those on the scene in the past. This assumption, however, obscures the actual process by which medical investigators first reach consensus that an innovative therapy is worth the risks and then later communicate with clinicians in the field on the need for its improvement. And, in denying the fundamental nature of medical progress – in which new knowledge inevitably repudiates old – fatal anachronisms are introduced into the narrative forms that are most often used to tell the story of medicine's evolution.

The next series of problems stem from the presumption within the laboratory model that what actually works in medicine possesses universal, timeless attributes that stand above the historical process. They do not. A second undertaking in this book, therefore, has been to explore how a therapy's usefulness is contingent upon a particular historical era. To ignore this is to overlook what was *at stake* in a given treatment – for the individual patient, the medical profession, or society – often the deciding factor in its viability. Which leads to a third, collateral issue: what works in medicine is also relative to a particular place, and to the specific characteristics of the individual patient as well as the prescribing physician. To ignore this is to overlook the human element in clinical practice, for the job of doctoring depends as much upon art as it does upon laboratory science. Doctors are thus routinely judged against the wrong sets of standards, to their detriment. And, ultimately, to ours. Once the matter of what works in medicine is resituated within the historical process, the tension between past and present perspectives will be resolved.

## Illusions about Success and Failure

The value of studying therapeutic failures also lies in the unique opportunity they provide for requestioning the way we tell our tales of scientific progress. As most stories focus only on science's celebrated *successes*, little effort has been spent on examining what really goes on at the core. Scientists themselves are expected to fill in this part, especially as they are engaged in work that, of all enterprises, seems the most insulated from broad historical currents. In fact, the traditional accounts have served as elaborate bits of misdirection, drawing our attention away from the more uncertain and unsavory aspects of medical advance. It is precisely in those moments when a wizard conspicuously fails, though, that we lose our spellbound innocence and are tempted to peek behind the curtain for a look at the machinery involved. But the urge does have its downside. Unless you have a strong stomach, someone warned long ago, don't inspect how sausages or treaties are made. Perhaps the making of scientific discoveries, too, is not as palatable as is generally thought. For our faith in the image of scientists as masters of reality has obscured a companion truth: in reality, they are masters of images too.[9]

The first illusion concerns the orderly, purely logical manner in which medical discoveries are thought to be produced. According to this model, any breaks in the rational chain of thought immediately stand out; the implication is that deviations from the normal path of scientific process are easily visible to observers in the past as well as the present. The familiar stories of scientific advance sustain this image by holding fast to a linear model of intellectual cause-and-effect in which an experimental or theoretical finding leads directly to a clinical innovation. In this manner, all existing tales of psychosurgery invariably trace the origins of the procedure back to the moment when Moniz first learned of the results of Fulton's experiments on chimpanzees; indeed, a credible source for this account was found in Fulton himself, the scientist closest to the scene. The story of Moniz's serendipitous discovery, then, was just like all the other such inspirational yarns that have been spun to recount the saga of medical progress – that is, of course, up until the time when lobotomy's reputation was savaged.

Interestingly, lobotomy's dramatic reversal in fortune did not imperil the usual mode of describing the rise of biomedicine. If anything, we have seen, its example was used as further confirmation. For the standard model contains, not one narrative frame, but two: one to exalt the successes of medical science and the other to explain away its failures. The logic is seductive: if valid ideas, properly applied, lead to medical progress, then surely medicine's monstrosities originate from ill-conceived or premature notions. And, applicable here: the closer historically minded investigators have inspected the data reported by Fulton and then Moniz, the less has been found to justify the procedure on intrinsically scientific grounds. In effect, the story of psychosurgery was simply shifted from Narrative One to Narrative Two, thereby shoring up, not undermining, medicine's reputation. And had the pair stayed true to the scientific method, it is further implied, the subsequent tragedy would not have ensued. The two frames represent opposite sides of the same coin.

I suggest, however, that this search for a valid scientific idea that alone might have legitimated the leap to psychosurgery – and the subsequent clinical trials – is nothing more than an elaborately staged wild-goose chase. There is none to be found; but not for the reason that psychosurgery's supporters were acting outside the boundaries of good science. Rather, it is often the case in *mainstream* science as well that such determinative data is lacking. Ever since the writings of Thomas Kuhn (and Ludwik Fleck before him), it has been evident that scientists, when choosing whether to invest in one line of research as opposed to another, often must act on the basis of information that is incomplete.[10] To deal with this overwhelming uncertainty, scientists draw upon an array of resources that are not usually thought to be consistent with proper experimental method, narrowly defined. They look within, to that haziest of personal qualities known as intuition, and they also look without, to trusted authorities and colleagues, for guidance. Thus, when investigators mull over which of the available research options is the best bet, the deciding factor is often contained not in the data alone but in the multidimensional filter applied to it: that is, in the amalgam of concerns, beliefs, and alliances that constitute the broader scientific culture itself. Indeed, history provides numerous examples of instances when the correctness of a scientific finding (as determined later) had little immediate consequence for its original rate of adoption; the key factor was not the quality of the data but the identity of the person reporting it.

In the present example, the successful germination of psychosurgery in America thus turned upon such matters as the perceived credibility of Moniz's findings and, subsequently, the ability of his followers to bring their results before prestigious academies and to publish them in influential journals. As described in Chapter 2, these positive circumstances followed from the belief among leading physicians and researchers that the procedure had in fact been justified on the basis of Fulton's findings. The ultimate source of their confidence, however, cannot be derived from the content of the scientific publications from Yale University. A more informative determinant is the social logic that prepared so many to believe Fulton when *he* stated that such a connection existed. The other origins of lobotomy, then, lie in reconstructing the many factors – personal, institutional, and professional – that had placed Fulton in a position of supreme trustworthiness within the medical and scientific communities. When Fulton spoke, others listened – and then acted. In following his counsel in the case of psychosurgery, this community acted no differently than it had in other such important circumstances.

The usual old chestnuts about the route to scientific innovation, which focus exclusively on the intellectual aspects of such events, thus often prove wrong when pressed on details. This is no accident. The fact that in crucial scientific decisions matters of professional trust and consensus – a thickly constructed social process – can overshadow what can be derived solely from the laboratory printout is one of science's dirty little secrets. Such parables, then, help ensure that our attention remains deflected away from the actual process by which investigators conclude that a new research venture is worth the risk, an often messy business rooted in factors better left unexamined (or so it is thought). It is not too surprising, therefore, that upon close inspection the oft-cited connection between Moniz's innovation and Fulton's discovery is found to be nothing more than a whole-cloth fabrication, spun after the fact by Fulton himself. Fulton's attempt to backdate the historical record so that his own ideas might be credited with precipitating an important medical discovery can be easily dismissed for what it manifestly is: a grab for personal aggrandizement. The latent content imbedded in the story, however, is not so readily ignored. With its narrative focus trained on the supposed intellectual effects of the Yale experiments, Fulton's tale successfully diverts our attention from the personal and professional arenas in which he *did* have a decisive influence. In short, this story, like the others upon which it was fashioned, was in fact an artful denial of the *social* process inherent in medical innovation, a means of perpetuating the familiar notion that in science only ideas matter.

This is not to say that ideas don't matter. They certainly do. Rather, the argument presented here concerns how we select *which* ideas were the influential ones, and to what we attribute their power. With benefit of hindsight, it may seem obvious how a scientist could logically have reached point C by first thinking of A and then B. When it comes to historical accuracy, however, hindsight is often more a hindrance than a help. For what looks logical and obvious today is something altogether different than what appeared rational and self-evident in the past. This truism applies to individual ideas as well as to entire frameworks of thought, or paradigms. In reviewing the publications or lab notebooks of yesterday's scientists, investigators have tended to skip over the notions that today appear foolish or nonsensical, believing that ideas whose substantive basis was so short-lived could not have had any long-lasting effects on the historical process. This habit, born out of deference to reason and logic, grossly distorts history. (It may be hard to believe that Darwin held Lamarckian beliefs or that Newton was also an alchemist, but it is nonetheless so.) In reconstructing the trains of thought of past medical scientists, the range of ideas in circulation and the ways in which they were connected is not something that can be deduced but is a matter of empirical investigation. In the present example, Fulton's emphasis on the Pavlovian model of experimental neurosis seems to us quirky and discountable; surely such a naive and implausible hypothesis was an improper basis upon which to weigh psychosurgery's merits. Yet within the inner circles of the day's prominent scientists, it was discovered, the model was considered to have profound implications for human welfare. In short, just because we happen to think that a particular model or hypothesis is patently absurd or without foundation is irrelevant. What matters is what our predecessors thought was important and compelling.

The point here is that the rush to fit the stories of scientific discoveries into linear, rational models of advance has stripped them of the richness of human thought and its complex links to action. What is later discovered to be an idea of stellar dimensions may have a very dubious pedigree; the path to the right answer may wander through areas that prove embarrassing or irrelevant. (As described in Chapter 7, for example, the modern neuroscientific understanding of the limbic system, the site of the brain involved with emotions, grew directly out of lobotomy research; this fact is not widely broadcast in science textbooks.) We often pride ourselves on our ability, in retrospect, to separate the intellectual content of a scientific model from the social context in which it was generated. In practice, though, the dichotomy is false. To working scientists, the attractiveness of a research venture *simultaneously* draws from its heuristic "puzzle-solving" utility, its fit within the existing institutional agenda, its resonance with currents at play within the broader disciplinary arena, and the like; these factors all merge together, eventually pushing one research venture to the foreground. In short, the power of a scientific idea reflects its inherent ability to unlock the secrets of nature – and its potential to alter human action.

Indeed, the professional stature of a scientist is often measured, not in his or her faculty for separating true ideas from untrue ones – something that might not be revealed for a generation or two later – but in a demonstrated capacity to valorize the research ahead, imbuing particular lines of investigation as worthy of pursuit. Thus, Fulton fulfilled his true role as a statesman of science when he successfully linked Moniz's findings to the contemporary forces, connecting neurophysiology and psychiatry, primate research and human well-being, and laboratory methods and social reality. In seeing the connections articulated by Fulton, others found in psychosurgery an exciting opportunity for medical advance. Psychosurgery now made sense to them.

The second illusion applies to the latter half of the story when the innovation was in wide use. When the reports of lobotomy's inadequacies and hazards first surfaced, and the original neurophysiological justification was found wanting, why didn't the enterprise as a whole grind to a halt? This kind of question – and the expected answer, that somewhere the system misfired – is also based on an unrealistic model of medical progress. Over the years, the usual stories of scientific advance have convinced us of a sort of trickle-down model of medical practice, in which the work of clinicians in the field necessarily remains subordinate to the guidance of their colleagues in the university laboratories who have direct access to scientific knowledge. If clinicians overstep their place, problems arise. Thus, the facts that the lobotomists continued on in spite of the paltry scientific support and conducted their trials without proper scientific protocols are considered to be evidence that they were working outside the boundaries of good medicine.

As described in Chapter 7, exactly this kind of controversy arose after World War II when Fulton (and other scientists) stepped forward to bring the corrective powers of experimental science to bear on the excesses of the lobotomists. In particular, antagonisms flourished when Freeman boldly introduced the "ice-pick" method of transorbital lobotomy, which was roundly condemned by university-based researchers as crude and unscientific; they offered instead more sophisticated, neurophysiologically based operations such as topectomy and gyrectomy. Here, then, is proof that the lobotomists were on the margins of medicine. If only they had followed the lead of the scientists, it is assumed, all would have been well.

Deductions such as this one, however, are based on a misconception of the actual relationship between laboratory science and clinical practice. In contrast to the impression produced by the customary stories, the connection is neither one-way nor unproblematic. As further discussed in Chapter 7, the heroes and the villains are not so easily distinguished; too much credence is given to the superiority of the laboratory. For what is considered worthwhile and acceptable in the laboratory and in the clinic are often at odds, and sometimes incommensurate. From Freeman's perspective in the field, the ice pick may have been missing the trappings of real science, but it was no less effective than some of the procedures developed in the universities, in spite of their pretensions; in this he was probably right. Moreover, just because the university trials were followed in line with scientific protocols did not make them any more certain or humane; the investigators themselves noted that the treatments and the patients were selected according to the interests of scientific knowledge, not necessarily those of the patients involved.

The continuing tensions between the laboratory and the clinic have been hard to see, for it has been in the interests of both sides to conceal this divide, presenting a unified front to the public upon whose trust and support both sides depend. Researchers must blot out any suggestion that they are engaged in the pursuit of idle phantasms, expending large resources on knowledge that we can live without. Clinicians, for their part, must avoid any appearance that their therapeutic practices are unbridled, resulting from simply hit-or-miss tactics. In what has been described as a model of "reciprocal legitimation," both parties thus agree to the fictions of the standard model whenever possible. Clinicians proclaim the putative ties between their treatments and recent laboratory findings; researchers in the laboratories back the physicians up, looking to justify their own spending of other people's money on the basis of the great clinical need that preliminary research has already addressed. Fulton and Freeman needed each other more than either ever cared to admit.

The third illusion relates to the ease with which we can judge, retrospectively, the incompetence of past practitioners. On the one hand, these earlier workers are granted certain allowances, as it is clear that they had to ply their trade at a comparative disadvantage to their peers today, who have at hand an immensely greater amount of information. Our faith in scientific progress, after all, rests largely upon the never-ending expansion of the existing knowledge base. On the other hand, this judiciousness is dissipated by a countervailing assumption – namely, that the *process* of scientific decision making remains remarkably stable. This or that fact may enlarge or disappear, but the core business of separating out good data from bad remains pretty much the same. The stench of bad science, then, is considered unmistakable regardless of when it appears. Indeed, upon close examination, virtually all of the lobotomy reports from this era appear crudely unscientific, comprised of mere clinical anecdotes or simplistic tallies. Without even a hint of good scientific method, there was surely nothing here that would pass the muster of a well-trained investigator. Perhaps the best evidence for this line of argument was provided by Freeman's own example in the late 1950s, when he brought his latest research data to scientific meetings; the summary rejection that his findings elicited is clear proof that those who claimed to have been convinced in the previous decade must have been acting outside the standards of quality science.

The assumed stability of scientific judgment, upon which such characterizations are made, is yet another fallacy. The reason Freeman's findings later seemed so unscientific was not because the facts reported by him had significantly changed, or that the research community had finally come to its senses; rather, the standards and methodology of what constituted valid science had significantly evolved from an earlier stage. It is this inherent instability implicit in the notion of scientific progress that has such dire consequences for the reputations of once esteemed scientists. To admit to this kind of change is to open up the possibility that our medical heroes were not just misinformed, but grossly incompetent, as judged by the latest standards. It is precisely this truth, that science itself is a historical phenomenon, which gave rise to Burlingame's apprehensions, and which the usual parables of scientific discovery work so hard to conceal.

The usual accounts tend to deny this historicity by distorting the record in two seemingly apposite ways. To begin with, they tend to insert temporal discontinuities where none existed, defending the notion that those who later rejected a failed therapy were more like us than were its original supporters. In this way, medicine is separated into cleanly defined epochs of bad and good practices, of ages of dark and then light. Transitions between newer and older are rarely this distinct and total, however. In practice, more continuities exist than we surmise.

In the example before us, the revolution of chloropromazine (CPZ) did not signal an outright break with past psychiatry; there were important continuities between its development and the prior era of psychosurgery.

When CPZ was first introduced, hospital psychiatrists described its beneficial effects through such signs as a noticeable reduction in disturbed
behavior, less destruction to hospital property, better worker morale, a
new therapeutic atmosphere, increased hopefulness in patients and families, and gains in public relations – that is, the very same terms used
previously to promote psychosurgery. Moreover, the framework used by
physicians on the wards to interpret the mode of action of CPZ was often
the same that had been constructed out of their experience with psychosurgery. The new drugs, some doctors explained, were simply a kind of
"chemical lobotomy." Lobotomy programs, furthermore, were not entirely repudiated by the advent of Thorazine. No treatment is successful in
all cases, and some hospitals would still consider lobotomy for those
patients who failed to respond to the pills.[11]

The adoption of the psychoactive drugs by American psychiatry can
also be linked directly to the personnel, facilities, and methods that had
been involved with lobotomy. When officials in New York in 1955, for
example, made the decision to expand the use of CPZ, an innovative
centralized program was set up to coordinate its introduction throughout
the state system. It was placed in the hands of Henry Brill, Pilgrim's
clinical director, who had supervised the largest lobotomy program in the
nation. As another example, the techniques used to establish the drugs'
efficacy had been adapted from those devised to evaluate lobotomy. One
particular study in this era stands out, an investigation sponsored by the
Collaborative Study Group of the NIMH that has since has been described as having signaled "a new era of methodological rigor." The
project, based on a collaborative study of nine hospitals, had as its direct
antecedent the VA cooperative studies that had begun as lobotomy investigations. And the major psychometric test used in this study to evaluate
the drug was none other than the IMPS, the scale designed by Maurice
Lorr specifically to measure the effects of psychosurgery.[12] The easy distinction between good and bad practitioners is not so easily made.

The other tactic found within the traditional accounts is to downplay
the degree of discontinuity between past and present science, an attempt
to establish that practitioners of the day were able to see what we do now
and thus should have known better. This belies several significant ways in
which medical science continually changes, altering the record from one
period to another. First, the very devices used by practitioners and researchers to diagnose or measure the human organism can change at any
time. As argued also in Chapter 7, a dominant reason why the deficits
associated with lobotomy were not paid much heed was not any conspiracy to ignore the scientific facts. Rather, the psychometric tools that
might have gauged these effects had not yet been created. This is one

instance of the generalizable case that every new drug or intervention may change the organism in a way that has not been experienced previously, necessitating the invention of a new kind of or more sensitive measuring device; there exists a coevolution between the introduction of new therapies and the tools necessary to assess them. Physicians may be staring directly at the effects of a new treatment but not yet be able to understand their significance until the tools catch up to the challenge.

Second, and more significantly, the standards of what is considered state-of-the-art scientific method also continuously evolve. Indeed, the assumed foundation of modern medical practice – the double-blind, controlled trial – is far more recent than we think, having become a dominant factor only within the last twenty years. Thus the reason why Freeman looked so unscientific at the end of his career: even by then, substantial changes in the standards of medical practice had occurred.

There is a substantial irony buried within the usual tales of psychosurgery that contrast the unscientific methods of the lobotomists to the scientific standards of their followers. In important ways, the psychopharmaceutical revolution of the late 1950s and early 1960s was dependent upon psychiatrists' ability to execute the kinds of experimental trials expected by peer reviewers at the NIH and the FDA. When the participants in these developments derided the lack of scientific rigor of their predecessors, there was a germ of truth in the comparison. The conclusion that later commentators have drawn from this comparison, however – that the psychiatrists' involvement with lobotomy somehow hindered the forward evolution of the profession – could not be more wrong. As mentioned in Chapter 8, this methodological sophistication of the psychiatrists was, in fact, a recent development. And it was mostly through the profession's confrontation with the clinical issues posed by psychosurgery that prominent psychiatrists became actively engaged in the problems of raising the scientific standards of psychiatric research. Thus, when histories of psychiatry lump all of the proponents of lobotomy into a single group and label them the antithesis of the new scientific psychiatry, they are actually pointing to some of its closest progenitors.

## Reconfiguring the Question

"What could they have possibly been thinking?" is often the first question that comes to mind when examining the actions of those who supported failed therapies such as lobotomy. And just as often it is the last, for it is used as a rhetorical slur, a measure of the contempt we have for those who acted in such an inexplicable manner. The answer is thus already contained in the question.

From today's perspective, it is indeed farfetched that these advocates could have believed such silly ideas, acted with so little restraint, or ignored basic rules of scientific methodology. When it comes to historical accuracy, however, what makes sense now is irrelevant to understanding the motivations and actions of our predecessors. Indeed, in judging these past actors on the basis of *today's* base of knowledge, clinical standards, and scientific methodology, such characterizations commit perhaps the cardinal sin of historical writing – namely, that of inserting anachronisms into the record.

There is certainly nothing wrong with the intellectual pursuit of perceiving connections between current triumphs of medical science and past research or clinical efforts. There is something intuitively satisfying about breaking up these brilliant discoveries into their constituent parts, then digging around in the past for who-got-which-piece-right-when, and putting the jigsaw puzzle back together again. The mistake is in assuming that such endeavors have anything to do with the practice of history, if by this we mean the study of how in the past individuals and circumstances interacted in the production of human events. For our predecessors broke up the world into jigsaw pieces that were differently shaped and fit them together with other sorts of pictures in mind.

To be fair, then, before any judgment can be made about the appropriateness of past medical doctors or researchers – regardless of how outlandish their actions or claims now appear – a considerable amount of historical investigation must first be conducted. At the minimum, this requires a full reconstruction of what was available at the time being studied in the way of facts, theories, instruments, and methodological tools of evaluation; the nature of the daily work performed in the laboratories and clinics; the lines that divided the discipline into various groups and factions; the professional hierarchies that placed on top particular individuals, institutions, and associations; and the social networks that generated ties of trust and loyalty. It also necessitates researching what were considered the primary challenges of the day, as set by the discipline and the larger society; the criteria of success and failure employed at the time; and the rewards, monetary or otherwise, that were thought to lie ahead. Only after this kind of sustained historical effort can a realistic assessment be made as to why certain lines of treatment or research were considered compelling and rational, and others not.

## Contingent to Time

Why a group of researchers and physicians formed the perception that clinical trials of psychosurgery made sense is one question; a separate one, though, is whether or not the treatment was actually viable. In the medicine-as-experimental-science model, a therapy's success ultimately hinges upon what can be determined by laboratory evaluation, the verdict rendered by test-tube reactions and machine printouts. Yet, as a generation of historians and sociologists of medicine has demonstrated, measures of clinical worthiness are not equivalent to such laboratory-based standards as those of length, weight, and power; what is regarded as health and well-being is not something that can be placed under a museum glass as can a meter rod, brass bearing, or amp meter. Thus, a treatment's utility is defined other than by just its inherent physical qualities and is established instead in the fit between a defined need and the particular solution it offers. Much as the evolutionary value of any anatomical structure is contingent upon the nature of a specific environmental challenge, so too are the products of medicine, *functionally* defined, open to continual reassessment whenever the world changes. And insofar as human beings must survive in complex social worlds as well as physiological ones, then in practice the full dimensions of this function escape definition by laboratory attributes alone; the problem of illness extends far beyond the boundary of the skin, representing a disruption in the larger social fabric as well.

Accordingly, the declaration "drug x is a valuable treatment" contains more than the fact that investigators can demonstrate, to a level of near-certainty, that a substance raises or lowers blood acidity. It includes assumptions about the urgency at hand, the acceptability of its risks, the availability of alternatives and their costs, what constitutes a return to health, and other such time-bound factors. When physicians work through the therapeutic calculus, balancing the benefits of a likely treatment against its detriments (often a matter more of salvage than of cure), the answer at which they arrive depends upon the marketplace values of a given moment. Moreover, exactly what is *at stake* in straightening spines, quieting the effects of menopause, or restoring mental well-being is formed within a larger social matrix. A treatment's worth is thus not limited to its effects on individual patients but also incorporates its secondary consequences for the patients' families who have to adapt to its results, the public who indirectly subsidizes its costs, and the physicians and administrators whose reputation it will affect. In short, the viability of a treatment is not a fixed quantity that exists independently of time; it is inextricably woven into the context of the day.

Accordingly, psychosurgery rose to prominence during the 1930s and 1940s for the very reason that it fulfilled a nexus of social, institutional, professional, and disciplinary interests specific to that time. The use of lobotomy subsequently declined because, when these underlying conditions changed, the procedure thereby became less relevant.

In the preceding chapters I have described some of these shifting currents. To wit: when Moniz made his startling claim that the solution to severe mental disturbances was to destroy large portions of the frontal lobes the research community in America was inclined to look favorably upon it for several reasons. To the neurophysiologists and neurological pioneers who had been mapping the frontiers of the brain, psychosurgery offered a unique opportunity for venturing into as yet unknown cerebral structures. Moniz's report also appeared as the first tangible proof of what they had been claiming all along, that developments in neurophysiology would someday pay off in significant clinical gains; indeed, a number of investigators were already exploring the relations between the frontal lobes and the emotions. Moreover, thanks to a reform movement sweeping through the universities and medical schools, as promoted by the calculated largesse of the major philanthropies, this interest was met by investigators in a broad array of disciplines whose work coincided in that portion of the research terrain formed at the intersection of brain and behavior. To a large extent, the belief in the potential of psychosurgery was an expression of the extraordinary faith of the 1930s that the walls between the laboratory and everyday life were finally collapsing.

The ultimate fate of any new treatment rests in the hands of the clinicians in the field. From the perspective of the physicians employed in the nation's vast system of mental hospitals, the innovation of lobotomy was judged to be a worthwhile addition to the therapeutic armamentarium. The considerations they used to reach this decision were not based on an absolute, timeless standard of clinical effectiveness, but a relative one: did this treatment work better than the other treatment options available to them at that specific moment, and if so, was its use preferable to the option of no treatment at all? Their answer was affirmative on both counts. In the experience of these doctors, the brain operations were the first treatment that made any significant change in the behavior of patients with chronic mental illness. They watched with their own eyes as some patients, previously tortured by bitter depressions, were transformed into a state of carefree jocularity, and as others, those once considered permanent residents on the wards, were eventually sent home. To be sure, even lobotomy's most fervent supporters noted that patients "paid a price" in diminished personality and intellect. When, however, these psychiatrists calculated what might befall these patients if no operation were performed, they decided that even a small chance of moderate improvement was better than the certain doom if they remained on the wards. The patients' families tended to agree, insisting that everything possible be done to return their loved ones home.

A treatment may be considered effective, but this does not insure that it will be used often. The importance of a therapy also depends on the *number* of patients for whom it appears appropriate. Consequently, it was hardly automatic that psychosurgery would take off into widespread practice, regardless of how effective it might be considered in the individual case. As a rule, lobotomy was described as a treatment of "last resort," by definition appropriate for a restricted pool of candidates. Thus, perhaps the most important factor in the rapid adoption of the brain operations – and the concomitant excitement they generated within the psychiatric profession – stemmed from the conjunction of historical circumstances that reconfigured this particular niche of medical practice into a problem of great consequence. During the Great Depression and after, patients had streamed into mental hospitals, filling the institutions far past their rated capacity and beyond what the public had been willing to pay for. As a result, hospital administrators were under enormous pressure to free up beds at any cost. At a time when as much as one-third of a state's budget was being spent on mental health care, psychosurgery thus appeared as the first technological solution available for what was becoming a grave social burden.

Lobotomy's importance was further heightened by the perception that a large portion of this growing population of uncured patients were in fact *incurable,* a belief whose origins also may be traced to the circumstances of the time. Ironically, the recent success of the other somatic treatments had raised expectations that the majority of the mentally ill were treatable but also lowered hopes for those patients who had not yet responded. The back wards filled up with countless thousands of individuals who were now seen to have failed in life and also to have failed modern medicine. For these patients who were doubly damned, lobotomy appeared both as a treatment of last resort and as their final hope. Normally, it is expected that the group of patients who fall into the category of last resort would represent a small residuum. This was not the case in psychiatry in the 1940s.

Furthermore, the benefits ascribed to psychosurgery were not limited to the immediate clinical gains observed in an individual patient. Lobotomies were also found to yield visible secondary gains for the institutions that offered them. In rendering the unmanageable more manageable, the brain operations were also discovered to restore order to the wards, a not insignificant matter in the understaffed facilities. Lobotomy programs were also touted by psychiatric leaders as showpieces in their campaign to transform custodial institutions into true hospitals and to upgrade the status of psychiatry as a medical specialty. Psychosurgery was thus valued as an "active" treatment effective both politically and clinically.

Finally, little or no conflict was seen to exist between the interests of the patient, society, and the profession, thanks to the prevailing conception of mental illness. Because of the long association of insanity with hospitalization, the single most important criterion of mental health was whether or not the patient had left the institution. The psychiatrist's primary objective was thus to get patients out of the hospital, by any means available. The recent infusion of the new maladaptive model of mental disorder had conceptualized this task as a matter of resocialization, with the goal of reestablishing an individual's ability to fulfill his or her social duties. Given lobotomy's purported ability to improve a patient's "adjustment" on the wards – and perhaps restore enough functioning to return the patient to an unskilled job if male, or to domestic work if female – the brain operations were thus seen as exactly fulfilling the mission of modern psychiatry.

Given the convergence of such currents, a great deal was found to be at stake in the success of the brain operations, for clinicians, researchers, and hospital administrators. And within the frameworks of the day, whatever it was that psychosurgery did to people was interpreted as an important gain. At multiple levels, psychosurgery worked – then.

The world of the 1950s, however, was already shifting. In neurology and neurophysiology, what once had looked like sophisticated research paled in comparison to more recent methods of exploration. Nobel prizes in the future would go to pioneers studying the physiology of the individual neuron and the subtleties of neurochemistry. Neurosurgeons, for their part, no longer needed to moonlight at state hospitals, having found an ample supply of clinical material in herniated discs, the victims of car accidents, and the tumors of an aging population. The taboo-laden domain of insanity was an area they could now afford to avoid.

From the viewpoint of hospital psychiatrists, the great necessity for the operations was declining. As was already mentioned, with the adoption of the drug therapies the population of patients who might fall into the category of last resort that had been earmarked for lobotomy was shrinking rapidly. And those who did remain on the wards were no longer thought to be in such drastic circumstances as to require immediate, desperate interventions. The campaigns to clean up the "shame of the states" had in fact led to increased state funding and better conditions (at least in the short run); the introduction of separate departments of social work and clinical psychology were additional signs of the easing strains. There was simply less need for active treatments, for the reason that the political campaign to sell psychiatry to the public had been won.

At the same time, less was now at stake in such dramatic therapies as psychosurgery because the battle to establish the state institutions as *medical* centers had been lost. From the perspective of hospital psychiatrists, the fault lay with the enactment of the wrong platform. In Adolf Meyer's vision of the new psychiatry, the world of the mental hospital and that of the academic medical center would one day merge. As it happened, however, the lure of university research and teaching came to overshadow the profession's original base. (The Rockefeller Foundation's deliberate policy of favoring university sites ultimately had undercut the work of those psychiatrists who desired to bring laboratories into the state hospitals.) "In seeking to integrate their specialty with scientific medicine," historian Gerald Grob has astutely observed, "psychiatrists were unaware that their efforts would lead them to modify their commitment to institutional care."[13]

Even as hospital administrators celebrated the arrival of the drug therapies into the wards, they decried the limited opportunities for medical research in the institutions. Their bitterest complaint, however, was their inability to convince young physicians to choose a career in hospital psychiatry. In the 1940s, the highest priority for a state hospital that styled itself progressive was to expand its residency program and to upgrade its status into a full three-year training site. (Hospitals often proved their readiness by establishing psychosurgery programs, which were viewed then as very sophisticated medical endeavors.) When the future finally arrived in the mid-1950s, hospital administrators were dumbfounded by a reversal of circumstances. The residency positions they had fought so hard to establish went unfilled. The only applicants were foreign-trained recent immigrants hoping to continue a career in medicine, even if it meant starting over again in the profession's cellar – which, at this time, was the state mental hospital.

At every level, psychiatry was moving away from its legacy of institutional care, and with this change the professional interest that once had promoted lobotomy was dissipating. The state hospital, Harry Solomon declared in his 1958 presidential address to the APA, was "antiquated, outmoded, and rapidly becoming obsolete." Administrators such as Robert Hunt were scandalized by this public airing of psychiatry's woes. He went so far as to deliver a scathing attack on Solomon at a private APA meeting. The problem, he outlined, was the pervasive stereotype of mental hospitals as places devoid of contact with medicine. Hunt saw two major threats. First, the drift away from the institutions he blamed on the likes of Mike Gorman and Albert Deutsch, populists who had carried the flag for GAP and its vision of a community-based psychiatry. Second, the plain reality was that a new image of the profession had supplanted the old:

public understanding of psychiatry now meant "the psychotherapy of one patient on a couch."[14]

Hunt's fears were well-founded. Grob has also recently described how, in the decades that followed World War II, a new era of mental health policy was germinating. In the previous century, the care of the mentally ill had been revolutionized when the states replaced the local townships as the major providers. In the modern postwar era, the national government superseded the role of the states, and the impetus shifted to federally funded community mental health centers. The new orientation was toward social psychiatry and preventative medicine; the belief was that community programs would so improve the mental health of the nation that asylums would become obsolete. At the same time, hospitals became the focus of withering critiques, such as that of sociologist Erving Goffman, whose landmark book *Asylums* (1961) turned the resocialization on the wards upside down. Patients in institutions, he argued, learned patterns of behavior that only further isolated them from normal living. Hospitals were no longer part of the solution, just more of a problem. Thus abandoned by the public, the profession, and academic leaders, the stage was set for the eventual deconstruction of the hospital system.

Hunt's second observation was also on target. In terms of clinical philosophy and practice, the most dramatic shift to occur in postwar psychiatry was clearly that of the turn to individual, psychoanalytically oriented psychotherapy. With the new emphasis on the academic basis of psychiatry, analysts took up residence in the university medical centers, thereby extending their reach over the growing army of social workers and clinical psychiatrists. The ranks of the analytic community swelled to meet the surging public and professional demand for psychotherapy.[15]

The relocation of the traditional center of the profession away from the state mental hospital to the individual consulting room profoundly affected every facet of American psychiatry – even altering at its core the public's understanding of what constituted mental health and of what looked like useful therapy. In particular, success in psychiatry no longer was defined solely in terms of discharging a person from a mental hospital to take up a role as taxpayer or keeper of the household. Rather, citizens who sought psychiatrists for psychotherapy were dissatisfied with their lives, hoping for more. Attainment of individual achievement – the era of "self-actualization" – was ushered in. In effect, the standard of mental health had changed from the stereotype of what a blue-collar citizen (the typical resident of the state hospitals) might want out of life to the upper-middle-class aspirations of the new clientele. A treatment like psychosurgery – which permanently lowered a patient's capacity to be all he or she could putatively be, and which was inextricably linked to the profession's institutional legacy – stuck out as incompatible with the new psychiatric worldview.

The internal changes within the field of psychiatry were further exacerbated by the deeply rooted political realignments then under way in America that eventually led to a reexamination of the psychiatrist's traditional social role. Here too the changes would bode ill for the future of lobotomy. As I have described earlier, psychiatry in the United States was in large measure originally constructed on Meyer's framework of maladjustment, a naturalistic model in which society's forward evolution depended upon the ability of each citizen to perform his or her respective duties. Of all medical specialists, it thus became the psychiatrist's primary responsibility to refit citizens to their tasks in life, delicately subordinating the interests of the individual to the demands of society. But in the reexaminations of 1960s politics, the faith that society's health was necessarily a higher priority than that of the individual was severely tested, and in the process the psychiatrist's primary social function was open to redefinition. As put by psychiatrist R. D. Laing, an often cited spokesman for the new criticism, "Psychiatry could be . . . on the side of transcendence, of genuine freedom, and of true human growth," yet "psychiatry can so easily be a technique of brainwashing, of inducing behaviour that is adjusted." He continued, "our 'normal', 'adjusted' state is too often the abdication of ecstasy, the betrayal of our true potentialities, so that many of us are only too successful in acquiring a false self to adapt to false realities."[16] I'm okay, you're okay – it's the world that's all screwed up. What had once been considered lobotomy's major asset – its celebrated ability to readjust citizens to modern life – was now a political liability.

By the 1980s, the future of psychiatry in America looked very different than it had in the 1930s. In the earlier period, psychiatric leaders had invested their hopes in the notion that a single medical expert might lay claim to the world of the seriously mentally ill as well as that of the worried neurotic, to the domain of consciousness as well as that of brain physiology, to the function of offering personal advice as well as that of performing laboratory research. Indeed, this unified vision, derived from Meyer's monistic doctrine of psychobiology, was used as a blueprint for many of the nation's premier psychiatric programs. The institutions at the vanguard of the new psychiatry in America (namely, The Institute of the Pennsylvania Hospital, The Institute of Living, Boston Psychopathic, The Menninger Foundation, and McLean Hospital) all vigorously espoused the new psychobiological agenda in which psychoanalysis and neurophysiology coexisted. It was no mere coincidence, nor a contradiction, that these same institutions offered brain operations alongside psychoanalysis. Lobotomy programs – an interdisciplinary endeavor that linked research with treatment, and the study of the brain with that of the emotions and intellect – were thus looked upon as a prime example of what modern-day psychiatry was all about.

A half-century later, however, the commitment to a unified psychiatric profession had withered away and the psychiatric domain splintered once again into a set of separatist camps, none of which had any further use for the brain operations. For those professionals who now worked entirely within the psychotherapeutic or community mental health model, psychosurgery certainly had little to offer to their particular clients. Its indirect benefits as a symbol of psychobiology also were no longer valued; this professional group had largely disavowed the notion that its own future was somehow joined to that of its colleagues in the laboratory. And at the other end of the spectrum, the laboratory-based neuropsychiatrists were all too happy to jettison yesteryear's concern with finding solutions to the immediate clinical problems in the state hospitals. An option which, thanks to generous NIMH funding, was now available.

In short, what were once the many compelling attractions of psychosurgery were reevaluated. The kinds of research opportunities presented by lobotomy no longer appealed to the community of scientists who once had gambled their careers upon it. The great need targeted by the operations had receded in parallel with the appearance of an alternative therapy. The secondary gains it once had offered the institutions either had vanished or were irrelevant. The new major concern of the profession was with a very different set of clinical problems. And the kinds of changes lobotomy produced in the individual were now viewed within a very different set of frames, and were interpreted as undesirable. The treatment thus came to symbolize the ideology of the discipline's past, seen now as a hindrance to future progress.

As a solution to the general problems confronting American psychiatry, psychosurgery no longer was viable. It had drifted in with the tide, and then it drifted out.

### But Did It Work?

Notwithstanding its temporary success in the medical marketplace, was lobotomy at any time actually effective for individual patients? In retrospect, what is our final judgment about those physicians in the 1940s who thought psychosurgery was the most appropriate choice of therapy for their own clients – were they right or wrong? In the final analysis, *did it work*?

At first impression this issue seems simple enough, a matter best left in the hands of present-day scientists to resolve, not historians. Establishing whether or not a treatment worked in the past, one may assume, is most easily determined by assessing its effectiveness today. For science, if anything, is contextless in its verdicts. (Indeed, it is the core principle of *ceteris paribus* – Latin for "other things being equal" – that provides scientists with their unique powers of generalization.)[17] Scientific findings automatically extend vertically and horizontally, across time as well as space. Thus, in synthesizing a compound, it makes no difference if a chemist performs the work in Bombay or New York, or in 1996 as opposed to 1942, so long as the laboratories are properly equipped and the same formulary is exactly followed. Everything is interchangeable. Derivative of this, within the laboratory-science model of medical practice, it is not just the medicaments that are thought to be standardized and fungible but the physicians and patients as well. When done right, the matching of treatment to disease proceeds in a manner similar to that of selecting the right chemical reagent for a desired product, in that it follows the guidelines of a standardized formula, the details of which make no mention of the specific identity of the individuals involved, or of any particular geographic locations in which the work is to be done. This kind of localized information – the stuff of historical inquiry – is simply considered not relevant.

But it is, very much so. Once again, the persistent habit of viewing medicine as a form of applied science has distorted our understanding of the complex nature of medical practice – as it was in the past or even as it functions today. In contrast to what is usually assumed, it has been argued in this monograph that what works in medicine is not an abstract, universal quality that transcends when and where. Rather, it is contingent upon the local circumstances in which physicians practice, characteristics that vary in place as well as time. The matter of judging the treatment decisions of physicians in the past thus becomes something for historical and not just scientific inquiry. When approached in this manner, new and different readings will be formed about what it means to be a physician.

To begin with, even in our own age of scientific medicine there are no easy recipes for success comparable to those found in chemistry. Human suffering is not something that appears in the well-controlled environs of the laboratory where a few variables at a time can be isolated, monitored, and manipulated at will. Indeed, the medical handbooks that specify which treatment to use for a particular condition are useful only to a point, as the recommendations refer to ideal-type patients, not to the kinds that walk in clinic doors or reside on hospital wards. There are no standardized patients as there are standardized weights or screws. Moreover, patients do not arrive prelabeled in the way reagents appear on a scientist's shelf, but have occult, heterogeneous qualities that can only be inferred. Some diseases and treatments, to be sure, do extend across virtually all peoples in similar ways. These are the exceptions, however. Physicians try the best they can to routinize their treatment decisions by developing indices – such as age, white-cell count, or blood pressure – that might hold true from place to place. Yet here, too, the complications posed by human variation and the intrusion of unforeseen or hidden variables tend to defeat such tactics. It is an uncomfortable fact of medical life that every encounter with a patient in itself constitutes a unique problem that is never fully generalizable to any other situation – past, present, or future.

This complex business of clinical decision making was explored in Chapter 6, through a re-creation of how physicians went about selecting lobotomy patients at a single institution, in this case McLean Hospital. It was found that such medical decisions are made in the juncture of what is learned, on the one hand, from scientific textbooks (which offer knowledge in the form of abstract generalized cases), and of what is gleaned, on the other hand, from the experience of personally treating a series of individual patients. To manage this difficult task of matching a specific patient to the right treatment, physicians thus work up what were termed *clinical frames:* a heuristic device that serves as a practical guidebook for care, tailored to fit the local medical ecology in which the physician plies his or her trade. Such frames necessarily reflect the interactions among the characteristics of the population native to that area, the range of therapeutic options locally available, and what are perceived as urgent problems – there. The tools of medical practice thus are not universally portable, but must be recalibrated with each shift in location. In short, the challenge of medicine is dissimilar to that of laboratory science, as no universal formulas can fully apply to the patient sitting in front of the doctor.

It was also emphasized that the kinds of variables that go into the clinical frame extend beyond a physiological understanding of the human body. The adept physician is also necessarily skilled at reading the social matrix, at understanding how the world in all its messy complexity works. For whether or not a treatment will be deemed successful for a given individual often depends on the circumstances of his or her employment, the demands of the domestic situation, personal aversions, and the like. At the same time, it was noted that the consequences of the decision to follow a particular course of treatment often involve extremely personal choices, heavily laden with individual values and morals; the matter of being a doctor inescapably involves consideration of factors often considered external to the proper business of medicine.

The distance from the original analogy to laboratory practice thus widens. Because every individual is comprised of a singular combination of physiology, social identity, and personal values, in effect *each patient constitutes a unique experiment.* Did the physician make the right choice for Mrs. Blythedale? It is often hard if not impossible to know the answer to such questions, as the experiment is not exactly repeatable. Moreover, as every doctor is ultimately responsible for constructing his or her own set of clinical frames, the end result is a uniquely determined product, representing individual talents, perspectives, values, and experiences. It is thus no contradiction that two different physicians can reasonably disagree about what is the best course of treatment for the same patient; or that two patients who otherwise match in exact physiological condition might receive two different treatment recommendations from the same physician. This kind of indeterminacy is not something usually associated with science.

This is not to argue that what works in medicine is a wholly relativistic quality. To the contrary, it is precisely the integration of knowledge of how the physical world works, seen through the filter of laboratory science, and taking into account the need to meet social strictures that makes medicine such a special challenge. In this, I want to suggest that the work of a physician is more akin to that of an architect than that of a physicist. In architecture, it is evident, buildings that do not adhere to the universal laws of physics will collapse, regardless of how aesthetically pleasing they are. Yet, as any architect knows all too well, it is equally true that buildings must also correspond to the realities of the local marketplace, conforming to the vagaries of human convention.

At a fundamental level, then, the challenges facing physicians as they go about their daily work are dissimilar to those facing the applied scientist, requiring a very different set of talents and temperaments. To fit the immediate clinical problem into the preexisting body of knowledge and experience that might be applicable, doctors must have a special mental flexibility allowing them to shift back and forth between the general law and the particular case; emotionally, they must also be willing to make fateful decisions on the basis of often incomplete or uncertain knowledge. And, as what works in medicine is often dependent upon the social context in which the patients are located, physicians cannot remain cloistered within the inner world of science but must also understand how the extramural world functions in all its complexity. Lastly, the task of constructing a treatment plan that is consistent with the values and expectations of a particular patient is not something that is decided through statistics or blood tests but has to be resolved using the personal resources of maturity and conscience. In sum, good medicine necessarily incorporates science, yet it also involves the clinical arts – in their most positive sense of intuition, craft, worldliness, and wisdom. And with the practice of medicine so deeply rooted in such human qualities, linear scales of progress become inappropriate or hard to define. Perhaps it is not so easy to judge our clinical forebears, after all.

## Psychosurgery in Context

Taken together, these reconsiderations lead to a new perspective from which to approach the rise and fall of medical innovations such as psychosurgery. It is now possible to solve the original puzzle, which was generated in the spectacle of the disagreement between past and present practitioners over the effectiveness of a given therapy. In short, the rift between then and now is revealed to be an artifact produced in the erroneous belief that medicine is a version of applied science. For within this model, efficacy is considered an absolute quality that exists independently of time and place, an attribute wholly inherent to the treatment itself; the historical subjects to be studied are thus divided up into good and bad ones, in the belief that separate kinds of narratives must apply. What results is an ahistorical, curiously static view of the past. Even before the historical investigations have begun, the essential narrative line has been formed, labeling some actors as virtuous and others as malevolent; and in fixing the matter of utility within the object, there is no room for the possibility of change. Here, then, is the source of the contradictions and confusions evident in the literature on psychosurgery. In contrast, a *contextual* reading implies that what works in medical practice reflects the particular circumstances of the time. Efficacy is not an inherent attribute, but is a functional quality produced in the fit between a treatment's action and the nature of the problem targeted at the time; and it is assessed using particular frames, which are themselves products of a historical time and place. The disjunction between past and present evaluations of lobotomy resulted, then, from shifts in the kinds of functions it was asked to perform, and in the overall frames from which it was being observed. As the world changed, so too did the environment and the frameworks.

Burlingame was right to worry about how he and his illustrious colleagues would be regarded in the future, for medical wisdom does not stand still, and neither does the world in general. In time, even the best of medical practices of today will eventually look outdated, perhaps inappropriate, and maybe even inhumane. At some point ahead, new knowledge will appear that will undermine the confidence once held in routine practices; different theories and modes of thought will come into favor; additional treatments will be devised that will render prior ones obsolete; and scientific methodology will be revamped, bringing about wholesale changes even in what is considered valid science. Concurrently, the kinds of health problems that individuals and society attend to will shift into other areas of concern; what is funded by institutions, agencies, or reimbursement plans will change; and different kinds of outcomes will be expected, valued, or tolerated. Also, dramatic changes in the social fabric may eventually work their way through the system, focusing attention on ethical or political considerations in treatment decisions that previously went unchallenged.

Some of these factors may change slowly, others fast; all interact together, creating waves that at first impel the use of a treatment and then recede. (Most therapies in fact do not stop abruptly, suddenly being deemed ineffective, but simply fade away.) Eventually, the medical practices that once made such good sense no longer will. Later observers will look back and wonder why the medical practitioners of the past did not know better. The answer is not found just in textbooks or publications, but in the richly woven context of the times. In short, what works in medicine is not simply about what we can do in bending nature to our will; it also concerns who we are.

## Conclusion: Medicine and Tragedy

In going about their work, historians, too, interweave the particular and the general. Seen from one perspective, this book is thus an intensive case study of the rise and fall of a single medical innovation, how at a particular moment of great social need medical research was recruited to provide a hopeful answer. From another viewpoint, it is also an extended musing on how we *tell* our stories of triumph and failure in science, and how we then use these lessons from history as a way of bracing for the future when such future needs arise.

"Prefrontal lobotomy," Walter Freeman and James Watts declared, "is the last resort, the end of the line."[18] The decision to operate was a measure of just how desperate things had become for the patients. "Most of all," Freeman and Watts continued, "they are failures in the place deep down where they live, unable to get along with themselves, harassed by doubts, fears, depression, suicidal ideas." Hope had also been lost that the usual methods of treatment might lead to further improvement. The determination that a particular patient was in special need of a treatment of last resort thus arose out of the grim confluence of two beliefs: first, that an impasse had been reached; and second, that such an impasse was unacceptable. In the clash of these two assessments, the usual rules of doing business in medicine no longer seemed to apply. Extreme risks became acceptable, disturbing side effects appeared bearable, and the achievement of even small gains was magnified in importance. The extraordinary became routine.

The case of psychosurgery was by no means the last time that psychiatrists faced a choice between letting a patient continue on as he or she was or, alternatively, placing hope in an uncertain new medical technology. An argument can be made that, even today, virtually *all* of psychiatry's severely impaired clients are already in a category of last resort. For psychiatry is a field defined not by reference to a specific part of the human body, like podiatry, or to a class of people, like gerontology, or even to a disease process, like oncology. Rather, it is a field demarcated by our collective helplessness in the face of problems that, to all appearances, should be solvable through medical science but as yet are not. (As in the case of syphilis and paresis, or vitamin deficiency and pellagrous insanity, at the precise moment when a psychiatric condition becomes fully explained by a somatic cause, both the disease and the patients are shifted to the province of a different specialty.) Put simply, psychiatry is the management of despair. This is the heart of the psychiatrist's social function: to care for those whose problems have no certain cure or satisfactory explanation. Hence, what comprises mental illness is fundamentally a moving target, a hazy area that is redrawn by every generation and local culture as new dilemmas arise.[19]

It is not just psychiatrists, of course, who must deal with such grim choices on a daily basis. At some point all physicians reach their limit, stymied by the problem in front of them. They too will have to decide if the time has come to reach for a desperate remedy, bringing to bear the latest weapon to emerge from the laboratory or clinic. The challenges facing the psychiatrists in the present story are thus fundamentally no different from those in any other area in medicine, past or present. Whether it is a cancer victim undergoing drastic chemotherapy, or a parent wondering if ritalin is appropriate for his kid, or an AIDS patient gambling on the latest designer protease, all face essentially the same kind of situation. They look to medical authority for guidance on what to do next.

In 1946, the mother of a schizophrenic daughter sought advice from Winfred Overholser, the director of a prestigious insane asylum. "I am trying to get the opinion of some outstanding doctors on the subject of lobotomy," her letter began. Already by the age of twenty-two, the daughter had been in and out of numerous institutions. Her condition had only worsened, even after trials of insulin and electric shock. The psychiatrists previously consulted had split into two camps. One group suggested a halt to the aggressive therapies, letting nature (and noninvasive psycho-therapy) take its course; the other camp, fearing that the daughter might sink further, thought instead that the right action was "to push on and see what else if anything can be done to help her." The mother explained to Overholser that she thus found herself "between 2 fires." She closed her letter with the poignant query, "I have been told that lobotomy operations should be considered a last resort but when does one reach the point when they consider they should use the last resort?"[20]

When indeed? Since the time of Hippocrates, we all know, the prime directive of medicine has been to "do no harm." If truth be told, however, physicians have always found themselves pincered between this and its opposite demand, the obligation – even in the face of hopeless odds – to "do something." Or, in the words of Harvard psychiatrist Harry Sol-omon, the physician's main responsibility "is to lead to improvement, not to become nihilistic because cure is not complete."[21] Thus beholden to the unruly duo of caution and bold intervention, physicians have looked to various systems of science and logic, belief and intuition, and ethics and values, to guide them in their difficult decisions. Sometime in the middle of the twentieth century, however, it is generally believed that this messy, haphazard process was regularized through the advent of controlled clini-cal trials, which provided the first truly defensible means of sorting the wheat from the chaff in therapeutics.

Unfortunately, this comforting image vastly overestimates the capa-bilities of modern medicine. Too much attention to those instances when science proved right has, over the years, led us to credit medical practi-tioners and investigators with fabulous talents and insights. We place great trust in their ability to foresee which avenue of research should be funded and which drug should enter clinical trials; to steer us to the therapy that offers the best hope of cure and the least chance of side effects; and to devise timely new remedies if one is not yet immediately available. These are all lovely, uplifting sentiments; but they often prove unfounded, for there are no guarantees in any of these activities. Science, it has been said, is a form of organized gambling. Investment of precious resources in a particular direction of research may indeed pay off in great success. However, as researchers do not have any special gift of foresight, it could just as well fail, ruining careers and laboratories in the process. More than a decade ago, for example, prominent scientists declared that an AIDS vaccine would be found shortly, and they were believed. Nor can trusted medical authorities know with any degree of certainty if a patient is best advised to wager on the available treatments or, instead, to hold out for what might lie ahead. In 1954, for illustration, in one of the first articles on chloropromazine, the authors noted its startling success with a patient who just recently had been considered in need of a treatment of last resort. "A lobotomy had been proposed but was rejected by her family," they noted, "who had more faith than we did."[22]

The constant retelling of such success stories has also diverted our attention away from the hazards always present in medicine and science. Indeed, the introduction of new kinds of therapies periodically results in the appearance of unforeseen dangers – hazards of a kind which previously were not even considered remotely possible. The medical literature is thus studded with moments of great tragedy, as when thalidomide led to birth defects or oxygen tents for premature babies induced permanent blindness. And, just yesterday, a promising new drug for hepatitis, fialuridine, was administered in a state-of-the-art clinical trial that boasted of every conceivable control and safety check. Massive liver failures and multiple deaths ensued nonetheless, terminating the study. The point is that such hidden land mines are not always detectable in advance. Science cannot be made accident-free; some measure of tragedy is inescapable.[23]

Of course, every now and then a failure does come to light. Yet, as I have argued throughout this book, the narrative forms that are typically applied to these unfortunate events do not substantially challenge our cheery illusions about biomedical progress. In fact, they reinforce them. That a particular mode of treatment crashed and burned is thus blamed not on any deficiencies inherent in the general process of medical advance but on the few participants in charge who pursued a course the pitfalls of which were obvious; the proximate cause of any and all such disasters is simply labeled pilot error, and filed away. My central aim in revisiting the story of psychosurgery has been to underscore the shortcomings of these narratives of blame.

Not all such stories are fictitious. There are indeed many occasions when scientists or physicians have acted irresponsibly, causing tremendous harm. This much is undeniable. Nevertheless, the lessons that have been selected from such accounts are not. As story after story of this kind has accumulated, in which bad medical practice or scientific research was followed by a conspicuous disaster, it has seemed prudent to presume a causal link: if smoke appears, it is because someone earlier must have started a fire. Thus, whenever a previously unrecognized medical calamity has come to light, the first place investigators have looked for its root causes is in this area of personal malfeasance, the instances when the participants must have strayed from the standards of good biomedicine. The other major lesson deduced from this model looks forward, not backward. The success of avoiding future such failures, history appears to teach, comes down to the extent to which scientists and physicians can be made to act responsibly.

In actuality, these kinds of stories instruct neither group. These deductions, which are based on a unidirectional causal model, simply cannot be made from this kind of limited data. For what is missing, as the scientists might say, are the necessary control cases. Perhaps a thousand instances can be found when biomedicine done badly led to the introduction of a procedure that turned out to be bad. Nonetheless, it would be wrong to conclude from this that the causal relationship is either sufficient or certain. There is nothing here that pertains to the likelihood that staying within the boundaries of proper scientific medicine will prevent similar disasters, or that allows one to deduce, from the mere fact that a widely used or investigated therapy becomes a notorious failure, that previously anyone did anything wrong. Yet such inferences are applied time and time again, almost reflexively, whenever stories like that of lobotomy arise.

The major significance of the psychosurgery story, I suggest, lies exactly in its value as this kind of historical control case. From its example – and from others out there like it – evidence begins to accumulate that contradicts the automatic deductions of the standard model. It appears increasingly likely, therefore, that medical scientists and practitioners who were involved in the development of a therapy that failed might have acted substantially no differently than their colleagues who were proponents of more positive ventures. The argument weakens, then, that the reason these treatments succeeded was because their advocates acted correctly. And, as the artificial barriers have been removed that once automatically separated good therapies from bad ones, there is no longer any reason to tell their stories separately. By and large, the story of psychosurgery has been interpreted as a routine example of an anomaly in medicine, another case of a worthless therapy being allowed to flourish; the story is thus held to be applicable only to other such anomalies. The strategy in this book, however, has been to look upon such events as a unique opportunity to examine the normal process of general medicine, moving the story from the periphery to the mainstream, where it is applicable everywhere.

How then *do* we confront the past? And how do we face the future? There is no clear moral here, other than that we must rethink the usual habits by which we parcel out praise and blame in medicine and medical science.[24] Scientists can be skilled or incompetent; they are also, it now seems, lucky or unlucky. Furthermore, there is no simple way to separate past villains from heroes without extensive historical investigation; this is not something that can be directly deduced from current perceptions. Any practitioner, regardless of his or her medical or scientific virtues, can one day end up looking quite foolish indeed. For there is no sure shield against future advances in knowledge, no bulwark that can stand against the changing circumstances of the world in which medical practices are judged. This is not to excuse instances of negligence or malicious conduct, but to remind us not to delude ourselves, either, into thinking that we ourselves are exempt from the historical process. Scapegoating our predecessors by presuming, whenever they engaged in medical practices that look dubious to us today, that such conduct must have resulted from bad science or immorality is not a helpful policy. Not only is it egregiously unfair to the original actors, but it instills a false sense of security and draws our attention even further away from dangers that are actually present.

In sum, in contrast to the lessons that have been customarily taught, there is no guarantee against a repetition of the kind of horror and tragedy associated today with the story of psychosurgery. *Medical science and practice done right is not enough.* Vigilance, of course, will always be necessary. But so too is humility – on the part of the participants in science as well as its observers.

Today when we confront circumstances similar to those which faced the lobotomists, will we make any wiser decisions? The headlines of our newspapers report the same kinds of situations that arose fifty years ago. "Surgery for Parkinson's Brings Success Stories in Face of Skepticism," reports a recent issue of the *Wall Street Journal,* under the banner "Hope from a Knife."[25] In considering the latest advance in the mechanical heart or treatment for hypertension, will we make better, more informed choices? In so doing, will we avoid facing the kinds of charges typically leveled at those who advocated psychosurgery? Only this is clear: the answer to present predicaments is not to be found on the microscope slide or in a statistical t-test, but in our hearts and minds, and in the dialogue between physicians and their patients as they decide *what works best for them.* In other words, to persist in the belief that medical practice must always have conformed to the ideals of laboratory science is to do a disservice to the practitioners of the past. And to insist on this ideal at present is also to do a serious disservice to ourselves; for it denies the very human elements that comprise medical practice, as well as the crucial part of it that remains an art. These lessons are too important to be ignored.

# Appendix

Statistical Portrait of Psychosurgery at McLean Hospital,
1938–1954

Table A.1. *Profile of Psychosurgery Patients at McLean Hospital,*
*1938–1954*

|  | Female | Male | All |
|---|---|---|---|
| *Lobotomy patients* | | | |
| Count | 66.0 | 14.0 | 80.0 |
| Percentage | 82.5 | 17.5 | 100.0 |
| *Age at operation* | | | |
| Mean | 50.1 | 45.9 | 49.4 |
| Median | 50.5 | 48.5 | 49.5 |
| *Length of stay, this admission (years)* | | | |
| Mean | 3.3 | 6.2 | 3.8 |
| Median | 1.2 | 3.0 | 1.3 |
| *Length of stay, all prior admissions (years)* | | | |
| Mean | 4.6 | 8.0 | 5.2 |
| Median | 1.8 | 6.6 | 2.1 |

*Source:* McLean Hospital, Belmont, Massachusetts.

Appendix

Table A.2. *Profile of All Residents at McLean Hospital on 1 January 1948*

|  | Female | Male | All |
|---|---|---|---|
| *Residents* | | | |
| Count | 133.0 | 62.0 | 195.0 |
| Percentage | 68.2 | 31.8 | 100.0 |
| *Age in 1948* | | | |
| Mean | 59.1 | 53.6 | 57.4 |
| Median | 61.0 | 54.5 | 60.0 |
| *Length of stay, this admission (years)* | | | |
| Mean | 8.6 | 7.6 | 8.3 |
| Median | 4.5 | 2.4 | 3.7 |
| *Length of stay, all prior admissions (years)* | | | |
| Mean | 10.3 | 9.7 | 10.1 |
| Median | 5.4 | 3.6 | 4.7 |

*Source:* McLean Hospital, Belmont, Massachusetts.

Table A.3. *Hospitalization Patterns of Patients in Residence at McLean Hospital on 1 January 1948. Percentage of Total Bed-Days Occupied by Each Sex during the Calendar Year, by Diagnosis; with Calculated Relative Ratios of Bed-Days (%) to Residents (%). (Total Female Bed-Days = 37,100, Male Bed-Days = 14,055; Female Residents = 133, Male = 62.)*

| Diagnosis | Bed-Days (%) | Residents (%) | Ratio |
|---|---|---|---|
| *Females* | | | |
| Paranoid schiz. | 28.9 | 25.6 | 1.13 |
| Senile | 17.3 | 15.0 | 1.15 |
| Manic-depressive | 16.1 | 16.5 | 0.97 |
| Catatonic schiz. | 11.3 | 11.3 | 1.01 |
| Paranoia | 6.1 | 5.3 | 1.15 |
| Involutional | 5.3 | 6.0 | 0.88 |
| Unspecified schiz. | 4.1 | 5.3 | 0.77 |
| Hebephrenic schiz. | 3.1 | 3.0 | 1.03 |
| Neuroses | 2.9 | 5.3 | 0.54 |
| Psychopathic | 2.4 | 2.3 | 1.06 |
| Organic | 2.0 | 2.3 | 0.90 |
| Other | 0.3 | 0.8 | 0.40 |
| Substance abuse | 0.2 | 1.5 | 0.13 |
| *Males* | | | |
| Hebephrenic schiz. | 17.4 | 11.3 | 1.54 |
| Senile | 16.1 | 14.5 | 1.11 |
| Manic-depressive | 14.4 | 16.1 | 0.89 |
| Paranoid schiz. | 14.2 | 11.3 | 1.26 |
| Organic | 11.8 | 8.1 | 1.46 |
| Neuroses | 8.1 | 12.9 | 0.63 |
| Catatonic schiz. | 6.5 | 8.1 | 0.81 |
| Other | 4.9 | 3.2 | 1.50 |
| Unspecified schiz. | 2.6 | 1.6 | 1.61 |
| Substance abuse | 2.2 | 8.1 | 0.27 |
| Psychopathic | 1.3 | 3.2 | 0.41 |
| Involutional | 0.7 | 1.6 | 0.42 |

*Source:* McLean Hospital, Belmont, Massachusetts.

*Appendix*

Table A.4. *Profile of Patients Admitted to McLean Hospital during 1948*

|  | Female | Male | All |
|---|---|---|---|
| *New Admissions* | | | |
| Count | 169.0 | 134.0 | 303.0 |
| Percentage | 55.8 | 44.2 | 100.0 |
| *Age in 1948* | | | |
| Mean | 46.6 | 43.6 | 45.3 |
| Median | 44.0 | 44.0 | 44.0 |

*Source:* McLean Hospital, Belmont, Massachusetts.

Table A.5. *McLean Hospital 1948. Comparison of Patients Admitted during the 1948 Calendar Year with Those in Residence on 1 January 1948, Diagnosis by Sex, with Calculated Ratio of Admissions to Residents (Excluding Diagnoses w/Admissions ≥ 5). Admissions n=298: 165 Females, 133 males; Residents n=184: 125 females, 59 males.)*

| Diagnosis | Admissions | Residents | Ratio |
|---|---|---|---|
| *Female* | | | |
| Paranoid schiz. | 15 | 34 | 0.44 |
| Catatoic schiz. | 11 | 15 | 0.73 |
| Paranoia | 6 | 7 | 0.86 |
| Senile | 19 | 20 | 0.95 |
| Unspecified schiz. | 10 | 7 | 1.43 |
| Involutional | 15 | 8 | 1.88 |
| Manic-depressive | 41 | 22 | 1.86 |
| Organic | 7 | 3 | 2.33 |
| Neuroses | 22 | 7 | 3.14 |
| Substance abuse | 19 | 2 | 9.50 |
| *Male* | | | |
| Senile | 5 | 9 | 0.56 |
| Hebephrenic schiz. | 6 | 7 | 0.86 |
| Paranoid schiz. | 11 | 7 | 1.57 |
| Catatonic schiz. | 8 | 5 | 1.60 |
| Neuroses | 14 | 8 | 1.75 |
| Organic | 10 | 5 | 2.00 |
| Manic-depressive | 24 | 10 | 2.40 |
| Psychopathic | 6 | 2 | 3.00 |
| Substance abuse | 34 | 5 | 6.80 |
| Unspecified schiz. | 10 | 1 | 10.00 |
| Paranoia | 5 | 0 | – |

*Source:* McLean Hospital, Belmont, Massachusetts.

448

## Appendix

### Codes of Patients and Physicians Cited in Chapters 3 and 6

| Patient Pseudonym | Code | Patient Pseudonym | Code |
|---|---|---|---|
| Regina Allen | PT11 | Emily Marr | PT341 |
| Abigal Banks | PT406 | Rosemary Merrill | PT228 |
| Catharine Birmingham | PT494 | Elizabeth Moorehouse | PT486 |
| William Brandford | PT374 | Mary Montero | PT244 |
| Jane L. Bremerton | PT138 | Maria Mulcahy | PT265 |
| Everett Daniels | PT139 | Claire Mulvahill | PT420 |
| Annete Draper | PT207 | Clara Northrup | PT119 |
| Joseph Eyler | PT602 | Miriam O'Connor | PT56 |
| Grace Farmer | PT462 | Harriet Palmer | PT461 |
| Jeanette Fehr | PT618 | Howard Peckler | PT434 |
| George Flannagan | PT13 | Robert Parkhurst | PT505 |
| Chauncey Fowler | PT610 | Anita Payne | PT363 |
| Fay Francis | PT120 | Gladys Randall | PT158 |
| Laura Gibbons | PT256 | Heloise Ann Rathburn | PT483 |
| Elizabeth Hanley | PT248 | Annabel Simms | PT609 |
| Adelaide Hitchcock | PT61 | Dora Singer | PT602 |
| Lenora Hutchins | PT266 | Anne Smith | PT165 |
| Ruth Ignatius | PT174 | Helen Stoddard | PT288 |
| Prudence Kinsella | PT93 | Pauline Stanton | PT129 |
| Frances Lee | PT39 | Helaine Strauss | PT394 |
| Kay Levitt | PT71 | Mary Sullivan | PT61 |
| Judith Loewy | PT185 | Eliza Wigglesworth | PT429 |
| Martha Loomis Jenkins | PT36 | Anna Winthrop | PT8 |
| Eleanor Lowell | PT35 | Hilary Wise | PT413 |
| | | Sarah Worthington | PT200 |

| Physician Pseudonym | Code | Physician Pseudonym | Code |
|---|---|---|---|
| William Addison | PH15 | Daniel Maddox | PH8 |
| Elliot Austin | PH3 | Donald Malenfant | PH13 |
| Herbert Averbuck | PH2 | Eugene Murphy | PH4 |
| Jackson Boyle | PH22 | Mitchell Norcross | PH16 |
| Arthur Burdett | PH5 | Samuel Partridge | PH10 |
| Roderick Caufield | PH21 | Julius Richardson | PH14 |
| Stanton Green | PH6 | Lester Rourke | PH11 |
| James Harmon | PH1 | James Simpson | PH12 |
| Kenneth Hollingshead | PH20 | Jonathan Swadley | PH7 |
| Harold Jaffe | PH19 | Joseph Taylor | PH17 |
| John Kellogg | PH9 | Hugh Thomason | PH18 |

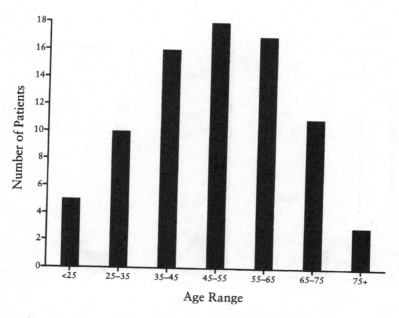

Figure A.1. Psychosurgery at McLean Hospital, 1938–1954. Age at operation, histogram (n = 80). (Source: McLean Hospital, Belmont, Massachusetts)

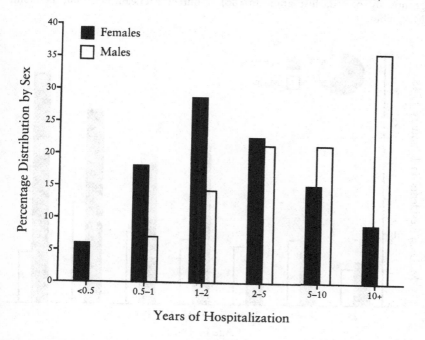

Figure A.2. Psychosurgery at McLean Hospital, 1938–1954. Hospitalization (all prior admissions) by sex, histogram (n = 80). (Source: McLean Hospital, Belmont, Massachusetts)

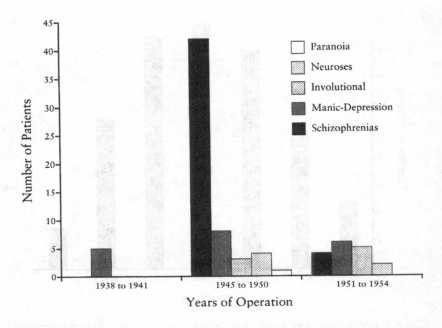

Figure A.3. Psychosurgery at McLean Hospital, 1938–1954. Major diagnostic groups by period, histogram (n=80). (Source: McLean Hospital, Belmont, Massachusetts)

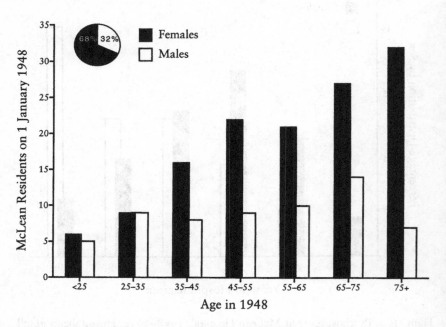

Figure A.4. Patients in residence at McLean Hospital on 1 January 1948. Age by sex, histogram (n=195: 133 females, 62 males). (Source: McLean Hospital, Belmont, Massachusetts)

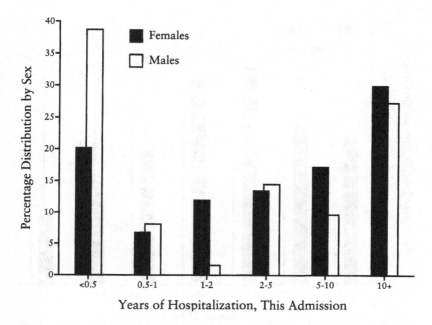

Figure A.5. Patients in residence at McLean Hospital on 1 January 1948. Hospitalization (all prior admissions) by sex, histogram (n=195: 133 females, 62 males). (Source: McLean Hospital, Belmont, Massachusetts)

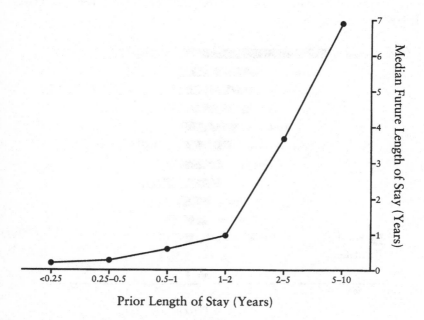

Figure A.6. Patients in residence at McLean Hospital on 1 January 1948. Future hospitalization plotted against past hospitalization, line-chart (n=195). (Source: McLean Hospital, Belmont, Massachusetts)

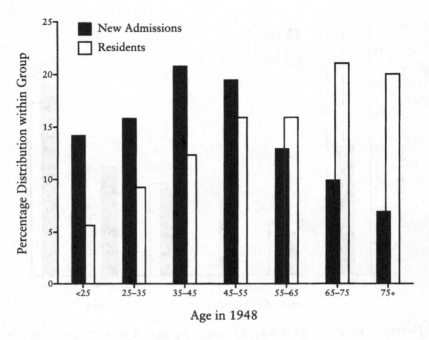

Figure A.7. McLean Hospital 1948. Comparison of patients in residence on 1 January 1948 with patients admitted during the calendar year, histogram (residents n = 195, admissions n = 303). (Source: McLean Hospital, Belmont, Massachusetts)

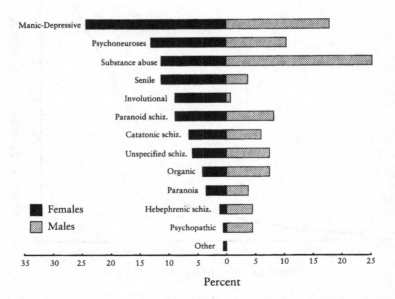

Figure A.8. Patients admitted to McLean Hospital during the 1948 calendar year. Diagnosis by sex, bar-chart (female n = 169, male n = 134). (Source: McLean Hospital, Belmont, Massachusetts)

# Notes

## Abbreviations for Books

F-W *PS1*  Walter Freeman and James Watts, *Psychosurgery; Intelligence, Emotion and Social Behavior following Prefrontal Lobotomy for Mental Disorders* (Springfield, Ill.: C. C. Thomas, 1942)

F-W *PS2*  Walter Freeman and James Watts, *Psychosurgery in the Treatment of Mental Disorders and Intractable Pain,* 2d ed. (Springfield, Ill.: C. C. Thomas, 1950)

Freeman *Auto*  Walter Freeman, "Autobiography," unpublished typescript, ca. 1970

Grob *Asylum*  Gerald Grob, *From Asylum to Community: Mental Health Policy in Modern America* (Princeton, N.J.: Princeton University Press, 1991)

Grob *IW*  Gerald Grob, *The Inner World of American Psychiatry, 1890–1940* (New Brunswick, N.J.: Rutgers University Press, 1985)

Grob *MI*  Gerald Grob, *Mental Illness and American Society 1875–1940* (Princeton, N.J.: Princeton University Press, 1983)

JF *Diary*  "The Diary of John Farquhar Fulton," Medical History Library, Sterling Hall of Medicine, Yale University Medical School, New Haven, Connecticut

Pressman *UP*  Jack Pressman, *Uncertain Promise: Psychosurgery and the Development of Scientific Psychiatry in America, 1935 to 1955.* Ph.D. diss., University of Pennsylvania, 1986 (Ann Arbor, Mich.: UMI, 1986). DAI No. 8624021

Valenstein *G&DC*  Elliot Valenstein, *Great and Desperate Cures: The Rise and Decline of Psychosurgery and Other Radical Treatments for Mental Illness* (New York: Basic Books, 1986)

## Abbreviations for Periodicals

AJI  *American Journal of Insanity*
AJP  *American Journal of Psychiatry*

# 454

*Notes*

| | |
|---|---|
| ANP | *Archives of Neurology and Psychiatry* |
| AR | *Annual Report* [generic] |
| ARNMD | *Research Publications – Association for Research in Nervous and Mental Disease* |
| BHM | *Bulletin of the History of Medicine* |
| BR | *Biennial Report* [generic] |
| JAMA | *Journal of the American Medical Association* |
| JHM | *Journal of the History of Medicine and the Allied Sciences* |
| JNMD | *Journal of Nervous and Mental Disease* |
| MHN | *Mental Hygiene News* |
| NEJM | *New England Journal of Medicine* |
| PSQ | *Psychiatric Quarterly* |
| SMJ | *Southern Medical Journal* |

## Abbreviations for Personal Names and Organizations

| | |
|---|---|
| AMA | American Medical Association |
| APA | American Psychiatric Association |
| ARNMD | Association for Research in Nervous and Mental Disease |
| CCB | C. Charles Burlingame |
| CSG | Council of State Governments |
| DMH | Department of Mental Hygiene (or Health) [generic] |
| EM | Egas Moniz |
| JF | John Farquhar Fulton |
| GAP | Group for the Advancement of Psychiatry |
| JW | James Winston Watts |
| NCMH | National Committee for Mental Hygiene |
| NIMH | National Institute of Mental Health |
| NRC | National Research Council |
| RF | Rockefeller Foundation |
| SH | State Hospital [generic] |
| USPHS | United States Public Health Service |
| WF | Walter Jackson Freeman |
| WM | William Menninger |

## Abbreviations for Archives

| | |
|---|---|
| APA | American Psychiatric Association |
| APB | Alfred P. Bay Papers |
| AR | Annual Report |
| BPH | Boston Psychopathic Hospital Papers |
| CCB | C. C. Burlingame Papers |
| EAS | Edward A. Strecker Papers |
| FG | Francis Grant Papers |

| | |
|---|---|
| GAP[MF] | Group for the Advancement of Psychiatry Papers, Menninger Foundation Corporate Records |
| GAP[NY] | Group for the Advancement of Psychiatry Papers, Archives of Psychiatry |
| GWU | Walter J. Freeman and James W. Watts Papers |
| HCS | Harry C. Solomon Papers |
| HPS | Helen P. Sargent Papers |
| HRV | Henry R. Viets Papers |
| HWB | Henry W. Brosin Papers |
| JF | John Farquhar Fulton Papers |
| JF[MED] | John Farquhar Fulton Collection |
| KAM | Karl A. Menninger Papers |
| LSH | Longview State Hospital Papers |
| McLH | McLean Hospital Archives |
| MG | Maxwell Gitelson Papers |
| NAMHC | National Advisory Mental Health Council Papers |
| NDCL | Nolan Don Carpentier Lewis Papers |
| NIMH | National Institute of Mental Health Papers |
| NRC | National Research Council Archives |
| OH | Ohio State Archives |
| PFL | Philadelphia Free Library, Government Documents Section |
| RF | Rockefeller Foundation Corporate Records |
| RMY | Robert M. Yerkes Papers |
| TMF | The Menninger Foundation Corporate Records |
| VA | Veterans Administration, Central Neuropsychiatric Research Laboratory Papers |
| VID | The Vidonian Club Papers |
| WCM | William C. Menninger Papers |
| WO | Winifred Overholser Papers |

## Introduction: A Stab in the Dark

1. Patient 303, neurosurgeon W. Jason Mixter's report 22 Jan. 1947, McLH; the use of patient files such as this one is discussed at greater length in Chapter 6. Some of the argument in this introduction has already been published as Jack Pressman, "Sufficient Promise: John F. Fulton and the Origins of Psychosurgery," *BHM* 62 (1988): 1–22; and Pressman *UP*.
2. [Editorial], "Topectomy – New Light on a Stab in the Dark," *PSQ* 23 (1949): 156–7.
3. Morton Kramer, "The 1951 Survey of the Use of Psychosurgery," in Winfred Overholser, ed., *Proceedings of the Third Research Conference on Psychosurgery*, USPHS pub. no. 221 (Washington, D.C.: GPO, 1954), 159–68.
4. The debate commenced with the publications of Vernon Mark and Frank Ervin, especially their *Violence and the Brain* (New York: Harper & Row, 1970), followed by Peter Breggin's response, "The Return of Lobotomy and

Psychosurgery," *Congress Record* 118 (24 Feb. 1972): 5567–77. Several books have since appeared on the conflict, most notably: Elliot Valenstein, ed., *The Psychosurgery Debate: Scientific, Legal, and Ethical Perspectives* (San Francisco: W. H. Freeman, 1980); Willard Gaylin, Joel Meister, and Robert Neville, eds., *Operating on the Mind: The Psychosurgery Conflict* (New York: Basic Books, 1975); and Mark O'Callaghan and Douglas Carroll, *Psychosurgery – A Scientific Analysis* (Ridgewood, N.J.: George A. Bogden, 1982). Elliot Valenstein has written the most informative accounts to date on the history of the operation; see his *Brain Control: A Critical Examination of Brain Stimulation and Psychosurgery* (New York: Wiley, 1973), and Valenstein *G&DC*. David Shutts's *Lobotomy: Resort to the Knife* (New York: Van Nostrand, 1982) is not reliable.

5. Valenstein *G&DC*, xi.
6. Roger Cooter, *The Cultural Meaning of Popular Science: Phrenology and the Organization of Consent in Nineteenth-Century Britain* (Cambridge University Press, 1984), 21.
7. Charles C. Burlingame, "Quacks But No Ducks," typescript of an after-dinner speech, Vidonian Club, 25 Jan. 1941, 4 (Box 2.1), VID.
8. Charles Rosenberg, "The Therapeutic Revolution: Medicine, Meaning, and Social Change in Nineteenth-Century America," in Morris Vogel and Charles Rosenberg, eds., *The Therapeutic Revolution: Essays in the Social History of American Medicine* (Philadelphia: University of Pennsylvania Press, 1979), 3–4. The paucity of studies of medical technology is documented in Joel Howell, *Machines' Meanings: British and American Uses of Technology 1880–1930* (Ph.D. diss., University of Pennsylvania, 1987; Ann Arbor: University of Michigan Press, 1987), 240; and Jonathan Liebenau, "Medicine and Technology," *Persp. Biol. Med.* 27 (1983): 76–92.
9. For examples of such studies by social scientists, see: Louise Russell, "The Diffusion of New Hospital Technologies in the United States," *Int. J. Health Serv.* 6 (1976): 557–80; idem, *Technology in Hospitals: Medical Advances and Their Diffusion* (Washington, D.C.: Brookings Institution, 1979); Ann Lennarson Greer, "Advances in the Study of Diffusion of Innovation in Health Care Organizations," *Milbank Mem. Fund Q.* 55 (Fall 1977): 505–32; Committee on Technology and Health Care (U.S.), *Medical Technology and the Health Care System: A Study of the Diffusion of Equipment-Embodied Technology* (Washington, D.C.: N.A.S., 1979); and H. D. Banta, Anne K. Burns, and Clyde J. Behney, "Policy Implications of the Diffusion and Control of Medical Technology," *Ann. AAPSS* 468 (1983): 165–81.
10. The electroencephalograph (EEG), e.g., was originally devised by its European inventor in the early 1930s as a noninvasive means of directly observing the soul in action. Imported into the U.S.A., the device first found favor in homes for disturbed children as a means of sorting out which mental disorders were due to errors of upbringing and which to an underlying brain pathology (epilepsy was still considered a psychiatric condition). Later, it gained a foothold in the general hospital as a confirmatory tool in the diagnosis of epilepsy and selected brain tumors. Currently, the EEG maintains a wide

usage mostly because of its ability to demonstrate when a patient is brain dead – the exact opposite function from where it began. Although a graphical plot of the rate of adoption of EEGs into American hospitals over the previous half-century traces out a straightforward mathematical equation, such an exercise obscures more than it illuminates. The EEG is simply a device that produces reams of squiggly lines; each shift in the interpretation of these lines started a different branch in its history. Thus, in spite of the fact that the underlying technology of the EEG has remained fundamentally unchanged, in truth there existed not one EEG but several. For a discussion of the multiple meanings of a medical technology, see Jack Pressman, "The EEG: A Medical Technology in Search of a Function," unpublished address to the "Conference on Twentieth-Century Health Sciences: Problems and Interpretations," 23 May 1988, University of California, San Francisco. For a detailed account of the relation between the EEG and the criteria of death, see Mita Giacomini, "Technological Imperatives and the Definition of Brain Death in 1968" (M.A. thesis, University of California, San Francisco, 1992).

11. See Jacques M. Quen, "Case Studies in Nineteenth-Century Scientific Rejection: Mesmerism, Perkinism, and Acupuncture," *J. Hist. Behav. Sci.* 11 (1975): 149–56.

12. Rosenberg, "Therapeutic Revolution," 3–25.

13. A 1982 survey of actively publishing historians of medicine identified this article by Rosenberg as the most influential in the previous decade; see Ronald Numbers, "The History of American Medicine: A Field in Ferment," *Rev. Am. Hist.* 10 (1982): 245–63. The best account of the transition of therapeutic modalities in this period is John H. Warner, *The Therapeutic Perspective: Medical Practice, Knowledge, and Identity in America, 1820–1885* (Cambridge, Mass.: Harvard University Press, 1986). See also idem, "Power, Conflict, and Identity in Mid-Nineteenth-Century American Medicine: Therapeutic Change at the Commercial Hospital in Cincinnati," *J. Am. Hist.* 73 (1987): 934–56; and "Science in Medicine," *Osiris* 1 (1985): 37–58. For a study of therapeutics in an earlier era, see Guenter Risse, *Hospital Life in Enlightenment Scotland. Care and Teaching at the Royal Infirmary of Edinburgh* (Cambridge University Press, 1986).

14. For examples of recent scholarship that have approached the history of technology or therapeutics in this manner, see Joel Howell, *Technology in the Hospital: Transforming Patient Care in the Early Twentieth Century* (Baltimore: Johns Hopkins University Press, 1995); idem, "Early Use of X-ray Machines and Electrocardiographs at the Pennsylvania Hospital, 1897 through 1927," *JAMA* 255 (1986): 2320–3; Judith Walzer Leavitt, *Brought to Bed. Child-Bearing in America, 1750–1950* (New York: Oxford University Press, 1986); idem, "The Growth of Medical Authority: Technology and Morals in Turn-of-the-Century Obstetrics," *Med. Anthrop. Q.* 1 (1987): 230–55; Allan Brandt, *No Magic Bullet: A Social History of Venereal Disease since 1880* (New York: Oxford University Press, 1985); Susan Bell, "A New Model of Medical Technology Development: A Case Study of DES," *Res. Soc. Health Care* 4 (1986): 1–32; Audrey Davis, "Life Insurance and the Physical

Examination: A Chapter in the Rise of American Medical Technology," *BHM* 55 (1981): 392–406. See also Sandra Harding, "Knowledge, Technology, and Social Relations," *J. Med. Phil.* 3 (1978): 346–58; and Melvin Kranzberg, "Presidential Address. Technology and History: 'Kranzberg's Laws,'" *Tech. Cult.* 27 (1986): 544–60.

15. H. D. Banta, "Embracing or Rejecting Innovations: Clinical Diffusion of Health Care Technology," in Stanley Reiser and Michael Anbar, eds., *The Machine at the Bedside: Strategies for Using Technology in Patient Care* (Cambridge University Press, 1984), 65–92.

16. See, e.g., Harry Collins and Trevor Pinch, *The Golem: What Everyone Should Know about Science* (Cambridge University Press, 1993); Simon Schaffer, "Scientific Discoveries and the End of Natural Philosophy," *Soc. Stud. Sci.* 16 (1986): 387–420; and Augustine Brannigan, *The Social Basis of Scientific Discovery* (Cambridge University Press, 1981).

17. Charles Rosenberg, "Toward an Ecology of Knowledge: On Discipline, Context, and History," in Alexandra Oleson and John Voss, eds., *The Organization of Knowledge in Modern America, 1860–1920* (Baltimore: Johns Hopkins University Press, 1979), 440–55. Rosenberg was applying the ecological model to disciplinary formation and the evolution of paradigms; the same model applies to conceptually embedded practices as well.

18. Talcott Parsons, "Illness and the Role of the Physician: A Sociological Perspective," *Am. J. Orthopsych.* 21 (1951): 452–60; and Charles Rosenberg, "Disease and Social Order in America," in Elizabeth Fee and Daniel Fox, eds., *AIDS: The Burdens of History* (Berkeley: University of California Press, 1988), 30.

19. This point has been well documented in historical studies of diseases that have since receded into the cultural landscape, or other instances of when "failed" products of medicine are useful subjects for analysis. See, e.g., Karl Figlio, "Chlorosis and Chronic Disease in Nineteenth-Century Britain: The Social Constitution of Somatic Illness in a Capitalist Society," *Soc. Hist.* 3 (1978): 167–97; Richard Gillespie, "Industrial Fatigue and the Discipline of Physiology," in Gerald Geison, ed., *Physiology in the American Context, 1850–1940* (Bethesda, Md.: American Physiological Society, 1987), 237–62; and Charles Rosenberg and Janet Golden, eds., *Framing Disease: Studies in Cultural History* (New Brunswick, N.J.: Rutgers University Press, 1992).

## Chapter 1. Psychiatry's Renaissance

1. Adolf Meyer, "The Contributions of Psychiatry to the Understanding of Life Problems" [1921], *The Collected Papers of Adolf Meyer*: vol. 4, *Mental Hygiene* (Baltimore: Johns Hopkins University Press, 1952), 1; Albert Barrett, "The Broadened Interests of Psychiatry," *AJP* 79 (1922): 1–13; Leslie Fishbein, "Freud and the Radicals: The Sexual Revolution Comes to Greenwich Village," *Canadian Rev. Amer. Stud.* 12 (1981): 173–89; John Burnham, "The Influence of Psychoanalysis upon American Culture," in Jacques Quen and Eric Carlson,

eds., *American Psychoanalysis: Origins and Development* (New York: Brunner/Mazel, 1978), 52–72; and idem, "From Avant-Garde to Specialism: Psychoanalysis in America," *JHBS* 15 (1979): 128–34. An account of the public reception of Freud in Britain is Dean Rapp, "The Early Discovery of Freud by the British General Educated Public, 1912–1919," *Soc. Hist. Med.* 3 (1990): 217–43. See also William Burgess Cornell, "The Broadening Field of Mental Medicine," *Med. Rec.* 94 (14 Aug. 1918): 329–31; L. Pierce Clark, "Extra Asylum Psychiatry," *AJI* 74 (1917–19): 425–9; Barrett, "The Broadened Interests of Psychiatry," 1–13; and William Healy, "The Newer Psychiatry. Its Field – Training for It," *AJP* 82 (1926): 391–401.

2. Cornell, "The Broadening Field," 329.

3. E. E. Southard declared in 1919 that "No greater power to change our minds about the problems of psychiatry has been at work in the interior of the psychiatric profession in America than the personality of Adolf Meyer"; cited in Leys, "Adolf Meyer: A Biographical Note," in Ruth Leys and Rand Evans, eds., *Defining American Psychology. The Correspondence between Adolf Meyer and Edward Bradford Titchener* (Baltimore: Johns Hopkins University Press, 1990), 39. For additional biographical accounts, see Gerald Grob, *The State and the Mentally Ill: A History of Worcester State Hospital in Massachusetts, 1830–1920* (Chapel Hill: University of North Carolina Press, 1966); Theodore Lidz, "Adolf Meyer and the Development of American Psychiatry," *AJP* 123 (1966): 320–32; and Eunice Winters, "Adolf Meyer's Two and a Half Years at Kankakee; May 1, 1893 – November 1, 1895," *BHM* 40 (1966): 441–58. David Tanner has argued for the identification of a distinct "American school" of psychiatry derivative of Meyer; see his *Symbols of Conduct: Psychiatry and American Culture, 1900–1935* (Ann Arbor: UMI [DA8217963], 1986; Ph.D. diss., University of Texas at Austin, 1981). Barbara Sicherman has provided the best overview of Meyer's contributions; see "The New Psychiatry: Medical and Behavioral Science, 1895–1921," in Quen and Carlson, *American Psychoanalysis.* Swiss born and trained, Meyer pursued postgraduate medical training in neuroanatomy and neuropathology in the workshops of the great European teachers such as J. H. Jackson in England, J. M. Charcot in France, and August Forel in Switzerland. European posts were tightly held, so in 1892, at the age of twenty-six, Meyer emigrated to the U.S.A. with the ambitious hope of directing one of the existing neuropathology centers. He began his career instead in a humble position as pathologist to the Eastern State Hospital, Kankakee, Ill. (1893–5), soon moving on, however, to a better post at Worcester State, Mass. (1895–1902). Meyer's achievements and shift in interests from neuropathology to mental illness led him to successive appointments as the director of the New York State Pathological Institute (1904–9), and then of the Phipps Psychiatric Institute in Baltimore (1910–41). At these institutes, which he established as the leading such programs in the nation, Meyer exerted great influence over the next generation of psychiatric leaders.

4. The most authoritative overview of the development of the American mental health care system is that found in the series of publications by Gerald Grob, especially: *The State and the Mentally Ill; Mental Institutions in America –*

*Social Policy to 1875* (New York: Free Press, 1973); *Mental Illness and American Society 1875–1940* (Princeton, N.J.: Princeton University Press, 1983); and *From Asylum to Community: Mental Health Policy in Modern America* (Princeton, N.J.: Princeton University Press, 1991). The best account of a nineteenth-century asylum is Nancy Tomes, *A Generous Confidence: Thomas Story Kirkbride and the Art of Asylum-Keeping, 1840–1883* (Cambridge University Press, 1984), and for a twentieth-century case study, see Lawrence Friedman, *Menninger: The Family and the Clinic* (New York: Knopf, 1990). For a portrait of American neurology, see Bonnie Bluestein, *Preserve Your Love for Science: Life of William A. Hammond, American Neurologist* (Cambridge University Press, 1991). An account of the uses of psychiatric conceptions in general practice is found in F. G. Gosling, *Before Freud: Neurasthenia and the American Medical Community, 1870–1910* (Urbana: University of Illinois Press, 1987).

Also helpful are Andrew Delano Abbott, "The Emergence of American Psychiatry, 1880–1930" (Ph.D. diss., University of Chicago, 1982); Bonnie Bluestein, "New York Neurologists and the Specialization of American Medicine," *BHM* 53 (1979): 170–83; John C. Burnham, *Psychoanalysis and American Medicine, 1894–1918: Medicine, Science, and Culture* (New York: International Universities Press, 1967); idem, "The Struggle between Physicians and Paramedical Personnel in American Psychiatry, 1917–1941," *JHM* 29 (1974): 93–106; idem, "The Founding of the *Archives of Neurology and Psychiatry;* or What Was Wrong with the *Journal of Nervous and Mental Disease?*" *JHM* 36 (1981): 310–24; idem, *Paths into American Culture: Psychology, Medicine, and Morals* (Philadelphia: Temple University Press, 1988); George E. Gifford, Jr., ed., *Psychoanalysis, Psychotherapy, and the New England Medical Scene, 1894–1944* (New York: Science History, 1978); Nathan G. Hale, *Freud and the Americans: The Beginnings of Psychoanalysis in the United States, 1876–1917* (New York: Oxford University Press, 1971); Constance McGovern, *Masters of Madness: Social Origins of The American Psychiatric Profession* (Hanover, N.H.: University of Vermont for the University Press of New England, 1985); John Pitts, "The Association of Medical Superintendents of American Institutions for the Insane, 1844–1892: A Case Study of Specialism in American Medicine" (Ph.D. diss., University of Pennsylvania, 1979); Jack Pressman, "Concepts of Mental Illness in the West," in *The Cambridge World History of Human Disease* (Cambridge University Press, 1993), 59–85; Charles Rosenberg, "The Place of George M. Beard in Nineteenth-Century Psychiatry," *BHM* 36 (1962): 245–59; idem, *The Trial of the Assassin Guiteau: Psychiatry and Law in the Gilded Age* (Chicago: University of Chicago Press, 1968); idem, "Body and Mind in Nineteenth-Century Medicine: Some Clinical Origins of the Neurosis Construct," *BHM* 63 (1989): 185–97; David Rothman, *The Discovery of the Asylum: Social Order and Disorder in the New Republic* (Boston: Little, Brown, 1971); idem, *Conscience and Convenience: The Asylum and Its Alternatives in Progressive America* (Glenview, Ill.: Scott, Foresman, 1980); Andrew Scull, *Social Order/Mental Disorder; Anglo-American Psychiatry in Historical Perspective* (Berkeley: University of California Press, 1989); and Barbara Sicherman, *The Quest for Mental Health in America, 1880–1917* (New York: Arno, 1980).

5. A recent exposition of Meyer's developmental psychiatry is Ruth Leys, "Types of One: Adolf Meyer's Life Chart and the Representation of Individuality," *Repres.* 34 (1991): 1–28. For a recent history of the Chicago school of sociology, see Dorothy Ross, *The Origins of American Social Science* (Cambridge University Press, 1991); see also Fred H. Matthews, *Quest for American Sociology: Robert E. Park and the Chicago School* (Montreal: McGill–Queen's University Press, 1977).

6. Adolf Meyer, "Insanity" [1926], Meyer *CP*, 2:405; emphasis mine.

7. For Meyer's role in the NCMH, see Grob *MI*, 144–78; Sicherman, *Quest for Mental Health;* and Christine Shea, "The Ideology of Mental Health and the Emergence of the Therapeutic Liberal State: The American Mental Hygiene Movement, 1900–1930" (Ph.D. diss., University of Illinois at Urbana, 1980). See also Norman Dain, *Clifford W. Beers, Advocate for the Insane* (Pittsburgh: University of Pittsburgh Press, 1980).

8. Thomas Salmon and Norman Fenton, "In the American Expeditionary Forces," in *The Medical Department of the United States in the World War: Volume 10, Neuropsychiatry* (Washington, D.C.: GPO, 1929), 293.

9. Adolf Meyer to Abraham Flexner, 20 Apr. 1927; cited in Grob *IW,* 178.

10. "Undoubtedly," Bond wrote, the two were "the leaders of American psychiatry – Salmon as a doer, Meyer as a thinker"; Earl Bond, "Seven Years of Awakening, 1906–1913," *AJP* 116 (1959): 112.

11. The psychiatrists' postwar success mirrored that of the psychologists who parlayed their introduction of the army intelligence test into a mental-testing industry in the coming decades. See Daniel Kevles, "Testing the Army's Intelligence: Psychology and the Military in World War I," *J. Am. Hist.* 55 (1968): 565–81; and Michael M. Sokal, ed., *Psychological Testing and American Society, 1890–1930* (New Brunswick, N. J.: Rutgers University Press, 1987). There are strong parallels between the response of the American medical establishment to shell shock and that of the British; I am indebted to Henrika Kuklick's invaluable *The Savage Within: The Social History of British Anthropology, 1885–1945* (Cambridge University Press, 1991).

12. The reversal in relations between neurology and psychiatry is described in Walter Bromberg, *Psychiatry Between the Wars, 1918–1945: A Recollection* (Westport, Conn.: Greenwood, 1982). Salmon's unique position is highlighted in Earl Bond, *Thomas W. Salmon, Psychiatrist* (New York: Norton, 1950), 205.

13. Thomas Salmon, *Mind and Medicine* (New York: Columbia University Press, 1924), 26; and Sidney Schwab, "Influence of War upon Concepts of Mental Diseases and Neuroses," *Mental Hygiene* 4 (1920): 661. After the war, ten regional government hospitals and 114 outpatient departments employed psychiatrists; Tanner, *Symbols of Conduct,* 66. As of 1920, 27 percent of all war-risk beneficiaries were awarded on the basis of neuropsychiatric disability; James May, "The Importance of Psychiatry in the Practice of Medicine," *BMSJ* 189, no. 24 (1923): 966. See also John Kindred, "The Neuro-

psychiatric Wards of the United States Government; Their Housing and Other Problems," *AJP* 78 (1921): 183–92; and Caroline Cox, "Bringing It All Back Home: The American Legion, Shell-Shocked Veterans and Mental Illness, 1919–1924" (unpublished seminar paper, University of California, Berkeley, 1992). Among other such activities, Salmon convinced the General Education Board of the Rockefeller Foundation (RF) to pay for full-time salaries of psychiatrists; Bond, *Salmon,* 199, 222.

14. Salmon turned down an offer to serve as dean and was generally credited with introducing psychiatry into university medical schools; ibid., 151, 204. J. K. Hall to H. B. Brackin, 19 Dec. 1929; cited in Grob *IW,* 94. For the significance of the redesigned Columbia Medical School, see Paul Starr, *The Social Transformation of American Medicine* (New York: Basic Books, 1982), 361.

15. In a letter written in 1925, Karl Menninger observed that before the war psychobiology and psychoanalysis had been generally unrecognized; cited in Tanner, *Symbols of Conduct,* 68. Paton cited in ibid., 30. Austen Fox Riggs, *Just Nerves* (Boston: Houghton Mifflin, 1922), 46.

16. Barrett, "The Broadened Interests of Psychiatry," 3, 13.

17. Healy, "The Newer Psychiatry," 391–3.

18. Percival Bailey quoted in Shea, *Ideology of Mental Health,* 170. Shepherd I. Franz, *Nervous and Mental Re-Education* (New York: MacMillan, 1923), v–vii, 202, 219. See also S. S. Colvin, "Education as the Modification of Behavior for Social Adaptation," in W. A. White and Smith Ely Jelliffe, eds., *The Modern Treatment of Nervous and Mental Diseases* (Philadelphia: Lea & Febiger, 1913), 1:56–99.

19. Salmon arranged for the first appointments of a psychiatrist in industry and a prison clinic; see Bond, *Salmon,* 187, 190. He also steered several foundations in their mental hygiene efforts, especially in regard to juvenile courts and demonstration clinics. See Margo Horn, *Before It's Too Late: The Child Guidance Movement in the United States, 1922–1945* (Philadelphia: Temple University Press, 1989); Komora, "The Late Dr. T. W. Salmon," 7.

20. Southard quoted in Shea, *Ideology of Mental Health,* 201.

21. For an excellent account of the origin and development of the "human relations" school of industrial sociology, see Richard Gillespie, *Manufacturing Knowledge: A History of the Hawthorne Experiments* (Cambridge University Press, 1991).

22. Henry Sigerist, "The History of Medicine and the History of Science. An Open Letter to George Sarton, Editor of *Isis*," *BHM* 4 (1936): 5.

23. Barrett, "The Broadened Interests of Psychiatry," 13; and William A. White, *Forty Years of Psychiatry* (New York: Nervous & Mental Disease Publ. Co., 1933), 114.

24. See Horn, *Before It's Too Late;* Grob *MI,* 163; Bond, *Salmon,* 196.

25. "Excerpt, Rockefeller Foundation meeting, 11 April 1933" (RG3 906 2 19), RFA. The foundation projected that through its long-term commitment to psychiatry it would achieve its "greatest single contribution to human welfare"; "Princeton Conference Report, Oct. 1930" (RG 3 906 2 19), RFA. For histories of the RF, see Robert Kohler, *Partners in Science: Foundations and*

*Natural Scientists* (Chicago: University of Chicago Press, 1991); Lily Kay, "'Social Control': Rockefeller Foundation's Agenda in the Human Sciences, 1913–1933," in *The Molecular Vision of Life; Caltech, The Rockefeller Foundation, and the Rise of the New Biology* (New York: Oxford University Press, 1993), 22–57; and Jack Pressman, "Human Understanding: The Rockefeller Foundation's Attempt to Construct a Scientific Psychiatry in America, 1930–1950," paper presented at the Mellon Symposium "Shifting Meanings and Representations of Life: What Defines 'Cutting Edge' Biology?" MIT Program in Science, Technology, and Society, 5 Apr. 1991, Boston, Mass.

26. The new departments were located at Yale, Rochester, Illinois, St. Louis, Duke, and Chicago; existing ones were strengthened at Colorado, New York, Tulane, Michigan, and the Institute of Pennsylvania. Large capital grants endowed research and training sites at Montreal, Harvard, Yale, Toronto, and the Chicago Institute of Psychoanalysis; Pressman, "Human Understanding."

27. Alan Gregg, "What Is Psychiatry?" 3 Dec. 1941 (RG 3 906 2 19), RFA; *RF AR* (1936), 23.

28. Lily Kay, "'Social Control,'" 28.

29. *RF AR* (1934), 78; and *RF AR* (1930), 210.

30. *RF AR* (1934), 78; and *RF AR* (1936), 24. In 1933, the RF announced that "the ultimate aim and the central problem" of the RF was the "analysis and rationalization of human behavior." The single most important focus would be "psychobiology," all "the other subjects being viewed as contributory." Cited from "The Medical and the Natural Sciences," 1933 Interim Report to the Trustees Meeting, 13 Dec. 1933 (RG 3 906 2 19), RFA.

31. See Grob *MI*, 293–6.

32. Dean David Edsall, "Memorandum Regarding Possible Psychiatric Developments," 3 Oct. 1930 (RG 3 906 2 19), RFA.

33. Theodore Brown, "Alan Gregg and the Rockefeller Foundation's Support of Franz Alexander's Psychosomatic Research," *BHM* 61 (1987): 155–82; Pressman, "Human Understanding"; and Wilder Penfield, *The Difficult Art of Giving: The Epic of Alan Gregg* (Boston: Little, Brown, 1967).

34. "Subject: Development of Psychiatry at Harvard Medical School and Massachusetts General Hospital," 31 Oct. 1933 (RG 1.1 200 90 1080), RFA; *RF AR* (1936), 135. The grants built and maintained a twenty-bed inpatient neuropsychiatric service, a bold move at a time when virtually all general hospitals refused to admit psychiatric patients for even routine medical care. So central was Harvard to Gregg's vision of how to reconstitute U.S. psychiatry that the foundation even paid for the direct costs of patient care on the ward – a gesture that violated a dearly held Rockefeller policy; "Funding resolution RF 37017, 19 Feb 1937" (RG 1.1. 200 90 1080), RFA. Benjamin White, *Stanley Cobb: A Builder of the Modern Neurosciences* (Boston: Countway Library, 1984). Here is Cobb's own approach to psychosomatic medicine: "When the connection of a frustration, a deeply rooted anxiety, or emotional problem to physical symptoms or social disability can be pointed out to the patient, and possibly help be given in adjusting mental attitude to

the problems of life and correcting the bad posture of the mind, symptoms and social maladjustments usually disappear"; *RF AR* (1940), 145–6. Cobb's interest in psychoanalysis stemmed from his own short-term analysis to deal with a life-long stutter. For further insight into Cobb's work, see his *Foundations of Neuropsychiatry*, 4th ed. (Baltimore: Williams & Wilkins, 1948); idem, *Borderlands of Psychiatry* (Cambridge, Mass.: Harvard University Press, 1943); and idem, *A Preface to Nervous Disease* (Baltimore: William Wood, 1936). Support eventually totaled $900,000; "Funding resolution RF 48055, 21 May 1948" (RG 1.1 200 91 1091), RFA. Gregg also funded similar programs of neuropsychiatry and psychobiology, though at a lower level, at university hospitals nationwide; thanks to these, e.g., "the concept of psychobiology has become a part of the teaching and clinical activities of medicine, surgery, obstetrics, and pediatrics in the School of Medicine and Colorado General Hospital"; *RF AR* (1939), 166–9.

35. Edward Taylor, "Types of Habit Neuro-psychoses," *BMSJ* 139 (21 July 1898): 62. James J. Putnam, "The Psychology of Health-II," *Psychotherapy* 1 (1909): 5. Llewellys Barker, "Psychotherapy," *JAMA* 51 (1 Aug. 1908): 371. Franz, *Mental Re-Education*, 18.

36. The importance of the Pavlovian model to psychiatry is discussed further in Chapter 2. See also *RF AR* (1936), 147–51.

37. Ibid.; and "Society Transactions," discussion of paper by C. F. Jacobsen, *ANP* 33 (1935): 886.

38. Adolf Meyer, "A Discussion of Some Fundamental Issues in Freud's Psychoanalysis" [1909–10], Meyer *CP*, 2:604. For a discussion of Meyer's reading of Freud, see Tanner, *Symbols of Conduct*, 102–3; Leys, "Adolf Meyer: A Biographical Note," 56 n. 19.

39. Jack Pressman, "Making Psychiatry Respectable: Earl Bond, Edward Strecker, Kenneth Appel and the Institute of Pennsylvania Hospital," *Trans. Stud. Coll. Phys. Phil.*, ser. 5, 13 (1991): 425–33.

40. Pressman, "Concepts of Mental Illness," 78–9.

41. Louis Casamajor, "Notes for an Intimate History of Neurology and Psychiatry in America," *JNMD* 98 (1943): 600–8; and Walter Freeman, Franklin Ebaugh, and David Boyd, Jr., "The Founding of the American Board of Psychiatry and Neurology, Inc.," *AJP* 115 (1959): 769–78. See also Bonnie Bluestein, "Percival Bailey and Neurology at the University of Chicago, 1928–1939," *BHM* 66 (1992): 90–113; and Percival Bailey, "The Practice of Neurology in the United States of America," *J. Assoc. Am. Med. Coll.* 21 (1946): 281–92.

42. Paula Fass illustrates the importance of the adjustment model to the articulation of social fears in the 1920s and 1930s in *The Damned and the Beautiful: American Youth in the 1920's* (New York: Oxford University Press, 1977).

43. J. C. Whitehorn and Gregory Zilboorg, "Present Trends in American Psychiatric Research," *AJP* 90 (1933): 303–12; Nolan Lewis, *Research in Dementia Praecox* (New York: NCMH, 1936); and William Malamud, "The History of Psychiatric Therapies," in J. K. Hall, ed., *One Hundred Years of American Psychiatry* (New York: Columbia University Press, 1944), 320.

44. For an account of the psychiatric significance of plastic surgery in this period, see Beth Haiken, "Plastic Surgery and American Beauty at 1921," *BHM* 68 (Fall 1994): 429–53.

45. Cobb, *Borderlands of Psychiatry*, ix.

46. Meyer suggested that the mental hygiene movement was oversold; Adolf Meyer to Abraham Flexner, 20 Apr. 1927; cited in Grob *IW*, 180.

47. The addresses from the conference were published in Madison Bentley and E. V. Cowdry, *The Problem of Mental Disorder: A Study Undertaken by the Committee on Psychiatric Investigations, National Research Council* (New York: McGraw-Hill, 1934).

48. Ibid., vii, 4, 6.

49. Ibid., 233.

50. Meyer to John Whitehorn, 12 Feb. 1932; cited in Grob *IW*, 219. Bentley and Cowdry, *Mental Disorder*, 96.

51. James May [1933], cited in Burnham, "Physicians and Paramedical Personnel," 102. See also idem, "Psychology and Counseling: Convergence into a Profession," in Nathan O. Hatch, ed., *The Professions in American History* (Notre Dame: University of Indiana Press, 1988), 181–98; and Donald Napoli, *Architects of Adjustment: The History of the Psychological Profession in the United States* (Port Washington, N.Y.: Kennikat, 1981). See also James Capshew, *Psychologists on the March* (Berkeley: University of California Press, in press).

52. Bentley and Cowdry, *Mental Disorder*, vii.

53. Ibid.

## Chapter 2. Sufficient Promise

1. The RF spent $4.5 million on the IHR; Jill Morawski, "Organizing Knowledge and Behavior at Yale's Institute of Human Relations," *Isis* 77 (1986): 219–42.

2. Milton Winternitz, "Yale University School of Medicine," *Methods and Problems of Medical Education* (1932), 20:2. Arthur Viseltear, "Milton Winternitz and the Yale Institute of Human Relations: A Brief Chapter in the History of Social Medicine," *Yale J. Bio. Med.* 57 (1984): 869–89. See also Yale University, *Report of the Dean of School of Medicine, 1931–2*; and John Fulton, "Medicine and the Infra-human Primates," 11, typescript of an address to the Association of Yale Alumni, 1933, JF. Unless otherwise indicated, letters, annual reports, and manuscripts cited in this chapter are from the Fulton papers (which were unprocessed at time of research).

3. In addition to Morawski, "Institute of Human Relations," see also Kay, " 'Social Control' " (Chap. 1, n. 25); and James Capshew, "Psychology, Yale University, and the Rockefeller Foundation: A Case Study in the Patronage of Science, 1920–1940," paper presented at CHEIRON (International Society for the History of the Behavioral and Social Sciences), Newport, R.I., June 1982.

4. Morawski, "Institute of Human Relations," 220.

5. Some of these complaints came from within the Nobel Committee itself. See the correspondence between Fulton, Yngve Zotterman, C. Olof Sjoqvist, and Nilson Rezende. Freeman electioneered the award; Valenstein *G&DC*, 224–6.

6. What actually occurred at the congress is uncertain, as only the session abstracts were published; John Fulton and Carlyle Jacobsen, "The Functions of the Frontal Lobes: A Comparative Study in Monkeys, Chimpanzees, and Man," Abstract, *Program of the Second International Neurological Congress*, 1 Aug. 1935, London, 70–1, JF[MED]. The paper eventually surfaced in a Russian journal after Fulton delivered the same paper in Moscow; *Adv. Mod. Biol.* (Moscow) 4 (1935): 359. Fulton had kept a daily journal of this excursion, but uncharacteristically lost it before returning home; JF *Diary*, vol. 9, 14 June 1935 – 1 Aug. 1936.

7. Carlyle Jacobsen, J. B. Wolfe, and T. A. Jackson, "An Experimental Analysis of the Functions of the Frontal Association Areas in Primates," *JNMD* 82 (1935): 10. The standard account is found in Fulton's William Withering Lectures, published as *Functional Localization in Relation to Frontal Lobotomy* (New York: Oxford University Press, 1949).

8. From *leuko*, Greek for *white*, as in the white matter of the brain. Egas Moniz, "Essai d'un traitement chirurgical de certaines psychoses," *Bulletin de l'Académie de Médecine* (Paris) 115 (1936): 385–92; idem, *Tentatives opératoires dans le traitement de certaines psychoses* (Paris: Masson, 1936). A translation of the first report, with a list of Moniz's other papers, can be found in Robert Wilkins, "Neurosurgical Classic-XXVI," *J. Neurosurg.* 21 (1964): 1109–14. Lima trained in neurosurgery under Hugh Cairns, England's leading neurosurgeon.

9. Valenstein *G&DC*, 113. An extensive bibliography of the literature during psychosurgery's first five years can be found in F-W *PS1*, 319–31.

10. JF *Diary*, 12 Mar. 1947; and Stanley Cobb, "Presidential Address," in the *Transactions of the American Neurological Association. Seventy-Fourth Annual Meeting* (Richmond, Va.: William Byrd, 1949), 3. JF to Stanley Cobb, 16 June 1949; and Yale Koskoff to JF, 15 Dec. 1947.

11. John Fulton, "The Physiological Basis of the Operation of Frontal Lobotomy," typescript of an address to the Harvey Cushing Society, 3–4 May 1940, Kansas City, Mo., 1–2. Fulton also notes in this account that Moniz was "button-holing" anyone "who was even remotely interested in the frontal lobes," and that he seemed particularly impressed by the clinical reports of Brickner (discussed below). See also JF to Waldemar Kaempffert, 12 Feb. 1941. The pair were in proximity at least once; in the official conference photograph, Fulton is situated next to Moniz.

12. Susan L. Star, *Regions of the Mind: Brain Research and the Quest for Scientific Certainty* (Stanford, Calif.: Stanford University Press, 1989); Anne Harrington, *Medicine, Mind, and the Double Brain: A Study in Nineteenth-Century Thought* (Princeton, N.J.: Princeton University Press, 1987); Edwin Clarke and L. S. Jacyna, *Nineteenth-Century Origins of Neuroscientific Concepts* (Berkeley: University of California Press, 1987); and Francis Schiller, "The Mystique of the Frontal Lobes," *Gesnerus* 42 (1985): 415–24.

13. The history of neurosurgery has received little attention from historians. The most informative accounts remain contemporary reviews, such as Cobb Pilcher, "Recent Advances in Neurosurgery," *Surg.* 1 (1937): 131–43, 290–313; J. Scarff, "Fifty Years of Neurosurgery," *Int. Abs. Surg.* 101 (1955): 417–513; William German, "Neurological Surgery; Its Past, Present, and Future," *J. Neurosurg.* 10 (1953): 526–37; and Ernest Sachs, *Fifty Years of Neurosurgery; A Personal Story* (New York: Vantage, 1958). See also David Reeves, "The Development of Neurological Surgery in the U.S.," *Int. Surg.* 52 (1969): 463–7; and Norman Dott, "The History of Surgical Neurology in the Twentieth Century," *Proc. Roy. Soc. Med.* 64 (1971): 1051–5.

14. Leonardo Bianchi, *The Mechanism of the Brain and the Function of the Frontal Lobes* (Edinburgh: E. & S. Livingstone, 1922).

15. Richard Brickner, "An Interpretation of Frontal Lobe Function Based upon the Study of a Case of Partial Bilateral Frontal Lobectomy," in *ARNMD* 13 (1934): 273, 336. This article also contains an excellent bibliography. R. G. Spurling, "Notes upon Functional Activity of the Prefrontal Lobes," *SMJ* 27 (1934): 4; Spafford Ackerly, "Instinctive, Emotional and Mental Changes following Prefrontal Lobe Extirpation," *AJP* 92 (1935): 717–29; Richard Brickner, *The Intellectual Functions of the Frontal Lobes: A Study Based upon Observation of a Man after Partial Bilateral Frontal Lobectomy* (New York: Macmillan, 1936); idem, "Brain of Patient A. after Bilateral Frontal Lobectomy; Status of Frontal-Lobe Problem," *ANP* 68 (1952): 293–313; and idem, "Modifications of Function Observed after Surgical Intervention on the Frontal Lobe," abstracted in *Neurological Congress,* 21, JF[MED].

16. Henri Claude, "Les Fonctions des lobes frontaux," *Revue Neurologique* 65 (1936): 523. Translation is courtesy of Caroline Acker. Fulton and Jacobsen's paper did not fit into the frontal lobe symposium, but was included in a section on experimental physiology; cited in note 6 above. For further details, see Valenstein *G&DC*, 77–9. The best entry into the literature on frontal lobe research in this period is John Fulton, *Physiology of the Nervous System* (London: Oxford University Press, 1938), 458–68.

17. For biographical account of Moniz, see Valenstein *G&DC*, 62–79.

18. For a sketch of earlier attempts at brain surgery for mental illness, see F-W *PS1.* Wilkins, "Neurosurgical Classic," 1112.

19. Ibid., 1111.

20. Moniz, *Tentatives opératoires,* 15; and Claude, "Lobes frontaux," 518–46.

21. Moniz, *Tentatives opératoires,* 5. See also Valenstein *G&DC*, 97–100.

22. Simon Schaffer, "Scientific Discoveries and the End of Natural Philosophy," *Soc. Stud. Sci.* 16 (1986): 387–420.

23. The classic tale of how Sir Alexander Fleming accidentally discovered penicillin in a petri plate provides a telling example of the way such stories mislead us. Fleming actually rejected the potential clinical significance of what he saw, and it was not until Howard Florey's work a decade later that penicillin was thought to have any actual medicinal value; see Gwyn MacFarlane, *Alexander Fleming: The Man and the Myth* (Cambridge, Mass.: Harvard University Press, 1984).

24. For an account of the first trials in other countries, see Valenstein *G&DC*, 161.

25. Solly Zuckerman, *From Apes to Warlords* (New York: Harper & Row, 1978), 73–7; and Lycurgus Davey, "Obituary: John Farquhar Fulton," *J. Neurosurg.* 17 (1960): 1119–26. For a list of Fulton's obituaries, see A. Earl Walker, "Fulton, John Farquhar," in Charles Coulston Gillispie, ed., *Dictionary of Scientific Biography* (New York: Scribner, 1970–80), 5:207–8. See also Paul Bucy, "John Fulton and the Frontal Lobes," *Int. J. Neurol.* 5 (1965): 239–46; idem, "The *Journal of Neurosurgery,* Its Origin and Development," *J. Neurosurg.* 21 (1964): 1–12; and Hebbel Hoff, "John Fulton's Contribution to Neurophysiology," *JHM* 17 (1962): 16–37. For Fulton's complete bibliography, see Madeline Stanton and Elizabeth Thomson, "Bibliography of John Farquhar Fulton, 1921–1962," *JHM* 17 (1962): 51–71.

26. Yale Department of Physiology, "AR," typescript, 1933, 9.

27. JF *Diary,* June 1935, 172; idem, *Physiology of the Nervous System;* Hebbel Hoff, "Fulton's Contribution," 36; Paul Bucy, "The *Journal of Neurosurgery,*" 1–12; and Walker, "Fulton," 208. Bucy to JF, 14 Dec. 1953. Upon his retirement in 1950 as a physiologist, Fulton was able to point to an extraordinary record of accomplishment: his laboratory group had produced more than 1,000 articles and books and filled more than 25 chairs in medical schools.

28. Hoff, "Fulton's Contribution," 16–37; Judith Swazey, *Reflexes and Motor Integration: Sherrington's Concept of Integrative Action* (Cambridge, Mass.: Harvard University Press, 1969). See also Roger Smith, *Inhibition: History and Meaning in the Sciences of Mind and Brain* (Berkeley: University of California Press, 1992). Fulton's early work included *Muscular Contraction and the Reflex Control of Movement* (Baltimore: Williams & Wilkins, 1926), and *The Sign of Babinski: A Study of the Evolution of Cortical Dominance in Primates* (Springfield, Ill.: C. C. Thomas, 1932). Walker, "Fulton," 207; and see also Donna Haraway, *Primate Visions: Gender, Race, and Nature in the World of Modern Science* (New York: Routledge, 1989).

29. John Fulton, E. Liddell, and D. Rioch, "'Dial' as a Surgical Anaesthetic for Neurological Operations," *J. Pharmacol.* 40 (1930): 423–32. Fulton pioneered the use of surgical anesthesia in primates and insisted upon utilizing the finest available operating equipment, as well as keeping typewritten notes for each animal similar to what one might find for a human patient at an elite hospital.

30. Fulton, "Medicine and the Infra-human Primates," 11, JF[MED]. Sherrington was referring to work by S. I. Franz, E. L. Thorndike, and Robert Yerkes; see a passage from his *The Integrative Action of the Nervous System* (1906), quoted in John Fulton, *Functional Localization in the Frontal Lobes and Cerebellum* (Oxford: Clarendon, 1949), xiii.

31. Fulton, "The Physiological Basis of Frontal Lobotomy," carbon copy of Henry A. Riley to Henri Claude, in JF *Diary,* 1 Feb. 1935.

32. Carlyle Jacobsen, "Recent Experiments on the Function of the Frontal Lobes," *Psychol. Bull.* 25 (1928): 6; idem, "A Study of Cerebral Function in

Learning; The Frontal Lobes," *J. Comp. Neurol.* 52 (1931): 271–340; and idem, "Studies of Cerebral Function in Primates," *Comp. Psych. Mono.* 13, no. 63 (1936): 7.

33. Jacobsen's theoretical position was a compromise between two warring schools of thought. According to one view, termed *mass action* by its developer Karl Lashley, intelligence was a function of the central nervous system as an integrated whole. Loss of intellect was correlated to the amount of brain tissue destroyed, not its location. Followers of S. I. Franz held the opposite view: that intelligence was localized in specific regions of the brain. Jacobsen's work prior to his arrival at Yale suggested that intelligence depended upon "equilibrated action" of the entire nervous system. However, Jacobsen shifted position as his experimental animals rose on the phylogenetic tree. His final conclusion was that, although specific areas of the cortex do have discrete functions, the amount of function lost was in direct proportion to the quantity of brain tissue destroyed. In effect, Jacobsen had integrated the approaches of Lashley and Franz. See his "Studies of Cerebral Function in Primates," 52, 55–7; idem, "Functions of Frontal Association Area in Primates," *ANP* 33 (1935): 558–69; and Jacobsen, Wolfe, and Jackson, "Experimental Analysis of Frontal Association Areas in Primates," 13. JF *Diary,* 4 Dec. 1933.

34. Jacobsen, "Studies of Cerebral Function in Primates," 52.

35. Jacobsen, "A Study of Cerebral Function," 337; idem, "Studies of Cerebral Function in Primates," 7, 52; Fulton and Jacobsen, "The Functions of the Frontal Lobes: A Comparative Study," 70; Richard Brickner, *Functions of the Frontal Lobes,* 26–7; and Jacobsen, "Recent Experiments on the Function of the Frontal Lobes," 1–11.

36. Carlyle Jacobsen, "Experimental Analysis of the Functions of the Frontal Association Area in Primates," *ANP* 34 (1935): 884–8.

37. I. P. Pavlov, "Neuroses in Man and Animals," *JAMA* 99 (1932): 1012–3. The latter half of Pavlov's career was devoted to problems of psychiatry; see his *Conditioned Reflexes and Psychiatry* (New York: International Publishers, 1941). Surveys of the literature on experimental neuroses are found in W. Horsley Gantt, "An Experimental Approach to Psychiatry," *AJP* 92 (1936): 1007–21; Harold S. Liddell, "Conditioned Reflex Method and Experimental Neurosis," in J. McV. Hunt, ed. *Personality and the Behavior Disorders; A Handbook Based on Experimental and Clinical Research* (New York: Ronald, 1944), 389–412; and Stuart Cook, "A Survey of Methods Used to Produce 'Experimental Neurosis'," *AJP* 95 (1939): 1259–76.

38. See the transcript of the "Conference on Experimental Neuroses and Allied Problems," 17–18 Apr. 1937, Inter-Divisional Committee on Borderland Problems of the Life Sciences, National Research Council (NRC); and "Problems of Neurotic Behavior. The Experimental Production and Treatment of Behavior Derangement . . . ," mimeographed report of the Committee on Problems of Neurotic Behavior, Division of Anthropology and Psychology, 1938, NRC. The committee's primary aim was to emulate, for the discipline of experimental psychopathology, the work of the highly regarded Committee

for Research in Problems of Sex. Its major finding was the need for a new journal. However, the committee was co-opted by the Josiah Macy, Jr., Foundation's desire to fund programs of psychosomatic research; thus *Psychomatic Medicine* became the title of the new journal. See also Glenn Bugos, "Managing Cooperative Research and Borderland Science in the National Research Council, 1922–1942," *Hist. Stud. Phys. Sci.* 20 (1989): 1–32.

39. Jacobsen, Wolfe, and Jackson, "Functions of the Frontal Association Areas," 9–10. Fulton stated that Moniz learned from his 1935 presentation to the Second Neurological Congress that the surgical intervention had rendered the animals "immune to experimental neurosis"; see Fulton, "The Physiological Basis of Frontal Lobotomy," 1–2. Without the experimental neurosis framework, the animal's behavior simply was described in terms of a cognitive deficit, i.e., its "distractibility."

40. See the correspondence between Fulton and Yerkes for 1931. JF to Dean Milton Winternitz, 17 Dec. 1932; and Yale University Department of Neurophysiology, 1931–5 (RG 1.1 200A 120 1480), RFA. Fulton, "Medicine and the Infra-human Primates," 11–12. Winternitz, "Yale University School of Medicine," 1–4; and John Fulton, "Yale University School of Medicine Department of Physiology," *Methods Probl. Med. Educ.* 20 (1932): 17–26. See also Robert Yerkes, "Yale Laboratories of Comparative Psychobiology," *Comp. Psych. Mono.* 8, no. 38 (1932); and Yale University Department of Physiology, "AR" (1935), 20.

41. The first meeting of the Committee on Problems of Neurotic Behavior, e.g., was held in New Haven in the office of Walter Miles, the director of the IHR. Yerkes made a strong claim for the use of primates to study psychiatric problems, in his "The Comparative Psychopathology of Infrahuman Primates," in Bentley and Cowdry, *Mental Disorder,* 327–38 (Chap. 1, n. 47). In 1935, Brickner, Watts, and others visited Jacobsen's chimpanzees to study their relevance to human pathology; JF *Diary,* vol. 9, 14 June 1933 – 1 Aug. 1936. Fulton's Neurological Study Unit in 1934 brought together faculty from the IHR, the medical school, and the New Haven clinics with a focus on psychiatry; see "Yale IHR Report of the Director, 1934–5," 4.

42. The RF (in conjunction with the resources of the General Education Board and the Laura Spelman Rockefeller Memorial) underwrote the reconstruction of Yale's medical school; it spent a total of $14 million between 1923 and 1939 on this program, which included the IHR and the founding of the psychiatry department. See "Exhibit A," Yale University Department of Psychiatry, 1937–41 (RG 1.1 200A 120 1484), RF. See also "Detail of Information," 9 Jan. 1934, 4 Jan. 1935, 17 Jan. 1936, Yale Neurophysiology, 1931–5 (RG 1.1 200A 120 1480), RF. The foundation emphasized the building of training centers for a new generation of psychiatrists; memoranda dated 7 Oct. 1930 and [?] Oct. 1943, Programs and Policy, Psychiatry, 1916–49 (RG 3 906 2 17–18), RF. Jacobsen acknowledged his debt to the RF in the foreword to his "Studies of Cerebral Function in Primates." See also Pressman, "Human Understanding" (Chap. 1, n. 25). Fulton, "Medicine and the Infrahuman Primates," 14; Yale University Department of Physiology, "AR"

(1933), 63; and see also John Fulton, "Remarks Concerning Yale Institute of Human Relations," typescript, 1 Apr. 1931.

43. Morawski, "Institute of Human Relations," 231; and Arthur Viseltear, "Milton Winternitz and the Yale Institute of Human Relations," 869–89. See also Yale University, *Report of the Dean of School of Medicine, 1931–2*, Sterling Archives, Yale University. "Society Transactions," discussion of paper by C. F. Jacobsen, ANP 33 (1935): 886.

44. JF to Alan Gregg, 20 Mar. 1933.

45. JW, résumé dated 4 Feb. 1935.

46. JF to Francis Grant, 8 Feb. 1933; see also JF to Daryl Hart, 12 June 1936. The allusion is to Dr. William S. Halsted of Johns Hopkins, America's preeminent teacher of surgery.

47. JW to JF, 11 Mar. 1935; and JF *Diary*, 14 June 1934.

48. JW to JF, 26 Feb. 1935; and WF to JF, 23 Feb. 1935.

49. Freeman's unpublished autobiography (cited as Freeman *Auto*) is invaluable for reconstructing the procedure's history. See also James W. Watts, "Neurology and Neurological Surgery: Its Story at George Washington University," *Med. Ann. D.C.* 34 (1965): 225–8.

50. Among his professional accomplishments, Freeman was secretary of the American Board of Psychiatry and Neurology, 1934–45, then president, 1946; chairman of the Section of Nervous and Mental Diseases, AMA, 1931; president of the Philadelphia Neurological Society, 1945; and president of the Medical Society of the District of Columbia, 1949. An advocate of often unpopular causes, Freeman was proudest of the moment when he presided over the admittance of the first black physicians into the D.C. Medical Society. Freeman, Ebaugh, and Boyd, "American Board of Psychiatry and Neurology" (Chap. 1, n. 41); Walter Freeman, *The Psychiatrist: Personalities and Patterns* (New York: Grune & Stratton, 1968), 184; idem, "George Washington University: 1924–1954," "Medical Societies, 1920–," and "The American Board of Psychiatry and Neurology," in Freeman *Auto*, chaps. 10, 12, 13.

51. For Keen's career, see Valenstein *G&DC*, 122–3; Freeman *Auto*, chaps. 1, 7, 8.

52. Freeman *Auto*; Zigmund Lebensohn, "Walter Freeman, 1895–1972," *AJP* 129 (1972): 356–7; and Valenstein *G&DC*, 122–6.

53. Freeman *Auto*, chap. 8.

54. Freeman, "St. Elizabeth's Hospital: 1924–1933," in his *Auto*, chap. 9; "The Pathology of Paralysis Agitans," *Ann. Clin. Med.* 4 (1925): 106–16; "Reactive Gliosis in a Case of Brain Tumor," ANP 14 (1925): 649–57; "Studies on the Etiology of Epidemic Encephalitis," *USPHS Rep.* (4 June 1926): 1095–117; "The Columnar Arrangement of the Primary Afferent Centers in the Brain-stem of Man," *JNMD* 65 (1927): 1–20, 149–70, 282–306, 378–97; and *Neuropathology: The Autonomic Foundation of Nervous Diseases* (Philadelphia: W. B. Saunders, 1933).

55. Walter Freeman, "The Psychological Panel in Diagnosis and Prognosis," *Ann. Int. Med.* 4 (1930): 29–38; and *Neuropathology*, 256. Freeman *Auto*, chap. 14.

56. It is possible that Freeman's sentiments about psychotherapy were influenced by an unfortunate experience during his internship, when a young woman suffering from an anal fistula was erroneously diagnosed as psychosomatic. Surgery cleared up the problem (ibid., chap. 22). The results of Freeman's autopsies were statistically analyzed by Raymond Pearl and published in an extensive monograph; Raymond Pearl, Walter Freeman, and Marjorie Gooch, *A Biometric Study of the Endocrine Organs in Relation to Mental Disease* (Baltimore: Johns Hopkins University Press, 1935).

57. Walter Freeman, "The Mind and the Body," GWU (italics added). See also Freeman *Auto,* ch. 9; and "Constitutional Factors in Mental Disorders," *Med. Ann. D.C.* 5 (1936): 334. Delivered in May and published in October, the text included references to the possibilities of Moniz's operation; in the same issue of this journal, Freeman and Watts published their first communication on the subject. See also his "Psychochemistry," *JAMA* 97 (16 June 1931): 293–6.

58. Freeman *Auto,* chap. 10. James Watts recalls that in his first year surgical fees were only $500, and in the next, $1,500; personal interview with the author, November 1984. When Lyerly set out to establish a neurosurgical practice in 1934, Fulton congratulated him on his "courage"; JF to J. Lyerly, 19 Oct. 1934. See also James Lyerly, Sr., "Pioneering Neurological Surgery in Florida," *J. Flor. Med. Assoc.* 63 (1976): 837–9.

59. Freeman, "International Congresses: 1931–1970," and "Prefrontal Lobotomy," in *Auto,* chaps. 14, 16; Valenstein *G&DC,* 73–8; WF to EM, 25 May 1936, GWU.

60. [Walter Freeman], "Review of *Tentatives opératoires* . . . , by Egas Moniz," in *ANP* 36 (1936): 1413. Walter Freeman, "International Congresses: 1931–1970," and "Prefrontal Lobotomy," in *Auto,* chaps. 14, 16.

61. Freeman and Watts described their first case in "Prefrontal Lobotomy in Agitated Depression," *Med. Ann. D.C.* 5 (1936): 326–8. Karl Menninger to WF, 22 Sept. 1936 (Pro/6.6), KAM. Valenstein reveals that in both Freeman's and Moniz's first series of patients the results were extremely problematic; Valenstein *G&DC,* 101–13, 142–5.

62. Freeman *Auto,* chap. 14.

63. Freeman and Watts, "Agitated Depression," 326–8. Karl Menninger to WF, 22 Sept. 1936. See also Friedman, *Menninger* (Chap. 1, n. 4).

64. WF to EM, 20 Oct. 1936, GWU.

65. The term *psychosis* often referred to any severe mental disorder, not just schizophrenia. Walter Freeman and James Watts, "Prefrontal Lobotomy in the Treatment of Mental Disorders," *SMJ* 30 (1937): 23–31.

66. Ibid. In spite of Meyer's assurances, Freeman already had arranged for considerable publicity. Freeman later reflected that Meyer's "accolade" had given him "a mission that has lasted for thirty years"; Freeman, *The Psychiatrist,* 122.

67. The incident created a rift between the two that later had important consequences within the profession; see Chapter 8.

68. WF to EM, 26 Nov. 1936, and WF to EM, 15 Jan. 1937, GWU.

69. The first indication of the brewing storm was Morris Fishbein's rejection of Freeman's translation of Moniz's work; see WF to EM, 5 Jan. 1937, GWU.

70. Walter Freeman and James Watts, "Subcortical Prefrontal Lobotomy in the Treatment of Certain Psychoses," ANP 38 (1937): 225–9.

71. Ibid.; and Valenstein *G&DC*, 145.

72. WF to EM 11 Aug. 1937, GWU; and Walter Freeman and James Watts, "Psychosurgery," *JNMD* 88 (1938): 589–601.

73. Walter Freeman and James Watts, "Some Observations on Obsessive Tendencies following Interruption of the Frontal Association Pathways," *JNMD* 88 (1938): 230–4. [W. S. Muncie], book review of Moniz's *Tentatives opératoires, JNMD* 87 (1938): 663.

74. Freeman and Watts, "Obsessive Tendencies," 230–4.

75. WF to JF, 8 June 1936, JF; Carlyle Jacobsen to WF, 26 Sept. 1934; and JF to WF, 12 Sept. 1936. Freeman *Auto*, chap. 16. Only a few months earlier, in an address on constitutional factors, Freeman speculated on the future of psychiatric research. A discussant noted that the physiological characteristics of personality had already been studied in depth by Pavlov, who showed that vulnerability to mental illness fell into two types. (1) Experimental neurosis is easily produced, as evidenced in hysterics and schizophrenics. (2) An experimental neurosis cannot be produced, which corresponded to "the majority of persons, who do not succumb to mental illness, despite many psychic and toxic traumas." A logical implication was that insusceptibility to experimental neurosis offered resistance to mental illness. See Walter Freeman, "Constitutional Factors in Mental Disease," ANP 37 (1937): 190–4.

76. The initial report was Freeman and Watts, "Agitated Depression," 326–8. Henry Viets, "Diary Entry," 11 Oct. 1936.

77. JF to Henry Viets, 16 Oct. 1936. JF to JW, 16 Oct. 1936; and Watts to JF, 19 Oct. 1936.

78. JW to JF, 19 Oct. 1936. JW to JF, 2 Nov. 1936; and JF to JW, 20 Oct. 1936, 4 Nov. 1936.

79. JF *Diary*, 10 Nov. 1936, and 16 Nov. 1936. JF to JW, 20 Nov. 1936; JW to JF, 23 Nov. 1936; and JF to (name withheld), 25 Nov. 1936. [Henry Viets,] "The Surgical Treatment of Certain Psychoses," *NEJM* 215 (3 Dec. 1936): 1088. Viets forwarded a manuscript copy of the editorial with the postscript "Boston conservatism!"; Henry Viets to JW, 3 Dec. 1936, GWU; and JW to Viets, 7 Dec. 1936, HRV.

80. Fulton, e.g., widely circulated a copy of Moniz's monograph. See Charles Lund to JF, 8 Dec. 1936; JF to R. G. Spurling, 8 Jan. 1937; and JF to Harry Solomon, 19 Jan. 1937. JF to Richard Brickner, 28 Oct. 1936. JF to Paul Bucy, 4 Nov. 1936.

81. Harry Solomon to JF, 9 Feb. 1937; and R. G. Spurling to JF, 5 Jan. 1937. Spurling, a neurosurgeon, performed the frontal lobe extirpations on Ackerly's famous case; see Ackerly, "Prefrontal Lobe Extirpation," 717.

82. R. Spurling to JF, 16 Jan. 1937. Fulton to Richard Brickner, 28 Oct. 1936; Paul Bucy, 4 Nov. 1936; Carlyle Jacobsen, 4 Nov. 1936; and Harry Solomon, 10 Feb. 1937.

83. JW to JF, 3 July 1937; and JF to JW, 6 July 1937. JF to JW, 12 May 1937, 27 May 1937; and JW to JF, 1 June 1937. See also JF *Diary*, 8 May 1937. JF to JW, 20 Jan. 1936[7]; and JW to JF, 2 Nov. 1936, and 21 Jan. 1937.
84. Spurling quoted in Thomas to JF, 11 June 1941.
85. Magnus C. Peterson and Harold F. Buchstein, "Prefrontal Lobotomy in Chronic Psychoses," *AJP* 99 (1942): 429.
86. JF to Alan Gregg, 25 Feb. 1933. Fulton believed that classical neurology had been at first modestly successful but more recently had both "bred contempt" for active therapy and perpetuated ignorance of physiological functions. By "dynamic" he meant "the analysis of neurological disturbances in terms of the brain reflex mechanisms responsible for the observed manifestations" – for him, the only basis for sound diagnosis and therapy. In substance, this involved neurology's incorporation of the physiological principles of Hughlings Jackson and Charles Sherrington, and of the clinical teachings of Ottfried Foerster.
87. The dedication in Fulton's *Physiology of the Nervous System* reads: "To students of medicine who must bridge the gap between the concepts of neurophysiology and the problems of clinical neurology." In Bucy's opinion, "Fulton's entire professional career was devoted to neurophysiology and its relation to neurosurgery. No man has ever done so much to bridge the gap between a clinical specialty and its basic scientific counterpart"; Bucy, "*Journal of Neurosurgery*," 1. Sherrington to JF, 27 May 1937, Letters of Charles Scott Sherrington to John Farquhar Fulton, 1923–1937, JF[MED].
88. JF to Alan Gregg, 25 Feb. 1933, 27 Feb. 1933. See also Howard Brown, "The Harvey Cushing Society. Past, Present and Future," *J. Neurosurg.* 15 (1958): 587–601. The society evolved into the American Assocation of Neurological Surgeons, the current national organization of neurosurgeons. See Robert H. Wilkins, ed., *History of the American Association of Neurological Surgeons, Founded in 1931 as the Harvey Cushing Society, 1931–1981* (Chicago: A.A.N.S., 1981); and Society of Neurological Surgeons, *The Society of Neurological Surgeons, 1920–1970* (privately printed, 1970).
89. JF *Diary*, "First International Congress."
90. JF to Alan Gregg, 27 Feb. 1933; Fulton, "Abstract of Presidential Address," typescript of an address delivered to the Harvey Cushing Society, St. Louis, 5 Apr. 1934, 1; and JF to W. P. Van Wagenen, 27 Feb. 1933.
91. Fulton, "Abstract," 2. William Livingston to JF, 12 Dec. 1932; JF to Livingston, 14 Dec. 1932; and Fulton, "Ivan Petrovich Pavlov," *NEJM* 214 (5 Mar. 1936): 487–9.
92. Minutes of the Harvey Cushing Society, Philadelphia, May 1937, 12. JF to Henry Viets, 10 Oct. 1936; and Charles Lund to JF, 8 Dec. 1936. JF to Viets, 10 Oct. 1936.
93. John Fulton, "Sigma Xi-Swarthmore," typescript of a speech delivered on a multicity tour, Feb. 1940, 8. Fulton wrote in his diary, "I am inclined to look upon Jacobsen's work as the most important development in experimental neurology that has taken place in recent years"; JF *Diary*, 14–20 June 1937.
94. EM to WF, 24 Dec. 1936, GWU.

95. Jack Pressman, "Reflections on Neurosurgery in Philadelphia: Oral Histories with Frederick Murtagh and Henry Shenkin," *Trans. Stud. Coll. Phys. Phila.* 12 (1990): 27–48.

96. See, e.g., the discussion in chapter 1 of Bentley and Cowdry, *Mental Disorder.*

97. In a circular form of anthropomorphism, in order to discuss the psychiatric problems of people, investigators projected human psychiatric conditions onto the behavior of animals so as to interpret, in turn, the original human problems.

98. Abraham Myerson, "Some Trends of Psychiatry," *AJP* 100 (1944): 161, 170.

99. Pavlov delivered a paper at the Ninth International Congress of Psychology held at Yale, 1–7 Sept. 1929.

100. This logical aversion to history is usually reinforced by one based on practical sentiment. Young scientists of today are universally taught that if they are to achieve anything professionally they must never look backward at a past strewn with errors and misadventures, but keep their eyes facing forward toward the current "cutting edge." History becomes, then, a room filled with decaying newspapers. (For an analysis of what is wrong with the concept of cutting edge, see Pressman, "Human Understanding.")

101. Isaac Newton to Robert Hooke, 5 Feb. 1675/76; *The Correspondence of Isaac Newton:* vol. 1, *1661–1675,* ed. H. W. Turnbull (Cambridge University Press, 1959), 416. Fulton, one of the last in a fading tradition of medical authors who wrote textbooks that encompassed an entire field, excelled at the ability to fit fast-breaking scientific news into the vast literature of prior research findings, constructing convincing narratives that reached centuries back; the chapters of his textbooks typically started with such encapsulated summaries. In Fulton's own life, history and experimental medicine were inextricably combined. In addition to his other accomplishments, Fulton established himself as one of the leading medical bibliographers of the day and created at Yale one of the centers of medical history. Upon his retirement as a scientist, he became Yale's first professor in the history of medicine and later was elected to the presidency of the American Association for the History of Medicine.

102. White suggests that the "value attached to narrativity in the representation of real events arises out of a desire to have real events display the coherence, integrity, fullness, and closure of an image of life that is and can only be imaginary"; Hayden White, *The Content of the Form: Narrative Discourse and Historical Representation* (Baltimore: Johns Hopkins University Press, 1987).

103. Walter Freeman and James Watts, "Subcortical Prefrontal Lobotomy in the Treatment of Certain Psychoses," *Med. Ann. D.C.* 6 (1937): 267–71.

104. This kind of symbiosis between laboratory and clinic – what I term *reciprocal legitimation* – is discussed further in Chapter 7.

105. Fulton, *Physiology of the Nervous System,* 465. Freeman and Watts's first paper underscored the connection; see "Surgical Treatment," 326. See also J. G. Lyerly, "Prefrontal Lobotomy in Involutional Melancholia" *J. Flor. Med. Assoc.* 25 (1938): 225; and E. Strecker, H. Palmer and F. Grant, "A Study of

Frontal Lobotomy; Neurological and Psychiatric Features and Results in 22 Cases with a Detailed Report on 5 Chronic Schizophrenics," *AJP* 98 (1942): 528, 532. M. Crawford et al., "Frontal Lobe Ablation in Chimpanzees: A Resume of 'Becky' and 'Lucy,'" *ARNMD* 27 (1948): 3–58.

106. It is suggestive that Jacobsen's full report on Becky was not published until 1947, when the ARNMD selected the frontal lobes – and especially their importance in psychosurgery – as that year's subject. Moniz's award was shared with Walter R. Hess (neurophysiology). The archival materials surrounding the decision are sealed until 1999. The text of the presentation can be found in Nobel Foundation, *Nobel Lectures, Including Presentation Speeches and Laureates' Biographies. Physiology or Medicine, 1942–1962* (Amsterdam: Nobel Foundation, 1964), 243–6. Some have stated, erroneously, that Moniz was given the Nobel Prize for his discovery of cerebral angiography; see, e.g., Sachs, *Fifty Years of Neurosurgery*, 142.

107. Edgar Congdon, "The Background of Present-Day Psychiatric Practice," *MHN* 24 (Feb. 1954): 5.

108. See Schaffer, "Scientific Discoveries."

109. I am paraphrasing Fleck: "In science, just as in art and in life, only that which is true to culture is true to nature"; Ludwik Fleck, *Genesis and Development of a Scientific Fact* (Chicago: University of Chicago Press, 1979 [1935]).

110. JF to R. G. Spurling, 20 Jan. 1937.

## Chapter 3. Certain Benefit

1. Folder of materials on the AMA, St. Louis Meeting, 15–19 May 1939; and John Fulton, Carlyle Jacobsen, and Margaret Kennard, "An Exhibition Illustrating the Functions of the Frontal Lobes," Ninetieth Annual Session of the AMA, St. Louis, 15–19 May 1939, privately printed, JF.

2. Lyerly was listed in *Who's Who in America, 1940–1941* (Chicago: Marquis, 1940), 1643; Lyerly, "Neurological Surgery in Florida" (Chap. 2, n. 58); and personal correspondence, James Lyerly to the author, 13 Apr. 1984. For more information on Orange Park, see also Haraway, *Primate Visions* (Chap. 2, n. 28); and Solly Zuckerman, *From Apes to Warlords* (New York: Harper & Row, 1978).

3. Lyerly, "Involutional Melancholia" (Chap. 2, n. 105). The names of all patients mentioned here are fictitious.

4. Ibid.; and James Lyerly, "Transsection of the Deep Association Fibers of the Prefrontal Lobes in Certain Mental Disorders," *South. Surg.* 8 (1939): 426–34. By 1941, Lyerly had operated upon forty-four cases; see AMA, Section of Nervous and Mental Diseases, "Neurosurgical Treatment of Certain Abnormal Mental States," panel discussion, *JAMA* 117 (16 Aug. 1941): 517–27.

5. J. G. Love, "Prefrontal Lobotomy in the Treatment of Mental Diseases: Surgical Technic," *Proc. Staff Meet. Mayo Clin.* 18 (1943): 372–3; and JF *Diary,* vol. 12, 2 Mar. 1939. Love was so impressed by Lyerly's paper at the Cushing Society that he traveled to Florida to learn the technique in person from Lyerly; Lyerly to author.

6. Grant, Watts, Tarumianz, and Freeman were in contact through the regular meetings of the Philadelphia Neurological Society, of which they were all active members. Patient E.W. fared poorly; Watts had to operate a second time, which also ended in failure. Bertrand G. Lawrence, "Prefrontal Lobotomy: Result in a Case of Agitated Depression," *Del. St. Med. J.* 10 (1938): 81–4; P. F. Elfeld, "Results of Lobotomies at Delaware State Hospital," *Del. St. Med. J.* 14 (1942): 81–3; and Tarumianz's discussion in AMA, "Neurosurgical Treatment."

7. The case descriptions that follow are drawn from the published report of Lawrence, "Prefrontal Lobotomy," and the original patient records in Grant's professional files, FG.

8. The "curiously" good results amazed Grant, as the operation had been botched.

9. Delaware State Hospital, AR (1936–8): 47.

10. Although the early patient records of Delaware State were reportedly destroyed in a hospital fire, some of the case notes survived in Dr. Grant's personal files.

11. AMA, "Neurosurgical Treatment," 520. As of 1942, nineteen patients had been operated upon, with most reported as improved, especially in cases of agitated depression and involutional melancholia; of ten of these, six returned home and were judged to have made excellent social recoveries. See Elfeld, "Lobotomies at Delaware State."

12. William Mixter, Kenneth Tillotson, and David Wies, "Reports of Partial Frontal Lobectomy and Frontal Lobotomy Performed on Three Patients: One Chronic Epileptic and Two Cases of Chronic Agitated Depression," *Psychosom. Med.* 3 (1941): 26–37.

13. The significance of the Rockefeller program is discussed in Chapter 1; the use of psychosurgery at McLean Hospital is examined at length in Chapter 6. For a recent biography of Cobb, see Benjamin V. White, *Stanley Cobb, A Builder of the Modern Neurosciences* (Boston: Countway Library, 1984).

14. Patient #612, McLH. All data that might be used to identify individual patients have been altered. The use of the McLean records is described in Chapter 6.

15. The names of all McLean doctors identified from unpublished sources, such as patient records and staff conference minutes, have also been altered. Drs. Thomason and Jaffe are thus pseudonyms.

16. Cobb no doubt learned about the operation from his good friend John Fulton; his own pioneering research on the physiological basis of the emotions also kept him abreast of related work. It is significant that, at this point, Cobb listed Watts's name first when referring to the operation.

17. A diagram representing the cut made was later published. See Mixter, Tillotson, and Wies, "Lobectomy and Frontal Lobotomy," 32.

18. Some years later, the hospital inquired about Arthur's condition. The brother wrote: "I am glad to tell you that my brother has, on the whole, been getting along very well. He is living quietly . . . , has a house, seems wholly to have lost his craving for alcohol, and has had no recurrence of the depression. . . .

On the other hand he has no initiative, seems to have little or no foresight about the future, and seems to have lost any capability of budgeting and husbanding his small income. And he seems not to realize that the operation did anything for him. He has spoken to me of you in a friendly way, I'll pass regards."A staff psychiatrist replied, "I think it is fair to assume from your letter that [Arthur] is better than he was prior to hospitalization." In 1957, Arthur was admitted to Taunton State Hospital.

19. Drs. Hollingshead, Rourke, Boyle, and Caufield are pseudonyms.
20. Phone call from sister, 12 Mar. 1945; and letter from nephew, 30 Oct. 1949.
21. Mixter, Tillotson, and Wies, "Lobectomy and Frontal Lobotomy."
22. Paul Flothow and Frederick Lemere, "Prefrontal Lobotomy in Mental Diseases," *West. J. Surg. Obs. Gyn.* 51 (1943): 1–3. Ralph Drake and James Hibbard, "Prefrontal Lobotomy in Certain Abnormal Mental States," *J. Kans. Med. Soc.* 43 (1942): 345–7. Other early sites of lobotomy included the Institute of Living in Hartford, Conn.; New York City, where Leo Davidoff performed the operation; and Rochester, N.Y., where Van Wagenen took it up. An extended list is included in F-W *PS1*, 16–17. McKenzie's use of the procedure in Toronto is mentioned in Kenneth McKenzie, "Results of Bilateral Frontal Leucotomies," *AJP* 101 (1944): 280–1.
23. A series of ten involutional melancholics and agitated depressives were operated upon at the Medical College of Virginia Hospital, Richmond, Va., beginning in 1941; R. Finley Gayle, Jr., and Claude Neale, "The Treatment of Certain Mental Disorders by Psycho-surgery," *Virg. Med. Monthly* 71 (1944): 361–5.
24. James Lyerly to JF, 22 Feb. 1940, JF; and J. G. Love, "Prefrontal Lobotomy," 372–3.
25. H. Woltman et al., "Prefrontal Lobotomy in the Treatment of Certain Mental Disorders," *Proc. Staff Meet. Mayo Clin.* 16 (1941): 200–1; and Love, "Prefrontal Lobotomy." See also William Peyton, John Haavik, and B. Schiele, "Prefrontal Lobectomy in Schizophrenia," *ANP* 62 (1949): 560–71, for another large trial.
26. George W. Gray, "The Attack on Brainstorms," *Harper's* 183 (1941): 366–76; and Edward Strecker, Harold Palmer, and Francis Grant, "Study of Prefrontal Lobotomy; Neurosurgical and Psychiatric Features in 22 Cases with Detailed Reports on 5 Chronic Schizophrenics," *AJP* 98 (1942): 530.
27. The stories of Strecker's and Grant's cases are reconstructed from information in Grant's patient files and published accounts that appeared in Gray, "The Attack on Brainstorms"; AMA, "Neurosurgical Treatment"; and Strecker, Palmer, and Grant, "Study of Prefrontal Lobotomy."
28. Strecker, Palmer, and Grant, "Study of Prefrontal Lobotomy," 528.
29. Ibid.; and AMA, "Neurosurgical Treatment."
30. AMA, "Neurosurgical Treatment," 521; and see also Pressman, "Making Psychiatry Respectable" (Chap. 1, n. 39).
31. Pressman, "Making Psychiatry Respectable," 437. The RF spent approx. $300,000 on the institute. Earl Bond to Alan Gregg, 8 Mar. 1939 (RG 1.1 200 150 1278), RF.

32. Edward A. Strecker, "Pharmacological and Surgical Approaches," in *Therapeutic Advances in Psychiatry* (Philadelphia: University of Pennsylvania Press, 1941); and Bicentennial Conference, University of Pennsylvania, "New Operation Improves Chronic Mental Patients" (press release for 17 Sept. 1940, abs. S. M. Spencer), EAS; and Greer Williams, "He Made Psychiatry Respectable," *Saturday Evening Post,* 18 Oct. 1947, 32. The APA address was published as Strecker, Palmer, and Grant, "Study of Prefrontal Lobotomy." A sketch of Strecker's career is found in Lauren Smith, "Edward A. Strecker, M.D.; President 1943–1944," *AJP* 101 (1944): 9–11. The allusions to Strecker's status are from "Madness, Measles, Metabolism," *Time,* 30 Sept. 1940, 36:49.

33. Strecker, Palmer, and Grant, "Study of Prefrontal Lobotomy," 531; Tarumianz's discussion in AMA, "Neurosurgical Treatment"; and Pressman, "Making Psychiatry Respectable."

34. A. Bennett, J. Keegan, and C. Wilbur, "Prefrontal Lobotomy in Chronic Schizophrenia," *JAMA* 123 (27 Nov. 1943): 809–13.

35. Heilbrunn and Hletko, "Disappointing Results," 569. Their high operative mortality led critics to wonder about the quality of the operative technique. In 1948, Freeman learned that even Heilbrunn had come round to supporting lobotomy; see Charles Jones to WF, 12 Dec. 1948, GWU.

36. See also F-W *PS2,* 488; and Strecker, Palmer, and Grant, "Study of Prefrontal Lobotomy," 531; Pressman, "Making Psychiatry Respectable."

37. Gray, "The Attack on Brainstorms," 370.

38. Petersen and Buchstein, "Prefrontal Lobotomy" (Chap. 2, n. 85); and F. Moersch, "Prefrontal Lobotomy in Treatment of Mental Diseases: Presentation of Four Cases," *Proc. Staff Meet. Mayo Clin.* 18 (1943): 368–71. Leopold Hofstatter et al., "The Results of Surgical Treatment in One Hundred Cases of Chronic Mental Illness," *SMJ* 38 (1945): 604–7; Hofstatter et al., "Prefrontal Lobotomy in Treatment of Chronic Psychoses with Special Reference to Section of the Orbital Areas Only," *ANP* 53 (1945): 125–30; and see also St. Louis City Hospital, *AR* (1942), 35, for a description of the new operative techniques. The results from these hospital series were published in the *Proc. Staff Meet. Mayo Clin.,* the *SMJ,* and the *ANP.*

39. Petersen and Buchstein, "Prefrontal Lobotomy," 370. Jacobsen won the bronze medal with Kennard and Fulton at the AMA meeting in St. Louis; he was also awarded the Warren medal for outstanding work in experimental psychology.

40. See the St. Louis City Hospital ARs for 1938 to 1942 for a description of the lobotomy program. Hofstatter noted that interest in psychosurgery was stimulated by Carlyle Jacobsen, then assistant dean of Washington University Medical School, and by Freeman's lecture to a neurosurgery conference in Barnes Hospital, ca. 1940; correspondence of Leopold Hofstatter to Elliot Valenstein, 1 Aug. 1983 (in author's possession, courtesy of Prof. Valenstein).

41. The first large program of psychosurgery was instituted at State Hospital #4 in Farmington, Mo., in 1939, when a young staff physician was given a leave of absence by the board of managers to learn enough neurosurgery to perform

lobotomies himself. Paul Schrader, between 1939 and 1942, operated on as many as 207 patients before leaving for the war. His contributions, however, were sui generis. Although partial accounts of his work were discussed with others in personal communications, Schrader himself never published these results; see, e.g., F-W *PS1*, 17, and Ziegler, "Bilateral Prefrontal Lobotomy," *AJP* 100 (1943): 178–9. See also Schrader to WF (16 Feb. 1942, GWU), in which he notes the less than satisfactory results with schizophrenics. Schrader's decision to take up the procedure, and to report his results directly to Freeman, might have been influenced by his plans to undergo the rigorous examination for board certification in psychiatry and neurology – a test administered by Freeman. At war's end, Schrader returned to a different state hospital, where he initiated a smaller lobotomy series in conjunction with psychologist Frances Robinson; the behavioral analyses were published as Paul Schrader and Mary F. Robinson, "Evaluation of Prefrontal Lobotomy through Ward Behavior," *J. Abn. Soc. Psych.* 40 (1945): 61–8. For brief accounts of the operations in Missouri, see Missouri SH #4 [Farmington] *BR* 20 (1939/40): 6–9, in Missouri Board of Managers of State Eleemosynary Institutions *BR* 20 (1939/40): 10; Missouri General Assembly, Committee on Legislative Research, Report No. 8, *The Mentally Ill: Their Care and Treatment in Missouri* (Jefferson City, Mo.: n.p., 1948), 17.

42. Sachs's ties to Fulton were strong; the two kept in constant correspondence on all matters of neurophysiology and neurosurgery. His son became a fellow in Fulton's lab and he himself retired there. Although Sachs personally was against lobotomy, many of his surgical fellows practiced it.

43. See "News and Notes. Neuropsychiatry at Washington University, St. Louis," *AJP* 95 (1938): 239; and Dean Philip Shaffer to Alan Gregg, 11 Feb. 1938 (RG 1.1 228 2 22), RF. The Department of Neuropsychiatry officially began in 1941, with the recruitment of J. C. Whitehorn from McLean, David Rioch from Harvard, and Jacobsen. The RF also forged similar innovative programs in Europe. The discipline of neurosurgery in Britain, e.g., was greatly influenced by the RF's support of Cairns, the country's leading practitioner of the specialty. Indeed, Cairns described himself as a "Rockefeller baby"; cited in Donald Fisher, "The Rockefeller Foundation and the Development of Scientific Medicine in Great Britain," *Minerva* 16 (Spring, 1948): 40. Lima, the young neurosurgeon who performed the operations for Moniz, trained with Cairns via a RF fellowship.

44. See Patient #7, FG.

45. See WF to EM, 15 Mar. 1938; EM to WF, 5 Apr. 1938; WF to EM, 12 Oct. 1940; and EM to WF, 30 Oct. 1940, GWU.

46. WF to (name withheld), 22 Sept. 1941, GWU.

47. Valenstein *G&DC*, 160.

48. See "Itinerary of Dr. J. F. Fulton; Sigma Xi Lectures – February 1940"; and "Brain Operations, Removing Parts of Frontal Lobes, Found to Aid Some Types of Hopeless Mental Patients" (Science Service Press Release, 8 Feb. 1940), JF. JF *Diary*, vol. 14, 31 Jan. 1940. For letters in response to his

lectures and newspaper accounts, see folder marked "Fan Mail, 1939–1941," JF.

49. Kaempffert had already communicated with Fulton about his Sigma Xi lecture; Waldemar Kaempffert to JF, 9 Feb. 1940; Kaempffert to JF, 9 Dec. 1940; JF to Kaempffert, 11 Dec. 1940; and Kaempffert to JF, 12 Dec. 1940, JF. The opposition that Freeman and Watts encountered is described in greater detail in Chapter 4. See also Valenstein *G&DC*, 144–6, 160, 180–8.

50. Waldemar Kaempffert to JF, 31 May 1941; JF to Kaempffert, 12 June 1941; JF to Charles C. Thomas, 27 May 1941; and JF to Henry Viets, 25 June 1941, JF.

51. [G. Stragnell], "The Lobotomy Delusion," *Med. Rec.* 151 (15 May 1940): 335.

52. Gregory Zilboorg, *A History of Medical Psychology* (New York: Norton, 1941); Stanley Cobb, "Review of Neuropsychiatry for 1940," *Arch. Int. Med.* 66 (1940): 1341–54.

53. AMA, "Neurosurgical Treatment," 87–8, 110–1, 116–19, 524–5, typescript, GWU.

54. See W. B. Saunders, Inc., to WF and JW, 10 Oct. 1940, GWU; and T. Myers [Macmillan] to Edward Strecker, 26 July 1940, EAS. Charles C. Thomas to JF, 26 May 1941; JF to Thomas, 27 May 1941; Thomas to JF, 4 June 1941; and JW to JF, 7 Sept. 1941, JF. The other informants who helped sway Thomas positively were Percival Bailey (Watts was his resident), Viets, and Spurling; copy of Thomas to Edward Lehman, 8 Apr. 1942, GWU. Spurling quoted in Thomas to JF, 11 June 1941, JF.

55. C. F. Williams to WF, 19 Feb. 1942, GWU.

56. Waldemar Kaempffert, "Science in the News. Psychosurgery," *New York Times*, 1 Nov. 1942, sec. II:7, col. 1.

57. M. Tarumianz to WF, 7 Jan. 1942, GWU. The impact on Europe would have to wait; the only shipment of the volume was torpedoed. C. C. Thomas to WF, 27 Feb. 1942; McKenzie to WF, 21 Apr. 1942; and JF to JW, 25 May 1942, GWU.

58. Early surveys of lobotomy are: George Kisker, "Remarks on the Problem of Psychosurgery," *AJP* 100 (1943): 180–4; Lloyd Ziegler, "Bilateral Prefrontal Lobotomy – a Survey," *AJP* 100 (1943): 178–9; McKenzie, "Frontal Leucotomies," 281; Schrader and Robinson, "Evaluation of Prefrontal Lobotomy," 61–8; and A. E. Walker, "Psychosurgery – Collective Review," *Int. Abs. Surg.* 78 (1944): 1–11.

59. Walker, "Psychosurgery," 10.

60. F. A. Carmichael and F. A. Carmichael, Jr., "Prefrontal Lobotomy in the Treatment of Malignant Mental Disorders," *J. Kans. Med. Soc.* 43 (1942): 200–2. No cases of their own were reported. Gayle and Neale, "Psychosurgery," 361.

61. F-W *PS2*, 381.

62. WF to EM, 17 Apr. 1944; and WF to EM, 18 Feb. 1946, GWU. Moniz had replied in June 1944: "Today you are the greatest pioneer of the method,"

and then he referred a case under his own care to travel to Freeman. Freeman did not present only the good side to Moniz, describing failures as well.

63. James Lyerly to JF, 22 Feb. 1940, JF. Kisker, "Remarks on Psychosurgery," 181.

64. "Society Transactions, . . . Discussion of Walter Freeman and James Watts, 'Psychosurgery: 1936–1946,' at the Boston Society of Neurology and Psychiatry, Kenneth Tillotson presiding, 17 January 1946," *ANP* 57 (1947): 771.

65. Hand-calligraphed poem, framed, signed by (name withheld), Freeman and Watts's 68th lobotomy patient, GWU.

66. F-W *PS1*, 294.

67. Bennett, Keegan, and Wilbur, "Lobotomy in Schizophrenia," 809.

68. Wilder Penfield to JF, 4 Jan. 1949, JF. For a description of when this gentlemen's agreement fails, see Andrew Scull, "Desperate Remedies: A Gothic Tale of Madness and Modern Medicine," *Psychol. Med.* 17 (1987): 561–77.

69. For an account of how middle- and upper-class patients often pave the way for the introduction of new technologies, see Judith Walzer Leavitt, *Brought to Bed. Child-Bearing in America, 1750–1950* (New York: Oxford University Press, 1986), 8.

70. JF to Henry Viets, 10 Oct. 1936 (see also Charles Lund to JF, 8 Dec. 1936); and JF to Harry Solomon, 10 Feb. 1937, JF.

71. Stanley Porteus and Richard De Monbrum Kepner, "Mental Changes after Bilateral Prefrontal Lobotomy," *Genetic Psychol. Mono.* 29 (Feb. 1944): 114–15. Cobb, "Neuropsychiatry for 1940," 1341–54; and idem, *Emotions and Clinical Medicine* (New York: Norton, 1950), 114.

## Chapter 4. Active Treatment

1. Morton Kramer, "The 1951 Survey of the Use of Psychosurgery" (Intro., n. 3); and *Patients in Mental Institutions 1949*, USPHS pub. no. 233 (Washington, D.C.: GPO, 1952), 14, 160. The survey was sent to all public and private asylums, veterans hospitals with neuropsychiatric facilities, and general hospitals with psychiatric wards; 897 replied, a 94 percent response rate. Between 1936 and 1950, 126 out of 201 state hospitals had used lobotomy; at the time of the survey, 106. Other surveys superseded by this study are Ziegler, "Bilateral Prefrontal Lobotomy," *AJP* 100 (1943): 178–9; Charles C. Limburg, "A Survey on the Use of Psychosurgery with Mental Patients," in Newton Bigelow, ed., *Proceedings of the First Research Conference on Psychosurgery*, USPHS pub. no. 16 (Washington, D.C.: GPO, 1951), 65–173; Council of State Governments (CSG), *The Mental Health Programs of the Forty-Eight States. A Report to the Governors Conference* (Chicago: CSG, 1950), 304–27, 346; and APA, *Better Care in Mental Hospitals; Proceedings of the First Mental Hospital Institute of the American Psychiatric Association*, held at the Institute of the Pennsylvania Hospital, Philadelphia, 11–15 Apr. 1949 (Washington, D.C.: APA, 1949), 183. The CSG survey is the only available source that identifies, by individual facility, where psychosurgery was used; it is not entirely accurate, however.

2. Harry Worthing, Henry Brill, and Henry Widgerson, "Evaluation of Immediate and Late Results of Prefrontal Lobotomy in 600 Cases, Including Case of Postencephalitis and Other Organic States," *AJP* 108 (1951): 328–36; and Board of Control, England and Wales, *Prefrontal Leucotomy in a Thousand Cases* (London: Her Majesty's Stationery Office, 1947). The appeals for a better lobotomy are discussed in Chapter 7. In 1946, Moniz confidentially asked Freeman to nominate him for the Nobel Prize. Freeman cheerfully complied, noting that he already had done so in the previous year; EM to WF, 4 Feb. 1946, and WF to EM, 18 Feb. 1946, GWU. Tracy Putnam, "Prefrontal Lobotomy – Its Evolution and Present Status," *Bull. Los. Ang. Neur. Soc.* 15 (1950): 225; and Robert Hyde and Harvey [*sic*] Solomon, "Clinical Management of Psychiatric Hospitals," *Conn. St. Med. J.* 15 (1951): 391–2.

3. Albert Q. Maisel, "Bedlam 1946, Most U.S. Mental Hospitals Are a Shame and a Disgrace," *Life* 20 (1946): 102–3. Maisel's comparison to concentration camps was echoed in other national publications; see, e.g., *Commonweal* 44 (17 May 1946): 107. The fullest description of mental hospital conditions and the resulting scandals is Grob *Asylum*, 70–92.

4. Frank L. Wright, Jr., ed., *Out of Sight, Out of Mind* (Philadelphia: National Mental Health Foundation, 1947), 35–7, 55, 64, 100, 107–12, 128–9. As strong as these stories were, Wright had refrained from publishing the most flagrant hospital abuses in order to preserve credibility. Its publisher, the NMHF, itself grew out of a group of concerned CO's; eventually the NMHF merged with the NCMH and exists today under the former's name. See also Robert Clark and Alex Burgess, Jr., "The Work of Conscientious Objectors in State Mental Hospitals during the Second World War," *PSQ Suppl.* 21 (1947): 128–40.

5. Albert Deutsch, *The Shame of the States* (New York: Harcourt, Brace, 1948); and Grob *Asylum*, 71, 73, 82. The title is a reference to Lincoln Steffens's *The Shame of the Cities* (New York: McClure, Phillips, 1904); Deutsch's *The Mentally Ill in America: A History of Their Care and Treatment from Colonial Times* (New York: Doubleday and Doran, 1937) was the leading work on the history of institutional psychiatry. See also idem, "The History of Mental Hygiene," in Hall, *American Psychiatry*, 325–65 (see above, Chap. 1, n. 43). Mary Jane Ward's *The Snakepit* (New York: Random House, 1946), a novel about a middle-class mental patient suffering the degradations of hospitalization, captured the public's imagination in this period. Even Ward, however, admitted that patients were often helped by hard-working, decent staff members who had the best interests of the inmates at heart. The story was further popularized by a movie version, which several mental hospitals showed to both patients and staff. Deutsch was eventually awarded the Lasker Prize.

6. Gerald Grob, "Abuse in American Mental Hospitals in Historical Perspective: Myth and Reality," *Int. J. Law Psychiat.* 3 (1980): 295–310.

7. Cherokee SH in Iowa Board of Control *BR* (1950): 117; and Pilgrim SH (N.Y.) *AR* 8 (1939): 36. These generalizations are based on annual reports from over 50 hospitals in 16 states for roughly 1935 to 1955. See Appendix for details.

8. Managers at a Missouri institution mentioned that effects of overcrowding

were "better left undescribed." CSG, *Mental Health,* 153; Longview SH "AR" (typescript, 1953), LSH; Marlboro SH (N.J.) (mimeo., 1949), 18, and (mimeo., 1951), 1, PFL; St. Louis City Sanitarium (Mo.) "AR" (typescript, 1947), 27 (St. Louis SH as of 1948); Connecticut SH (Middletown) *BR* 51 (1945/6): 18, and 52 (1947/8): 11.

9. Norristown SH (Pa.) *AR* (1948): 12. See also Mount Pleasant SH in Iowa Board of Control of State Institutions *BR* 25 (1945/66): 84; and Deutsch, *Shame,* 43–5. West Virginia Board of Control *BR* (1945/8): 11, 14. Due to lack of funds, state hospitals in this period often had to submit their annual reports in the form of carbon copies.

10. Connecticut SH *AR* (1946): 11, 18; Topeka SH (Kans.) *BR* 37 (1949/50): 3; and Wladimir Eliasberg, "Institutionalizing the Obsessive Psychopath," *PSQ* 19 (1945): 697–701.

11. For an entry into the sizable literature on the history of the American insane asylum, see Chap. 1, n. 4. Each state hospital's opening date is in Samuel Hamilton, "The History of American Mental Hospitals," in Hall, *American Psychiatry,* 153–60. Statistics on patient populations in American mental hospitals from 1904 to 1946 were compiled and published by the U.S. Bureau of the Census under varying titles; thereafter, the NIMH Biometrics Branch assumed the responsibility.

12. CSG, *Mental Health,* 31–2; *Mental Institutions 1949,* 14; and "Hospital Statistics," *Hosp.* 23, no. 6 (June 1949): 22. Figures exclude tuberculosis sanatoria.

13. NYS DMH *AR* (1950): 80; NCMH, *State Hospitals in the Depression: A Survey . . .* (New York: NCMH, 1934); and Harold Dern, "The Incidence and Future Expectancy of Mental Diseases," *USPHS Rep.* 53 (1938): 1991. The rise in mental hospitals has been attributed to a shift in social welfare policy in the late nineteenth century, when responsibility for the care of dependent classes shifted from local county and city agencies to state authorities. In the twentieth century, the institutions swelled further when the elderly poor were diagnosed as "senile" or "cerebral arteriosclerotic." See Grob *MI,* 72–107, 179–233; and John M. Grimes, *Institutional Care of Mental Patients in the United States* (Chicago: privately printed, 1934).

14. NYS DMH *AR* (1950): 150–1; and CSG, *Mental Health,* 36; and Richard H. Hutchings, "The President's Address," *AJP* 96 (1939): 5–6.

15. Hutchings, "President's Address," 5. Superintendents monitored essential aspects of hospital life in terms of "patient movement."

16. Ibid., 3; Hamilton, "The History of American Mental Hospitals," 153–60; Horatio Pollock, "The Depression and Mental Disease in New York State," *AJP* 91 (1935): 763–71; and Komora, *State Hospitals in the Depression,* 1–5.

17. Albert Deutsch, "Psychiatry as State Medicine," *AJP* 100 (1944): 184.

18. "Comment. Psychiatry in Delaware," *AJP* 98 (1941): 304.

19. Deutsch, "State Medicine," 189.

20. Other techniques included phlebotomy, fever, freezing, fasting, fattening, prolonged narcosis, carbon dioxide inhalation, and oxygen deprivation; see Karl Bowman, "Review of Psychiatric Progress 1941 – Shock Therapy," *AJP* 98

(1942): 590–1. Psychiatry has had a long history of resorting to chemical, electrical, surgical, and other such physical treatments. The new shock therapies, however, transformed the nature of institutional practice and enjoyed unprecedented professional support. Since the mid-nineteenth century, various drugs had been available for sedative purposes, but these were admitted to afford only symptomatic relief. Useful overviews are Grob *MI*, 296–304; idem, *Asylum*, 124–56; Valenstein *G&DC*, 23–61; Judith Swazey, *Chlorpromazine in Psychiatry: A Study of Therapeutic Innovation* (Cambridge, Mass.: MIT Press, 1974), 11–14; Arthur Sackler, ed., *The Great Physiodynamic Therapies in Psychiatry: An Historical Reappraisal* (New York: Hoeber-Harper, 1956); Malamud, "Psychiatric Therapies," 273–323 (Chap. 1, n. 43); M. Fink, "A History of Convulsive Therapy," *Psychiat. J. Univ. Ottawa* 4 (1979): 105–10; Lucie Jessner and V. Ryan, *Shock Treatment in Psychiatry* (New York: Grune & Stratton, 1941); Joseph Wortis, "The History of Insulin Shock Treatment," in Max Rinkel and Harold Himwich, *Insulin Treatment in Psychiatry* (New York: Philosophical Library, 1959), 19–41; and Lothar Kalinowsky, "The Discoveries of Somatic Treatments in Psychiatry: Facts and Myths," *Comp. Psychiat.* 21 (1980): 428–35. Unlike the case of paresis, the cause of which was attributable to an identifiable neurological disorder, most of the serious psychiatric conditions had no identifiable physiological basis; these were known as "functional" as opposed to "organic" maladies.

21. Benjamin Malzberg, "Outcome of Insulin Treatment of One Thousand Patients with Dementia Praecox," *PSQ* 12 (1938): 528–53; L. Kolb and V. Vogel, "The Use of Shock Therapy in 305 Mental Hospitals," *AJP* 99 (1942): 90–100; Grob *MI*, 301; and Valenstein *G&DC*, 52. See also NYS DMH, Temporary Commission on State Hospital Problems, *Insulin Shock Therapy* (New York: n.p., 1944).

22. Jessner and Ryan, *Shock Treatment*, xv.

23. Deutsch popularized this phrase to describe the faith mid-nineteenth-century asylum superintendents had placed in their ability to treat mental illness. See Albert Deutsch, *The Mentally Ill in America; A History of Their Care and Treatment from Colonial Times*, 2d ed. (New York: Columbia University Press, 1946), 132–57. For a list of popular articles on shock treatment, see Grob *MI*, 392, n. 21.

24. NYS DMH, *Insulin Shock*, 18.

25. CSG, *Mental Health*, 227. AMA, "Neurosurgical Treatment," 520 (Chap. 3, n. 4); F. Haas and D. Williams, "Transorbital Lobotomy; A Preliminary Report in Twenty-four Cases," *S.D. J. Med. Pharm.* 1 (May 1948): 192; and St. Louis SH (Mo.) "AR" (typescript, 1944), 21.

26. J. Pool, "Topectomy: A Surgical Procedure for the Treatment of Mental Illnesses," *JNMD* 110 (1949): 167, 171.

27. "Dewey Sees Gain in Mental Hygiene," *New York Times*, 20 July 1949, 27.

28. C. C. Burlingame, "Can the Point of View and Technique of Private Practice Be Carried into the Mental Hospital?" typescript of a paper delivered at the Southern Psychiatric Association, 9 Oct. 1937, San Antonio, Tex., CCB.

29. St. Louis City Hospital "AR" (mimeo., 1947), 27.
30. Cherokee SH in Iowa Board of Control *BR* (1950): 117; and Pilgrim SH (N.Y.) *AR* 8 (1939): 36. Connecticut SH (Middletown) *AR* (1946): 18, 22–3; Cherokee SH in Iowa Board of Control *BR* (1950): 116; and Rochester SH (N.Y.) *AR* (1949): 11.
31. Topeka SH (Kans.) *BR* (1950): 3. NYS Commission to Investigate the Management and Affairs of the Department of Mental Hygiene . . . , *The Care of the Mentally Ill in the State of New York* (Albany: n.p., 1944), 94.
32. Deutsch, *Shame*; Wright, *Out of Sight*; and Maisel, "Bedlam 1946," 102–10.
33. Committee on Psychiatric Standards and Policies (CPSP), "Preliminary Report," mimeo., 18 Dec. 1944, Box 200-10, CPSP, 1941–5, APA.
34. Ellen Philtine, *They Walk in Darkness* (New York: Liveright, 1945), 83.
35. Alan Gregg, "A Critique of Psychiatry," *AJP* 101 (1944): 285–91; and S. Weir Mitchell, "Address before the Fiftieth Annual Meeting of the American Medico-Psychological Association . . . 1894," *JNMD* 21 (1894): 413–37. Gregg recounted how Mitchell's talk criticized psychiatry's isolation from the rest of medicine. For an account of the profession's response to Mitchell's original speech, see Grob *MI*, 61.
36. Pepper's findings were included in a survey done by William Menninger, "Research in Mental Health in the National Perspective," typescript of an address to the Third Annual Coordinating Conference of the Western State Psychiatric Institute and Clinic, Pittsburgh, Pa., 1 Apr. 1948, WCM; "Statistics Pertinent to Psychiatry in the United States," *GAP Rep.* no. 7 (March 1949): 7; GAP, "Research in State Hospitals," Circular Letter no. 108, 17 Sept. 1948, MG; and Richard Shryock, *American Medical Research Past and Present* (New York: Commonwealth Fund, 1947), 232. See also CSG, *Training and Research in State Mental Health Programs; A Report to the Governors' Conference* (Chicago: CSG, 1953), 122–5, 188, 326; and Stella Deignan and Esther Miller, "The Support of Research in Medical and Allied Fields for the Period 1946 through 1951," *Science* 115 (1952): 321–43.
37. *Elgin Papers* 3 (1939): 1.
38. For a brief history of these facilities, see Deutsch, *Mentally Ill*, 2d ed., 291–9. In 1949, a dozen such research institutes existed, most notably the New York State Psychiatric Institute, Boston Psychopathic Hospital, Langley Porter Institute, Illinois Neuropsychiatric Institute, Western Psychiatric Institute, and State University of Iowa Psychopathic Hospital.
39. David Rothman, *Conscience and Convenience: The Asylum and Its Alternatives in Progressive America* (Boston: Little, Brown, 1980), 331–2, 329; William Sandy, "The President's Address," *AJP* 97 (1940): 11; and William Bryan, *Administrative Psychiatry* (New York: Norton, 1936), 242.
40. Franklin Ebaugh and Charles Rymer, "Teaching and Research in State Hospitals," *AJP* 96 (1939): 535–49; idem, *Psychiatry in Medical Education* (New York: Commonwealth Fund, 1942); Franklin Ebaugh, "The History of Psychiatric Education in the United States from 1844 to 1944," *AJP* 100 (1944): 151–60; Herbert Modlin, "Integration of Educational and Administrative Psychiatry," *PSQ* 25 (1951): 475–83; "Statistics Pertinent to Psychiatry," 6;

CPSP, "Report" (mimeo., Jan. 1944), Box 200-10, CPSP, 1941–5, APA; and Gregg, "A Critique of Psychiatry," 287.

41. Franklin Ebaugh, "The Care of the Psychiatric Patient in General Hospitals," *Official Bulletin of the American Hospital Association,* no. 207 (Chicago: A.H.A., 1940), 35. In 1950, only 181 general hospitals had psychiatric wards; Kramer, "The 1951 Survey of Psychosurgery," 159.

42. Ebaugh, "The Care of the Psychiatric Patient in General Hospitals," 75; and Alfred Bay, typescript of an untitled address to the Volunteer Services Institute, 29 Jan. 1952, Illinois State Hospital, APB; and "Through the Years – Pilgrim," 8.

43. The phrase was used by William A. White in his 1925 presidential address to the APA and reaffirmed by William L. Russell in his 1932 address; *AJP* 82 (1925): 4 and 89 (1932): 4, respectively.

44. CPSP, "Preliminary Report"; and "Report" (mimeo., 26 May 1946), Box 89, General Correspondence – APA, MG.

45. CPSP, "Report" (mimeo., 26 May 1946); "Preliminary Report" (mimeo., 18 Dec. 1944); and "Report" (mimeo., 13 Dec. 1947), Box 200-10, CPSP, 1946–7, APA.

46. Maisel, "Bedlam 1946"; and letter (mimeo.) from Samuel Hamilton, APA President, to APA Membership, 26 May 1946, Box 200-10, CPSP, 1946–7, APA. The CPSP findings were also quoted in Deutsch, *Mentally Ill,* 2d ed., 452.

47. CPSP, "Report" (mimeo., 26 May 1946); "Preliminary Report" (mimeo., 18 Dec. 1944); and "Report" (mimeo., 13 Dec. 1947), Box 200-10, CPSP, 1946–7, APA.

48. This incompatibility of missions was later described by Robert Hunt, "APA Standards for Public Mental Hospitals; History, Development and Present Status" (mimeo., 3 June 1959), Box 200-10, Standards and Policies of Hospitals and Clinics, APA; Ebaugh, "The Care of the Psychiatric Patient in General Hospitals," 75; and Bay, (untitled address), 29 Jan. 1952 (Illinois SH), 2, APB; and Calif. DMH *BR* (1950–2): 5.

49. Missouri SH #4 (Farmington) *BR* 21 (1941/2): 3, in Missouri Board of Managers of the State Eleemosynary Institutions *BR* (1941/2): 10. The reform of uses of new therapies has a long tradition in psychiatry. The statement "active treatment as contrasted with custodial care," e.g., was the rallying cry of Thomas Salmon and his neuropsychiatrists in World War I; see Pearce Bailey, Frankwood Williams, and Paul Komora, "In the United States," in *Neuropsychiatry,* 92 (chap. 1, n. 8).

50. Calif. DMH *Stat. Rep.* (1948): 21. An earlier parallel can be seen in the story of the use of surgery for focal infections at Trenton SH in the 1920s, a procedure that for a time brought national attention within the psychiatric profession to the institution's director, Henry Cotton. No less a figure than Adolf Meyer wrote a foreword to Cotton's treatise on the subject, the 1921 Vanedecum lectures, *The Defective, Delinquent and Insane: The Relation of Focal Infection to Their Causation, Treatment and Prevention* (Princeton, N.J.: Princeton University Press, 1921). "The work for mental health," Meyer

declared, "must be carried on where active and determined work is the order of the day." Cotton's work demonstrates that "an important experiment is being carried out there," and thus, Meyer concluded, "The New Jersey State Hospital at Trenton has proved to be such a place." For details of the story of focal infection and Cotton, see Grob *MI,* 124–6, and Scull, "Desperate Remedies" (Chap. 3, n. 68).

51. Deutsch, *Mentally Ill,* 2d ed., 259–61, 285, 298. For further analysis of New York's mental health care and policy before World War II, see Grob *MI.* See also "Your State Department of Mental Hygiene; Through the Years – Part III," *MHN* 21 (June 1951): 6–8, 10; NYS DMH, *Five Years of Progress in Mental Hygiene* (Utica, N.Y.: State Hospitals Press, 1949).

52. NYS DMH *AR* (1950): 146–7. New York's ratio of hospital residents to civilian population in 1947 was 1:152 and the national average was 1:263; Illinois Department of Finance, *A Budget Survey of State Mental Hospitals Presenting the Replies from the 48 States* (Springfield, Ill.: Department of Finance, 1948), 23. See also Benjamin Malzberg, "A Comparison of First Admissions to the New York Civil State Hospitals during 1919–1921 and 1949–1951," *PSQ* 28 (1954): 312–19; and "A Statistical Study of Patients in the New York Civil State Hospitals, April 1, 1950," *PSQ Suppl.* 26 (1952): 70–85.

53. NYS DMH, *Five Years of Progress,* 7. Between 1943 and 1950 state appropriations rose 257 percent; "State's Mental Aid Reported at Peak," *New York Times,* 11 June 1950, 66; and "Your State Department of Mental Hygiene," 10. New York's operating budget for 1950–1 was $323 million, with 104 million spent on asylums; *McKinney's Session Laws of New York 1952* (Brooklyn, N.Y.: Edward Thompson, 1952), 1558.

54. The system's evolution into a modern medical enterprise, the commission revealed, had been hindered by its civil service structure – a set of rules and guidelines that, ironically, had originally been instituted to protect the hospitals from political influence; NYS Commission, *Care of the Mentally Ill,* 7, 16, 20–1, 103.

55. Ibid., 22.

56. "Your State Department of Mental Hygiene," 7; Deutsch, *Shame,* 162; Grob *MI,* 300–2; and NYS DMH, *Insulin Shock.*

57. The first operations were performed at Brooklyn SH on 16 May 1946, and at Binghamton SH on 27 May; see Brooklyn SH *AR* (1947): 18, and Binghamton SH *AR* (1947): 10–11. See also NYS DMH *AR* (1951): 13.

58. Pilgrim SH *AR* 17 (1948): 14.

59. Background on Pilgrim can be found in Verne Dyson, *A Century of Brentwood* (n.p.: Brentwood Village Press, 1950), 263–90; Robert Kessler, "50 Years of Mental Care," *Newsday,* 17 Dec. 1981; and "Your State Hospitals – Pilgrim," *MHN* 20 (March 1950): 6–8, 11. Philtine's novel, *They Walk in Darkness,* depicts Pilgrim in the late 1930s and early 1940s. See also Morton Hunt's profile of Henry Brill, "Pilgrim's Progress, Part I," *New Yorker,* 30 Sept. 1961, 37:51; and "Pilgrim's Progress, Part II," *New Yorker,* 7 Oct. 1961, 37:67.

60. Pilgrim SH *AR* 13 (1944): 19; and "Your State Hospitals – Pilgrim," 6.
61. Pilgrim SH *AR* 17 (1948): 7, 14–19, and 18 (1949): 7, 12. See also Worthing, Brill, and Widgerson, "350 Cases," 616, 644. Worthing was attracted to lobotomy by published accounts and personal communications. The first 100 cases yielded a 29 percent rate of remission.
62. Pilgrim SH *AR* 19 (1950): 17 and 20 (1951): 7. Worthing, Brill, and Widgerson, "350 Cases"; see also: idem, "Evaluation of Prefrontal Lobotomy in 600 Cases," 328–36; Henry Brill, "The Place of Neurosurgery in the Treatment Program of a Department of Mental Hygiene," *N.Y. St. J. Med.* 52 (15 Oct. 1952): 2503–7; and H. S. Barahal, "1,000 Prefrontal Lobotomies – A Five-to-Ten-Year Follow-up Study," *PSQ* 32 (1958): 653–78. A progress report on the first 100 cases was read to the New York Academy of Medicine, 19 Oct. 1948; Pilgrim SH *AR* 18 (1949): 16.
63. Harry Worthing et al., "The Organization and Administration of a State Hospital Insulin-Metrazol-Electric Shock Therapy Unit," *AJP* 99 (1943): 692–7; and Pilgrim SH *AR* 16 (1947): 34.
64. Brill, "The Place of Neurosurgery," 2503–4.
65. Worthing et al., "Shock Therapy Unit," 692–7.
66. Pilgrim SH *AR* 17 (1948): 22.
67. Worthing boasted that the rise in the hospital's residency program to a full three-year accreditation was due to such efforts; Pilgrim SH *AR* (1952): 35.
68. The CSG survey listed eight New York institutions as not using the procedure in 1950 (*Mental Health*, 308). However, annual reports of four of these indicate that either they did eventually use the procedure or they were having their patients operated on elsewhere. Buffalo State Hospital was the only facility reporting unsatisfactory results. Critics might raise doubts about the quality of their neurosurgery, as four of fifteen patients died, an unusually high mortality rate; Buffalo SH *AR* (1950): 14.
69. Central Islip SH *AR* (1953): 17; Utica SH *AR* (1949): 7, (1950): 12–13, and (1951): 10; Harlem Valley SH *AR* (1948): 11 and (1951): 10; Gowanda SH *AR* (1952): 17; and Rochester SH *AR* (1951): 13.
70. Herman Snow, "A Review of 27 Prefrontal Lobotomy Patients," *PSQ* 23 (1949): 33; Binghamton SH *AR* (1948): 11, 13–14, (1950): 10–11, (1952): 9; and (1954): 8. In fiscal year 1956, 12 operations were performed. Middletown SH *AR* (1952): 12–13; St. Lawrence SH *AR* (1946): 8–9; Gowanda SH *AR* (1948): 8.
71. Binghamton SH *AR* (1945): 5, (1946): 6, and (1949): 6. "Through the Years – Binghamton," *MHN* 19 (Jan. 1949): 7–8; NYS DMH *AR* (1947): 13. Central Islip SH *AR* (1952): 6–7, and (1954): 8; Rochester SH *AR* (1951): 5; Utica SH *AR* (1949): 7; and Brooklyn SH *AR* (1950): 7–9, 18, 20. Photos of lobotomy operations also appeared in NYS DMH *AR* (1948): 9, (1949): 15, and (1953): 16.
72. Central Islip SH *AR* (1952): 17; Rochester SH *AR* (1949): 6–7, 11, and (1954): 15; Binghamton SH *AR* (1950): 11; Brooklyn SH *AR* (1950): 8; Brill, "The Place of Neurosurgery," 2507; and Irving Cooper, Francis O'Neill, and

Thomas Hoen, "State Hospital as University Teaching Center (for Neurology and Neurosurgery)," *PSQ Suppl.* 29 (1955): 308–13.

73. Rochester SH *AR* (1951): 9, and (1953): 15; "Rochester Neurosurgical Film Takes Top Photography Award," *MHN* 21 (March 1951): 2; and B. Pollack, "Psychosurgery; 5 Year Follow-up Report on 200 Patients," *Med. Times* 83 (1955): 370.

74. [Bigelow], "Topectomy," 163 (Intro., n. 2). Publications by the Columbia-Greystone Associates and the NYS Brain Research Project include Fred Mettler, ed., *Selective Partial Ablation of the Frontal Cortex* (New York: Paul Hoeber, 1949); idem, *Psychosurgical Problems* (Philadelphia: Blakiston, 1952); Fred Mettler et al., "Factors . . . Considered to be of Significance in Influencing Outcome Following Psychosurgery," *PSQ* 28 (1954): 549–606; and Nolan Lewis, Carney Landis, and H. E. King, *Studies in Topectomy* (New York: Grune & Stratton, 1956). See also "Surgery Restores 'Incurably Insane'," *New York Times*, 19 March 1948; "Topectomy Project Explained," *MHN* 18 (June 1948): 5, 12; and "Columbia Associates Issue 2nd Report on Psychosurgery," *MHN* 22 (April 1952): 2, 14. The significance of these experiments is discussed in later chapters. The Columbia-Greystone Project was a joint undertaking of the university and Greystone Park SH (N.J.), and was supervised by Mettler, a professor of neuroanatomy at Columbia. In discussion with Rockefeller Foundation officials, Mettler stated that Governor Dewey had asked him to develop a large-scale project, with the assurance that $200,000 would be available. Mettler noted Dewey's enthusiasm and his pressuring of New Jersey officials to cede authority to New York State. See interview notes of Robert Morison, "Meeting of the Columbia-Greystone Collaborators, Greystone Park, New Jersey, Monday December 1, 1947"; and "Dr. Frederick A. Mettler Phone," 4 Dec. 1947, Columbia University, Brain Surgery (RG 1.2 200 121 1070), RFA.

75. "Your State Department," 10; Newton Bigelow, "Clinical Progress in State Hospitals," *MHN* 24 (Sept. 1953): 4, 7, and 24 (Oct. 1953): 4, 6.

76. "Dewey Sees Gain in Mental Hygiene," 27; see also *MHN* 20 (Dec. 1949): 1; and "For the Mentally Ill," (editorial) *New York Times*, 19 Apr. 1949, 24.

77. "Governor Reports Department Needs," *MHN* 22 (Jan. 1952): 7.

78. [Margaret Farrar], "Two Shining Decades," *MHN* 20 (June 1950): 2; Bigelow, "Clinical Progress in State Hospitals;" and "Your State Department," 7.

79. Lucy Freeman, "State Mental Care Entering New Era," *New York Times*, 14 Sept. 1948, 31, 34. Brooklyn SH *AR* (1951): 8; Clarence Bellinger and Christopher Terrence, "Insulin Shock at Brooklyn State Hospital," in NYS DMH Commission, *Insulin Shock*, 83–7; Deutsch, *Shame*, 151; and "Christopher F. Terrence," *PSQ Suppl.* 25 (1951): 153.

80. *MHN* 18 (Jan. 1948): 3, 7–8; Pilgrim SH *AR* 23 (1954): 27. The broadcast occurred 24 Apr. 1953 on WNYC, the municipal radio station.

81. To illustrate, at Longview SH (Ohio) lobotomy operations were paid for through a special voluntary "Hypoglycaemic Fund" that had been collected from the families of patients undergoing insulin treatments; Longview SH

"AR" (typescript, 1949), 26, LSH. "Downing Radio Program Script" (typescript, 19 Nov. 1948), 6, GWU; the show was broadcast on 27 Nov. 1948, on KIRO.

82. Longview SH "AR" (typescript, 1937), 12–13; (1940), 12; and "AR" (1942), 7, LSH. Calif. DMH *AR* (1948): 93–4; and William Stewart and John Stewart, *"Let Me Not Be Mad, Sweet Heaven!" Dr. Emmett F. Hoctor's Years at Missouri State Hospital No. 4* (St. Louis, Mo.: Fireside, 1968), 96.

83. Kenneth Appel and James Flaherty, "Modern Trends in Psychiatric Therapy," *Del. St. Med. J.* 11 (1939): 196–7; "Comment: Psychiatry in Delaware," 304–5; and CPSP, "Report" (1948), APA.

84. "A Measure of Progress" (editorial), *MHN* 23 (June 1953): 2, 7; the piece referred to psychosurgery in conjunction with the other somatic therapies. Creedmoor SH (N.Y.) *AR*, cited in Susan Sheehan, *Is There No Place on Earth for Me?* (New York: Vintage, 1983), 10. Buffalo SH *AR* (1946): 24, and *AR* (1947): 14. Austin SH (Tex.) "AR" (typescript, 1949), 45.

85. See, e.g., Pilgrim SH *AR* (1948): 7; Calif. DMH *BR* (1949): 120; and Cherokee SH (Iowa) *AR* (1950): 115. Longview SH *AR* (typescript, 1950), 3, LSH. In his famous exposé, Maisel listed eight psychiatric therapies the use of which might serve as an index of an institution's therapeutic efforts; Maisel, "Bedlam 1946," 112.

86. CSG, *Mental Health,* 225. The extraordinary range of cooperative projects connecting state hospitals and the larger medical community are profiled in Philip Sapir, "Survey of Current Research in Psychosurgery," in *First Research Conference,* 143–56. See also Winfred Overholser, ed., *Proceedings of the Second Mental Hospital Institute,* held under the auspices of the Mental Hospital Service of the APA, St. Louis Medical Society Auditorium (Washington, D.C.: APA, 1951), 80. An interesting parallel can be found in the nation's system of TB sanatoria, which were also trying to upgrade their status from custodial institutions to places for active treatment through an emphasis on a new surgical therapy; see Richard Overholt, "The Role of the General Hospital in the Control of Tuberculosis from the Standpoint of the Thoracic Surgeon," *Trans. A.H.A.* 42 (1940): 482–94. In 1910, Bernard Hollander, one of the last serious phrenologists, published a book suggesting that mental disease could be treated by surgical removal of specific brain lesions. In the preface, a psychiatrist from the Belgian State Commission on Lunacy looked to men of "true scientific and humanitarian spirit" to reform the asylums, which currently were "for custody more than hospitals for scientific study and treatment of the insane"; J. Morel, "Preface," in Hollander, *The Mental Symptoms of Brain Disease; An Aid to the Surgical Treatment of Insanity . . .* (New York: Rebman, 1910), v.

87. CSG, *Mental Health,* 225–6. See, e.g., Longview SH (Ohio) "AR" (typescript, 1952), 12, LSH. Lobotomy programs were useful vehicles for residency training.

88. Pilgrim SH *AR* (1944): 19.

89. Karl Bowman, "Presidential Address," *AJP* 103 (1946): 1–17.

90. "Through the Years – Pilgrim," 8; see also Henry Brill, "The Personality Factor in Mental Illness," *MHN* 21 (Feb. 1951): 10.
91. Esta Carini et al., *The Mentally Ill in Connecticut: Changing Patterns of Care and the Evolution of Psychiatric Nursing 1636–1972* (Hartford, Conn.: DMH, 1974), 52; Worthing et al., "Shock Therapy Unit," 695; and A. Stearns, "Report on Medical Progress: Psychiatry," *NEJM* 220 (1939): 709–10, cited in Valenstein *G&DC*, 61.
92. Marcus Curry and Henry Cotton, Jr., "Institutional Management and Social Implications," in Mettler, *Partial Ablation*, 33; and CSG, *Mental Health*, 28.
93. Overholser, *Second Mental Hospital Institute*, 12.
94. "Lobotomy," *Time*, 30 Nov. 1936, 28: 66–8; and "Explorers of the Brain" (editorial), *New York Times*, 30 Oct. 1949, sec. IV, 8.
95. Pool, "Topectomy," 167–9.
96. Deutsch, "State Medicine," 189.
97. Worthing et al., "Shock Therapy Unit," 695; Bernard Moore, "Report of the Connecticut Cooperative Lobotomy Study 1946–1949" (mimeo., Dec. 1949), 1, JF; and Worthing, Brill, and Widgerson, "350 Cases," 625.
98. Harry Solomon, "Treatment of the Psychoses," *PSQ* 25 (1951): 16–17; see also Harry Solomon, interview (Tape 2.1), 18, HCS; and "Anglo-American Symposium on Psychosurgery, Neurophysiology and Physical Treatments in Psychiatry," *Proc. Roy. Soc. Med. Suppl.* 42 (1949): 52.
99. Middletown SH AR (1948): 10. See also Isadore Spinka, Milton Tinsley, and George Genyes, "Psychosurgery in a State Hospital," *Ill. Med. J.* 102 (1952): 201–4; and Worthing, Brill, and Widgerson, "350 Cases," 624–5.
100. Wright, ed., *Out of Sight*, 135–6.
101. Wilson et al., "Transorbital Lobotomy"; and Solomon, "Treatment of Psychoses," 16.
102. Pennsylvania Department of Public Welfare, *A Pictorial Report on Mental Institutions in Pennsylvania* (n.p.: D.P.W., 1947), 31.
103. Curry and Cotton, "Institutional Management," 33.
104. St. Lawrence SH (N.Y.) AR (1946): 8–9.
105. Brooklyn SH AR (1951): 8. CSG, *Recent Progress in the States in the Field of Mental Health* (Chicago, Ill.: CSG, 1954), 28, 38. See also Hudson Valley SH (N.Y.) AR (1953): 6; and Deutsch, *Shame*, 185. Moore's report, e.g., stated that psychotherapy was the "cornerstone" of hospital psychiatry, with shock therapy and psychosurgery completing the program; Moore, "Cooperative Lobotomy Study," 1. Another example of psychosurgery earning a favorable recommendation alongside a statement of psychotherapy as the "cornerstone" is [Alexander Simon], "Drastic Therapies," *Calif. Med.* 68 (1948): 308–9. A distinction should be made between psychotherapy and psychoanalysis.
106. Herbert Modlin, "Integration of Educational and Administrative Psychiatry," 476; and Kramer, "The 1951 Survey," 160, 166. Texas was one of three states with the highest rate of operations per thousand resident patients; and each of the 37 VA hospitals with neuropsychiatric services employed the procedure.

107. [Bigelow], "Topectomy – New Light," 163. Casamajor, "Neurology and Psychiatry" (Chap. 1, n. 41). Gray, "Brainstorms," 376 (Chap. 3, n. 26).
108. W. Keller to J. Evans, 12 Feb. 1948 (copy); C. Jones to WF, 23 Apr. 1948, GWU.
109. Deutsch, *Shame*, 14.

## Chapter 5. Human Salvage

1. Untitled poem printed in the patient newsletter of the Boston Psychopathic Hospital; *Boston Psycho. News* (20 Oct. 1950), MMHC.
2. CSG, *Mental Health Programs*, 346 (Chap. 4, n. 1); and David Wilson, "Role of Lobotomy in Psychiatric Management," *SMJ* 45 (1952): 695.
3. Roy Porter notes that even psychiatry's most trenchant critics often assume that what is "good" scientific medicine is easily known; he calls this the "agonistic double." See his "The Patient's View: Doing Medical History from Below," *Theory and Society* 14 (1985): 175–98.
4. Brooklyn SH (N.Y.) *AR* (1950): 8, 18; and Isadore Spinka, Milton Tinsley, and George Fenyes, "Psychosurgery in a State Hospital," *Ill. Med. J.* 102 (1952): 203.
5. An account of earlier "heroic" therapies is Scull, "Desperate Remedies" (Chap. 3, n. 68); and discussion by Kurt Goldstein of Freeman and Watts, "Obsessive Tendencies," 226 (Chap. 2, n. 73).
6. Freeman and Watts, "Obsessive Tendencies," 642.
7. One physician wrote, e.g., "The best we can hope for is that she quiets down and accepts a protective existence in an institution or perhaps a nursing home"; see patient #378, "Case Presentation," 21 Sept. 1938, McLH (see below, Chapter 6).
8. A "career" of insanity is illustrated in Sheehan, *No Place* (Chap. 4, n. 84).
9. "Surgery Aid to Mentally Ill Discussed," *Cincinnati Times-Star*, 13 May 1954.
10. Harry J. Worthing, Henry Brill, and Henry Widgerson, "350 Cases of Prefrontal Lobotomy," *PSQ* 23 (1949): 639; and Boston Psychopathic Hosital "AR" (typescript, 1944), BPH.
11. Snow, "Lobotomy Patients" (Chap. 4, n. 72). Shock therapies similarly were described as "a more humane alternative to physical restraint and seclusion"; Calif. DMH *AR* (1953): 140. James L. Pool, "Topectomy: A Surgical Procedure for the Treatment of Mental Illnesses," *JNMD* 110 (1949): 172.
12. F-W *PS2*, 377; Stanley Cobb, "Review of Neuropsychiatry for 1940," *Arch. Int. Med.* 66 (1940): 1354; and the Yale University News Bureau, Press Release No. 671, statements made by F. Redlich during the radio show "Yale Interprets the News," 31 May 1948, JF. See also Lothar Kalinowsky and John Scarff, "The Selection of Psychiatric Cases for Prefrontal Lobotomy," *ANP* 62 (1949): 698.
13. P. Elfeld, "Results of Lobotomies at Delaware State Hospital," *Del. St. Med. J.* 14 (1942): 82; F-W *PS2*, 503–10; and Walter Freeman and James Watts, "Prefontal Lobotomy. The Problem of Schizophrenia," *AJP* 101 (1945): 741.

14. "Your State Hospitals – Pilgrim," *MHN* 20 (1950): 8; C. C. Burlingame, "Advances in Psychiatry – 1946," typescript of a radio broadcast on the International Broadcasting Service, 7 Mar. 1946, CCB; and Worthing, Brill, and Widgerson, "350 Cases," 644.

15. Longview SH (Ohio) "AR" (typescript, 1951), 6, LSH. The word *salvaging* frequently appears in reference to psychosurgery cases. See, e.g., Boston Psychopathic "AR" (typescript, 1946), 44, BPH. "Minutes of Meeting," Medical and Surgical Staff, Illinois Neuropsychiatric Institute, 17 Mar. 1947, 2, Minutes of Illinois State Hospital Superintendent 1945–9, BAY.

16. Husband of (name withheld) to Grant, 14 May 1940, FG.

17. Elfeld, "Lobotomies at Delaware State," 82; Gayle and Neale, "Psychosurgery" (Chap. 3, n. 23); and Freeman and Watts, "Prefrontal Lobotomy," 748.

18. NYS Commission, *Care of the Mentally Ill*, 94 (Chap. 4, n. 31); and Frank Leon Wright, Jr., *Out of Sight, Out of Mind* (Philadelphia: National Mental Health Foundation, 1947), 148. G. Weickhardt and A. Duval, "Adjustment Levels in Hospitalized Schizophrenic Patients following Prefrontal Lobotomy," *Dis. Nerv. Sys.* 10 (1949): 306–7.

19. Worthing, Brill, and Widgerson, "350 Cases," 641.

20. W. Wilson et al., "Transorbital Lobotomy in Chronically Disturbed Patients," *AJP* 108 (1951): 445; and Mt. Pleasant SH in Iowa Board of Control *BR* (1946): 83.

21. Brooklyn SH *AR* (1948): 18; L. Hohman et al., "Preliminary Report on Follow-up of Prefrontal Lobotomies Performed by Duke Neurosurgical Staff," *N.C. Med. J.* 12 (1951): 533; Wilson et al., "Transorbital Lobotomy," 447–8; Rochester SH (N.Y.) *AR* (1952): 10; and St. Louis SH (Mo.) "AR" (typescript, 1953), 35.

22. AMA, "Neurosurgical Treatment," 520 (Chap. 3, n. 4); Wilson et al., "Results of Transorbital Lobotomy in 400 State Hospital Patients," *Neur.* 3 (1953): 884; F. Haas and D. Williams, "Transorbital Lobotomy; A Preliminary Report in Twenty-four Cases," *S. Dak. J. Med. Pharm.* 1 (May 1948): 192; and St. Louis SH "AR" (typescript, 1944), 21. J. Freed and E. Burn, "Electro Shock Therapy and Lobotomy Program in State Hospitals," *J. S.C. Med. Assoc.* 48 (1952): 262.

23. AMA, "Neurosurgical Treatment," 520; and F-W *PS2*, 89, 218, 221, 238, 467.

24. Huntington SH in West Virginia Board of Control, *Rep.* 15 (1945–8): 33; Norristown SH (Pa.) *AR* (1954): 13; and Brooklyn SH *AR* (1948): 12.

25. Freeman and Watts, "Prefrontal Lobotomy," 748.

26. J. Hetherington et al., "Psychosurgery in Logansport State Hospital," *J. Ind. Med. Assoc.* 47 (1954): 1097.

27. Strecker, Palmer, and Grant, "Study of Prefrontal Lobotomy," 524 (Chap. 3, n. 26). W. Kane, H. Hurdum, and J. Schaerer, "Prefrontal Lobotomy; Analysis of Results in 122 Cases in a State Hospital," *ANP* 68 (1952): 206; Worthing, Brill, and Widgerson, "350 Cases," 623; Calif. DMH *Statist. Suppl.* (1948),

106; Freeman and Watts, "Prefrontal Lobotomy," 741. See also Snow, "Lobotomy Patients," 26–34.

28. Hohman et al.,"Preliminary Report," 531; and Snow, "Lobotomy Patients," 32.

29. Worthing, Brill, and Widgerson, "350 Cases," 621; Snow, "Lobotomy Patients," 26–34; Wilson et al., "Transorbital Lobotomy," 444–9; and Pilgrim SH (N.Y.) *AR* (1948): 18. See also St. Louis City Sanatarium "AR" (1947), 23.

30. Hohman et al., "Preliminary Report," 529–34; Marlboro SH "AR" (mimeo., 1953), 3, PFL; Milton Greenblatt and Harry Solomon, *Frontal Lobes and Schizophrenia* (New York: Springer, 1953), 6; Milton Greenblatt, Richard York, and Esther Brown, *From Custodial to Therapeutic Patient Care in Mental Hospitals; Explorations in Social Treatment* (New York: Russell Sage Foundation, 1955), 103; and Worthing, Brill, and Widgerson, "350 Cases," 625.

31. Binghamton SH (N.Y.) *AR* (1947): 10. Nurses who had been attacked hoped that lobotomy might make their jobs easier; see Carini, *Mentally Ill in Connecticut*, 386–7 (Chap. 4, n. 91). Walter Freeman, "Psychosurgery," in Silvano Arieti, ed., *American Handbook of Psychiatry* (New York: Basic Books, 1959), 2:1532–3. Milton Greenblatt and Paul Myerson, "Medical Progress; Psychosurgery," *NEJM* 240 (1949): 1014.

32. Connecticut SH (Middletown) *AR* (1946): 26. A labor-intensive treatment, hydrotherapy was difficult to maintain during the war shortages. Rebekah Wright, *Hydrotherapy in Psychiatric Hospitals for Mental Diseases* (Boston: Tudor, 1932); and Pilgrim SH *AR* 1 (1932): 25.

33. Ellen Philtine, *They Walk in Darkness* (New York: Liveright, 1945), 44, 50.

34. Thomas A. C. Rennie, "Use of Insulin as Sedation Therapy in Control of Basic Anxiety in the Psychoses," *ANP* 50 (1943): 697–705; and Phillip Polatin, Hyman Spitnitz, and Benjamin Wiesel, "Effects of Intravenous Injections of Insulin in Treatment of Mental Disease," *ANP* 43 (1940): 925–31.

35. Louis Cohen, "The Early Effects of Metrazol Therapy in Chronic Psychotic Over-activity," *AJP* 95 (1938): 327–8; Harrisburg SH (Pa.) *BR* (1948–50): 26; Pilgrim SH *AR* 16 (1947): 12, 15, and *AR* 18 (1949): 13. See also Brooklyn SH *AR* (1949): 17; Norristown SH *AR* (1946): 14; Calif. DMH (1953): 140, and (1949): 121; and Marlboro SH (N.J.) "AR" (mimeo., 1949), 4, PFL.

36. J. Koenig and H. Feldman, "Nonstandard Method of Electric Shock Therapy," *PSQ* 25 (1951): 65–72; Norristown SH *AR* (1946): 14, and (1948): 12; James Brussell and Jacob Schneider, "The B.E.S.T. in the Treatment and Control of Chronically Disturbed Mental Patients – A Preliminary Report," *PSQ* 25 (1951): 55–64; Kings Park SH (N.Y.) *AR* (1949): 12. The B.E.S.T. was developed as an emergency measure to subdue violent psychotics onboard navy hospital ships.

37. Some hospitals identified prospects for lobotomy by their response to ambulatory shock. Pilgrim SH *AR* 17 (1948): 18, and 19 (1950): 13; and W. Peyton, J. Haavik, and B. Schiele, "Prefrontal Lobectomy in Schizophrenia," *ANP* 62

(1949): 562. Paul Hoch, "Evaluations of the Results of Topectomy Operations," *Surg. Gyn. Obs.* 92 (1951): 610; St. Louis City Sanatorium "AR" (typescript, 1947), 23; Wilson et al., "Transorbital Lobotomy," 447; and Norristown SH *AR* (1951): 12. William A. White, "Presidential Address," *AJP* 82 (1925): 11.

38. Philtine, *They Walk in Darkness*, 73.
39. Ironically, the "ambulatory" insulin technique was in fact pioneered by the husband of novelist Ellen Philtine, Phillip Polatin, whose experiences at Pilgrim provided a model for the character of Peter Carson; see n. 34 above.
40. W. Malamud, quoted in *First Research Conference*, 16 (Chap. 4, n. 1).
41. Philtine's novel vividly depicts the incompatibility between the psychiatrists' daily work and their emerging sensibility as medical scientists. Dr. Carson, e.g., ruminates: "throughout the building patients of all types were mingled indiscriminately in 'good' or 'bad' wards. Surely he must replace those purely disciplinary standards by a more humane and scientific classification. Yet such reorganization required an intimate knowledge of all his patients – and for that the day had not enough hours" (Philtine, *They Walk in Darkness*, 72).
42. *First Research Conference*, 18.
43. In the nineteenth-century asylum, ward placement constituted a major part of a patient's medical status; Tomes, *A Generous Confidence*, 204 (Chap. 1, n. 4).
44. Rothman describes the ward hierarchies as akin to the internal logic of prisons, but he does not consider their putative therapeutic structure; Rothman, *Conscience and Convenience*, 340 (Chap 1., n. 4).
45. William L. Russell, "Presidential Address," *AJP* 89 (1932): 17. The argument here is not to deny that occupational therapy was ever used as a form of behavioral control but to emphasize that at times it was also more than this.
46. NYS Commission, *Care of the Mentally Ill*, 19.
47. See Chapter 1, especially the discussions of Albert Barrett and Austen Fox Riggs.
48. See the patient file of Helaine Strauss (pseudonym), McLH.
49. Paul Howard, "Staff Conference, Pre-'drug' Treatment," corrected typescript, n.p, n.d, (1949?); in the author's possession thanks to the generosity of Dr. Howard.
50. F-W *PS2*, 398–9. A table that aggregated the pounds gained by patients after lobotomy is in Lyerly, "Involutional Melancholia," (Chap. 2, n. 105). For a history of anorexia, see Joan Jacobs Brumberg, *Fasting Girls: The Emergence of Anorexia Nervosa as a Modern Disease* (Cambridge, Mass.: Harvard University Press, 1988).
51. Calif. DMH *AR* (1953): 139; and "Your State Hospital – Pilgrim," *MHN* 20 (March 1950): 8; Worthing, Brill, and Widgerson, "350 Cases."
52. J. Farmer, "Program of Postlobotomy Reeducation and Rehabilitation," *N.C. Med. J.* 9 (1948): 287–91; Pilgrim SH (N.Y.) *AR* 21 (1952): 13; and Worthing, Brill, and Widgerson, "350 Cases," 626.
53. Worthing, Brill, and Widgerson, "350 Cases," 626.

54. A popular mid-nineteenth-century belief was that "the brain is formed by bad habits" (Tomes, *A Generous Confidence*, 82). The "experimental neurosis" model, covered in Chapter 2, was used to justify the initial trials, but the cerebral "reorganization" model was more commonly used to explain everyday hospital results. The two models were not incompatible.

55. C. C. Burlingame, "Psychiatry in 1950," typescript of a paper presented at the AMA annual meeting, San Francisco, 27 June 1950, 12, CCB; Worthing, Brill, and Widgerson, "350 Cases," 644; Missouri General Assembly, *The Mentally Ill*, 17 (Chap. 3, n. 41); Petersen and Buchstein, "Prefrontal Lobotomy," 428 (Chap. 2, n. 85); Walter Freeman and James Watts, "Prefrontal Lobotomy; Convalescent Care and Aids to Rehabilitation," *AJP* 99 (1943): 798–806; "Value of Rorschach Test and Prefrontal Lobotomy Discussed at Binghamton Institute for Social Workers," *MHN* 18 (December 1947): 8; Freeman quoted in *Third Research Conference*, 151 (Intro., n. 3); F. Ewald, Walter Freeman, and James Watts, "Psychosurgery; The Nursing Problem," *Am. J. Nurs.* 47 (1947): 211; and Evelyn Friedman, "Nursing Aspects of the Treatment of Lobotomized Patients," *Bull. Menn. Clin.* 14 (1950): 138–42.

56. "Your State Hospital – Pilgrim," 8; Worthing, Brill, and Widgerson, "350 Cases," 634; and Pilgrim SH AR 18 (1949): 15. See also "Your State Hospital – Binghamton," *MHN* 19 (January 1949): 7.

57. Weickhardt and Duval, "Adjustment Levels," 306.

58. J. Mulvaney, "Results of 160 Prefrontal Lobotomies," unpublished research summary, September 1951, sent to the author through the courtesy of Winnebago SH. See also Schrader and Robinson, "Prefrontal Lobotomy" (Chap. 3, n. 41); and Weickhardt and Duval, "Adjustment Levels," 306–9.

59. Malamud, n. 40 above.

60. See the patient file of Mary Sullivan (pseudonym), McLH.

61. Freed and Burn, "Shock Therapy," 259–63; and Henry Brill, "The Place of Neurosurgery in a Treatment Program of a Department of Mental Hygiene," *N.Y. St. J. Med.* 52 (1952): 2506. The VA Central Office appointed a special committee to draw up specific guidelines for the selection of lobotomy patients. "Patients falling into the following diagnostic groups should not be considered for the operation: (a) Alcoholic and drug addicts. (b) Psychopaths. (c) Homosexuals or other sexual deviates"; "Criteria to Guide in the Selection of Patients for Prefrontal Leukotomy," 3, included within Milton Wexler to B. E. Boothe, Office Memo., 25 Sept. 1947, Lobotomy Research Winter VA Hospital 1947–51, MSP[MF].

62. Some attempts had been made to use psychosurgery for these purposes. See, e.g., R. S. Banay and L. Davidoff, "Apparent Recovery of a Sex Psychopath after Lobotomy," *J. Crim. Psychopath.* 4 (1942): 59–66; and Robert Jennings, Aage Nielsen, and Milton Erickson, "Prefrontal Lobotomy for Severe Conduct Disorder," Proceedings of the Michigan Society of Neurology and Psychiatry, 5 Dec. 1946, *ANP* 58 (1947): 244–5. A review by Kalinowsky and Scarff stated that the treatment was not useful for psychopaths; idem, "Selection of Psychiatric Cases," 700. For a finding that criminals were only made worse by the operation, see Flothow and Lemere, "Prefrontal Lobot-

omy," 3 (Chap. 3, n. 22). Perhaps the most publicized case of a criminal being lobotomized is that of Millard Wright, a habitual burglar in Pittsburgh who after an operation subsequently resumed his old habits. Upon recapture he committed suicide. A biography was written by the neurosurgeon who performed the lobotomy; see Yale Koskoff and Richard Goldhurst, *The Dark Side of the House* (New York: Dial, 1968). For further details of the case, see Valenstein *G&DC*, 191.

63. Freeman quoted in "Anglo-American Symposium," 1 (Chap. 4, n. 98).
64. Moore, "Cooperative Lobotomy Study" (Chap. 4, n. 97).

## Chapter 6. Localizing Decisions

1. "Discussion of . . . 'Psychosurgery'" (Chap. 3, n. 64). Staff conference discussion of Mary Montero (pseudonym), 9 Mar. 1948, McLH.
2. The file of a single patient may include 200 pages of handwritten entries. For a description of the McLean Archives, see Terry Bragg, *Guide to the Archives of the McLean Hospital Corporation* (Belmont, Mass.: McLean Hospital, 1984). In the interest of strict confidentiality, any patient name that appears in this and other chapters is fictitious; names of physicians cited in conjunction with any confidential patient record or staff conference meeting are also inventions. The real identity of any individual can be reconstructed only by finding the code number for the pseudonym that appears in the *Appendix* and then comparing this to a master list that is on deposit in the McLean Office of the Registrar. Access to this master list is subject to the same regulations that cover any other hospital records; the author does not have a personal copy.
3. The term *clinical frame* is an elaboration of a theme explored by Charles Rosenberg, "Disease in History: Frames and Framers," *Milbank Mem. Fund Q.* Suppl. 1, 67 (1989): 1–15.
4. The best account of McLean Hospital to date is S. B. Sutton, *Crossroads in Psychiatry: A History of the McLean Hospital* (Washington, D.C.: APA, 1986). In 1939, the standard weekly rate for hospital care was $75. In the 1938 *Annual Reports* of McLean Hospital (hereafter *AR*), administrators complained that patients of "moderate means," those who could only afford a rate of $25, were currently forced to enter state hospitals; *AR* (1938): 148. Following in the nineteenth-century tradition of charitable stewardship, McLean Hospital absorbed the not inconsiderable costs of a number of patients who could only pay below standard rates. In 1946, e.g., one out of three inmates paid less, and seven were maintained free; *AR* (1946): 172, 178. It was also the stated hospital policy never to refuse admission on the basis of "race, creed, or color"; *AR* (1948): 206. Such lofty aims notwithstanding, most patients came from a class of individuals the hospital staff described as "old New England stock."
5. In a cruel twist of fate, Olmsted too eventually suffered a "breakdown." His last five years were spent as an inmate at McLean; Sutton, *Crossroads*, 131.
6. Ibid., 130, 143.
7. Sutton noted that the nurses would arrange every year for the patients' minks to go in and out of storage; Sutton, *Crossroads*, 251.

8. Physicians spent as much as one-third of their time on such administration; *AR* (1951): 188. "The patient is not an isolated unit but lives in complicated social connections, and much thought and time of the physician and nurses extends the hospital service to interested family physicians, psychiatrists, legal advisors, friends, employers, and a host of relatives." *AR* (1948): 217.

9. The rich social dimensions of the nineteenth-century asylum are depicted in Tomes, *A Generous Confidence* (Chap. 1, n. 4).

10. Although McLean was mostly a "locked hospital," the staff noted that "There is enough individual care so that activities and personal preferences need not be too much regimented, and the individual, often ashamed of his illness, preserves a sense of his own value, rather than feeling dominated by the institution." *AR* (1949): 220.

11. Sutton, *Crossroads*, 185, 251. In 1932, Psychiatrist-in-Chief Kenneth Tillotson described what the hospital did to combat the usual syndromes of "depersonalization"; Tillotson, "Some Newer Trends in Psychiatry," *NEJM* 207 (7 July 1932): 10. McLean's indulgence of patients went so far as to allow separate cottages to be constructed on the grounds for their personal use.

12. For a contemporary description of elite asylum care, see "The 'Nervous Breakdown,'" *Fortune* 11 (1935): 84. The histories of these kinds of middle-range institutions (the records of which contain a rich source of materials for reconstructing the social history of the elite) have yet to be written. Little is also known about the farms and seaside villas in which the mildly disturbed lived under the care of personal caretakers or nurses (what later were termed "halfway" facilities). The records at McLean suggest that such arrangements often resulted from negotiations between patients and their families, in which the former would agree to a form of voluntary exile rather than face commitment proceedings.

13. Bloomingdale Hospital, another well-respected private charitable facility, provides a helpful comparison. In 1938, of 500 cases previously admitted, only 6 percent had been hospitalized more than three years. Schizophrenics were admitted, but they did not remain long. According to hospital policy, it "not infrequently asks for the removal of a patient when it is felt that the patient will receive no further benefit in this hospital"; C. Cheney and P. Drewry, Jr., "Results of Non-specific Treatment in Dementia Praecox," *AJP* 95 (1938): 208.

14. There was some overlap; Codman House III, e.g., was also an open ward.

15. Cowles had been recruited from his post as superintendent of Boston City Hospital, where he previously had set up a training program for nurses. For Cowles's story, see Sutton, *Crossroads*, 91–133. Edward Cowles, "The Seminary Method in Asylum and Hospital Work," *AJI* 48 (1892): 365–72; and idem, "The Laboratories of the McLean Hospital for Research in Pathological Psychology and Biochemistry," in Henry Hurd, ed., *The Institutional Care of the Insane in the United States and Canada* (Baltimore: Johns Hopkins University Press, 1916), 618–36. C. MacFie Campbell, "History of Insanity during the Past Century with Special Reference to the McLean Hospital," *BMSJ* 185 (3 Nov. 1921): 538–44. See also Terry Bragg, "Scientific Laboratories at

McLean Hospital: A Legacy of Edward Cowles, M.D. and a Focus for Progress (1888–1943)," unpublished paper.

16. Tillotson, "Trends in Psychiatry," 8–12; idem, "Sociological Implications in Modern Psychiatric Thought," *AJP* 93 (1936): 503–11; and idem, "Psychobiology in General Medicine," *NEJM* 215 (23 July 1936): 146–9. In 1934, e.g., three patients had been treated by orthodox psychoanalysis. Tillotson assumed the post of medical superintendent in 1930. Wood was hired in 1932, and responsibilities for running the hospital were split between them. Tillotson was forced to resign in 1948 following a scandal; see Sutton, *Crossroads*, 210, 246–8. Paul Howard replaced Tillotson as acting psychiatrist-in-chief, a post that he held for the next seven years. Wood retired in 1956.

17. *AR* (1945): 186. When Tillotson was hired he was also appointed as Psychiatrist to Massachusetts General, charged with reconstituting its mental hygiene clinic. And when Cobb became director of the neuropsychiatric service at Harvard, he continued the exchange of personnel between the two institutions. The new research building was opened in 1946. For more details, see Sutton, *Crossroads*, 219, 242–4. When Altschule was hired, the *AR* noted that "this is the first time that a full-time internist and clinical physiologist of professorial rank has been added to a psychiatric hospital staff in this country" (1947): 199. Altschule also received an appointment at Harvard Medical School.

18. Tillotson, "Trends in Psychiatry," 10. Sutton notes that in 1930 all but one admission was for psychosis. By 1937, the "non-insane" accounted for as much as 20 percent of all admissions; Sutton, *Crossroads*, 211.

19. *AR* (1945): 187.

20. Sutton, *Crossroads*, 224; and *AR* (1938): 158.

21. *AR* (1939): 162. These cases were described in Mixter, Tillotson, and Wies, "Lobectomy and Frontal Lobotomy" (Chap. 3, n. 12); see also Chapter 3.

22. *AR* (1938): 158. The method was developed by Abraham Myerson at the nearby Boston SH; see his "Theory and Principles of the 'Total Push' Method in the Treatment of Chronic Schizophrenia," *AJP* 95 (1939): 1198–204. See also Kenneth Tillotson, "The Practice of the Total Push Method in the Treatment of Chronic Schizophrenia," *AJP* 95 (1939): 1205–13.

23. *AR* (1938): 156, and (1939): 162.

24. *AR* (1946): 181; Sutton, *Crossroads*, 237; and *AR* (1945): 187. Physical treatments consumed only 2 percent of the physicians' working hours; *AR* (1951): 188.

25. For an overview of the first few years of McLean's shock-therapy program, see Kenneth Tillotson and Wolfgang Sulzbach, "A Comparative Study and Evaluation of Electric Shock Therapy in Depressive States," *AJP* 101 (1945): 455–9.

| From the Annual Reports: | *1945* | *1946* | *1947* | *1948* | *1949* | *1950* |
|---|---|---|---|---|---|---|
| ECS | 74 | 75 | 101 | 11 | 103 | 88 |
| Insulin | 10 | 18 | 0 | 0 | 0 | 0 |

| Sub-Coma Insulin | 0 | 8 | 75 | 100 | 77 | 93 |
|---|---|---|---|---|---|---|

26. The figure reported is for all prior hospitalizations, including institutions other than McLean. Lobotomy patients were identified by reconciling names of the thirty-six patients listed in a letter from J. Butler Tompkins to Paul [Howard], ca. 1947, with those found in the "Operating room log book, 16 January 1946 – 22 August 1960." *AR* (1945): 187.

27. At the Boston Psychopathic, 100 patients were operated upon between October 1943 and April 1946; a follow-up report is Milton Greenblatt, Marie Wingate, and Harry Solomon, "Work Adjustment Five to Ten Years after Bilateral Prefrontal Lobotomy," *NEJM* 250 (20 May 1954): 856–60. For an analysis of the first 250 cases, see *Studies in Lobotomy*, Milton Greenblatt, R. Arnot, and H. Solomon, eds. (New York: Grune and Stratton, 1950). Fay Francis, clinical note, 25 Sept. 1945.

28. "Discussion of 'Psychosurgery,'" 772.

29. *AR* (1936): 182, and (1947): 200. There are some discrepancies between the number of lobotomies reported in the *AR*s, the operating room log, and the individual patient records. Some of these inconsistencies are due to oversight, and others represent differences in fiscal year reporting. These additional sources indicate that fourteen were performed in the calendar year of 1947.

30. J. Butler Tompkins, "A Summary of Thirty-Six Cases of Lobotomy," *AJP* 105 (1948): 443–4; and *AR* (1948): 218.

31. *AR* (1948): 218, and (1949): 219; J. Butler Tompkins, "Penis Envy and Incest: A Case Report," *Psych. Rev.* 27 (1940): 319–25; and *AR* (1949): 219.

32. Howard, "Staff Conference" (Chap. 5, n. 49). This patient is most likely Sarah Worthington, described later.

33. Materials used in the preparation of these narratives (e.g., clinical notes, nursing records, staff conference transcripts, and correspondence) were drawn from the original patient files housed at McLean.

34. Another middle-aged woman with manic-depression who seemed to do quite well was a nun, Sister Miriam O'Connor; her Mother Superior reported that all the other sisters were thrilled with her new condition.

35. After another year went by, the husband noted that she regained her fussiness and had become a "shrewish wife"; on the other hand, she was an excellent and meticulous housekeeper, free from delusions, and able to take care of herself. She was just impossible to live with.

36. The patient later was reported as severely deteriorated and entered the Boston Psychopathic Hospital in 1949. She returned to McLean in 1954, in poor shape, and eventually was transferred to Medfield SH.

37. The possibility of lobotomy was first mentioned in September 1941.

38. Rose's main goal was to obtain control of her trust fund so that she might buy a house and invite her son to move in. Austin was deeply afraid that her poor judgment would result in all of her money being squandered, and that, on the basis of her current positive appearance, a court might erroneously judge her sufficiently competent to handle her affairs.

39. Thorner returned to McLean in the early 1960s, now elderly. From the clinical

note it appears that she coped until just a year before admission, which was apparently caused by alcohol abuse. After a brief stay she went home.

40. This patient was lobotomized because her sisters had inspected the results of the procedure on Lenora Hutchins and liked what they saw.

41. See the files of Dora Singer, Maria Mulcahy, Jeanette Fehr, and Laura Gibbons.

42. This is not to say that the staff was unanimous in its support of the procedure; there often were heated debates in the staff conferences.

43. Although Howard does not name the patient in this paper, the operation date, period of residency, and clinical description all fit Thorner uniquely.

44. Paul Howard, "Staff Conference."

45. Tompkins, "Thirty-Six Cases of Lobotomy," 444.

46. See also the files of Adelaide Hitchcock and Sandra Jordan.

47. This patient was transferred to Butler, where the superintendent noted the resistance of the family to the brain operation. He feared that "later they will have to come to the frontal lobotomy or let her continue to suffer from mental symptoms." It is significant that although Cobb was at this time publicly critical of the lobotomists, he was still recommending the procedure for his private patients; see the files of Howard Peckler and Martha Jenkins.

48. "Discussion of 'Psychosurgery.'" Solomon, Poppen, and Mixter were also in attendance; Watts was not present.

49. See the examples of Anita Payne and Anne Smith.

50. Tompkins, "Thirty-Six Cases of Lobotomy," 443.

51. See Erwin Ackerknecht, "A Plea for a Behaviorist Approach in the History of Medicine," *JHM* 22 (1967): 211–14.

52. This figure does not include second operations, or patients transferred to McLean after a lobotomy elsewhere, or patients recommended for lobotomy at McLean who received one after discharge to a different institution.

53. See Appendix, Table A.1 and Figure A.1.

54. See Appendix, Table A.1. Of the first 36 patients, my own analysis of the patient records indicates a mean age of 46 and a median age of 44.5; and a mean total length of hospitalization of 5.7 years but a median of only 3.2 years.

55. See Appendix, Table A.1 and Figure A.2. An independent t-test shows a weak level of significance ($p < 0.1$) due to wide variance.

56. See Appendix, Figure A.3. This crossover was discussed in Chapters 3 and 5. The 5 patients between 1938 and 1941 had a median age at operation of 61, and a length of stay of 4.1 years; the 58 lobotomy patients between 1945 and 1950 were 46.5 and 2.1, respectively. Patients who exhibited forms of agitated depression were generally lumped into the manic-depressive diagnosis.

57. Published hospital statistics for 1948 record 228 patients who either were in the hospital on 1 Jan. 1948 or placed "on leave"; see *AR* (1948): 213. The sample population reconstructed for this study identified 227 individuals, a capture rate of 99.6 percent. The names were checked against the hospital's master card index, and then each patient's original patient file was abstracted. I am indebted to Jeff Mifflin for assisting me with data collection. An alternate

strategy of reconstructing a hospital population is to add and then subtract from sixty or so years' worth of admission/discharge books – a formidable undertaking indeed, even for a small facility like McLean.

58. See Appendix, Table A.2. An independent t-test of the two populations shows a faint significance, $p = .058$.

59. See Appendix, Figures A.4, A.5. The proportion of males with hospitalizations longer than one year but less than two is less than 2 percent.

60. Of the 195 patients in residence, 80 were 65 years of age or older; 59 of these were female, representing 30 percent of the total ward population (as opposed to the 21 males, or 11 percent.) Of these elderly women, 37 (one-fifth of the total resident population) had been hospitalized more than five years.

61. Patients who died at McLean within five years of admission were removed from the sample, leaving a population of 165. A regression analysis resulted in a $p < .001$, with an F-ratio of 36.0.

62. See Appendix, Figure A.6. There was a wide difference in their fates, depending upon diagnosis. Of the 7 patients admitted for alcohol or drug abuse, all lived to witness their discharge, and so did 13 out of 15 psychoneurotics, and 4 out of 5 psychopathics. As might be expected, the seniles fared the worst, as only 9 out of 29 survived. Of the hebephrenic schizophrenics, 55 percent did not outlive their stay.

63. See Appendix, Table A.3.

64. Ibid.

65. Of the seven male hebephrenics, only one had a hospitalization of less than ten years.

66. William Brandford was rejected on clinical grounds.

67. *AR* (1951): 186.

68. See Appendix, Figure A.7. The *Annual Reports* for 1948 state that 304 patients were admitted; this indicates a capture rate of 99.7 percent for this sample.

69. The ratio calculates as 1.26 : 1. See Appendix, Table A.4.

70. Compare Appendix, Figure A.8, to Figure 6.8.

71. See Appendix, Table A.5.

72. An appropriate analogy might be to think in terms of total *exposure* that year.

73. This is not an unduplicated count, as the same patient might have been discharged and later readmitted; they are handled as separate persons. The assumption is also made that the characteristics of the hospital population did not significantly vary in the two years before and after 1948. This five-year window in fact corresponds to the peak years of the psychosurgery program, a time when the clinical frame had settled into its most expansive form. In this period, 49 patients were chosen for operation, which amounts to 61.3 percent of the total 80 lobotomies; 42 were female, and 7 male. As the age and length of stay of the psychosurgery patients were calculated on the basis of the actual date of operation, which ranged over a five-year period, the statistical effect of comparing the two populations is the same as if their true date had been shifted to that of 31 Dec. 1948, and their dates of admission adjusted accordingly. In addition, as the purpose here is to compare the lobotomized and

nonlobotomized patients, those individuals who had had an operation prior to 31 Dec. 1948 were removed from the hospital-year sample.

74. Those patients in the hospital sample who had a lobotomy prior to 1950 were removed, yielding a population size of 458. Contour maps were generated through the statistical device known as density estimation. Historically, density estimation derived from the search for nonparametric forms of discriminant analysis, and is a useful technique for letting the data describe themselves, as no prior distribution pattern is assumed. These plots were generated using SYSTAT, which employs the popular Epanechicov kernel as the density estimator; see B. W. Silverman, *Density Estimation for Statistics and Data Analysis* (New York: Chapman and Hall, 1986.)

75. Note that the point outside the box is in fact much farther away, representing over thirty years of hospitalization.

76. Adolf Meyer, architect of the new psychiatry, thus also pioneered the development of psychiatric social work.

77. Tompkins complained of the lack of social-support mechanisms for the newly released patients; see idem, "Thirty-Six Cases of Lobotomy," 443.

78. Limburg, "A Survey," in *First Research Conference,* 169 (Chap. 4, n. 1).

79. See, e.g., Andrew Scull and Diane Favreau, " 'A Chance to Cut is a Chance to Cure': Sexual Surgery for Psychosis in Three Nineteenth-Century Societies," *Res. Law Deviance Soc. Control* 8 (1986): 3–39.

80. Freeman and Watts, "Subcortical Prefrontal Lobotomy," 229 (Chap. 2, n. 70).

81. Interview of Dr. Paul Howard by the author, 11 May 1987. Howard noted that upper-class men with severe mental problems were apt to end up less well off financially than women, and thus had less chance of becoming long-term residents at McLean.

82. Psychosurgery was by no means the only treatment that was experimented with during this period at McLean. A partial list includes: shock treatments, sodium amytal, electronarcosis, hypothermia, benzedrine, thyroid operations, hormone extracts, steroids, and zinc. McLean also used EEGs much earlier than most other places, thanks to the proximity of the Davises, who were on staff at Harvard.

83. In arriving at the decision to operate upon Loewy, e.g., Rourke noted that "We might . . . also learn something ourselves about its reaction on a girl of this type."

84. See, e.g., Chauncey Fowler, Lenora Hutchins, and Grace Farmer.

85. An operation was performed in January 1949.

86. See, e.g., the cases of Joseph Eyler and Patricia Lewinger.

87. E.g., the case of Jane L. Bremerton.

88. Care must be taken when assessing the role that behavioral factors played in influencing the McLean physicians. As discussed in the previous chapter, there was less tension than might be supposed between the administrative perspective and the clinical one, for the single most important standard of mental health at this time was that of a person's social adjustment or adaptation. Lobotomy was perceived to be of great *clinical* benefit precisely for the reason

that it potentiated the resocialization of the patient. Seen through the maladjustment framework, the torments of the patients' private world were translated into the same coinage as the disruptions they caused in the social one. Robert Parkhurst's family, e.g., was informed that, although the operation "does not offer complete recovery," it does have a benefit: "the patient is more comfortable and is more easily trained to live a more social life."

89. William Brandford, e.g., posed extreme behavioral problems for the hospital staff. Yet he was the only male hebephrenic on the ward on January 1 who did *not* receive a lobotomy; he too was ruled out of bounds for lack of emotional tone.

90. See the records of Anita Payne. Only one paranoid patient was ever lobotomized.

91. Sutton, *Crossroads*, 255.

92. For returnees, see, e.g., Mary Sullivan, Kay Levitt, and Grace Farmer.

93. Howard, "Staff Conference."

## Chapter 7. The Politics of Precision

1. This chart represents a count of the publications reported in the *Quarterly Cumulative Index Medicus*, the bibliographic files of Freeman and Watts (GWU), and other items encountered in preparation of this manuscript. The chart is offered not as an exact representation but as a relative indicator of the changing level of research and clinical interest in the subject. Nolan Lewis, "Review of Psychiatric Progress 1948 – Psychosurgery," *AJP* 105 (1949): 515.

2. In 1949 *Newsweek* quoted Lewis as stating that lobotomy produced more "zombies" than it cured patients; see Valenstein *G&DC*, 254. Lewis did not repudiate lobotomy, however. He remarked in private that the comment was partly facetious and taken out of context; see Lewis to Irving Wallace, 28 June 1951, NDCL. In any event, he continued to recommend the operation, believing that in many cases of deteriorated psychosis, its benefits outweighed the negative consequences.

3. The array of side effects and possible complications is described in F-W *PS2*, 487–513. Statements about the need to lower lobotomy's deficits are scattered throughout the "Anglo-American Symposium," 1–95 (Chap. 4, n. 98). Jan Frank, "Some Aspects of Lobotomy (Prefrontal Leucotomy) under Psychoanalytic Scrutiny," *Psychiatry* 13 (1950): 35–42; and Lawson Lowrey, "Quo vadis, Psychiatry? Our Profession at the Crossroads," *PSQ* 24 (1950): 448–61. The perception of personality damage following lobotomy may have been heightened by its use on terminal patients with intractable pain who were otherwise psychiatrically normal; their postoperative behavior clearly changed for the worse, as opposed to psychotics, whose postoperative effects were judged against a far more negative baseline; see MacDonald Tow in "Anglo-American Symposium," 40.

4. [Editorial], "Topectomy – New Light on a Stab in the Dark," *PSQ* 23 (1949): 156–7; and discussion of Pool, "Topectomy," 169, 171 (Chap. 4, n. 26).

5. Overviews of the many variant lobotomies can be found in O'Callaghan and Carroll, *Psychosurgery*, 27–38 (Intro., n. 4); and Valenstein *G&DC*, 167–98. In general, the innovations were based on attempts to interrupt the connections between the thalamus and the frontal lobes. Scoville summarized: "Let us compare the frontal lobes and their thalamic connexions to a telephone switchboard with its connecting cable to various telephones. Pool with his topectomy actually cuts out sections of the switchboard proper. Smith, Dax and Reitman with their superior and orbital leucotomies have cut parts of the telephone cable. Wycis and Spiegel with their thalamotomy have cut out a considerable number of the telephones and the speaker with his selective undercutting has stepped behind the switchboard and cut the wires connecting various portions of it to the cable"; "Anglo-American Symposium," 4. See, e.g., the proceedings of the 1st International Conference on Psychosurgery, 4–7, August 1948, Lisbon; published as *Psychosurgery* (Lisbon: Livraria Luso-Espanhola, 1949).

6. [Editorial], "Functional Localisation in the Frontal Lobes," *Lancet* 1 (26 June 1948): 994. The quotation is from Wiley McKissock, "The Technique of Prefrontal Leucotomy," *J. Ment. Sci.* 89 (1943): 194–8. A prominent British neurosurgeon, McKissock eventually performed as many as 1,400 lobotomies.

7. Karl Pribram described a similar model of medical progress into which he placed lobotomy's development; see his "Psychosurgery in Midcentury," *Surg. Gyn. Obs.* 91 (1950): 365.

8. Bitter disagreements arose concerning the validity of each proponent's technique. Scoville was skeptical of the precision Pool claimed to obtain through his topectomies, as damaged blood vessels led to secondary-tissue death beyond the immediate operative site; Pool and Scoville had only contempt for Freeman's blind operative procedure; and Freeman and Watts derided the false superiority of seeing what you cut but not knowing what you see.

9. Stanley Cobb to JF, 21 Jan. 1952, JF. (Unless otherwise indicated, letters, annual reports, manuscripts, etc., cited in this chapter are from the John F. Fulton Papers, JF.) Cobb described the give-and-take between clinicians and researchers in ambivalent terms: "one might mention the rise of a therapeutic procedure started by physiologists, taken up wholesale by therapists, and already returning great dividends to the physiologists. But how great the return is to the patient is still to be evaluated"; Cobb, "Presidential Address," 2–3 (Chap. 2, n. 10). Idem, "Review of Neuropsychiatry for 1940" *ANP* 66 (1940): 1340; and *Emotions and Clinical Medicine* (New York: Norton, 1950), 114.

10. Fulton was quoted in a newspaper interview as saying, "Some day we hope to have a tailor-made operation for each individual"; "Brain Surgery Might Save Fourth of Mental Patients, Doctor Says," *Pittsburgh Press*, 5 Nov. 1948, 20.

11. Freeman *Auto*, chap. 14.

12. From the dust-jacket of W-F *PS1*; a facsimile is in Valenstein *G&DC*, 166.

13. Karl Pribram to JF [Oct.] 1952.

14. John Fulton, "Lobotomy in Man," typescript of an address to the Milwaukee Academy of Medicine, 20 Feb. 1951; published as same title in *Wisc. Med. J.* 50 (1951): 387, 389. John Fulton, *Functional Localization in Relation to*

Frontal Lobotomy (New York: Oxford University Press, 1949), vi; and Frontal Lobotomy and Affective Behavior: A Neurophysiological Analysis (New York: Norton, 1951), 129. Fulton informed an administrator at GWU, Freeman and Watts's home institution, that lobotomy was attracting wider notice than "almost anything that has happened in clinical medicine since the advent of insulin"; JF to Thomas Perry, 9 Mar. 1947. JF *Diary,* 30 Nov. 1948, 26:262.

15. John Fulton to NRC, Division of Medical Sciences, Committee on Veterans Medical Affairs, "Grant Application," 5 Feb. 1948; *Functional Localization,* vi; and "Historical Contributions of Physiology to Neurology," typescript of an address to the AMA, Section of Nervous and Mental Disease, 12 June 1947.

16. John Fulton, "Grant Application"; and "Progress Report: Lobotomy Project, VAm-23379," 10 Oct. 1950.

17. JF to John Eccles, 5 Feb. 1947.

18. John Fulton, "An Experimental Approach to the Problem of Lobotomy," typescript of a paper given at the Harvey Cushing Society, New Haven, 3 June 1948. During the war, Fulton developed a large program of research on the effects of decompression on primates, which yielded direct practical applications for aviation medicine, and served on several NRC committees. For these and other contributions, he was decorated by France, Belgium, Bulgaria, and Cuba, and in Britain was made an O.B.E. He also served as an important liaison between the European medical-scientific community and its American counterpart; with contacts in the highest centers of power and access to diplomatic pouches, Fulton acted as a facilitator and an important conduit of information. His scholarly works during this period included: *A Bibliography of Aviation Medicine* (Springfield, Ill.: C. C. Thomas, 1942); *Physiology of the Nervous System,* 2d ed. (New York: Oxford University Press, 1943); *Howell's Textbook of Physiology,* 15th ed. (Philadelphia: W. B. Saunders, 1946); and his 750-page *Harvey Cushing, A Biography* (Springfield, Ill.: C. C. Thomas, 1946).

19. John Fulton, R. B. Livingston, and G. D. Davis, "Ablation of Area 13 in Primates," *Fed. Proc.* 6 (1947): 108; JF, "Christmas Letter" (sent to family, friends, and alumni of the Laboratory), 18 Nov. 1946; JF to Murray Falconer, 25 Sept. 1946; and "Department of Physiology, Yale University, 1930–1951," typescript (1953), 16; "An Experimental Approach"; and JF *Diary,* 18 Dec. 1946, 23:196. Fulton was prodded by Burness Moore, chairman of Yale's psychiatry department, to become actively involved in lobotomy research; see Moore to JF, 12 Sept. 1946; JF to Moore, 16 Sept. 1946; and Moore to JF, 7 Apr. 1947.

20. John Fulton, "Physiological Basis of Frontal Lobotomy," typescript of early draft with corrections of paper presented to the House Officer Association, Boston City Hospital, 14 Jan. 1947; later published as same title in *Acta Med. Scand. Suppl.* 196 (1947): 617–25. See also JF *Diary,* 14 Jan. 1947. Fulton had last broached the subject of lobotomy in a paper delivered at the Harvey Cushing Society, 3 May 1940, Kansas City, Mo.; see "The Physiological Basis

of the Operation of Frontal Lobotomy," typescript of an address to the Brooklyn Society of Internal Medicine, 18 May 1949. Lobotomy and its relations to frontal-lobe research was by no means Fulton's only focus, but it was clearly dominant; see JF to Captain Ashton Graybiel, 30 Jan. 1947. The more significant lectures and publications of Fulton's on this topic include: the 27th annual meeting of the ARNMD, 12–13 Dec. 1947, New York, published as John Fulton, Charles Aring, and S. Bernard Wortis, eds., *The Frontal Lobes* (Baltimore: Williams & Wilkins, 1948), also cited as *ARNMD* (1948), vol. 27; the Alpha Omega Alpha Lecture of the McGill University Medical School, "The Surgical Approach to Mental Disorder," 8 Jan. 1948, published in *McGill Med. J.* 17 (1948): 133–45 (see also JF *Diary*, same date, vol. 26); the William Withering Memorial Lectures of the Birmingham Medical School, England, 7–10 June 1948, published as *Functional Localization*. Fulton's most important contribution to the literature on psychosurgery was his Thomas Salmon Lecture, 9–11 Jan. 1951, New York, published as *Frontal Lobotomy and Affective Behavior*. For further details of this address, see JF *Diary*, same dates, vol. 32; "Big Advance Seen in Brain Surgery; Prof. Fulton Cites Techniques Developed from Knowledge Gained in Experiments," *New York Times*, 12 Jan. 1951; and "Brain Surgery Urged as Aid in Mental Illness," *New York Herald Tribune*, 14 Jan. 1951.

His later efforts included: "The Physiological Basis of Psychosurgery," *Proc. Amer. Phil. Soc.* 95 (1951): 538–41; "Lobotomy and Affective Behavior," Norwegian Neurological Association, Oslo, 11 May 1951, described in JF *Diary*, 10 May 1951, vol. 32; the 2d Sherrington Lecture of the University of Liverpool, England, 11 Oct. 1951, published as John F. Fulton, *The Frontal Lobes and Human Behaviour* (Liverpool: University of Liverpool Press, 1952); and Visiting Lectureship, Conférences de la Fondation Francqui et de la Belgian-American Foundation, Louvain, Belgium, Sept.–Dec. 1951, published as *Physiologie des Lobes Frontaux et du Cervelet. Etude Experimentale et Clinique* (Paris: Masson, 1953).

21. At the Huggins Lecture in Pittsburgh, e.g., six hundred people attended; Fulton was extensively interviewed by radio and newspaper reporters (JF *Diary*, 26 Nov. 1948, vol. 26). See, e.g., "Brain Surgery Declared Remedy for Mentally Ill; and Restores Some Patients to Useful Lives, Says Yale Specialist Here for Address," *Post-Gazette* (Pittsburgh), 5 Nov. 1948, 1. The flier for the Salmon Lectures identified Fulton as the foremost authority on lobotomy.

22. JF to Russell Garton, 21 Feb. 1949.

23. Fulton, "Physiological Basis of Frontal Lobotomy," 621; and idem, *Functional Localization*, 87–9. Fulton's calculations were based on a combination of Karl Menninger's somewhat overinflated accounting of the costs of psychiatric illness in America; the results of the first large-scale survey of lobotomy (published as Board of Control, *Pre-Frontal Leucotomy in a Thousand Cases* [London: Her Majesty's Stationery Office, 1947]); and a comment by Aneurin Bevan, Britain's controversial minister of health, who was presiding over sweeping changes in the British health care system. In June 1948, Fulton had the opportunity to chat with Bevan at a private dinner in the minister's house.

Fulton reported in his diary that, after a spirited interrogation by Bevan on the American attitude toward the Health Act, "Finally we became switched to lobotomy and to my surprise he was completely informed concerning recent developments and was particularly interested in the considerable economic significance of the operation. He stated that there are 330,000 beds for mental cases in Great Britain and that if, through lobotomy, we could empty even ten percent of them it could alter the whole hospital organization problem under the new Act" (JF *Diary,* 28 June 1948, 26:134). This figure of 10 percent stuck in Fulton's mind; see, e.g., his "Preface" to *The Frontal Lobes,* xii, written a fortnight after the dinner.

24. Fulton, "Preface." The study of functional localization in the human brain had been a haphazard affair, restricted by the scarcity of patients who exhibited either a well-defined tumor or discrete epileptogenic scar tissue that might provide justification for surgical exploration and evaluation. Even rarer, however, was the appearance of such damage bilaterally (equally mirrored on both sides of the brain) – a necessary condition for the production of many cortical deficits that otherwise remain masked if one side is left intact. Surgery on mental patients vastly increased the occasion for study of cerebral function. In addition, because the surgery was performed on brains free of visible tissue pathologies, such material was greatly superior to the "accidents of nature," which had more diffuse effects.

25. This was a somewhat disingenuous remark, as Fulton himself had urged the neurosurgeons forward to experiment with psychosurgery; see Chapter 2.

26. Fulton, *Functional Localization,* vi; Yale Department of Physiology, "AR," typescript, 1951; "Surgical Approach to Mental Disorder," 137; and *Frontal Lobes and Human Behaviour,* 7. Fulton joked, in the original version of his Boston City Hospital address, that when Moniz inquired about a potential operation, "Dr. Jacobsen and I had not then had as much experience with neurosurgeons as has since been my fate, and we rather incautiously agreed with him." This remark was deleted in the printed version.

27. Fulton, "Grant Application"; and JF to John Ransmeier, 14 Jan. 1948.

28. JF, "Christmas Letter," 18 Nov. 1946; JF to Murray Falconer, 25 Sept. 1946; JF to Percival Bailey, 23 Sept. 1946, JF; and "Department of Physiology, Yale University, 1930–1951," 16; and JF *Diary,* 18 Dec. 1946, 23:196. Theodore Ruch and Henry Shenkin, "The Relation of Area 13 on the Orbital Surface of Frontal Lobes to Hyperactivity and Hyperphagia in Monkeys," *J. Neurophys.* 6 (1943): 349–60; and Fulton, "Physiological Basis of Frontal Lobotomy," 622–4. For an oral history of Shenkin's career, see Jack Pressman, "Reflections on Neurosurgery in Philadelphia: Oral Histories with Frederick Murtagh and Henry Shenkin," *Trans. Stud. Coll. Phys. Phila.,* ser. 5, 12 (1990): 27–48.

29. Fulton, "Preface," xi; and JF *Diary,* 12 Dec. 1948, vol. 25.

30. JF to John Eccles, 5 Feb. 1947; see also the correspondence on this meeting filed under "Clubs and Societies"; and Charles Aring to JF, 3 Feb. 1947.

31. Fulton, *ARNMD* 27 (1948): 830.

32. Gosta Rylander, "Personality Analysis Before and after Frontal Lobotomy," *ARNMD* 27 (1948): 691–705. Fulton honored Rylander with an invitation to the conference at the suggestion of Carl Olof Sjoqvist, a distinguished Swedish neurosurgeon who had been an RF Fellow at the Yale laboratory. Rylander was well known for his earlier clinical study of patients operated on for tumors of the frontal lobes; see his *Personality Changes after Operations on the Frontal Lobes; A Clinical Study of 32 Cases* (London: Oxford University Press, 1939).

33. Rylander, "Personality Analysis," 702.

34. JF *Diary*, 10 Dec. 1947, vol. 25.

35. Rylander, "Personality Analysis," 702.

36. Ibid., 703.

37. Fulton declared the paper to have been the best presentation at the meeting and later termed it a "classic." JF to Gosta Rylander, 21 Dec. 1951; JF to Torsten Sjogren, 26 Jan. 1948; and JF to Rylander, 26 Jan. 1952. Paul Bucy informed Fulton that Rylander's findings were "so obviously correct that no intelligent person who was not blinded by his own enthusiasm could not doubt them." The slur was aimed at Freeman (Bucy to JF, 26 Dec. 1948). The tenor of Rylander's comments was that of a loyal opposition. Indeed, Rylander himself soon became a prominent supporter of modified lobotomies and remained so for the following twenty years. See his "The Renaissance of Psychosurgery," in L. Laitinen and K. Livingston, eds. *Surgical Approaches in Psychiatry* (Baltimore: University Park, 1973), 3–12. Allusions to the patient who "lost his soul" or to Rylander's other criticisms can be found, e.g., in *Time*, 25 Oct. 1948, 69; GAP, "Research on Prefrontal Lobotomy," *GAP Report* No. 6 (June 1948): 1; and Kenneth Livingston, "Cingulate Cortex Isolation for the Treatment of Psychoses and Psychoneuroses," *ARNMD* 31 (1951): 374. At the meeting, Rylander also presented a case of a politically active patient whose communist activities ceased after an operation. A local daily newspaper in New York sensationalized this remark as an announced cure for communism, a story which created an international scandal at the very moment Rylander was being considered for an important medical post in Sweden; see JF to The Medical Editor, *Time*, 17 Dec. 1947; Gosta Rylander to JF, 29 Apr. 1948; and JF to Murray Falconer, 19 Dec. 1947.

38. Arthur A. Ward, "The Anterior Cingulate Gyrus and Personality," *ARNMD* 27 (1948): 443. See also W. Smith, "The Results of Ablation of the Cingular Region of the Cerebral Cortex," *Fed. Proc.* 3 (1944): 42.

39. Ward, "Cingulate Gyrus," 443–4.

40. Yale Koskoff to JF, 15 Dec. 1947; and JF to WF, 5 Feb. 1947.

41. J. Pool to JF, 10 Dec. 1948; Henry Viets to JF, 27 Apr. 1948; and JF to Viets, 28 Apr. 1948.

42. Fulton reported to Howard Florey on the results of the first clinical use of penicillin in the U.S.A. – an event which Fulton himself had staged; see JF to Florey, 17 Apr. 1942. Fulton played a crucial role in orchestrating governmental and scientific support for Florey when the British penicillin team visited America in 1941. See George Dohrmann, "Fulton and Penicillin," *Surg. Neur.*

3 (May 1975): 277–80; and Robert Gwyn Macfarlane's biography, *Howard Florey, The Making of a Great Scientist* (Oxford: Oxford University Press, 1979), 339–40, 342, 364.

43. Fulton belonged to sixty-three societies; committee posts included Trustee of the Institute for Advanced Study and Vice-Chairman, NRC Division of Medical Sciences. He was the founding editor of the *Journal of Neurophysiology* and was on the editorial board of the *NEJM*. In 1947, the British Society of Neurosurgeons elected him to an honorary membership. Paul Bucy has written that Fulton "made all neurosurgeons conscious of neurophysiology"; see Lycurgus Davey, "Obituary" (Chap. 2, n. 25). See also Bucy to JF, 14 Dec. 1953. Walter Freeman III, himself a Fulton alumnus, notes that "During the 1940's and 1950's almost every chair in Neurosurgery around the world was held by someone with one or more years of postdoctoral experience in his group"; Freeman to the author, 18 Apr. 1985.

44. See, e.g., the correspondence between Fulton and Harold Buchstein, 1942–3.

45. His confidants on this subject also included Karl Menninger, Leo Davidoff, Fred Mettler, Joseph Siris, Percival Bailey, Walter Freeman, S. D. Porteus, Kenneth McKenzie, Asenath Petrie, Wiley McKissock, Alfred Meyer, and Hidezo Nakagawa.

46. For a list of Fulton's "alumni," see "Research Fellows, 1930–1951." For a detailed list of such discussions, see Pressman *UP*, 305 n. 59. Fulton maintained his ties to Watts. Indeed, Peter Murphy, whom Fulton described as his brightest medical student, went to work with Watts in Washington, D.C., following his graduation from Yale; see JF *Diary*, 13 Nov. 1948, vol. 26. Those from the Yale Lab who later published on lobotomy include Henry Shenkin, Abraham Wikler, and Arthur Ward, as well as the foreign guests Jose Delgado, S. O. Alcalde, Robert Messimy, and Carl Sjoqvist.

47. Watts to JF, 29 Jan. 1951. Fulton, e.g., received many requests for advice on lobotomy from families in New York, whom he referred to Pool, Davidoff, Mahoney, and Scarff; those in Philadelphia he sent to Nulsen; in Pittsburgh, to Koskoff; in Washington, D.C., to Watts; in Minnesota, to Buchstein; in Oregon, to Livingston; in Kentucky, to Grantham; in Texas, to D'Errico; and one patient in England was referred to Cairns. A single lecture in Pittsburgh, e.g., resulted in Fulton sending seven such inquiries to Koskoff.

48. Fulton pointed to eighteen years of primate experience, with operations on a hundred chimps and five thousand monkeys; Fulton, "Grant Application."

49. These included Karl Pribram, Patrick Wall, James Stevenson, R. Livingston, Paul MacLean, Sylvan Kaplan, and H. Rosvold, as well as graduate students George Davis and Mortimer Mishkin.

50. JF *Diary*, 30 July 1950; JF to Theodore Moise, 29 Sept. 1953; and "Department of Physiology, Yale University, 1930–1951," 14, 18. In the first renewal of the VA contract, the NRC oversight committee recommended the addition of clinical trials. Fulton was not averse to this notion, believing that the primate research already had yielded ideas for improved operations. Through such a hybrid project, he felt, "the investigative facilities of the university" might be brought to "the vast clinical material of the state institutions." Yale's

psychiatry department, headed by Burness Moore, took on the responsibility for this portion of the VA grant, selecting a small series of patients from local state hospitals. Operations were performed by Yale's neurosurgeon William German, and the patients were hospitalized and studied at the Yale Psychiatric Clinic. The arrangement formalized an intricate set of ties that had already been established between Fulton and the Connecticut Cooperative Lobotomy Project (CCLP). This group, also directed by Moore, included the Yale psychiatry department, local neurosurgeons, Connecticut's three state hospitals, and the Institute of Living. The VA grant provided research funds for extensive psychological testing and medical analyses that the CCLP had lacked and also financially rescued the psychiatry department. The strong connection between Fulton's group and psychiatric research in Connecticut was illustrated best by Fulton himself, when he described the Institute of Living as an "outpost" of Yale. See Fulton, "Progress Report," 10 Oct. 1950, 5 Jan. 1951; Moore to JF, 12 Sept. 1946, 12 Dec. 1949; JF to Moore, 16 Sept. 1946; and JF to Pat Wall, Sept. 1949. The CCLP's report on two hundred patients was the only major clinical study presented at the 1947 ARNMD meeting. See also William Scoville to JF, 12 Nov. 1948, 15 Nov. 1948; and JF to Scoville, 29 Dec. 1950.

51. See note 14 above for full cites. These celebrated works represented, respectively, an early report and a summation of his VA contract. Fulton termed the latter his "swan song" as professor of physiology; see JF to Harold Wolff, 17 Jan. 1951. The Salmon Lecture in particular exemplified Fulton's reliance upon his extended network to obtain the most recent research findings. No less than thirty-four papers cited (representing 17 percent of the total) were either in preparation or in press. Freeman remarked, in his review of the Withering Lectures, that many of Fulton's conclusions were based on research from his Yale group; in *AJP* 108 (1952): 877–8.

52. Fulton described how Scoville developed three different kinds of improved lobotomy and yet his patients had not been preselected to match the operations; Fulton, *Frontal Lobotomy and Affective Behavior*, 105.

53. W. Smith, "The Functional Significance of the Rostral Cingular Cortex as Revealed by its Responses to Electrical Excitation," *J. Neurophys.* 8 (1945): 241–55; Ward, "Cingulate Gyrus"; idem, "The Cingular Gyrus: Area 24," *J. Neurophys.* 11 (1948): 13–23; and Fulton, *Frontal Lobotomy and Affective Behavior*, 95.

54. The exact beginnings of cingulectomy are unknown. What is clear is Fulton's crucial role as inspirator and then legitimator. Ralph Bailey, e.g., a British neurosurgeon, stated that his "scruples of conscience" had previously dampened his enthusiasm for psychosurgery, but his mind changed when he heard Fulton suggest that the effects of cingulotomy in monkeys implied new operative possibilities in man; see Bailey to JF, 30 Apr. 1949. Fulton spoke on the subject at the 1947 meeting of the Society of British Neurological Surgeons. Sir Hugh Cairns to JF, 28 Nov. 1950; JF to Cairns, 23 Jan. 1950, JF; and JF *Diary*, 30 July 1950. See also Paul Glees et al., "The Effects of Lesions in the Cingular Gyrus and Adjacent Areas in Monkeys," *J. Neur. Neurosurg. Psy-*

*chiat.* 13 (1950): 178–90; Hugh Cairns, "A Symposium on the Operative Treatment of Mental Disorders," *Oxf. Med. Sch. Gaz.* 3 (1951): 3–7; and C. Whitty et al., "Anterior Cingulectomy in the Treatment of Mental Disease," *Lancet* 1 (8 March 1952): 475–81. Fulton's ideas about the potential of Area 24 for limited lobotomies, as stated in the 1948 Withering Lectures, were publicized in a leading English medical journal; see (Editorial) "Functional Localisation," 994.

Kenneth Livingston to JF, 4 Jan. 1951; cited in *Frontal Lobotomy and Affective Behavior*, 142. Earlier, Livingston had been directly involved in a joint lobotomy study involving Yale, Harvard, and the Lahey Clinic (where he was a neurosurgeon); his brother, Robert, was Fulton's junior research associate. See Robert Livingston et al., "Stimulation of Orbital Surface of Man Prior to Frontal Lobotomy," in *Frontal Lobes*, 421–32. See also Livingston, "Cingulate Cortex," 374.

William Scoville, who selected the cingulate areas as one of three regions he experimented on with his new undercutting technique, claims to have persuaded Cairns and LeBeau; see O'Callaghan and Carroll, *Psychosurgery*, 36. Nevertheless, Scoville himself was influenced by Fulton's interpretation of the animal findings. See Scoville, "Proposed Methods of Cortical Undercuttings of Certain Areas of the Frontal Lobes as a Substitute for Prefrontal Leucotomy," in International Conference, *Psychosurgery*, 191–204; "Selective Cortical Undercutting," in "Anglo-American Symposium," 3–8; and Scoville to JF, 12 Nov. 1948. Pool, after hearing Fulton's Salmon Lecture, took exception to the reports of Cairns and Livingston, claiming priority himself, as one patient (case #40, 1947) in the Columbia-Greystone series had Area 24 removed; see Pool to JF, 17 Jan. 1951. Fulton duly reported this case in the published version (p. 118). Pool's claim was rather weak, however, being based on a single case and lacking any overall theoretical conception; also, the topectomy removals had had severe sequelae. For further evidence of Fulton's impact, see J. Siris, "Thalamo-Cingulate Fasciculotomy," *PSQ* 25 (1951): 252; and M. B. Parhad, "Bilateral Cingulo-Tractotomy," *J. Neurosurg.* 10 (1953): 483–9. For additional discussions of the early cingulectomy trials, see Kenneth Livingston, "The Frontal Lobes Revisited; The Case for Second Look," *Arch. Neurol.* 20 (1969): 90–5; Valenstein *G&DC*, 327 n. 22; O'Callaghan and Carroll, *Psychosurgery*, 36, 210–13; and W. Cassidy, H. Ballantine, and N. Flanagan, "Frontal Cingulotomy for Affective Disorders," *Rec. Adv. Biol. Psychiat.* 8 (1965): 269–75.

55. JF to Grantham, 3 Jan. 1951, 7 Jan. 1951; and JF to Rylander, 16 Jan. 1951. See also Fulton, *Frontal Lobotomy and Affective Behavior*, 123–4; F. Reitman, "Orbital Cortex Syndrome following Leucotomy," *AJP* 103 (1946): 238–41; and William Scoville, "Proposed Methods of Cortical Undercutting . . . ," *Dig. Neur. Psychiat.* 16 (1948): 433; T. McLardy and A. Meyer, "Anatomical Correlates of Improvement after Leucotomy," *J. Ment. Sci.* 95 (1949): 182–96, 403–17. Electrocoagulation involved insertion of a thin needle followed by its electrification, which slowly destroyed tissue discretely and without as much incidental damage to brain tissue as in the other surgical

techniques; Fulton hoped that cingulectomies would also be performed using this method. Grantham originally used it for treatment of intractable pain. See E. Grantham, "Prefrontal Lobotomy for the Relief of Intractable Pain," *South. Surg.* 16 (1950): 181–90; idem, "Prefrontal Lobotomy for Relief of Pain: With a Report of a New Operative Technique," *J. Neurosurg.* 8 (1951): 405–10; and E. Grantham and L. Segerberg, "Experiences with Frontal Lobotomy," *Am. Surg.* 22 (1956): 242–8.

56. Fulton, *Frontal Lobotomy and Affective Behavior,* 124–8; "Grant Application"; A. Earl Walker to JF, 19 Jan. 1951; and JF to J. Ransmeier, 14 Jan. 1948.

57. Fulton, "Physiological Basis of Psychosurgery," 539.

58. JF to Stanley Cobb, 20 Dec. 1952; and JW to JF, 29 Jan. 1951. P. K. Bridges and J. R. Bartlett state that Fulton "pointed the way forward"; in "Psychosurgery: Yesterday and Today," *Brit. J. Psychiat.* 131 (1977): 251. Siris, e.g., attributed the inspiration behind his own surgical innovation to Fulton's comments at the 1947 ARNMD; Siris, "Thalamo-Cingulate Fasciculotomy," 252.

59. [Name withheld] to JF, 22 Oct. 1951; and JF's reply, 1 Nov. 1951. There is no indication that an operation was ever performed.

60. Howard McIntyre to JF, 24 Aug. 1954; JF to McIntyre, 30 Sept. 1954; and McIntyre to JF, 5 Oct. 1954. See also H. McIntyre, F. Mayfield, and A. McIntyre, "Ventromedial Quadrant Coagulation (Electrocoagulation) in Treatment of the Psychoses and Neuroses," *AJP* 111 (1954): 112–20; and F. J. Ayd, Jr., "Grantham Lobotomy for Relief of Neurotic Suffering," *Dis. Nerv. Sys.* 17 (1956): 132–5.

61. [Name withheld] to JF, 20 Jan. 1951; Fulton recommended that he contact a former Yale Fellow, neurosurgeon C. G. Mahoney, at St. Vincent's Hospital.

62. See note 12 above. F-W *PS2,* 53–7; and Freeman, "Anglo-American Symposium," 42. Most of the comments in this section on Freeman are based on his "Autobiography" and an interview of James Watts by the author, 14 Nov. 1984.

63. Amarro Fiamberti, "Proposta di un tecnica operatoria modificata e semplificata per gli interventi alla Moniz sur lobi prefrontali in malati di mente," *Rassegna Stud. Psichi.* 26 (1937): 797–806. Fiamberti's technique was itself a variant of A. M. Dogliotti's method of injecting opaque substances for ventriculography. For more details, see Valenstein *G&DC,* 118, 163, 201.

64. Freeman *Auto,* chap. 14. The blunt tip helped to lower the risk of nicking blood vessels. Even so, fatal hemorrhages occasionally occurred. For patients with thick orbits, Freeman designed a heavier leucotome, forbiddingly called an "orbitoclast"; see his "Transorbital Lobotomy; The Problem of Thick Orbital Plate (with Description of Orbitoclast)," *AJP* 108 (1952): 825–8. On occasion the instruments would break, leaving tips that had to be neurosurgically removed; see Valenstein *G&DC,* 231, 235.

65. Freeman *Auto,* chaps. 13, 14; and Valenstein *G&DC,* 256. The knowledge that Freeman was now operating on his own with the transorbital method was more than his partner Jim Watts could stomach, causing a breach in their

relations; Watts's dissent is found in F-W *PS2*, 57–61. Watts later suspected that Freeman always "wanted to be the surgeon himself," in order to live up to the tradition of his grandfather, the eminent surgeon W. W. Keen. Watts, "Psychosurgery: The Story of the 20-Year Follow-up of the Freeman and Watts Lobotomy Series," typescript of a paper presented at the Tenth Anniversary Meeting of the Instituto Nacional de Neurologia, Mexico, 4 Nov. 1974, 21, GWU.

66. Freeman, "Transorbital Leukotomy: Deep Frontal Cut," in "Anglo-American Symposium," 8–12. In the comment, a British neurosurgeon charged that, on occasion, little if any brain material was actually cut, as the brain merely had been pushed aside by the instruments.

67. Walter Freeman, "Transorbital Lobotomy," *AJP* 105 (1949): 734–40; and idem, "Psychiatric Evaluation of Psychosurgery; Lobotomy; A Comparison of Prefrontal Lobotomy with Transorbital Lobotomy," *Surg. Gyn. Obs.* 92 (1951): 603–6.

68. Freeman *Auto*, chap. 18. Walter Freeman and James Watts, "Transorbital Lobotomy," *Med. Ann. D.C.* 17 (May 1948): 257; and see also Walter Freeman, "Transorbital Lobotomy. Survey after from One to Three Years," *Dis. Nerv. Sys.* 10 (1949): 360–3; idem, "Clinical Aspects of Psychosurgery; Theoretic and Clinical Consideration of Various Leukotomy Technics," in "Anglo-American Symposium," 28–31; idem, "Transorbital Lobotomy in State Mental Hospitals," *J. Med. Soc. N.J.* 51 (1954): 148–50; "Frontal Lobotomy 1936–1956: A Follow-up Study of 3000 Patients from One to Twenty Years," *AJP* 113 (1957): 877–86; and "West Virginia Lobotomy Project: A Sequel," *JAMA* 181 (1962): 1134–5. "Mass Lobotomies," *Time*, 15 Sept. 1952, 60:86.

69. Freeman *Auto*, chap. 14. Freeman recounted that many medical students (and even some experienced practitioners) fainted when witnessing the procedure. An eyewitness to one of Freeman's transorbital clinics likened it to a medical "circus act"; see Alan Scheflin and Edward Opton, Jr., *The Mind Manipulators* (New York: Paddington, 1978), 247–9.

70. Percival Bailey, e.g., in an annual review of neurosurgery, stated that the transorbital method "violates all surgical instincts"; see Roland MacKay, Nolan D. C. Lewis, and Percival Bailey, eds., *The 1949 Yearbook of Neurology, Psychiatry and Neurosurgery* (Chicago: Yearbook, 1950), 542.

71. Pool, "Topectomy," 171.

72. *Third Research Conference*, 66; and Freeman, "Psychiatric Evaluation," 604–5.

73. "Downing Radio Program Script," typescript, 19 Nov. 1948, 2, GWU; the show was broadcast on 27 Nov. 1948, on KIRO. See also the correspondence between Freeman and Charles Jones, 1947–8, GWU.

74. Initial reports on transorbital lobotomy in America include: F. Hass and D. Williams, "Transorbital Lobotomy; A Preliminary Report in Twenty-four Cases," *S. Dak. J. Med. Pharm.* 1 (May 1948): 191–2; C. Jones and J. Shanklin, "Transorbital Lobotomy. A Preliminary Report of 40 Cases," *Northwest. Med.* 47 (1948): 421–7; and C. Jones, "Social Adjustment fol-

lowing Transorbital Lobotomy," *Post-Grad. Med.* 6 (1949): 392–7. A detailed list of subsequent articles can be found in Pressman *UP*, 311–12 n. 91.

75. *Third Research Conference,* 164; and *First Research Conference,* 168. See also Tracy Putnam, "Prefrontal Lobotomy. Its Evolution and Present Status," *Bull. Los Ang. Neur. Soc.* 15 (1950): 229.

76. JF to WF, 2 Oct. 1947; and WF to JF, 6 Oct. 1947.

77. WF to JF, 31 Oct. 1947.

78. Discussion of Crawford, " 'Becky' and 'Lucy,' " 58 (Chap. 2, n. 105). Discussion of Walter Freeman and James Watts, "The Thalamic Projection to the Frontal Lobe," in *Frontal Lobes,* 209.

79. Discussion of Ward, "Cingulate Gyrus," in *Frontal Lobes,* 443.

80. Discussion of S. Spafford Ackerly and Arthur Benton, "Report of Bilateral Frontal Lobe Defect," in ibid., 504; see also Freeman's discussion of Ward Halstead, "Specialization of Behavioral Functions and the Frontal Lobes," in ibid., 64.

81. See the letters between JF and WF, January 1950.

82. Although Fulton retired from physiology in 1951, he continued teaching full-time as the university's first professor of the history of medicine.

83. William G. Spiller, the eminent Philadelphia neurologist, was Freeman's primary role model in medical school; Freeman *Auto,* chap. 5. His life's most gratifying work, Freeman also wrote, were the transorbital efforts which allowed him "to have been the means of relieving suffering and restoring a goodly number of patients to their homes"; ibid., chap. 8.

84. Fulton, "Surgical Approach to Mental Disorder," 144. Wilder Penfield wryly commented to Fulton that, unlike chimps, "my subjects for physiological observations not only do not cost me six hundred dollars, but I can hardly keep them out of the operating room! I grow more impressed by the courage, not to say the foolhardiness, of the human race"; Penfield to JF, 4 Jan. 1949.

85. [Editorial] "Topectomy – New Light," 159; and Pool, "Topectomy," 171.

86. Fulton, *Functional Localization,* 85.

87. WF to JF, 21 Dec. 1949, GWU; and L. Kalinowsky and P. Hoch, *Shock Treatments and Other Somatic Procedures in Psychiatry* (New York: Grune & Stratton, 1946), 6.

88. Freeman, "Transorbital Lobotomy," 734.

89. "Anglo-American Symposium," 20.

90. John H. Warner argues that the arrival of the medical laboratory in the nineteenth century did not introduce science into medicine so much as it occasioned a redefinition of what was considered "scientific"; see works cited in Intro., n. 13 above. See also Christopher Lawrence and Richard Dixey, "Practising on Principle: Joseph Lister and the Germ Theories of Disease," in C. Lawrence, ed., *Medical Theory and Surgical Practice: Studies in the History of Surgery* (New York: Routledge, 1992), 153–215; G. Geison, "Pasteur, Roux, and Rabies: Scientific versus Clinical Mentalities," *JHM* 45 (1990): 341–65; idem, " 'Divided We Stand': Physiologists and Clinicians in the American Context," in Vogel and Rosenberg, *Therapeutic Revolution,* 67–90 (Intro., n.

8); L. S. Jacyna, "The Laboratory and the Clinic: The Impact of Pathology on Surgical Diagnosis in the Glasgow Western Infirmary, 1875–1910," *BHM* 62 (1988): 384–406; C. Lawrence, "Incommunicable Knowledge: Science, Technology and the Clinical Art in Britain 1850–1914," *J. Contemp. Hist.* 20 (1985): 503–20; S. E. D. Shortt, "Physicians, Science, and Status: Issues in the Professionalization of Anglo-American Medicine in the Nineteenth Century," *Med. Hist.* 27 (1993): 51–68; and Russell Maulitz, " 'Physician versus Bacteriologist': The Ideology of Science in Clinical Medicine," in ibid., 91–107.

91. L. L. Bernstein, a neurosurgeon who performed lobotomies at the Menninger Clinic, quoted Sherrington in a review of F-W *PS2*, in *Bull. Menn. Clinic* 16 (1952): 33. The full statement can be found in Fulton, *Functional Localization*, viii. Sherrington was paraphrasing Keats's notion of "busy common sense."

92. Fulton's departmental budget in 1931 was an adequate $50,000; in 1951, his allotment had increased to only $51,000, and he was forced to underwrite the costs of a much larger teaching load through misappropriation of research funds. See "History of the Department of Physiology," 9–10.

93. University research was supported during the war by the Office of Scientific Research and Development (OSRD) and afterward by the Office of Naval Research (ONR); these dominated the scene until the NSF and the NIH were fully operational. See Harvey Sapolsky, "Academic Science and the Military: The Years Since the Second World War," in Nathan Reingold, ed., *The Sciences in the American Context: New Perspectives* (Washington, D.C.: Smithsonian, 1979), 379–99. See also J. Capshew, "Big Science: Price to the Present," *Osiris* 7 (1992): 3–25. Fulton's own laboratory mirrored this pattern. In 1941, Fulton described the financial woes of his laboratory to Alan Gregg; JF to Gregg, 4 Feb. 1941. During the war, however, the OSRD underwrote the costs of aviation research in amounts that were massive in proportion to Fulton's previous departmental budgets. In 1942, his department's total research funds amounted to $11,000, comprised of a patchwork of small individual grants from private philanthropies. Three years later, the OSRD contributions to Fulton's Aeromedical Unit amounted to over $100,000; after the war, the ONR contributed over $30,000 annually, for several years. (See Yale Department of Physiology, "AR," for these years.) Fulton had anticipated that public support of science would grow increasingly important. This thought lay behind his decision to side with Freeman and Watts when Kaempffert's *Saturday Evening Post* article was viewed as a form of medical advertising, almost causing the professional censure of the two physicians (these events are described in Chapter 3). Fulton had been convinced by Kaempffert that the medical profession could ill afford the luxury of insularity from public inspection; money for medical research was obtainable only if the public were educated about what might be accomplished through research. Fulton afterward made a point of helping science journalists, defending them from often harsh criticisms. The upbeat tone of Fulton's campaign to reform psychosurgery also followed this scheme. He thus trumpeted not just the benefits of this particular line of research, but the general principle of medical

research as well. See Waldemar Kaempffert to JF, 31 May 1941; JF to C. C. Thomas, 27 May 1941, 5 June 1941; and Yale Department of Physiology, "AR," typescript, 1949, 26a.

94. Kramer, "The 1951 Survey," 160 (Introduction, n. 3); and JF to John Ransmeier, 5 Feb. 1948, 14 Jan. 1948. It was particularly appropriate for the VA to sponsor the project, Fulton noted, because the procedure was "looming large" as a therapeutic measure for severe cases of war neurosis; "Grant Application."

95. Open letter of James Krauss, in "Notes and Comment," *AJI* 66 (1909): 320–2.

96. Freeman often pointed to his isolation from the research community as the reason he was turned down nine times by foundations; Freeman *Auto*, chap. 14.

97. Fulton's neurophysiological model is discussed at greater length in Chapter 2.

98. Fulton, *Frontal Lobotomy and Affective Behavior,* 32, 94; see also W. E. Le Gros Clark, "The Connexions of the Frontal Lobes of the Brain," *Lancet* 1 (3 June 1948): 353–6; and (editorial) "Functional Localisation," 994–5.

99. A good overview of the dramatic reconception of the frontal lobe and its autonomic connections is Fulton, "Somatic Functions of the Central Nervous System," *Ann. Rev. Physiol.* 15 (1953): 305–28. See also his revised chap. 22, "Cerebral Cortex: The Orbitofrontal and Cingulate Regions," in *Physiology of the Nervous System,* 3d ed. (1949), 447–67. Fulton described how the interconnections were newly mapped by three routes of investigation: localized electrical stimulation, such as Livingston et al., "Stimulation of Orbital Surface"; evoked potential studies; and physiological neuronography, such as Ernest Sachs, Jr., S. Brendler, and J. Fulton, "The Orbital Gyri," *Brain* 72 (1949): 227–40, and A. Ward and W. McCulloch, "The Projection of the Frontal Lobe on the Hypothalamus," *J. Neurophys.* 10 (1947): 309–14. See his *Frontal Lobotomy and Affective Behavior,* 51–68.

100. James W. Papez, "A Proposed Mechanism of Emotion," *ANP* 38 (1937): 725–43. In 1981, Kenneth Livingston conducted a series of oral histories concerning the origin and impact of this paper; see Robert Livingston, "Epilogue: Reflections on James Wenceslas Papez, according to Four of His Colleagues (Compiled by Kenneth Livingston)," in Benjamin Doane and Kenneth Livingston, eds., *The Limbic System: Functional Organization and Clinical Disorders* (New York: Raven, 1986), 317–34. Papez wrote the paper in response to a challenge from an English philanthropy that offered $150,000 for the best paper on emotions. Papez was irked by the dearth of reprint requests, yet at first he too failed to cite this article.

101. Paul MacLean, "Psychosomatic Disease and the 'Visceral Brain': Recent Developments bearing on the Papez Theory of Emotion," *Psychosom. Med.* 11 (1949): 338–53. Paul Yakovlev devised the new cerebral trinity of entopallium, mesopallium, ectopallium, as being the structural bases for the three spheres of thought: "visceration," "expressions," and "effectuation." See his "Motility, Behavior and the Brain," *JNMD* 107 (1948): 313–35.

102. The Rockefeller Foundation's program of psychosomatic medicine is discussed in Chapter 1. Fulton had read Papez's article in manuscript in 1937, but its significance had escaped him at the time. In even the last (3d) edition of *Physiology of the Nervous System,* Fulton ignored this article, a piece which only one year later he would describe as a "classic work." See Doane and Livingston, *Limbic System,* 330; and Fulton, *Frontal Lobotomy and Affective Behavior,* 67.

103. Fulton, "The Limbic System: A Study of the Visceral Brain in Primates and Man," *Yale J. Bio. Med.* 26 (1953): 107–18. Fulton's discourse in his Salmon Lecture on the limbic lobe was built upon the previous such address delivered by Stanley Cobb; see Cobb, *Emotions and Clinical Medicine,* 35–47, 82–8, 113–26. On a number of earlier occasions, the results of the psychosurgery operations led to speculations about the exact structural location of the emotions, a distinct shift in emphasis from the usual concern with intellect, behavior, or some generalized "mind." As early as 1937, Freeman himself postulated that the operation cut unknown tracts between the hypothalamus and the frontal lobes; see Freeman and Watts, "Subcortical Prefrontal Lobotomy," 270 (Chap. 2, n. 103). Brickner, e.g., stated in the discussion of an early paper of Freeman and Watts that he thought their work brought new insight to the relations between the intellect and the "feeling tone" in the brain; see comments by Brickner in "Society Transactions. New York Neurological Society, 2/1/38. Discussion of Paper by Walter Freeman and James Watts," *ANP* 40 (1938): 203. Fulton was intrigued by this notion that one of the most primitive structures and one of the most recently advanced might in fact be directly connected; Fulton, *Physiology of the Nervous System* (1938), 273. In 1939, Lyerly, too, speculated about the role of the thalamus; Lyerly, "Deep Association Fibers" (Chap. 3, n. 4). By 1942, commentators on psychosurgery might cite as scientific explanation for the procedure the need to "disconnect the diencephalon"; Carmichael and Carmichael, Jr., "Malignant Mental Disorders," 200 (Chap. 3, n. 60). See also Hofstatter, "Orbital Areas" (Chap. 3, n. 38).

104. Fulton, "The Limbic System," 107–18; Paul MacLean, "Some Psychiatric Implications of Physiological Studies on Frontotemporal Portion of Limbic System (Visceral Brain)," *EEG Clin. Neurophys.* 4 (1952): 407–18. See also his "Neurophysiological Symposium. Limbic System and Its Hippocampal Formation: Studies in Animals and Their Possible Implications in Man," *J. Neurosurg.* 11 (1954): 29–44. The current status of limbic system research can be surveyed in Doane and Livingston, *The Limbic System,* especially Paul MacLean, "Culminating Developments in the Evolution of the Limbic System: The Thalamocingulate Division," 1–28, and Benjamin Doane, "Clinical Psychiatry and the Physiodynamics of the Limbic System," 285–315. The quotation is of K. Livingston, cited by Doane, ibid., 286. See also Livingston, "Frontal Lobes Revisited," 90–5. Paul Yakovlev, "Recollections of James Papez and Comments on the Evolution of Limbic System Concept," in K. E. Livingston and O. Hornykiewicz, eds., *Limbic Mechanisms: The Continuing Evolution of the Limbic System Concept* (New York:

Plenum, 1978); and Paul MacLean, *A Triune Concept of the Brain and Behavior* (Toronto: University of Toronto Press, 1969). For an overview of recent research on the prefrontal lobe that incorporates earlier studies, see Joaquin Fuster, *The Prefrontal Cortex; Anatomy, Physiology and Neurophysiology of the Frontal Lobe* (New York: Raven, 1980).

105. A. Meyer and T. McLardy, "Posterior Cuts in Prefrontal Leucotomy: A Clinico-Pathological Study," *J. Ment. Sci.* 94 (1948): 555; Gerhardt von Bonin, *Essay on the Cerebral Cortex* (Springfield, Ill.: C. C. Thomas, 1950), 123; and Pool, "Topectomy," 164–73. Fulton, *Physiology of the Nervous System*, 3d ed., 451.

106. This line of discussion is similar to that in the conclusion to Chapter 2. My argument is an extension of Shapin's anti-Mertonian analysis of the impact that phrenology had on the development of early theories of cerebral localization, and of Fleck's framework for understanding the evolution of scientific concepts. See Steve Shapin, "The Politics of Observation: Cerebral Anatomy and Social Interests in the Edinburgh Phrenology Disputes," in Roy Wallis, ed., *On the Margins of Science: The Social Construction of Rejected Knowledge* (London: Sociological Review, 1979), 139–78. (There are, of course, many strong parallels between the phrenology scenario and that of psychosurgery, which Freeman himself once likened to "surgical phrenology.") Fleck suggested that every significant step forward in science contains one dimension that may indeed be thought of in terms of inner-directed puzzle solving, what he terms *passive* knowledge, as well as a second dimension that addresses its perceived social value or effect, what he terms *active* knowledge. Neither factor ever fully vanishes from the scene, though the proportional influence of each may fluctuate depending upon local circumstance. Fleck, *Scientific Fact* (Chap. 2, n. 109).

107. In the case of such reversals, researchers later tend to deny that they thought a justification ever existed. Fulton himself was not immune from such whiggish reconstructions; see JF to WF, 1 Oct. 1954. Variants of the procedure did survive, though with much more restrictive uses; this is discussed further in the Epilogue.

108. Myerson, " 'Total Push,' " 1199 (Chap. 6, n. 22).

109. The search by Fulton and others for a physiologically justified lobotomy rested upon an assumption that selection of operative site was more important than the extent of tissue destroyed – that brain function was divisible into discrete, localizable units. It was hardly inevitable that such an assumption would prove correct. Indeed, a growing body of evidence indicated that the relevant variable in lobotomy's success on the wards was in fact quantity of brain material sectioned, not just location. W. Scoville, "Psychosurgery and Other Lesions of the Brain Affecting Human Behavior," in Edward Hitchcock, Lauri Laitinen, and Kjeld Vaernet, eds., *Psychosurgery* (Springfield, Ill.: C. C. Thomas, 1972), 18; and "Anglo-American Symposium," 54. Freeman's original psychosurgical strategy was largely based on the "mass action" model, where he cut as much tissue as was necessary for "remission."

110. Science's power, Latour argues, derives from its unique privilege of making its mistakes in private. See Bruno Latour, "Give Me a Laboratory and I Will Raise the World," in Karin Knorr-Cetina and Michael Mulkay, eds., *Science Observed: Perspectives on the Social Study of Science* (Beverly Hills, Calif.: Sage, 1983), 141–70.

111. See O'Callaghan and Carroll, *Psychosurgery;* and Valenstein *G&DC,* 167–98.

112. Carlyle Jacobsen to JF, 2 May 1940.

113. Susan Bell analyzes the problems medical regulatory agencies faced when monitoring field-workers. Even though treatments were labeled "for experimental uses only," general practitioners had great latitude in their choice and application of therapies. See Bell, "Medical Technology" (Intro., n. 14).

## Chapter 8. Medicine Controlled

1. Kalinowsky and Scarff, "Selection of Psychiatric Cases," 81 (Chap. 5, n. 12).

2. Samuel Hamilton, "Presidential Address. Our Assocation in a Time of Unsettlement," *AJP* 104 (1947): 1–12; and Lawson G. Lowrey, "Quo vadis, Psychiatry? Our Profession at the Crossroads," *PSQ* 24 (1950): 448–61; and Grob *Asylum,* 3. In 1947, APA membership reached 4,341. William Menninger, "President's Page. Membership," *AJP* 105 (1949): 625. From 1944 to 1957, APA membership tripled; Harry Solomon, "Presidential Address," *AJP* 115 (1958): 1–9. Statistics for APA membership are scarce; the USPHS performed this survey at Menninger's request, using the sometimes inaccurate 1947–8 APA Membership Directory. For full findings, see: Robert Robinson to APA President, "Interoffice Memorandum," 4 Dec. 1948; and Robert Felix to WM, 2 Dec. 1948, Comm. on Membership, Box 200-5, APA.

3. An excellent account is Nathan Hale, Jr., *The Rise and Crisis of Psychoanalysis in the United States: Freud and the Americans, 1917–1985* (New York: Oxford University Press, 1995).

4. These attacks are described in Chapter 3. "Proceedings of the First Postgraduate Course in Psychosurgery," *Dig. Neur. Psych.* 17 (1949): 426–9; and Harry S. Sullivan, *Conceptions of Modern Psychiatry; The First William Alanson White Memorial Lectures* (Washington, D.C.: White Memorial, 1940), 73. Little overlap existed between formal psychosurgical and psychoanalytic investigations. An exception is Elizabeth Zetzel, "Psychoanalytic Observations Regarding the Dynamic Effects of Frontal Lobe Surgery," in Greenblatt and Solomon, *Frontal Lobes,* 185 (Chap. 5, n. 30).

5. Freeman and Watts, "Subcortical Prefrontal Lobotomy" (Chap. 2, n. 103). The psychoanalytic and the somatic domains were often interwoven, as evidenced by a scene in the 1948 movie *The Snakepit.* The afflicted heroine, sitting in her psychiatrist's office, listens to an explanation of how electroshock therapy works; in view of a picture of Sigmund Freud, she learns that such treatments help the psychiatrists "regain contact" with patients. The patient recovers after a session of narcosynthesis, in which a sodium pentothal–induced hypnosis

enables her to remember a repressed trauma. On occasion, popular magazines would explain lobotomy by applying elaborate Freudian models; see, e.g., "Psychosurgery," *Life,* 3 Mar. 1947.

6. "Proceedings of Societies," *AJP* 105 (1949): 859, 863; and Dexter Bullard, "Interview," 5 Aug. 1964, Oral History 148, APA. I am grateful to Gerald Grob for directing my attention to this document.

7. Although the two were once on cordial terms, they had clashed on professional issues in the recent past. Freeman traced the antagonism to the time when, in his role as examiner for the Board of Neurology and Psychiatry, he failed Bullard on the neurology section of the exam; Freeman *Auto,* chap. 13. Bullard, "Interview." Chestnut Lodge and Bullard were central to the development of American psychoanalysis; see David McK. Rioch, "Dexter Bullard, Sr., and Chestnut Lodge," *Psychiat.* 47 (February 1984): 1–8.

8. See Friedman's excellent *Menninger* (Chap. 1, n. 4).

9. WM to Albert Deutsch, 7 Oct. 1957; and Sol Ginsburg to Deutsch, 15 Oct. 1957, Box 15, GAP[NY]. See also John Romano to Leo Bartemeier, 9 Aug. 1945, Correspondence, GAP[MF]. Grob has reconstructed the postwar battles within the APA; see "The Reorganization of Psychiatry," chap. 2, in *Asylum,* 24–43.

10. Albert Deutsch offers a somewhat whitewashed organizational history in *The Story of GAP* (New York: G.A.P., 1959). The infamous "smoke-filled room" included Daniel Blain, Henry Brosin, Norman Brill, Roy Grinker, Robert Felix, Ralph Kaufman, and John Romano. WM to Mildred Scoville, 20 Apr. 1948, GAP–Commonwealth Fund, HWB; Albert Deutsch, " 'Young Turks in Psychiatry May Rebel against Old Guard," *PM* (29 May 1946): 13; and "New Group of Psychiatrists Formed to Speed up War on Mental Ills," *PM* (18 Nov. 1946): 24.

11. WM to Mildred Scoville, 20 Apr. 1948, GAP–Commonwealth Fund, HWB.

12. Dale E. Cameron to WM, 28 Mar. 1949, CCB/APA vs. GAP 1947–49, WCM; and Gerald Grob, "Psychiatry and Social Activism: The Politics of a Specialty in Postwar America," *BHM* 60 (1986): 477–501. CCB to Winfred Overholser, 26 Apr. 1945, Series 54, CCB/1939–1950, WO.

13. See the exchange of letters in C. B. Farrar Papers, APA, described in Grob, "Psychiatry and Social Activism," 477–501; "Shock Therapy," *GAP Rep.* 1 (15 Sept. 1947): 1–2; Lothar Kalinowsky to Robert Knight, 3 May 1949, MG; "Research on Prefrontal Lobotomy," *GAP Rep.* (June 1948): 6; and Circular Letter #78, 27 Feb. 1948, Comm. on Research, 1948–9, Box 200-8, APA. For an attack on psychosurgery which made reference to this report, see S. A. Robins, "Letter to the Editor," *AJP* 105 (1948): 387.

14. Clarence Cheyney to Douglas Thom, cited in Grob, "Psychiatry and Social Activism," 490; and A. A. Brill, "Samuel Hamilton, President 1946–1947," *AJP* 104 (1947): 13. Burlingame's name was raised by Vidonian Fred Parsons, a retired psychiatrist who had served as commissioner of the NYS DMH; Cheney seconded. See Vidonian Club, "Minutes," 25 Oct. 1947, 9 June 1948, Box 3–5, VID. Bowman, relocated to California, had become an inactive member.

15. WM to Ralph Kaufman, 20 Jan. 1948, Shock Therapy–Report #1, GAP[MF]. For details surrounding the nomination and responses, see Pressman *UP*, 369 n. 18. The events were so sensitive, Smith suggested that all correspondence be destroyed; copy of Lauren Smith to Norman Brill, 1 Mar. 1948. Menninger felt that his own role must remain "passive" lest internal strife consume the APA; WM to Morse, 4 Mar. 1948, CCB/APA vs. GAP 1947–49, WCM.
16. T. H. Robie to CCB, 21 May 1948, Series 54, CCB/1939–1950, WO.
17. Vidonian Club, "Minutes," 9 June 1948, VID.
18. CPMSP, Newsletter #1 (Jan. 1949), #2 (Mar. 1949), #4 (May 1949), Box 15/CPMSP, GAP[NY]; and a copy of a Newsletter (Feb. 1950), CPMSP, GAP[MF]. See also a copy of minutes of CPMSP meeting, 6 Nov. 1949, that Brosin happened to obtain for WM, CPMSP, GAP[MF].
19. CPMSP, Newsletter #1, #4.
20. See copy of Jesse Arnold to Hugh Carmichael, 13 Jan. 1948, CCB/APA vs. GAP 1947–49, WM Foster Kennedy, "In Memoriam. C. Charles Burlingame," *AJP* 107 (1950): 399. In the 1920s, Burlingame had been instrumental in the design of the Columbia-Presbyterian Medical Center; "Dr. Burlingame Dies, Noted as Psychiatrist," *Hartford Times*, 23 July 1950, 1.
21. C. C. Burlingame, "Report of the Physician-in-Chief," Institute of Living *AR* 108 (1932): 8–9, and 124 (1948): 10–11; and idem, "Can the Point of View and Technique of Private Practice be Carried into the Mental Hospital?" typescript of address to the Southern Psychiatric Association, San Antonio, Texas, 9 Oct. 1937, CCB.
22. Institute of Living, *The Story of the Institute of Living* (Hartford, Conn.: Institute of Living, 1946), 7. The institute's psychosurgery program exemplified this dual philosophy, stressing postoperative reeducation; C. C. Burlingame, "Rehabilitation after Leucotomy," *Proc. Roy. Soc. Med. Suppl.* 42 (1949): 31–42.
23. For the effects of a speech by "Burly," see, e.g., H. Carmichael to WM, CCB/APA vs. GAP 1947–49, WCM Tomes, *A Generous Confidence* (Chap. 1, n. 4).
24. C. C. Burlingame, "Psychiatric Sense and Nonsense," *JAMA* 133 (5 Apr. 1947): 971–2; CCB to Winfred Overholser, 12 May 1947, Series 54, CCB/1939–50, WO; and C. C. Burlingame, "The Psychiatrist-in-Chief reports to the Board of Directors," Institute of Living *AR* 124 (1948): 11.
25. Albert Deutsch, "Revolt May Split Ranks in Psychiatry," *Compass* (24 May 1949): 3, 21; Will Menninger's series of editorials, "President's Page," *AJP* 105 (1949): 704, 870. Copy of Karl Bowman to WM, 9 May 1949; WM to Karl Bowman, 2 July 1948; WM to Bowman, 16 Jan. 1950; Bowman to Max Gitelson, 11 Jan. 1950; WM to Gitelson, 16 Jan. 1950, Shock Therapy–Report #1, GAP[MF]; Bowman to Bob McGraw, 17 Mar. 1949, CPMSP, GAP[MF]; Henry Brosin to WM, 22 Feb. 1949, Brosin (Sec'y) 1949, GAP[MF]; and WM to D. Ewen Cameron, 21 Apr. 1949, CCB/APA vs. GAP 1947–49, WCM. See also Lucy Freeman, "Dr. Knight Assails 'Strong-Arm' Cure," *New York Times*, 6 June 1948, 48; and response, T. H. Robie, "Letter to the Editor," ibid., 12 July 1948, 18. The Committee on Therapy's second

electroshock report incorporated the views of GAP opponents McGraw, Bowman, and Kalinowsky; see "Revised Electroshock Report," *GAP Rep.* No. 15 (August 1950). See also Lothar Kalinowsky to Robert Knight, 3 May 1949, MG.

26. WM to Deutsch, 7 Oct. 1957; Box 10, Comm. on Therapy, GAP[NY]. Perhaps the most extreme example of anti-GAP sentiment was J. O'Connor, "Thought Control – American Plan," which derided GAP members as "shock troops of Sigmund Freud," *The Sign* (November 1949): 23. See, e.g., "Confidential Agenda," GAP Meeting, 7 Apr. 1949, Asbury Park, N.J., Meeting, 1949, GAP[MF].

27. Copy of Karl Bowman to WM, 9 May 1949; Bowman to Max Gitelson, 11 Jan. 1950, Shock Therapy–Report #1, GAP[MF]; and Robert Knight to GAP Comm. on Therapy, "Memo–communication #5," 1 Nov. 1948, Comm. on Therapy, APA.

28. Burlingame, "Report of the Physician-in-Chief" (1948): 11.

29. "The Social Responsibility of Psychiatry, a Statement of Orientation," *GAP Rep.* No. 13 (July 1950), cited in Grob, "Psychiatry and Social Activism."

30. CPMSP Newsletter #1. Samuel Orton, in his 1929 APA presidential address, had already observed such "dislocations." Orton commented that the success of the mental hygiene movement had forced the psychiatrist to become an "arbiter of questions of behavior and of social relations." Because the new role contained little actual medical content, Orton feared, psychiatry was thus withdrawing from medicine in order to gain popularity – a losing proposition. Orton urged a return to brain research. Samuel Orton, "Presidential Address," *AJP* 86 (1929): 1–16.

31. Robert Morse to WM, 25 Feb. 1948, CCB/APA vs. GAP 1947–49, WCM.

32. Kalinowsky to Robert Knight, 3 May 1949, MG. The strategy of reforming the state hospitals through "active treatments" is the subject of Chapter 4.

33. Sam Feigin and Lewis Sharp to James Wall, 13 Mar. 1950; Box 2-10, VID.

34. Sydney Margolin to WM, 27 Mar. 1951; and Margolin to Members of the Committee on Therapy, 15 Dec. 1952, Box 10, Comm. on Therapy, GAP[NY].

35. R. Morison, "Memo.," 30 Sept. 1948, Programs and Policy (RG3 906 2 18), RFA.

36. Ibid.; Sandor Rado to Nolan D. C. Lewis, 12 Mar. 1940; George Daniels to Lewis, 28 July 1944; and Arcangelo D'Amore, "Oral History Interview with Nolan D. C. Lewis" (23 Sept. 1972), 95, NDCL. The RF's role in the development of American psychiatry is described in Chapter 1.

37. J. Berkeley Gordon to Leo Bartemeier, 23 June 1948 (copy); and "Report on the Orgone Therapy of Dr. Wilhelm Reich," prepared by Jacob Finesinger, Research Committee Chair, n.d., Comm. on Research, 1948–1949, Box 200-8, APA.

38. WM to J. B. Gordon, 30 June 1948, 9 July 1948; WM to D. Flicker, 22 July 1948; Jacob Finesinger to WM, 11 Aug. 1948; WM to Finesinger, 13 Aug. 1948; and Finesinger to WM, 27 Sept. 1948, Comm. on Research, 1948–1949, Box 200-8, APA.

39. Copy of J. Berkeley Gordon to WM, 24 June 1948, Comm. on Research, 1948–1949, Box 200-8, APA. The FDA eventually served Reich with a complaint in 1954; in 1957 he was imprisoned in a federal penitentiary and died shortly thereafter. Jerome Greenfield, in *Wilhelm Reich vs. The U.S.A.* (New York: Norton, 1974), recounts Reich's ill-fated battles with the government and details the construction and operation of orgone boxes. Reich is possibly the only person in history to have been on the run from the Nazis, the secret police of the USSR, *and* the FBI. The U.S. government publicly burned Reich's books.

40. Paul Jordan to WM, 22 Oct. 1947, Shock Therapy–Report #1, GAP[MF]; and Henry Brosin "Historical Remarks on the First Five Years of GAP," speech to GAP, Asbury Park, N.J., 1 April 1951, HWB.

41. Stella Deignan and Esther Miller, "The Support of Research in Medical and Allied Fields for the Period 1946 through 1951," *Science* 115 (28 Mar. 1952): 321–43. See also Jeanne Brand, *Private Support for Mental Health* (Washington, D.C.: USDHEW, 1961), USPHS Pub. no. 838. The 1946 National Mental Health Act established the NAMHC under the authority of the USPHS (no funds were appropriated until 1948). The NAMHC administered the federal mental health grants program until 1949, when the NIMH was formed within the NIH. The NAMHC'S first board were all ardent members of GAP.

42. The origins of the lobotomy report are found in the report itself, "Research on Prefrontal Lobotomy," *GAP Rep.* No. 6; "Report of the Committee on Research to the Council of the American Psychiatric Association" (1948), submitted by Thomas French, Chairman, pp. 2–4, Comm. on Research, 1948–1950, Box 200-8, APA; Roy Grinker to Nolan Lewis, 6 Sept. 1947; Lawrence Kolb to Lewis, 8 Sept. 1947, NDCL; and Thomas French to WM, 23 Apr. 1948, Comm. on Research, 1948–1949, Box 200-8, APA. See also a prior version, GAP Circular Letter #78, 27 Feb. 1948, MG.

    Accounts of the NAMHC's Research Study Section and its Sub-Committee on Lobotomy are in "The Organization and Functions of the National Institute of Mental Health," 15 Aug. 1950, orientation pamphlet for new members of advisory groups, 2, 9, and 15; "Classified Digest, 15 Aug. 1950," 3, 35–43, NAMHC. Between 1947 and 1950, the council received 14 psychosurgery applications, of which 4 were accepted for a total of $152,000; in comparison, all 7 applications for shock-therapy investigations were rejected. In its first year, NAMHC disbursed $373,000 over 38 research grants; NIMH Progress Report (July 1949), 1. Mettler claimed that grant MH-118, $53,000 to his Columbia topectomy studies, was the largest of these early awards; Fred Mettler to Robert Morison, 23 Aug. 1948; Columbia University–Brain Surgery, (RG1.2 200 121 1070), RFA. The sponsored survey was Lawrence Kolb, "An Evaluation of Lobotomy and Its Potentialities for Future Research in Psychiatry and the Basic Sciences," *JNMD* 110 (1949): 112–49.

43. The three "Research Conferences on Psychosurgery" were held in New York City, 17–18 Nov. 1949, 2–3 June 1950, and 19–20 Oct. 1951. Transcripts were published as: *First Research Conference* (Chap. 4, n. 1); Winfred Over-

holser, ed., *Proceedings of the Second Research Conference on Psychosurgery,*
USPHS Pub. no. 156 (Washington, D.C.: GPO, 1952); and *Third Research
Conference* (Intro., n. 3).

44. *Third Research Conference,* 4.
45. *First Research Conference,* 123–4.
46. *Third Research Conference,* 65.
47. *First Research Conference,* 92; *Second Research Conference,* 58; and I. W.
Scherer, "Prognoses and Psychological Scores in Electroconvulsive Therapy,
Psychosurgery and Spontaneous Remission," *AJP* 107 (1951): 927
48. Gosta Rylander, "Personality Analysis before and after Frontal Lobotomy,"
*ARNMD* 27 (1948): 702, 704.
49. "Proceedings of the Conference on the Development of a Research Program
for the Evaluation of Psychiatric Therapies" (Princeton, N.J., 20–2 Mar.
1952, transcript), 444. I would like to express my special thanks to the late Dr.
Joseph Wortis, Brooklyn, N.Y., for allowing me access to his personal copy; it
appears to be the only extant transcript of the full proceedings. See also Kolb,
"An Evaluation of Lobotomy," 132, which contains a good overview of
psychological tests in lobotomy. The definitive work on psychosurgery and
personality tests is Mary Robinson and Walter Freeman, *Psychosurgery and
the Self* (New York: Grune & Stratton, 1954).
50. Capshew, *Psychology on the March* (Chap. 1, n. 51) and John Reisman, *A
History of Clinical Psychology* (New York: Irvington, 1976).
51. E.g., a thesis by a clinical psychologist on lobotomy is George W. Kisker, "The
Behavioral Correlates of Neurosurgical Transsection of the Prefrontal Association Areas in the Psychoses," (Ph.D. diss., Ohio State University, 1943).
Kisker also published several important articles on psychosurgery. The
development of hospital rating scales is described in Maurice Lorr, "Rating
Scales, Behavior Inventories, and Drugs," in Leonard Uhr and James Miller,
eds., *Drugs and Behavior* (New York: John Wiley, 1960), 519–39. In the
same volume, see also Julian Lasky, "Veterans Administrative Cooperative
Chemotherapy Projects and Related Studies," 540–4. Lorr, "Ratings Scales
and Check Lists for the Evaluation of Psychopathology," *Psych. Bull.* 51
(1954): 119–27. Lorr's Multidimensional Scale for Rating Psychiatric Patients (MSRPP) was especially significant. It began as the "Northport Record," a rating system devised at the Northport VA Hospital for the study of
lobotomized patients; the MSRPP was used as the core of the VA Lobotomy
Study's attempt to establish a standardized behavioral measurement that was
practical for hospitalized psychotics (see Pressman *UP,* 374 n. 59, which also
lists other rating scales developed in conjunction with lobotomy). In 1966, the
MSRPP evolved into the Inpatient Multidimensional Psychiatric Scale, one of
the major hospital scales; see Oscar Buros, ed., *Personality Tests and Reviews*
(Highland Park, N.J.: Gryphon Press, 1970), xxiv–v, 124–5.
52. Joseph Zubin, "Evaluation of Therapeutic Outcome in Mental Disorders,"
*JNMD* 117 (1953): 109.
53. "An Investigation of the Effectiveness of Psychiatric Therapies . . . ," grant
application, Research Pro–Comm. on Therapy, Box 200-10, APA.

54. "Conference on the Development of a Research Program for the Evaluation of Psychiatric Therapies"; and "Summary Data concerning Grant M-579," application, 9 Oct. 1952, Research Pro–Comm. on Therapy, Box 200-10, APA. See also the notice in *APA Newsletter* 5, no. 5 (1953): 1.
55. "Conference on . . . evaluation of psychiatric therapies," 19–20, 376–7.
56. Ibid., 379, 384–5.
57. Ibid., 283–5, 327.
58. Ibid., 8–10, 234.
59. Ibid., 320–1, 370; and "Preliminary Notes," IV, 8, Box 200-1, APA.
60. "Conference on . . . Evaluation of Psychiatric Therapies," 388; "Summary Report, Conference on . . . Evaluation of Psychiatric Therapies," Box 200-10, Comm. on Therapy, APA.
61. For background on the VA psychiatry program, see Daniel Blain, "Program of Veterans Administration for Physical and Mental Health of Vets," *Bull. Menn. Clin.* 10 (1946): 33–46; P. Hawley, "Neuropsychiatric Program of Veterans Administration," *Mil. Surg.* 99 (1946): 759–62; idem, "The Place of Psychiatry in VA," *AJP* 104 (1947): 16–19; Karl Menninger, "Mental Patients Predominate at This General Hospital," *Hospitals* 20 (October 1946): 44–6; Florence Powdermaker, "The Neuropsychiatric Training Program of the VA," *AJP* 103 (1947): 470–2; Blain, "Priorities in Psychiatric Treatment," *Mil. Surg.* 102 (1948): 85–97; and Harry Solomon, prep., "Prefrontal Leukotomy, an Evaluation," *Tech. Bull.* (VA) #10–46 (21 May 1948). A partial list of publications from the VA Lobotomy Study is: Josephine Ball, C. James Klett, and Clement Gresock, "The Veterans Administration Study of Prefrontal Lobotomy," *J. Clin. Exp. Psychopath.* 20 (1959): 205–17; Richard Jenkins and James Holsopple, "Criteria and Experimental Design for Evaluating Results of Lobotomy," *ARNMD* 31 (1953): 319–27; Jenkins, Holsopple, and Lorr, "Effects of Prefrontal Lobotomy." See also "Report on History and Present Status of the Lobotomy Project" (October 1956, typescript); and J. Q. Holsopple, "Improvement of Chronic Schizophrenic Patients Attributable to Prefrontal Lobotomy," typescript of a paper presented at the VA Annual Medical Research Conference, Memphis, Tenn., 13 Dec. 1955, VA. Later development of psychosurgery within the VA can be ascertained from VA, Department of Medicine and Surgery, *Cooperative Studies in Mental Health & Behavioral Sciences,* prepared by Susan Abrams and Sandra Ciufo (Perry Point, Md.: VA, 1975); and Committee on Labor and Public Welfare and Committee on Veterans' Affairs, subcommittee on Health, U.S. Senate, *Psychosurgery in Veterans Administration Hospitals,* Joint Hearing, 93d Congress, 1st session, 18 June 1973 (Washington, D.C.: GPO, 1973), 6–17. C. James Klett, interview with the author, 14 Nov. 1984, Perry Point, Md.
62. John Gronvall, "The VA's Affiliation with Academic Medicine: An Emergency Post-War Strategy Becomes a Permanent Partnership," *Acad. Med.* 64 (1989): 61–6; and Capshew, *Psychology on the March.*
63. John Barnwell, "The Value of Cooperative Research," in VA Department of Medicine and Surgery, *Transactions of the First Research Conference on*

Notes to Pages 396–401

*Chemotherapy in Psychiatry,* 26–7 Apr. 1956, Downey, Ill. (Washington, D.C.: VA, 1956), 1:4.

64. Accounts of these studies are found in Harry Marks, "Notes from the Underground: The Social Organization of Therapeutic Research," in Russell Maulitz and Diana Long, eds., *Grand Rounds: One Hundred Years of Internal Medicine* (Philadelphia: University of Pennsylvania Press, 1988), 297–336; and Abraham Lilienfeld, "Ceteris paribus: The Evolution of the Clinical Trial," *BHM* 56 (1982): 1–18.

65. Ball, Klett, and Gresock, "Veterans Administration Study"; and Holsopple, "Improvement of Chronic Schizophrenic Patients," 5.

66. Valenstein *G&DC*, 261; and O'Callaghan and Carroll, *Psychosurgery,* 191 (Intro., n. 4).

67. For example, a retrospective study of clinical reports in major medical journals determined that even as late as 1976, only 5 percent might be considered true double-blind controlled trials; R. H. Fletcher and S. W. Fletcher, "Clinical Research in General Medical Journals: A 30-Year Perspective," *NEJM* 301 (1979): 180–3. The history of experimental design has yet to be studied in depth. The best account is Marks, "Notes from the Underground." See also Marcia Meldrum, "'Departures from the Design': The Randomized Clinical Trial in Historical Context, 1946–1970" (Ph.D. diss., SUNY, Stony Brook, 1994); and Lilienfeld, "Ceteris paribus." Also helpful is John Burnham, "The Evolution of Editorial Peer Review," *JAMA* 263 (9 Mar. 1990): 1323–9.

68. Cooter, *Phrenology* (Intro., n. 6).

### Epilogue. The New Synthesis

1. Ken Kesey, *One Flew Over the Cuckoo's Nest* (New York: Viking, 1973 [1962]), 38.

2. Marlboro SH "AR," typescript (1960), 1, PFL; H. Brill and R. Patton, "Analysis of 1955–56 Population Fall in New York State Mental Hospitals in First Year of Large-scale Use of Tranquilizing Drugs," *AJP* 114 (1957): 509–17; and Hunt, "Pilgrim's Progress [II]," 84, 89 (Chap. 4, n. 59). At the VA, e.g., within two years of CPZ's arrival, ECS use lowered 77 percent, insulin 73 percent, and hydrotherapy 90 percent; Swazey, *Chlorpromazine,* 220 (Chap. 4, n. 19). For further history of the psychotropic drugs, also see Anne Caldwell, *Origins of Psychopharmacology: From CPZ to LSD* (Springfield, Ill.: C. C. Thomas, 1970); and A. Hordern, "Psychopharmacology: Some Historical Considerations," in C. R. B. Joyce, ed., *Psychopharmacology; Dimensions and Perspectives* (London: Tavistock, 1968), 95–148. In 1961, the Joint Commission on Mental Illness and Health published its now famous blueprint for psychiatric reform, *Action for Mental Health* (New York: Basic Books, 1961). In a section titled, "The Tranquilized Hospital," it was noted that the new drugs "have largely replaced the various forms of shock, as well as surgery on the prefrontal lobes of the brain" (p. 39). The annual decline in hospital numbers caused by the new drugs was about 2 percent, at the time a dramatic reversal. The later,

more rapid deinstitutionalization of the asylums resulted from explicit policy decisions (such as the transfer of the elderly to nursing homes); see William Gronfein, *From Madhouse to Main Street: The Changing Place of Mental Illness in Post World War II America* (Ph.D. diss., SUNY, Stony Brook, 1984; Ann Arbor: UMI, 1985). For the impact of the drugs on mental hospital care and policy, see Grob *Asylum*, 146–56.

3. Irrespective of the success of the chemotherapies, the psychosurgery programs by this time were already losing their impetus (Figure 4.1.) One explanation is that the search for more limited and precise lobotomies had inadvertently marginalized the procedure. As the operations became more sophisticated, being targeted to ever smaller areas of brain tissue, clinical indications of when to use the procedures also narrowed. Thus, fewer types of patients seemed appropriate. And, as the overall behavioral effects of the newer operations were less pronounced, the threshold was raised for when it appeared permissible to subject a patient to such a risk. In 1973, Gosta Rylander reflected that, for the past generation of psychiatrists, lobotomy was attractive precisely because its crude, broad cuts had yielded such dramatic effects on patients whose behavior had been unmodifiable by other means; see Laitinen and Livingston, *Surgical Approaches*, 4 (Chap. 7, n. 37). The primary diagnostic category operated upon reverted back to the non-schizophrenic population, i.e., the agitated depressives and obsessive-compulsives, where the procedure had begun.

4. Kesey, *Cuckoo's Nest*, 16.

5. Valenstein *G&DC*, 284–90; National Commission for the Protection of Human Subjects . . . , *Psychosurgery: Report and Recommendations*, DHEW Pub. (OS) 77-0001 (Bethesda, Md.: The Commission, 1977); and Peter Breggin, "Psychosurgery for Political Purposes," *Duq. Law Rev.* 13 (1975): 841–62.

6. John Fulton, "Brain as Matrix of Mind: An Historical Approach," typescript of an address to the St. Vincent's Psychiatric Clinic, New York, 19 Nov. 1959, JF.

7. Freeman *Auto*, chap. 17. Zigmund Lebensohn, Paul Chodoff, and Oscar Legault were the three he cited. The costs of a training analysis were restrictive. Thanks to the liberal interpretations of the G.I. Bill, however, the profession of psychoanalysis was made affordable even to middle-class entrants. The roadtrips and professional difficulties Freeman encountered are described in *Auto*, chaps. 19, 21.

8. Watts, "20-year Follow-up" (Chap. 7, n. 65); Freeman, "Lobotomy 1936–1956" (Chap. 7, n. 68); and idem, "With Camera and Ice-Pick in Search of the Super Ego," typescript, April 1960, GWU.

9. On the theatrical performances of scientists, see Latour, "Give Me a Laboratory" (Chap. 7, n. 110).

10. Thomas Kuhn, *The Structure of Scientific Revolutions*, 2d ed. (Chicago: University of Chicago Press, 1970); and Fleck, *Scientific Fact* (Chap. 2, n. 109).

11. Swazey, *Chlorpromazine*, 105, 155, 201–7, 215–24. Marlboro SH "AR," typescript 1957, 4, PFL; St. Louis SH "AR," typescript (1955), 50; and Nor-

530

Notes to Pages 422–40

ristown SH AR (1957): 18. See also Benjamin Pollack, "Preliminary Report on 500 Patients Treated with Thorazine at Rochester State Hospital," PSQ 29 (1955): 39–57.

12. Henry Brill, "Analysis of 1955–6 Population Fall in New York State Mental Hospitals in First Year of Large-scale Use of Tranquilizing Drugs," AJP 114 (1957): 509–17; Swazey, Chlorpromazine, 236–58. NIMH, "Phenothiazine Treatment in Acute Schizophrenia; Effectiveness," Arch. Gen. Psychi. 10 (1964): 246–61; and Maurice Lorr, "Problems in the Controlled Study of Drug-Modified Patient Behavior," in VA, Chemotherapy, 2:44–6 (Chap. 8, n. 63). The development of Lorr's IMPS test is described in Chapter 8. As another example, prior to the first clinical trial of CPZ in the U.S.A., a landmark study on a related class of drugs was conducted at Rockland SH in an unusual research unit established by the NYS DMH. The facilities were a direct conversion of those the hospital had constructed for its psychosurgery studies. Nathan Kline, director of the new unit and author of the experiment, had earlier proven his potential as a research administrator in the New York State Brain Research Project. See Swazey, 191; Rockland SH AR (1953): 703; and "News and Comment; and New York Launches New Interdisciplinary Research Project," PSQ (1952): 26. Mettler later reflected that the Rockland chemotherapeutic program grew out of the brain research project, which he had directed; Fred Mettler, letter to the author, 19 Nov. 1983. Kline's now classic article is "Use of rauwolfia serpentina benth. in Neuropsychiatric Conditions," Ann. N.Y. Acad. Sci. 59 (1954): 107–32.

13. Grob MI, xi.
14. Solomon, quoted in Grob Asylum, 165; and Robert Hunt, "The State Hospital Stereotype," typescript of address before the APA Commission on Long Term Policies, 30 October 1959, Detroit; Mental Health Subject Files 1957–60, Box 2, NIMH. The author thanks Professor Grob for bringing this document to his attention.
15. Grob Asylum; Erving Goffman, Asylums: Essays on the Social Situation of Mental Patients and Other Inmates (Garden City, N.Y.: Doubleday, 1961); and Hale, Jr., Psychoanalysis (see Chap. 8, n. 3). The vast social problem posed by severe mental illness did not simply vanish. Rather, in the course of 1980s politics, it was reclassified as a subset of the welfare issue and was thus effectively abandoned.
16. R. D. Laing, The Divided Self (New York: Penguin, 1965), 12.
17. Lilienfeld, "Ceteris paribus" (Chap. 8, n. 64).
18. F-W PS2, 203.
19. This paragraph is condensed from the conclusion of Jack Pressman, "Concepts of Mental Illness in the West," in Kenneth Kiple, ed., The Cambridge World History of Human Disease (Cambridge University Press, 1992), 82.
20. [Name withheld] to Winfred Overholser, 6 Sept. 1946, in Administrative Files, Box Legislation-Lobotomy/Lobotomy (1944–1956), WO.
21. Solomon, "Introduction," in Studies in Lobotomy, 3 (Chap. 6, n. 27).
22. Paul Feyerabend, Against Method: Outline of an Anarchistic Theory of Knowledge (London: Verso, 1978). Hamilton Ford and Grace Jameson,

"Chlorpromazine in Conjunction with Other Psychiatric Therapies: A Clinical Appraisal," *Dis. Nerv. Sys.* 16 (1955): 179–85.

23. Sunday Times of London, The Insight Team, *Suffer the Children. The Story of Thalidomide* (New York: Viking, 1979); Robert Jacobson and Alvan Feinstein, "Oxygen as a Cause of Blindness in Premature Infants: 'Autopsy' of a Decade of Errors in Clinical Epidemiologic Research," *J. Clin. Epid.* 45 (1992): 1265–87; and Institute of Medicine, *Review of the Fialuridine (FIAU) Clinical Trials* (Washington, D.C.: N.A.S., 1995).

24. On the need for demystification, see Harry Collins and Trevor Pinch, *The Golem: What Everyone Should Know about Science* (Cambridge University Press, 1993).

25. David Stipp, "Hope from a Knife," *Wall Street Journal,* 22 Feb. 1995, 132:1, 36.

# Sources

## Collections Cited

American Psychiatric Association. Archives. Washington, D.C., including:
Committee on Hospitals
Committee on Research
Committee on Standards
Committee on Therapy
Office of the Medical Director (Daniel Blain)
Office of the Secretary (C. B. Farrar)
American Psychopathological Association. Papers. Archives of Psychiatry, New York University–Cornell Medical Center, New York.
Archives of Psychiatry. New York University–Cornell Medical Center, New York.
Bay, Alfred P. Papers. The Menninger Foundation Archives, Topeka, Kansas.
Boston Psychopathic Hospital (now Massachusetts Mental Health Center). Papers. Boston, Massachusetts.
Bowman, Karl. Papers. Columbia University Manuscripts, New York, New York.
Brosin, Henry W. Papers. The Menninger Foundation Archives, Topeka, Kansas.
Burlingame, C. C. Papers. Institute of Living Archives, Hartford, Connecticut.
Central Neuropsychiatric Research Laboratory. Papers. Veterans Administration, Perry Point, Maryland.
Freeman, Walter J., and James W. Watts. Papers. Himmelfarb Library, George Washington University, Medical School, Washington, D.C.
Fulton, John Farquhar. Collection. Medical Historical Library, Sterling Hall of Medicine, Yale University Medical School, New Haven, Connecticut.
Fulton, John Farquhar. Papers. Archives and Manuscripts, Sterling Memorial Library, Yale University, New Haven, Connecticut.
Gitelson, Maxwell. Papers. Library of Congress, Washington, D.C.
Goldstein, Kurt. Papers. Columbia University Manuscripts, New York, New York.
Grant, Francis C. Papers. College of Physicians, Philadelphia, Pennsylvania.
Harrisburg State Hospital. Papers. Pennsylvania State Archives. Allentown, Pennsylvania.
Illinois Department of Mental Hygiene. Director's Files. Illinois State Archives, Springfield, Illinois.
Jelliffe, Smith Ely. Papers. Library of Congress, Washington, D.C.

Kolb, Larry C. Papers. Columbia University Manuscripts, New York, New York.

Levy, David M. Papers. Archives of Psychiatry, New York University–Cornell Medical Center, New York, New York.

Lewis, Nolan Don Carpentier. Papers. Carrier Foundation, Belle Meade, New Jersey.

Liddell, Howard S. Papers. Cornell University, Ithaca, New York.

Longview State Hospital Papers. Ohio State Historical Library, Columbus, Ohio.

McLean Hospital Archives, McLean Hospital, Belmont, Massachusetts.

Manhattan State Hospital (now Manhattan Psychiatric Center). Papers. Wards Island, New York.

The Menninger Foundation Archives, Topeka, Kansas.

Menninger, Karl A. Papers. The Menninger Foundation Archives, Topeka, Kansas.

Menninger, William C. Papers. The Menninger Foundation Archives, Topeka, Kansas.

National Advisory Mental Health Council. Papers. Record Group 90 and Record Group 443, USPHS, National Archives, Washington, D.C.

National Institute of Mental Health. Papers. Record Group 90 and Record Group 443, National Archives, Washington, D.C.

National Research Council. Archives, National Academy of Sciences, Washington, D.C.: Committee on Borderland Problems in the Life Sciences Committee on the Problem of Neurotic Behavior

Ohio State Archives. Ohio State Historical Library, Columbus, Ohio.

Overholser, Winifred. Papers. Record Group 418, St. Elizabeth's Government Hospital for the Insane, National Archives, Washington, D.C.

Philadelphia Free Library, Government Documents Section. Philadelphia, Pennsylvania.

Rockefeller Foundation Corporate Records. Rockefeller Archive Center, Tarrytown, New York.

St. Elizabeth's Government Hospital for the Insane. Papers. Record Group 418, National Archives, Washington, D.C.

Sargent, Helen P. Papers. The Menninger Foundation Archives, Topeka, Kansas.

Solomon, Harry C. Papers. Countway Library, Harvard Medical School, Boston, Massachusetts.

Strecker, Edward A. Papers. Institute of Pennsylvania Hospital, Philadelphia, Pennsylvania.

Toledo State Hospital Papers. Ohio State Historical Library, Columbus, Ohio.

Veterans Administration Cooperative Research Group. Central Neuropsychiatric Research Laboratory. Papers. Perry Point, Maryland.

The Vidonian Club. Papers. Archives of Psychiatry, New York University–Cornell Medical Center, New York, New York.

Viets, Henry R. Papers. Countway Library, Harvard Medical School, Boston, Massachusetts.

Western Psychiatric Institute. Papers. Pittsburgh, Pennsylvania.

Winter Veterans Hospital. Papers. The Menninger Foundation Archives, Topeka, Kansas.

Yerkes, Robert. Collection. Archives and Manuscripts, Sterling Memorial Library, Yale University, New Haven, Connecticut.

## Annual Reports Examined

I have examined reports from the following institutions and agencies for roughly the years 1935 to 1955:

| | |
|---|---|
| CA | Department of Mental Hygiene |
| | Agnews State Hospital |
| | Camarillo State Hospital |
| | DeWitt State Hospital |
| | Langley Porter Clinic |
| | Mendocino State Hospital |
| | Modesto State Hospital |
| | Napa State Hospital |
| | Norwalk State Hospital |
| | Patton State Hospital |
| | Stockton State Hospital |
| CT | Connecticut State Hospital (Middletown) |
| | Institute of Living (Hartford) |
| DE | Delaware State Hospital |
| DC | St. Elizabeth's Government Hospital for the Insane |
| FL | Florida State Hospital (Chattahoochee) |
| IL | Department of Public Welfare |
| | Chicago State Hospital |
| | Elgin State Hospital |
| | Illinois Neuropsychiatric Institute |
| | Kankakee State Hospital |
| | Manteno State Hospital |
| IA | Board of Control |
| | Cherokee State Hospital |
| | Clarinda State Hospital |
| | Independence State Hospital |
| | Mount Pleasant State Hospital |
| KS | The Menninger Foundation |
| | Topeka State Hospital |
| MA | Department of Mental Health |
| | Boston Psychopathic Hospital |
| | Worcester State Hospital |
| MI | Kalamazoo State Hospital |
| MO | State Hospital Number 4 (Farmington) |
| | St. Louis State Hospital |

NV    Nevada State Hospital

NJ    New Jersey State Hospital (Greystone)
New Jersey State Hospital (Marlboro)

NY    Department of Mental Hygiene
Binghamton State Hospital
Brooklyn State Hospital
Buffalo State Hospital
Central Islip State Hospital
Creedmoor State Hospital
Gowanda State Hospital
Harlem Valley State Hospital
Hudson River State Hospital
Kings Park State Hospital
Manhattan State Hospital
Marcy State Hospital
Middletown State Hospital
Pilgrim State Hospital
Psychiatric Institute
Rochester State Hospital
Rockland State Hospital
St. Lawrence State Hospital
Syracuse Psychopathic Hospital
Utica State Hospital
Willard State Hospital

OH    Department of Public Welfare
Longview State Hospital

PA    Department of Welfare
Harrisburg State Hospital
Norristown State Hospital
Western Psychiatric Institute

TX    Austin State Hospital

WV    Board of Control

# Index

Continued from the front of the book